Contraception for the Medically Challenging Patient

Rebecca H. Allen • Carrie A. Cwiak
Editors

Contraception for the Medically Challenging Patient

Springer

Editors
Rebecca H. Allen, MD, MPH
Department of Obstetrics and Gynecology
Warren Alpert Medical School of Brown University
Providence, RI, USA

Carrie A. Cwiak, MD, MPH
Department of Gynecology and Obstetrics
Emory University School of Medicine
Atlanta, GA, USA

ISBN 978-1-4939-1232-2 ISBN 978-1-4939-1233-9 (eBook)
DOI 10.1007/978-1-4939-1233-9
Springer New York Heidelberg Dordrecht London

Library of Congress Control Number: 2014945758

Springer is part of Springer Science+Business Media (www.springer.com)

To Dr. Uta Landy and Dr. Philip Darney, whose dedication to women's reproductive health and a new generation of providers has established and fostered an incredible community of experts through the Fellowship in Family Planning, of which we are proud graduates.

And to our families, who patiently endured all the hours we spent planning, writing, and editing.

Foreword

Family planning saves lives and improves women's health and well-being by delaying childbearing, spacing pregnancies, reducing unintended pregnancies and abortions, and allowing women to choose when and how often pregnancy is desired [1]. In 2014, women, men, and couples in the United States have more Food and Drug Administration (FDA)-approved contraceptive methods available to them that at any time in the past. However, around half of pregnancies in the United States are unintended—a percentage that has not change in the last two decades [2, 3]. Further, half of unintended pregnancies occur among women not using contraception, demonstrating that there remains an unmet need for contraception in the United States [4]. Overall, contraceptive use in the United States is fairly high; in 2006–2010 (the most recent national data available), 62 % of women ages 15–44 reported current use of contraception [5]. However, 11 % of women determined to be at risk of unintended pregnancy were not using any method of contraception [5]. Among those using contraception, only a small percentage (~6 %) used the most highly effective, long-acting, reversible methods—intrauterine devices and implants [5, 6].

While unintended pregnancies themselves can lead to negative consequences for both mother and infant [7], risks may be compounded in women who have medical conditions. Certain medical conditions, such as diabetes, hypertension, and obesity, are increasing in prevalence among US women of reproductive age [8]. For many women with medical conditions, unintended pregnancies may worsen the condition and involve particularly high maternal and perinatal risks. There is a critical need to avoid or delay pregnancy until disease management is optimal.

Most women, even those with chronic medical conditions, can safely use most methods of contraception. All women should be able to choose from the complete range of FDA-approved methods to find one that best fits their needs. Health care providers caring for women with medical conditions may be concerned about the effects of contraception on the medical condition, and therefore may avoid providing contraception or addressing family planning needs. However, this must be balanced against the fact that certain adverse outcomes and disease progression are likely to be greater during pregnancy than during contraceptive use [9]. To address these concerns, the World Health Organization (WHO) in 1996 published the first evidence-based guidance on *Medical Eligibility Criteria for Contraceptive Use*, which provided recommendations for safe use of contraceptive methods for women with medical conditions [10]. The goal of this guidance is to maximize access to the full range of contraceptive methods, while keeping necessary safety restrictions in place, based on the best available scientific evidence. The US Centers for Disease Control and Prevention has adapted the WHO guidance to create the *US Medical Eligibility Criteria for Contraceptive Use, 2010* (US MEC) for best implementation by US health care providers [11]. The US MEC includes recommendations for over 60 characteristics and conditions. For medical conditions where there is a safety concern about a specific method, there are most often several other methods that are safe. The US MEC also highlights certain conditions, such as diabetes, hypertension, human immunodeficiency virus (HIV), and lupus, for which unintended pregnancy may lead to a high risk of adverse health events, and therefore use of highly effective contraception is particularly encouraged.

Contraception for the Medically Challenging Patient expands the concepts of the MEC and provides a comprehensive discussion of contraceptive management among women with medical conditions of many organ systems, including cardiovascular, endocrine, neurologic, hematologic, rheumatologic, gastrointestinal, and psychiatric. This textbook also includes a discussion of the assessment of women with medical conditions, management in perimenopause, and interactions between contraception and certain medications. The purpose of this textbook is to provide a complement to the US MEC, with detailed explanation of the safety classifications and how they can be used in practice.

For many women in the United States, there remains an unmet need for family planning. It is our hope that this textbook will help demystify the provision of contraception among women with medical conditions. We anticipate that this information will be useful not only to specialists in obstetrics/gynecology and women's health, but by all health care providers, including primary care providers and the specialists who take care of women with the medical conditions described here. Finally, we hope that this textbook will encourage health care providers to address the critical need for family planning among all female patients of reproductive age.

Disclaimer: The findings and conclusions in this report are those of the authors and do not necessarily represent the official position of the Centers for Disease Control and Prevention.

Atlanta, GA, USA

Kathryn M. Curtis
Naomi K. Tepper

References

1. Population Reference Bureau. Family Planning Saves Lives, 4th ed. 2009; http://www.prb.org/pdf09/familyplanningsaveslives.pdf. Accessed 26 Dec 2013.
2. Finer LB, Zolna MR. Shifts in intended and unintended pregnancies in the United States, 2001–2008. Am J Public Health. 104 Suppl 1:S43–8.
3. Henshaw SK. Unintended pregnancy in the United States. Fam Plann Perspect. 1998;30(1):24–29, 46.

4. Finer LB, Henshaw SK. Disparities in rates of unintended pregnancy in the United States, 1994 and 2001. Perspect Sexual Reprod Health. 2006;38(2):90–6.
5. Jones J, Mosher WD, Daniels K. Current contraceptive use in the United States, 2006–2010, and changes in patterns of use since 1995. National health statistics reports; No. 60. Hyattsville, MD: National Center for Health Statistics. 2012. http://www.cdc.gov/nchs/data/nhsr/nhsr060.pdf. Accessed 7 Jan 2014.
6. Guttmacher Institute. Contraceptive use in the United States. 2013; http://www.guttmacher.org/pubs/fb_contr_use.html Accessed 8 Jan 2014.
7. Gipson JD, Koenig MA, Hindin MJ. The effects of unintended pregnancy on infant, child, and parental health: a review of the literature. Stud Fam Plann. 2008;39(1):18–38.
8. Hayes DK, Fan AZ, Smith RA, Bombard JM. Trends in selected chronic conditions and behavioral risk factors among women of reproductive age, behavioral risk factor surveillance system, 2001–2009. Prev Chronic Dis. 2011;8(6):A120.
9. Jensen JT, Trussell J. Communicating risk: does scientific debate compromise safety? Contraception. 2012;86(4):327–9.
10. World Health Organization. Medical eligibility criteria for contraceptive use, 4th ed. Geneva: WHO; 2009: http://www.who.int/reproductivehealth/publications/family_planning/9789241563888/en/.
11. Centers for Disease Control and Prevention. U.S. Medical Eligibility Criteria for Contraceptive Use, 2010. MMWR Recomm Rep. 2010;59(RR-4):1–86.

Preface

As is the case for many of the chapter authors in this book, we have spoken to groups of providers numerous times about increasing contraceptive access to women with complex medical conditions. The audience has ranged in their expertise, from medical students to professors, and in their focus, whether Family Planning or Internal Medicine. The evidence-based resource, the *Centers for Disease Control and Prevention's United States Medical Eligibility Criteria for Contraceptive Use* (*USMEC*), has provided an excellent cornerstone for such discussions. Inevitably, these presentations end similarly, with thought-provoking questions from the audience, considerate discussion, and requests for even more information.

This book was borne from those lectures, in order to continue the conversation. The various chapters answer key questions (i.e., The What? How? Who? Why?) generated by the USMEC: (1) **what** are the studies that have led to the category ratings for various methods and conditions, (2) **how** does a provider incorporate that information into daily clinical practice, (3) **who** do you turn to when the answer is not in the USMEC, and (4) **why** is this so important to women's lives.

For the family planning or women's health practitioner, we anticipate that you, like we, will turn to individual chapters from time to time as patients present to your practice. For our colleagues in other fields of medicine, we offer individual chapters in your respective fields that will illustrate the importance for contraceptive discussions and shared decision-making for all your female reproductive-aged patients and provide insight into how we navigate those discussions. Finally, the chapter authors represent a rich collaboration so vital to the success of health care today, with a depth and breadth of expertise and practical experience from which we can draw to improve the lives of our patients.

Enjoy!

Providence, RI, USA — Rebecca H. Allen, MD, MPH

Atlanta, GA, USA — Carrie A. Cwiak, MD, MPH

Contents

Contributors

Rebecca H. Allen, MD, MPH Department of Obstetrics and Gynecology, Warren Alpert Medical School of Brown University, Providence, RI, USA

Deborah Bartz, MD, MPH Department of Obstetrics, Gynecology, and Reproductive Biology, Harvard Medical School, Brigham and Women's Hospital, Boston, MA, USA

Joan Briller, MD Division of Cardiology, Department of Medicine, University of Illinois Medical Center, Chicago, IL, USA

Anne E. Burke, MD, MPH Departments of Gynecology and Obstetrics/ Population, Family, and Reproductive Health, Johns Hopkins Bayview Medical Center, Bloomberg School of Public Health, Johns Hopkins University School of Medicine, Baltimore, MD, USA

Ronald T. Burkman, MD Department of Obstetrics and Gynecology, Baystate Medical Center, Tufts University School of Medicine, Springfield, MA, USA

Angela Chen, MD, MPH Department of Obstetrics and Gynecology, David Geffen School of Medicine at UCLA, UCLA Health System, Los Angeles, CA, USA

Julie Chor, MD, MPH Department of Obstetrics and Gynecology, The University of Chicago, Chicago, IL, USA

Jennifer Corbelli, MD, MS Division of General Internal Medicine, University of Pittsburgh Medical Center, Pittsburgh, PA, USA

Kelly R. Culwell, MD, MPH Planned Parenthood of the Pacific Southwest, San Diego, CA, USA

Kathryn M. Curtis, PhD U.S. Centers for Disease Control and Prevention, Atlanta, GA, USA

Carrie A. Cwiak, MD, MPH Department of Gynecology and Obstetrics, Emory University School of Medicine, Atlanta, GA, USA

Autumn Davidson, MD Department of Obstetrics and Gynecology, The University of Chicago, Chicago, IL, USA

S. Lindsey Davis, MD Department of Hematology and Medical Oncology, University of Colorado Denver, Aurora, CO, USA

Anne R. Davis, MD, MPH Department of Obstetrics and Gynecology, Columbia University Medical Center, New York, NY, USA

Amanda Dennis, DrPH, MBE Ibis Reproductive Health, Cambridge, MA, USA

Monica Dragoman, MD, MPH Department of Obstetrics and Gynecology, Albert Einstein College of Medicine and Montefiore Medical Center, Bronx, NY, USA

Alison Edelman, MD, MPH Department of Obstetrics and Gynecology, Oregon Health and Science University, Portland, OR, USA

Andrea G. Edlow, MD, MSc Division of Maternal-Fetal Medicine, Department of Obstetrics and Gynecology, Tufts Medical Center, Boston, MA, USA

Lisa B. Haddad, MD, MS, MPH Department of Gynecology and Obstetrics, Emory University School of Medicine, Atlanta, GA, USA

Sadia Haider, MD, MPH Department of Obstetrics and Gynecology, University of Illinois at Chicago, Chicago, IL, USA

Kelli Stidham Hall, PhD, MS Department of Obstetrics and Gynecology, Institute for Social Research, University of Michigan, Ann Arbor, MI, USA

Elizabeth Harleman, MD Department of Internal Medicine, San Francisco General Hospital, University of California, San Francisco, San Francisco, CA, USA

Wendy Ho, MD, MPH Division of Digestive Diseases, Department of Medicine, University of California Los Angeles, Los Angeles, CA, USA

Melody Y. Hou, MD, MPH Department of Obstetrics and Gynecology, Davis School of Medicine, University of California, Sacramento, CA, USA

David R. Kattan, MD, MPH Department of Obstetrics and Gynecology, Baystate Medical Center, Tufts University School of Medicine, Springfield, MA, USA

Andrew M. Kaunitz, MD, FACOG Department of Obstetrics and Gynecology, University of Florida College of Medicine-Jacksonville, Jacksonville, FL, USA

Colleen M. Krajewski, MD, MPH Department of Obstetrics and Gynecology, Magee Womens Hospital, University of Pittsburgh School of Medicine, Pittsburgh, PA, USA

Allison Lange, MD Department of Gynecology and Obstetrics, Emory University School of Medicine, Atlanta, GA, USA

Sheila M. Marcus, MD Department of Psychiatry, University of Michigan, Ann Arbor, MI, USA

Michael R. McClung, MD, Founding Director Oregon Osteoporosis Center, Portland, OR, USA

Elizabeth Micks, MD, MPH Department of Obstetrics and Gynecology, University of Washington Medical Center, Seattle, WA, USA

Geraldine M. Navarro, MD Division of Rheumatology, Department of Medicine, Ronald Reagan Medical Center, UCLA David Geffen School of Medicine, Porter Ranch, CA, USA

M. Angela O'Neal, MD Department of Neurology, Brigham and Women's Hospital, Boston, MA, USA

Erica O'Neill, MD, MPH Division of Family Planning Services, Department of Obstetrics and Gynecology, John H. Stroger, Jr. Hospital of Cook County, Chicago, IL, USA

Ighovwerha Ofotokun, MD, MSc Division of Infectious Diseases, Department of Medicine, Emory University School of Medicine, Atlanta, GA, USA

Alison M. Pack, MD, MPH Department of Neurology, Columbia University Medical Center, New York, NY, USA

Ashlesha Patel, MD, MPH Division of Family Planning Services, Department of Obstetrics and Gynecology, John H. Stroger, Jr. Hospital of Cook County, Chicago, IL, USA

Ashok R. Patel, MD Rush Medical College, Chicago, IL, USA

Anish Vinit Patel, MD Department of Internal Medicine, Cedars Sinai Medical Center, Los Angeles, CA, USA

Rachel Perry, MD Department of Obstetrics and Gynecology, University of Illinois Hospital and Health Sciences System, Chicago, IL, USA

Tina Rizack, MD, MPH Program in Women's Oncology, Women and Infants Hospital, Alpert Medical School of Brown University, Providence, RI, USA

Alicia Roston, MPH Division of Family Planning Services, Department of Obstetrics and Gynecology, John H. Stroger, Jr. Hospital of Cook County, Chicago, IL, USA

Jennifer Salcedo, MD, MPH, MPP, FACOG Department of Obstetrics and Gynecology, John A. Burns School of Medicine, University of Hawaii at Manoa, Honolulu, HI, USA

Eleanor Bimla Schwarz, MD, MS Women's Health Services Research Unit, Center for Research on Health Care, University of Pittsburgh, Pittsburgh, PA, USA

Anandi N. Sheth, MD Division of Infectious Diseases, Department of Medicine, Emory University School of Medicine, Atlanta, GA, USA

Katharine Simmons, MD Department of Obstetrics and Gynecology, Oregon Health and Science University, Portland, OR, USA

Aparna Sridhar, MD, MPH, FACOG Department of Obstetrics and Gynecology, University of California Los Angeles, Los Angeles, CA, USA

Julie M. Sroga, MD Section of Reproductive Endocrinology and Infertility, Department of Obstetrics and Gynecology, University of Cincinnati College of Medicine, West Chester, OH, USA

Jody Steinauer, MD, MAS Department of Obstetrics, Gynecology and Reproductive Sciences, San Francisco General Hospital, San Francisco, CA, USA

Julia R. Steinberg, PhD, MA Department of Psychiatry, University of California, San Francisco, San Francisco, CA, USA

Kelly Stempinski, MPH Division of Family Planning Services, Department of Obstetrics and Gynecology, John H. Stroger, Jr. Hospital of Cook County, Chicago, IL, USA

Rebecca H. Stone, PharmD, BCPS College of Pharmacy, University of Illinois Hospital and Health Sciences System, University of Illinois at Chicago, Chicago, IL, USA

Jessica Tarleton, MD, MPH Department of Gynecology and Obstetrics, Emory University School of Medicine, Atlanta, GA, USA

Naomi K. Tepper, MD, MPH Division of Reproductive Health, U.S. Centers for Disease Control and Prevention, Atlanta, GA, USA

Michael A. Thomas, MD Section of Reproductive Endocrinology and Infertility, Department of Obstetrics and Gynecology, University of Cincinnati College of Medicine, West Chester, OH, USA

Kristina Tocce, MD, MPH Department of Obstetrics and Gynecology, Anschutz Medical Campus, University of Colorado, Aurora, CO, USA

Tram T. Tran, MD Department of Gastroenterology, Liver Transplant, Cedars Sinai Medical Center, Los Angeles, CA, USA

Meredith Macrae Warden, MD, MPH Department of Obstetrics, Gynecology and Reproductive Sciences, San Francisco General Hospital, University of California, San Francisco, San Francisco, CA, USA

Lindsay Zimmerman, MPH Division of Family Planning Services, Department of Obstetrics and Gynecology, John H. Stroger, Jr. Hospital of Cook County, Chicago, IL, USA

Abbreviations

ACOG	American College of Obstetricians and Gynecologists
AIDS	Acquired immunodeficiency syndrome
ANA	Antinuclear antibodies
APS	Antiphospholipid syndrome
ARV	Antiretroviral
AUC	Area under the curve
BMD	Bone mineral density
BMI	Body mass index
BP	Blood pressure
CDC	Centers for Disease Control and Prevention
CHC	Combined hormonal contraception
COC	Combined oral contraceptive
CRP	C-reactive protein
Cu-IUD	Copper IUD
CVD	Cardiovascular disease
DM	Diabetes mellitus
DMPA	Depot-medroxyprogesterone acetate
DVT	Deep vein thrombosis
EC	Emergency contraception
EE	Ethinyl estradiol
ELISA	Enzyme-linked immunosorbent assay
ENG	Etonogestrel
ESR	Erythrocyte sedimentation rate
FDA	Food and Drug Administration
FSH	Follicule stimulating hormone
GI	Gastrointestinal
HCG	Human chorionic gonadotropin
HDL	High-density lipoprotein
HIV	Human immunodeficiency virus
HSV	Herpes simplex virus
HT	Hormone therapy
HTN	Hypertension
IBD	Inflammatory bowel disease
ICU	Intensive care unit
IUD	Intrauterine device
IUGR	Intrauterine growth restriction
LARC	Long-acting reversible contraception

LNG	Levonorgestrel
LNG-IUD	Levonorgestrel IUD
MAOI	Monoamine oxidase inhibitor
MEC	Medical eligibility criteria
OC	Oral contraceptive
OR	Odds ratio
PE	Pulmonary embolism
PHQ	Patient health questionnaire
PID	Pelvic inflammatory disease
POP	Progestin-only pill
RA	Rheumatoid arthritis
RCT	Randomized controlled trial
RF	Rheumatoid factor
SHBG	Sex hormone binding globulin
SLE	Systemic lupus erythematosus
SNRI	Serotonin norepinephrine reuptake inhibitor
SPR	Selected practice recommendations
SSRI	Selective serotonin reuptake inhibitor
STI	Sexually transmitted infection
TCAs	Tricyclic antidepressants
TSH	Thyroid-stimulating hormone
UPA	Ulipristal acetate
US	United States
USMEC	United States Medical Eligibility Criteria for Contraceptive Use
USSPR	United States Selected Practice Recommendations for Contraceptive Use
VMS	Vasomotor symptoms
VTE	Venous thromboembolism
WHO	World Health Organization

Patient Assessment and Counseling for Contraceptive Care

1

Melody Y. Hou and Elizabeth Micks

The typical woman spends about 5 years of her reproductive life trying to get pregnant, and the other three decades trying to avoid it [1]. Nearly half of all pregnancies are unintended, and 40 % of these end in abortion [2]. Fortunately, the medical community has acknowledged the importance of contraception over the last few decades as contraceptive innovations such as novel intrauterine devices, implants, and sterilization methods have been introduced [3]. As long-term data have been amassed on the use of contraceptive methods among women with chronic medical conditions, guidance on contraceptive use has also blossomed, which has benefited both patients and clinicians [4, 5].

Certain populations have not fully benefited from this contraceptive evolution. With the development of novel contraceptive methods has come uncertainty regarding the safety of these methods for women with coexisting medical conditions. Historically, clinicians did not give much consideration to contraception for these women, citing that they may not survive to sexual maturity, or their medical problems may preclude sexual intercourse or cause infertility [6–8]. However, as medical care in the USA continues to improve, the population of women with medical comorbidities who reach and retain their fertility, and who are fully realized sexual beings, is growing. Pregnancy and contraceptive methods can have important health implications for women with medical conditions. Thus, reproductive health and access to safe and effective contraception should be of vital importance to these women and their clinicians.

M.Y. Hou, M.D., M.P.H. (✉)
Department of Obstetrics and Gynecology, Davis School of Medicine, University of California, Sacramento, CA, USA
e-mail: melody.hou@ucdmc.ucdavis.edu

E. Micks, M.D., M.P.H.
Department of Obstetrics and Gynecology, University of Washington Medical Center, Seattle, WA, USA
e-mail: emicks@uw.edu; emicks@gmail.com

Efficacy Versus Effectiveness, Perfect Use Versus Typical Use

The best method for any woman is the most effective method that is safe for her and one that she will use consistently and correctly. Selecting this contraceptive method is an important process that should involve shared decision-making between a woman and her clinician. Understanding and assessing contraceptive efficacy and effectiveness is an important part of that counseling.

Contraceptive efficacy is assessed by measuring the number of unplanned pregnancies that occur during a specified period of use of a particular contraceptive method. Contraceptive efficacy is often presented as a Pearl Index, or number of failures per 100 woman-years of exposure, but may be more usefully illustrated by a life-table analysis, or failure rate for each month of use.

R.H. Allen and C.A. Cwiak (eds.), *Contraception for the Medically Challenging Patient*, DOI 10.1007/978-1-4939-1233-9_1, © Springer Science+Business Media New York 2014

$$\text{Effectiveness} \approx \frac{\text{Efficacy x Adherence* x Continuation*}}{\text{Fecundity x Coital Frequency and Timing*}}$$

Fig. 1.1 The relationship between effectiveness and efficacy. *Asterisk* denotes patient-dependent variables. Adapted from [9]

However, efficacy does not necessarily equate to effectiveness. The relationship between efficacy and effectiveness can be visualized in (Fig. 1.1) [9]:

Efficacy best describes how well the method itself works to prevent pregnancy. Patient use and continuation translate contraceptive efficacy into effectiveness. High adherence and continuation increase effectiveness, while high fecundity (the probability of pregnancy in one menstrual cycle) and high coital frequency and timing decrease effectiveness. A low-efficacy method for a particular woman can lead to an unintended pregnancy. However, a high-efficacy method that a woman does not use correctly can lead to the same outcome. Incorrect use can result from flawed counseling, user error, user non-adherence, or external factors such as insurance limitations that may hamper access or continuation. Further, as personal considerations, medical conditions, and reproductive health goals change over time, efficacy, method use, and baseline fertility may also fluctuate.

Understanding the relationship between effectiveness and efficacy, often portrayed as "typical use" versus "perfect use," can help guide clinicians and patients in their contraceptive selection (Table 1.1) [10]. Pregnancy rates with perfect use refer to the lowest rates that can be achieved with the use of the method under controlled circumstances (i.e., women in a clinical trial), while pregnancy rates with typical use are rates actually observed with the use of the method by adherent as well as non-adherent users. Typical and perfect use in this chart is presented as the percentage of women experiencing an unintended pregnancy during the first year of typical use and first year of perfect use of contraception, respectively, followed by the percentage of women continuing use at the end of the first year.

Correct use and adherence play major roles in contraceptive effectiveness. They are critically important in the counseling of women with coexisting medical conditions given the risks pregnancy may pose. Establishing the safety of a specific contraceptive method for any particular patient is important, but clinicians should also understand how a contraceptive method may fit into the woman's reproductive goals and her lifestyle to maximize effectiveness.

Determining Contraceptive Safety

Clinicians often recognize that their patients are sexually active and have contraceptive needs. However, they may be unfamiliar or uncomfortable with contraceptive assessment, counseling, and management for women with coexisting medical conditions. This discomfort may stem from uncertainty about the safety of a contraceptive method with an existing medical condition, or the potential effect of a medical condition on contraceptive effectiveness. However, unintended pregnancy itself can pose serious health risks to women who have particular medical conditions (Table 1.2) [11]. The task of making an evidence-based recommendation regarding contraception and a medical condition at the point of care can be overwhelming to any individual clinician.

In 1996 the World Health Organization (WHO), in collaboration with a large number of international family planning agencies, published the first edition of the Medical Eligibility Criteria for Contraceptive Use (MEC) [12]. Built on a structured systematic evaluation of available evidence, these regularly updated guidelines provide guidance to clinicians and health care organizations on the safety of contraceptive methods for persons with specific medical conditions worldwide.

Table 1.1 Percentage of women experiencing an unintended pregnancy during the first year of typical use and the first year of perfect use of contraception and the percentage continuing the use at the end of the first year, USA

	% of Women experiencing an unintended pregnancy within the first year of use		% of Women continuing use at 1 year[a]
Method	Typical use[b]	Perfect use[c]	
(1)	(2)	(3)	(4)
No method[d]	85	85	
Spermicides[e]	28	18	42
Fertility awareness-based methods	24		47
Standard Days method[f]		5	
TwoDay method[f]		4	
Ovulation method[f]		3	
Symptothermal method		0.4	
Withdrawal	22	4	46
Sponge			36
Parous women	24	20	
Nulliparous women	12	9	
Condom[g]			
Female (fc)	21	5	41
Male	18	2	43
Diaphragm[h]	12	6	57
Combined pill and progestin-only pill	9	0.3	67
Evra patch	9	0.3	67
NuvaRing	9	0.3	67
Depo-Provera	6	0.2	56
IUD			
ParaGard (copper T)	0.8	0.6	78
Mirena (LNG-IUD)	0.2	0.2	80
Implanon	0.05	0.05	84
Female sterilization	0.5	0.5	100
Male sterilization	0.15	0.10	100

Emergency contraceptive pills: Treatment initiated within 72 h after unprotected intercourse substantially reduces the risk of pregnancy[i]
Lactational amenorrhea method: LAM is a highly effective, *temporary* method of contraception[j]

Reprinted with permission from Trussell J. Contraceptive Efficacy. In: Hatcher RA, Trussell J, Nelson AL, Cates W, Kowall D, Policar MS, editors. Contraceptive Technology, 20th ed. Atlanta, GA: Contraceptive Technology Communications, Inc.; 2011

[a]Among couples attempting to avoid pregnancy, the percentage who continue to use a method for 1 year

[b]Among *typical* couples who initiate the use of a method (not necessarily for the first time), the percentage who experience an accidental pregnancy during the first year if they do not stop use for any other reason. Estimates of the probability of pregnancy during the first year of typical use for spermicides and the diaphragm are taken from the 1995 National Survey of Family Growth corrected for underreporting of abortion; estimates for fertility awareness-based methods, withdrawal, the male condom, the pill, and Depo-Provera are taken from the 1995 and 2002 National Survey of Family Growth corrected for underreporting of abortion. See the text for the derivation of estimates for the other methods

[c]Among couples who initiate the use of a method (not necessarily for the first time) and who use it *perfectly* (both consistently and correctly), the percentage who experience an accidental pregnancy during the first year if they do not stop use for any other reason. See the text for the derivation of the estimate for each method

[d]The percentages becoming pregnant in columns (2) and (3) are based on data from populations where contraception is not used and from women who cease using contraception in order to become pregnant. Among such populations, about 89 % become pregnant within 1 year. This estimate was lowered slightly (to 85 %) to represent the percentage who would become pregnant within 1 year among women now relying on reversible methods of contraception if they abandoned contraception altogether

[e]Foams, creams, gels, vaginal suppositories, and vaginal film

[f]The Ovulation and TwoDay methods are based on the evaluation of cervical mucus. The Standard Days method avoids intercourse on cycle days 8 through 19. The Symptothermal method is a double-check method based on the evaluation of cervical mucus to determine the first fertile day and evaluation of cervical mucus and temperature to determine the last fertile day

[g]Without spermicides

[h]With spermicidal cream or jelly

[i]Plan B One-Step and Next Choice are the only dedicated products specifically marketed for emergency contraception. The label for Plan B One-Step (one dose is one white pill) says to take the pill within 72 h after unprotected intercourse. Research has shown that all of the brands listed here are effective when used within 120 h after unprotected sex. The label for Next Choice (one dose is one peach pill) says to take one pill within 72 h after unprotected intercourse and another pill 12 h later. Research has shown that both pills can be taken at the same time with no decrease in efficacy or increase in side effects and that they are effective when used within 120 h after unprotected sex. The Food and Drug Administration has in addition declared the following 19 brands of oral contraceptives to be safe and effective for emergency contraception: Ogestrel (one dose is two white pills); Nordette (one dose is four light-orange pills); Cryselle, Levora, Low-Ogestrel, Lo/Ovral, or Quasense (one dose is four white pills); Jolessa, Portia, Seasonale, or Trivora (one dose is four pink pills); Seasonique (one dose is four light-blue-green pills); Enpresse (one dose is four orange pills); Lessina (one dose is five pink pills); Aviane or LoSeasonique (one dose is five orange pills); Lutera or Sronyx (one dose is five white pills); and Lybrel (one dose is six yellow pills)

[j]However, to maintain effective protection against pregnancy, another method of contraception must be used as soon as menstruation resumes, the frequency or duration of breastfeeds is reduced, bottle feeds are introduced, or the baby reaches 6 months of age

Table 1.2 Conditions associated with increased risk for adverse health events as a result of unintended pregnancy

Breast cancer
Complicated valvular heart disease
Diabetes: insulin dependent; with nephropathy/retinopathy/neuropathy or other vascular disease; or of >20 years' duration
Endometrial or ovarian cancer
Epilepsy
Hypertension (systolic >160 mmHg or diastolic >100 mmHg)
History of bariatric surgery within the past 2 years
HIV/AIDS
Ischemic heart disease
Malignant gestational trophoblastic disease
Malignant liver tumors (hepatoma) and hepatocellular carcinoma of the liver
Peripartum cardiomyopathy
Schistosomiasis with fibrosis of the liver
Severe (decompensated) cirrhosis
Sickle cell disease
Solid organ transplantation within the past 2 years
Stroke
Systemic lupus erythematosus
Thrombogenic mutations
Tuberculosis

Reprinted from [11]

In 2010 the Centers for Disease Control and Prevention (CDC) adapted the WHO MEC for use in the USA [11]. The CDC MEC are very similar to those of the WHO, since the CDC contributed substantially to the evidence base for the WHO MEC. However, small modifications were made with the CDC MEC to accommodate specific health care circumstances, medical conditions, and contraceptives that are relevant to medical practice in the USA. The contraceptives evaluated in the CDC MEC include combined hormonal contraceptive (CHC) methods, including low-dose (≤35 mcg ethinyl estradiol) combined oral contraceptive pills (COC), combined hormonal patch (P), and combined hormonal vaginal ring (R); progestin-only methods including progestin-only pills (POP), depot medroxyprogesterone acetate (DMPA) injection, and etonogestrel implant; intrauterine devices (IUD), including the copper IUD (Cu-IUD) and the levonorgestrel IUD (LNG-IUD), as well as emergency contraception, barrier methods, lactational amenorrhea, sterilization, withdrawal, and fertility awareness-based methods.

New evidence for these recommendations is reviewed and the CDC MEC are updated on a regular basis. The CDC MEC are meant to provide general guidance for clinicians in the USA when they counsel patients about safe contraceptive choices. The most recent CDC MEC document can be found at www.cdc.gov/reproductivehealth/UnintendedPregnancy/USMEC.htm. There is also a free app version of the CDC MEC that is downloadable for use from iTunes.

Clinicians should be aware that the CDC MEC recommendations are meant to guide the selection of a contraceptive method used for pregnancy prevention, and not for the treatment of other medical disorders. However, clinicians may reference the other chapters in this book for guidance on conditions such as menorrhagia, leiomyoma, or endometriosis, for which certain contraceptives may provide benefit.

Understanding the CDC Medical Eligibility Criteria for Contraceptive Use

The CDC MEC use four categories to classify conditions affecting eligibility for the use of each contraceptive method (Table 1.3). For most clinicians, the categories can be divided into a dichotomy—a contraceptive is safe to recommend in medical conditions categorized as 1 or 2, and not recommended for category 3 or 4 conditions. This may be particularly helpful for settings like Title X-funded family planning clinics, in which the primary providers are advanced practice clinicians (i.e., nurse practitioners or physician assistants). Many medical conditions, such as obesity or thyroid disease, are considered a category 1 or 2 for all or most contraceptive methods. Category 3 conditions should not be considered absolutely unsafe. However, making a recommendation in this situation requires careful clinical judgment, with detailed counseling and

Table 1.3 Categories of medical eligibility criteria for contraceptive use

Category 1	A condition for which there is no restriction for the use of the contraceptive method
Category 2	A condition for which the advantages of using the method generally outweigh the theoretical or the proven risks
Category 3	A condition for which the theoretical or proven risks usually outweigh the advantages of using the method. Use of this method is not usually recommended unless other more appropriate methods are not available or acceptable
Category 4	A condition that represents an unacceptable health risk if the contraceptive method is used

Adapted from [11]

evaluation. The risks of unintended pregnancy and possible complications that may result when an effective method is not initiated must be considered. Therefore, if alternative methods are not available or acceptable to a patient, a contraceptive for a category 3 condition may be initiated with caution, preferably in consultation with a specialist. These subtleties are explored in detail by family planning experts in the subsequent chapters of this book, many of whom made significant contributions to the CDC MEC.

Few medical conditions are considered category 4, and these largely pertain to estrogen-containing hormonal contraceptive methods and their potential effect on cardiovascular health and thromboembolic disease (Table 1.4). The recommendation of a contraceptive method for a category 4 condition is rare, as in the case of a patient with breast cancer and tamoxifen therapy, and should be left to a specialist. Clinicians may consult the chapters in this book for examples of when this may be appropriate for various conditions.

For fertility awareness-based methods, the CDC MEC use a different classification system (Table 1.5), since no medical conditions would be worsened with fertility awareness-based method use. However, certain conditions may make fertility awareness-based methods more difficult to use, and the CDC MEC provide guidance on this topic.

An important point to keep in mind is that the CDC MEC guidelines are based on evidence regarding safety, and they do not take effectiveness into account. These guidelines are meant to assist in making contraceptive recommendations that should also take into consideration individual clinical circumstances.

Assessing a Patient's Medical Eligibility

Clinicians should be aware that assessing a woman for eligibility for a specific contraceptive can be done primarily by taking a detailed medical history. Formal screening for all possible category 3 or 4 conditions in a woman who is interested in a specific method is expensive, unnecessary, and acts as an additional barrier to accessing effective contraception. The CDC Selected Practice Recommendations (SPR), published in 2013, provide guidance regarding the circumstances under which screening should take place [4]. For example, women with complicated diabetes are considered category 3 or 4 for CHCs, depending on the severity of their disease. However, according to the CDC SPR, screening for diabetes for any woman interested in starting hormonal contraceptives is not necessary because of the low prevalence of undiagnosed diabetes among reproductive-aged women, and the high likelihood that women with complicated diabetes would have already been diagnosed prior to presenting for contraceptive counseling. Although hormonal contraceptives can have some adverse effects on glucose metabolism in diabetic women, the overall clinical effect is minimal, and so requiring screening for diabetes prior to starting hormonal contraception is not recommended.

Additional testing for category 3 or 4 conditions via advanced exam or diagnostic tests is generally not necessary, and should only be done if history-taking yields information that requires further investigating. For example, a woman who reports a history of systemic lupus erythematosus would require testing for antiphospholipid antibodies before initiating combined hormonal contraceptives. Further details are described in

Table 1.4 Category 4 conditions that pose an unacceptable health risk for use of a specific contraceptive

Contraceptive method	Condition	Subcategory
Combined hormonal contraceptives	Smoking	Age ≥35 yo, ≥15 cigarettes/day
	Multiple risk factors for arterial cardiovascular disease	–
	Hypertension	Systolic ≥ 160 mmHg or diastolic ≥ 100 mmHg
		Vascular disease
	Deep venous thrombosis (DVT)/ pulmonary embolism (PE)	Higher risk for recurrent DVT/PE (≥1 risk factors)
		Active DVT/PE
		DVT/PE and established on anticoagulant therapy for ≥3 mo: Higher risk for recurrent DVT/PE (≥1 risk factors)
		Major surgery with prolonged immobilization
		Known thrombogenic mutations
	Current and history of ischemic heart disease	–
	Stroke	–
	Valvular heart disease	Complicated (pulmonary hypertension, risk for atrial fibrillation, history of subacute bacterial endocarditis)
	Peripartum cardiomyopathy	Normal or mildly impaired cardiac function <6 mo
		Moderately or severely impaired cardiac function
	Systemic lupus erythematosus	Positive (or unknown) antiphospholipid antibodies
	Migraines	Without aura ≥35 yo (continuation only)
		With aura any age (initiation and continuation)
	Current breast cancer	–
	Diabetes	Severe nephropathy/retinopathy/neuropathy
		Other severe vascular disease or diabetes of >20-year duration
	Viral hepatitis	Severe acute or flare episode
	Severe cirrhosis	–
	Liver tumors	Hepatocellular adenoma
		Malignant liver tumors
	Complicated solid organ transplant	–
Progestin-only contraceptives (not including LNG-IUD)	Current breast cancer	–
Intrauterine device	Current pregnancy	–
	Puerperal sepsis	–
	Immediate postseptic abortion	–
	Unexplained vaginal bleeding (initiation only)	–
	Gestational trophoblastic disease	Persistently elevated HCG levels or malignant
	Cervical cancer	Awaiting treatment (initiation)
	Current breast cancer (LNG-IUD only)	–
	Endometrial cancer (initiation only)	–

(continued)

Table 1.4 (continued)

Contraceptive method	Condition	Subcategory
	Distorted uterine cavity that interferes with IUD insertion	–
	Pelvic infection	Current pelvic inflammatory disease (initiation only)
		Current purulent cervicitis or chlamydial infection or gonorrhea (initiation only)
		Pelvic tuberculosis (initiation only)
Barrier methods	High risk for contracting HIV (spermicide, ±diaphragm/cap)	–

Adapted from [11]

Table 1.5 Categories of medical eligibility criteria for fertility awareness-based contraceptive methods

A = Accept	No medical reason to deny the particular method to a woman in this circumstance.
C = Caution	The method can be normally provided in a routine setting but with extra preparation and precautions.
D = Delay	Use of this method should be delayed until the condition is evaluated or corrected. Alternative temporary methods of contraception should be provided.

Adapted from [11]

Table 1.6 Scenario 1

Postpartum	Combined hormonal contraceptives
Breastfeeding	
<1 month postpartum	3
≥1 month postpartum	2
Non-breastfeeding	
<21 days postpartum	3
>21 days postpartum	1

Adapted from [11]

the "Initiating a New Method of Contraception" section of this chapter, in the subsequent chapters of this book for specific medical conditions, and in the CDC SPR (found at http://www.cdc.gov/reproductivehealth/UnintendedPregnancy/USSPR.htm).

The following are clinical scenarios to help you understand how to use the CDC MEC to determine the safety of a particular method for your patient, or to select an array of safe contraceptive options for her.

Initiating a Method

Clinical Scenario 1

A 32-year-old healthy woman who had an uncomplicated vaginal delivery 2 days ago is interested in restarting COCs. She is breastfeeding and plans to do so for about a year (Table 1.6).

Whether she is breastfeeding or not, her status on postpartum day 3 is considered category 3 for COCs due to the elevated risk of thrombosis during the postpartum period. She should consider alternate methods until at least 1 month postpartum if she is still breastfeeding, or 21 days if she is not, and may then safely switch to COCs. The CDC MEC recommendations were updated in 2011 to include considerations for other risk factors for thrombotic events during the postpartum period [13].

Continuing a Method

For certain contraceptive methods, recommendations are subdivided into two CDC MEC subcategories: initiation (I) of a new contraceptive method and continuation (C) of a currently used contraceptive method. If a woman develops a health condition while using a contraceptive method, then her risk profile may be different, and so the recommendation for continuation should be followed.

Clinical Scenario 2

A 24-year-old woman who was started on COCs 5 months ago now presents with worsening headaches. Prior to initiating contraception, she had mild infrequent headaches with no associated symptoms. In the last 3 months, her headaches have become regular and more severe. They are now associated with nausea and photophobia, which drive her to dark, quiet places to alleviate some of her symptoms. She denies any auras (Table 1.7).

Although this patient was safe to initiate COCs with her non-migrainous headache history (category 1), her headaches have since developed migrainous characteristics. The initiation of a COC is considered relatively safe with migraines at her age (category 2), but since she has developed these migraines since starting the pills, she is now considered category 3 for continuing with this method. She should be counseled to switch to a different method at this point, unless another method is not available or acceptable to her. If this patient had also developed any associated auras with her migraines, continuing COCs would be considered an unacceptable health risk, or category 4. Clinicians may consult Chap. 7 for further details.

Table 1.7 Scenario 2

	Combined hormonal contraceptives	
	Initiation	Continuation
Headaches: non-migrainous	1	2
Migraine without aura, <35 yo	2	3
Migraine with aura, any age	4	4

Adapted from [11]

If a Patient Has Two or More Medical Conditions

A patient may present with two or more medical conditions that have implications for her contraceptive choices. Although the effort to unify various recommendations may seem challenging, combining multiple CDC MEC categories for different conditions can often be straightforward. Generally, the condition with the highest category number will dictate the safety of a contraceptive choice for a patient.

Clinical Scenario 3

A 28-year-old obese woman smokes a quarter pack of cigarettes (five cigarettes) per day. She underwent bariatric surgery via laparoscopic gastric banding 1 year ago. Her blood pressure today is 144/88; at her primary care visit 3 months ago, her blood pressure was 138/90. She wants to use the contraceptive vaginal ring (Table 1.8).

Table 1.8 Scenario 3

	Contraceptive vaginal ring (combined hormonal method)
Age <40 yo	1
Smoking <35 yo	2
Hypertension: systolic 140–159 or diastolic 90–99	3
Obesity	2
Bariatric surgery: restrictive	1

Adapted from [11]

Since the patient is less than 35 years old, smoking and obesity are each considered category 2 for the contraceptive vaginal ring. A restrictive bariatric surgery procedure is category 1. However, she can be given a diagnosis of hypertension based on her elevated blood pressure at two visits, which is considered a category 3 condition for this method. Thus, this patient as a whole should be considered a woman with a category 3 condition for the ring. She may use the ring if and only if she has access to no other alternatives or will accept no other alternatives. This patient should be carefully counseled about the risks and benefits of using the ring compared to other methods. In many cases, with proper counseling, the patient may accept an alternative method that is not only safer (category 2 or less for all her conditions), but also more effective, such as the implant or the IUD.

Clinical Scenario 4

A 23-year-old woman with a history of end-stage renal disease due to systemic lupus erythematosus

Table 1.9 Scenario 4

	CHC (COC/P/R)	POP	Injection	Implant	LNG-IUD	Cu-IUD	Barrier
Systemic lupus erythematosus: negative for antiphospholipid antibodies	2	2	2	2	2	1	1
Solid organ transplant: uncomplicated	2	2	2	2	2	2	1
Hypertension: adequately controlled	3	1	2	1	1	1	1

Adapted from [11]

underwent a renal transplant 2 months ago. Laboratory analysis is negative for antiphospholipid antibodies. Her hypertension persisted after her transplant, but is well controlled with lisinopril. She is interested in effective contraception because she has been counseled to wait at least 1 year after her transplantation before attempting pregnancy, which she desires to do within the next 2 years. She is taking mycophenolate (CellCept), a known teratogen, to prevent organ rejection (Table 1.9).

This patient's controlled hypertension is considered category 3 for CHCs, so these are not recommended unless she cannot or will not accept any other method. All other methods are considered medically safe for her to use. However, since they do not provide equal effectiveness, these methods should not be recommended equally. Pregnancy would be very high risk for her at this time, so she needs highly effective contraception. Of these safe methods, the implant and IUDs would be significantly preferable to progestin-only pills and barrier methods based on their effectiveness.

Careful consideration is required to evaluate more complicated medical conditions and clinical scenarios, as this book will describe in the subsequent chapters. However, clinicians should feel reassured that most contraceptives are safe in most medical conditions, without the need for an extensive work-up prior to initiation.

General Approach to Contraceptive Counseling

Gynecologists and reproductive health care providers are often the first to discuss pregnancy and contraception with women. However, pregnancy has profound health and social implications for all women, and thus primary care and specialty providers who have patients of reproductive age should regularly assess pregnancy intention and discuss family planning. Contraceptive counseling is a critical component of preventive health care, and must not be limited to those women actively seeking contraception. Establishing reproductive goals is of paramount importance for women with medical conditions. Such women may have limited options for safe and effective contraception, may be taking teratogenic medications, or may face serious health consequences if unintended pregnancy occurs. Optimal opportunities for assessment of pregnancy intention and contraceptive counseling include preventive visits, annual examinations, and prenatal care visits. In addition, these topics must be addressed at any visit in which a woman is given a new diagnosis or medication that may affect the safety of her current or desired method of contraception (such as a woman on combined oral contraceptives who is newly diagnosed with hypertension), or if a new diagnosis or medication could affect her fertility or the safety of pregnancy. These interventions are important in the preconception care paradigm established by the CDC, since improving a woman's health before conception can improve pregnancy outcomes for women and infants [14].

Patients have a wide variety of personal beliefs, experiences, goals, and motivations that they bring to their health care visits, and contraceptive decision making is complex. Nonetheless, contraceptive counseling works. Patients who receive contraceptive counseling are more likely to use contraception [15]. When women receive contraceptive counseling that highlights the most effective methods, they are highly likely to use such effective methods, particularly when barriers such as cost and access are removed [16]. Some patients may be ambivalent about pregnancy or resistant to contraceptive counseling. However, as with other preventive topics such as smoking cessation, contraceptive education and counseling by health care providers have positive impacts on behavior [17].

Because of the potential health implications of a patient's contraceptive choice, health care providers should approach contraceptive counseling in a standardized fashion, emphasizing the most effective methods that are medically appropriate. Contraceptive specialists often use the analogy of a cardiologist prescribing medications to a patient with high blood pressure. In this setting, few physicians would present all available medications equally, regardless of the efficacy in clinical trials, and then simply ask the patient to choose. Similarly, patients should know that some methods of contraception work better than others. Providers should feel comfortable making strong recommendations while using an evidence-based approach and avoiding their personal biases or anecdotes regarding methods.

Step 1: Review All Medically Eligible Methods, Emphasizing the Most Effective Options

After a patient has been assessed for medical eligibility, she must be informed of all available safe options, with emphasis on the most effective methods. This is particularly important for a patient who comes to the visit requesting a specific method. Many women make assumptions regarding contraceptive methods or have received erroneous information from family, friends, and other nonmedical sources such as the Internet. Clinicians should take the time to explore the reasons for a woman's desired method and educate her about more effective options that she may not be aware of or has not considered.

Many health care providers, particularly those who provide specialty care outside the realm of women's reproductive health, are not trained in procedures such as IUD placement, contraceptive implant insertion, or permanent sterilization. However, an individual provider's lack of experience with and access to these procedures should not affect contraceptive recommendations. Women who select these methods can be referred to other providers. However, they must be instructed to use another contraceptive as a bridging method while awaiting referral. When contraceptive provision is delayed, as is often seen in the postpartum and post-abortion settings, many women either fail to return for contraception or become pregnant in the interim. Providers have a duty to help women develop a feasible contraceptive plan that starts on the day of their visit [18, 19].

Step 2: Discuss Future Pregnancy Plans

Patients should be queried regarding interest in future childbearing and planned pregnancy timing or birth spacing. In general, shorter acting methods are preferable for women who are planning to conceive within a year. Long-acting reversible contraceptive (LARC) methods such as the IUDs and contraceptive implant generally provide more effective pregnancy prevention, but may be less appealing to some women due to procedural discomfort and higher up-front costs. However, the IUD and contraceptive implant are highly cost-effective after just 1 year of use [20, 21]. All women should be assured that these methods can easily be removed at any time for any reason, with rapid return to fertility [22]. In fact, all contraceptive methods have a rapid return to fertility except for DMPA, which has a mean return to ovulation of 10 months [23, 24]. Thus, an individual's possible desire for pregnancy within 1 year should not preclude the use of these LARC methods, especially for women with medical comorbidities.

Conversely, women who do not desire future fertility should also be counseled regarding permanent methods, including vasectomy and tubal occlusion. Providers should emphasize that there are reversible alternatives to sterilization that are equally or more effective, such as the IUD and implant, which may also have noncontraceptive benefits that sterilization cannot provide. Women considering permanent methods should be counseled regarding the risk of regret, which varies depending on several factors but is higher among women less than age 30 [25].

Step 3: Consider Adherence Behaviors

Contraceptive adherence is a critical aspect of counseling. Most women have a reasonable assessment of what they can manage, given their history and prior use. It is important to help patients realistically decide which method they can use consistently and correctly. Any gap between perfect-use and typical-use failure rates should be clearly described.

In general, patients should be counseled regarding the typical-use failure rates. Those who opt for user-dependent methods should be informed that effectiveness depends on how consistently the method is used. Many patients have a difficult time understanding a chart such as Table 1.1 on the perfect- versus typical-use effectiveness, but have an easier time comparing effectiveness when contraceptive methods are illustrated and arranged in contraceptive effectiveness tiers from least effective to most effective (Fig. 1.2). Clinicians have found the accompanying contraceptive counseling tool and other similar charts helpful during counseling.

In the case of COCs, women need to know that effectiveness decreases if they miss pills or delay starting a new pill cycle. It is important to put the long-term magnitude of this risk in perspective: preventing pregnancy for 3 years requires a woman to take over a 1,000 pills. Almost everyone forgets to take medications as instructed from time to time. But in the case of contraceptives, a woman risks unintended pregnancy if she misses her pills, which is a much greater health consequence than that of the occasionally missed cholesterol-lowering pill. Because of this risk, reproductive health professionals have been moving away from recommending COCs in favor of the more effective LARC methods as first-line contraceptive methods for nearly all women, including adolescents and nulliparous women.

Step 4: Weigh the Noncontraceptive Benefits and Bleeding Profiles

For women with chronic medical conditions, choice of contraceptive method may depend more on noncontraceptive factors (potential side effects, medication interactions, and uterine bleeding profile) than on efficacy, convenience, or other characteristics. For instance, in a woman with catamenial epilepsy (i.e., seizures that increase in frequency or severity during menses), DMPA may be a preferred option because it may increase the seizure threshold while also leading to amenorrhea [26, 27]. This discussion is also an opportunity to review the many health benefits of contraceptives, even for women with certain medical conditions. These benefits vary considerably by method and may be of short term, such as a reduction in acne and decreased dysmenorrhea, or of long term, such as decreased risk of ovarian or uterine cancer. Patients can decide how important these factors are for their particular situation.

The uterine bleeding profile of contraceptive methods, particularly hormonal methods, must be highlighted because menstrual blood loss may affect the health status of women with certain medical problems. For instance, decreased blood loss with menses or amenorrhea may be beneficial in women with anemia or on anticoagulation therapy. For some women, however, changes in menstruation or the cessation of uterine bleeding may be unacceptable. Bleeding irregularity is an important cause for early discontinuation of contraceptive methods [28]. Proper counseling prior to method initiation will provide realistic expectations of a contraceptive method and potentially improve contraceptive continuation.

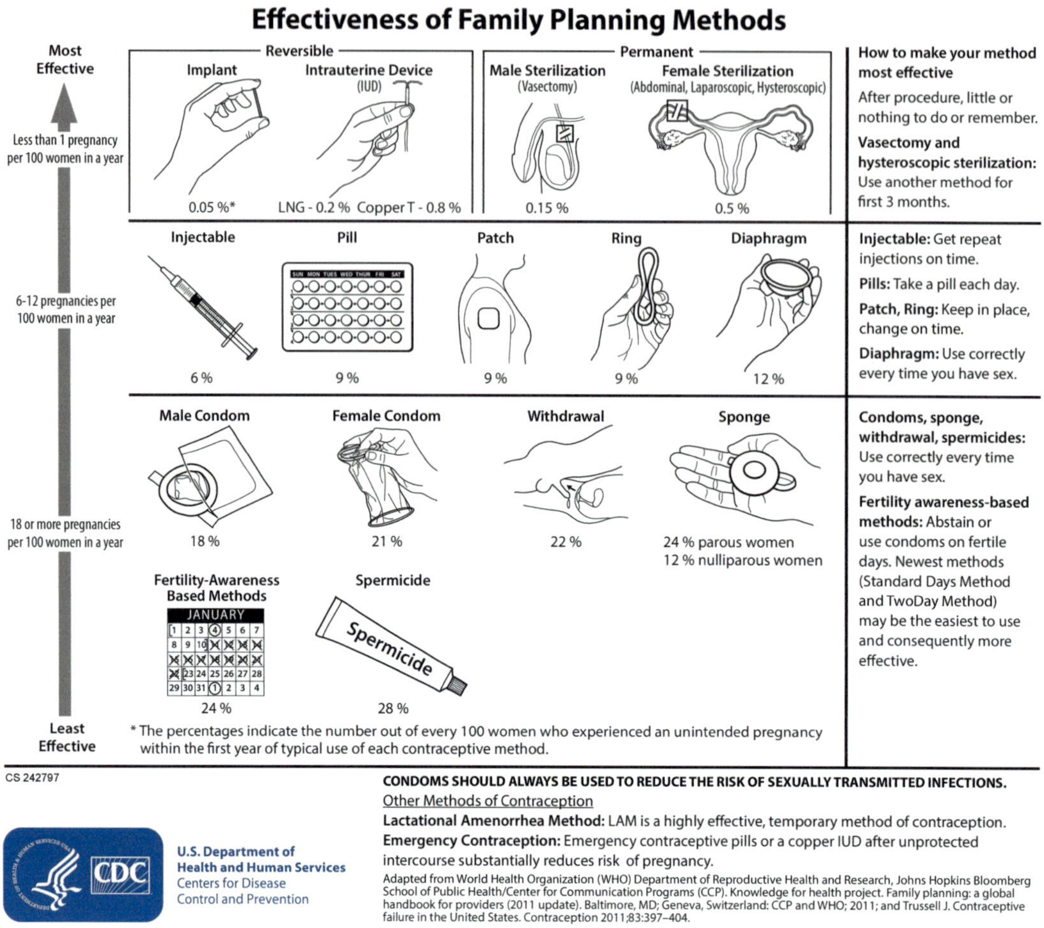

Fig. 1.2 Effectiveness of family planning methods. Reprinted from [34]

Step 5: Assess Need for Dual Protection

Clinicians must assess the risk of exposure to sexually transmitted infections (STIs) among patients who are initiating contraception. For patients who engage in sexually risky behaviors, such as those who are not in mutually monogamous relationships, have a new partner, or have multiple partners, dual-protection strategies should be considered. Male condoms must be used with every act of intercourse for optimal STI prevention, but should not be used as a sole contraceptive method due to their high contraceptive failure rates with typical use. Combining condoms with another form of contraception is an excellent strategy for maximizing contraceptive efficacy and preventing STIs.

Initiating a New Method of Contraception

When initiating a contraceptive method, most women do not require any additional evaluation. However, clinicians should assess contraceptive needs in the context of other health matters. In healthy patients, most components of routine health maintenance such as blood pressure assessment, weight, lipid panel, Pap test, and breast exam are not necessary for contraception commencement, but may be performed if otherwise indicated. Importantly, clinicians should not hold contraceptive provision hostage to other health maintenance recommendations. Women should not be denied contraception if they decline health maintenance exams or are noncompliant with other care recommendations.

The CDC SPR can provide guidance on how to initiate contraceptive methods and how to manage common issues that arise, in addition to screening recommendations as described earlier [4]. Similarly to the MEC, the SPR were adapted from WHO guidelines, but are tailored to the US medical practice. While the MEC describe which patients can safely use the various methods of contraception, the SPR provide guidance on actual use of the methods: how to initiate and optimally use methods of contraception, management of common side effects and problematic bleeding profiles, when to initiate methods in certain clinical settings, and when it is appropriate to discontinue contraception. The SPR also counsel on ways to optimize contraceptive use in special patient populations including adolescents. The SPR document can be found at http://www.cdc.gov/reproductivehealth/UnintendedPregnancy/USSPR.htm.

Table 1.10 Using the SPR when initiating a contraceptive method

SPR provides the following guidelines for each contraceptive method:
– Timing of initiation
– Need for backup contraception after initiation
– Special considerations: – Amenorrhea (not postpartum) – Postpartum (breastfeeding) – Postpartum (not breastfeeding) – Postabortion (spontaneous or induced) – Switching from another contraceptive method
– Examinations and tests needed before initiation of the method (*varies by method*) – Weight (BMI) – Bimanual examination and cervical inspection – Blood pressure – Glucose – Liver enzymes – Clinical breast examination – Other screening: testing for cervical intraepithelial neoplasia or cervical cancer, HIV or other STDs, hyperlipidemia, anemia, thrombogenic mutations
– Routine follow-up after method initiation
– Bleeding irregularities – Spotting or light bleeding – Heavy or prolonged bleeding – Amenorrhea
– Additional guidelines provided for specific methods: management of missing IUD strings, timing of repeat injection, number of pill packs to provide, missed or late doses

Ensuring That a Woman Is Not Pregnant

Prior to initiating any method of contraception, it is important to assess for possible pregnancy by taking a menstrual history, inquiring about recent sexual intercourse, and assessing the current use of contraception (Table 1.10). If pregnancy cannot be reasonably ruled out by the patient's history, urine pregnancy tests can be used, but may be limited due to the interval between fertilization and HCG detection within the urine. It generally takes more than 2 weeks after ovulation before a negative urine or serum pregnancy test can effectively rule out pregnancy, due to the time it takes for a fertilized egg to implant in the uterus and produce detectable levels of HCG. Of note, human chorionic gonadotropin (HCG) is typically detectable in blood and urine for several weeks after a spontaneous or an induced abortion or delivery.

Most contraceptive methods can be initiated immediately even if there is uncertainty regarding possible pregnancy. There is no evidence that methods such as CHCs or progestin-only methods are harmful to a developing fetus [29]. If the benefits of immediate contraceptive initiation outweigh any theoretical risks, clinicians may recommend that a patient start the method and check a urine pregnancy test 2–4 weeks later. Same-day initiation of contraception, originally developed with COCs, can initially improve continuation rates of hormonal contraception [30–32]. Although this advantage disappears over time, "quick start" initiation can be applied to initiation of nearly any hormonal contraceptive method.

IUDs, on the other hand, can lead to serious complications if placed during pregnancy. According to the SPR, clinicians must ensure that patients are not pregnant before placing the device. Once a clinician is reasonably certain that a woman is not pregnant, IUDs can be safely initiated at any time of the menstrual cycle [33].

As noted above, all methods of contraception can be initiated immediately, at any time in the menstrual cycle, provided that the clinician can be reasonably certain that the patient is not pregnant. If a patient is switching from another method, there should be no break prior to initiating a new method. Waiting for onset of menses prior to contraceptive initiation is unnecessary and possibly harmful as it creates an unnecessary barrier to contraceptive provision. In the case of IUD placement, clinicians do not need to wait until menstruation to place an IUD, as there is no evidence that menstruation increases the rate of successful placement.

Routine physical examination and screening laboratory studies are not recommended prior to initiating most contraceptive methods. Exceptions include CHC and IUD initiation. Prior to initiation of CHC, blood pressure should be measured (either by a health care provider or in a nonclinical setting such as a pharmacy) to screen for hypertension. Prior to IUD placement, clinicians should perform bimanual examination and inspect the cervix. This practice allows clinicians to assess for uterine size and position, and for certain cervical or uterine conditions that may make IUD placement unsafe. Measuring weight prior to initiation of hormonal methods is suggested, but not medically necessary, in order to detect any subsequent changes in weight and aid in future counseling.

Routine follow-up is not necessarily required after initiation of any contraceptive method, though a woman should be advised to contact her clinician if problems arise or if she is considering discontinuing or switching her method. At routine health visits, including those scheduled with other clinicians, each patient should be assessed for changes in health status or the use of new medications that may not be compatible with her current contraceptive method according to the MEC. In addition, particular medical conditions may warrant additional follow-up with the use of certain contraceptive methods. Details regarding follow-up recommendations for various medical conditions can be found in the corresponding chapters of this book.

Despite the potential interaction between medical conditions and certain contraceptive methods as described in the MEC, such conditions have generally low prevalence and do not justify routine screening of healthy patients, for example, for hyperlipidemia or thrombophilia. The high costs of screening, and additional barriers that these tests would represent for women seeking contraception, outweigh any marginal increase in safety. However, women with medical problems require individualized counseling and assessment. If there is clinical suspicion for a condition that would cause a contraceptive method to be risky, then screening may be indicated.

This book, when used in conjunction with the CDC publications, provides thorough guidance for clinicians who care for women with complex medical conditions. Once they have the willingness and ability to offer safe and effective contraception, clinicians can help patients achieve their reproductive goals while maximizing their health and well-being.

References

1. The Alan Guttmacher Institute (AGI). Fulfilling the promise: Public Policy and U.S. Family Planning Clinics. New York: The Alan Guttmacher Institute; 2000.
2. Finer LB, Zolna MR. Unintended pregnancy in the United States: incidence and disparities, 2006. Contraception. 2011;84(5):478–85.
3. Hou MY, Creinin MD. Update on contraception. OBG Manage. 2013;25(8):22–9.
4. Centers for Disease Control and Prevention. United States Selected Practice Recommendations for Contraceptive Use. MMWR Morb Mortal Wkly Rep. 2013;62(RR-5):1–60.
5. American College of Obstetricians and Gynecologists. ACOG Practice Bulletin. No. 73: Use of hormonal

contraception in women with coexisting medical conditions. Obstet Gynecol. 2006;107(6):1453–72. PubMed PMID: 16738183.
6. Wald RM, Sermer M, Colman JM. Pregnancy and contraception in young women with congenital heart disease: general considerations. Paediatr Child Health. 2011;16(4):e25–9.
7. Nagelkerke NJ, Bernsen RM, Sgaier SK, Jha P. Body mass index, sexual behaviour, and sexually transmitted infections: an analysis using the NHANES 1999–2000 data. BMC Public Health. 2006;6:199.
8. McKay DB, Josephson MA, Armenti VT, August P, Coscia LA, Davis CL, et al. Reproduction and transplantation: report on the AST Consensus Conference on Reproductive Issues and Transplantation. Am J Transplant. 2005;5(7):1592–9. PubMed PMID: 15943616.
9. Grimes DA. Intrauterine devices. In: Hatcher RA, Trussell J, Nelson AL, Cates W, Kowall D, Policar MS, editors. Contraceptive technology. 19th ed. Atlanta, GA: Contraceptive Technology Communications, Inc.; 2007.
10. Trussell J. Contraceptive efficacy. In: Hatcher RA, Trussell J, Nelson AL, Cates W, Kowall D, Policar MS, editors. Contraceptive technology. 20th ed. Atlanta, GA: Contraceptive Technology Communications, Inc.; 2011.
11. Centers for Disease Control and Prevention. United States medical eligibility criteria for contraceptive use. MMWR. 2010;59(RR04):1–6.
12. World Health Organization. Medical eligibility criteria for contraceptive use. 4th ed. Geneva, Switzerland: WHO; 2010.
13. Centers for Disease Control and Prevention. Update to CDC's U.S. medical eligibility criteria for contraceptive use, 2010: revised recommendations for the use of contraceptive methods during the postpartum period. MMWR. 2011;60(26):878–83.
14. Centers for Disease Control and Prevention. Recommendations to improve preconception health and health care—United States. MMWR. 2006; 55(RR06):1–23.
15. Lee JK, Parisi SM, Akers AY, Borrero S, Schwarz EB. The impact of contraceptive counseling in primary care on contraceptive use. J Gen Intern Med. 2011;26(7):731–6.
16. Madden T, Mullersman JL, Omvig KJ, Secura GM, Peipert JF. Structured contraceptive counseling provided by the Contraceptive CHOICE Project. Contraception. 2013;88(2):243–9.
17. Atrash HK, Johnson K, Adams M, Cordero JF, Howse J. Preconception care for improving perinatal outcomes: the time to act. Matern Child Health J. 2006;10(5 Suppl):S3–11.
18. Thurman AR, Janecek T. One-year follow-up of women with unfulfilled postpartum sterilization requests. Obstet Gynecol. 2010;116(5):1071–7.
19. Bednarek PH, Creinin MD, Reeves MF, Cwiak C, Espey E, Jensen JT. Immediate versus delayed IUD insertion after uterine aspiration. N Engl J Med. 2011;364(23):2208–17.
20. Mavranezouli I. The cost-effectiveness of long-acting reversible contraceptive methods in the UK: analysis based on a decision-analytic model developed for a National Institute for Health and Clinical Excellence (NICE) clinical practice guideline. Hum Reprod. 2008;23(6):1338–45.
21. Lipetz C, Phillips CJ, Fleming CF. The cost-effectiveness of a long-acting reversible contraceptive (Implanon) relative to oral contraception in a community setting. Contraception. 2009;79(4):304–9.
22. Hov GG, Skjeldestad FE, Hilstad T. Use of IUD and subsequent fertility–follow-up after participation in a randomized clinical trial. Contraception. 2007;75(2):88–92.
23. Mishell Jr DR. Pharmacokinetics of depot medroxyprogesterone acetate contraception. J Reprod Med. 1996;41(5 Suppl):381–90.
24. Schwallie PC, Assenzo JR. Contraceptive use—efficacy study utilizing medroxyprogesterone acetate administered as an intramuscular injection once every 90 days. Fertil Steril. 1973;24(5):331–9.
25. ACOG. ACOG Practice Bulletin No. 133: benefits and risks of sterilization. Obstet Gynecol. 2013;121(2 Pt 1):392–404.
26. Mattson RH, Cramer JA, Caldwell BV, Siconolfi BC. Treatment of seizures with medroxyprogesterone acetate: preliminary report. Neurology. 1984;34(9): 1255–8.
27. Mattson RH, Cramer JA. Epilepsy, sex hormones, and antiepileptic drugs. Epilepsia. 1985;26 Suppl 1: S40–51.
28. Edelman AB, Gallo MF, Jensen JT, Nichols MD, Schulz KF, Grimes DA. Continuous or extended cycle vs. cyclic use of combined oral contraceptives for contraception. Cochrane Database Syst Rev. 2005;3, CD004695.
29. Wilson JG, Brent RL. Are female sex hormones teratogenic? Am J Obstet Gynecol. 1981;141(5):567–80.
30. Westhoff C, Heartwell S, Edwards S, Zieman M, Cushman L, Robilotto C, et al. Initiation of oral contraceptives using a quick start compared with a conventional start: a randomized controlled trial. Obstet Gynecol. 2007;109(6):1270–6.
31. Westhoff C, Osborne LM, Schafer JE, Morroni C. Bleeding patterns after immediate initiation of an oral compared with a vaginal hormonal contraceptive. Obstet Gynecol. 2005;106(1):89–96.
32. Murthy AS, Creinin MD, Harwood B, Schreiber CA. Same-day initiation of the transdermal hormonal delivery system (contraceptive patch) versus traditional initiation methods. Contraception. 2005;72(5):333–6.
33. Turok DK, Godfrey EM, Wojdyla D, Dermish A, Torres L, Wu SC. Copper T380 intrauterine device for emergency contraception: highly effective at any time in the menstrual cycle. Hum Reprod. 2013; 28(10):2672–6.
34. Centers for Disease Control and Prevention. Effectiveness of family planning methods. Atlanta, GA: Centers for Disease Control and Prevention; 2013.

2 Contraceptive Management of Women with Cardiac Disease

Autumn Davidson, Joan Briller, and Julie Chor

Introduction

Early twentieth-century physicians recognized cardiac disease as an indication for contraception and sterilization out of concern for high maternal mortality rates. Though contraceptive methods were largely illegal at the time, physicians were able to prescribe contraception for women with medical conditions such as cardiac disease [1]. Whereas early twentieth-century physicians painted cardiac disease risk in pregnancy with broad strokes, contemporary physicians take a more nuanced approach to risk stratification. This type of approach is essential to appropriately counsel high-risk women to prevent unintended pregnancy and to avoid inappropriate recommendations for termination of pregnancy in women with conditions that pose little or no pregnancy risk.

Reproductive health for women with cardiac disease is becoming an increasingly important topic because the prevalence of cardiac disease in reproductive-aged women is on the rise. Berg et al. compared national intrapartum maternal morbidity rates in 1993–1997 and 2001–2005 and found that 33,800 women with cardiac disease (distinct from chronic hypertension) delivered per year during the 2001–2005 period [2]. Data from Washington State demonstrated a 224 % increase in the proportion of births to women with heart disease (congenital and acquired) between 1987–1994 and 2002–2009 [1]. Increases in acquired heart disease in reproductive-age women reflect rising rates of obesity, diabetes, and advanced maternal age, while increases in maternal congenital heart disease are largely attributed to medical and surgical advancements for these conditions that allow women to live longer and reproduce [1, 2].

The rise in maternal cardiac disease has significant maternal, perinatal, and neonatal implications. In their evaluation of "near-miss" maternal mortality, Small et al. identified maternal cardiac disease as the leading cause of ICU admission (36 %) [3]. Compared to women without these conditions, women with chronic heart disease (including congenital heart disease, ischemic heart disease, heart failure, or pulmonary hypertension) are more likely to experience a maternal death, small-for-gestational age neonate, or perinatal or postnatal death [1].

The increased prevalence and the associated sequelae of heart disease in reproductive-aged women should motivate practitioners of diverse specialties to have an appreciation of the importance of appropriate contraceptive management

A. Davidson, M.D. • J. Chor, M.D., M.P.H. (✉)
Department of Obstetrics and Gynecology,
The University of Chicago, Chicago, IL, USA
e-mail: davidson.autumn@gmail.com;
jchor@bsd.uchicago.edu

J. Briller, M.D.
Division of Cardiology, Department of Medicine,
University of Illinois Medical Center,
Chicago, IL, USA
e-mail: briller@uic.edu

R.H. Allen and C.A. Cwiak (eds.), *Contraception for the Medically Challenging Patient*,
DOI 10.1007/978-1-4939-1233-9_2, © Springer Science+Business Media New York 2014

for these women. In this way, we can help women with cardiac disease avoid unintended pregnancies and/or optimize preconception cardiac health. Despite the important role of contraception for women with heart disease, there is limited published literature regarding contraceptive safety and efficacy in this population and even fewer prospective studies on this topic [4]. In this chapter, we focus on contraceptive management for women with cardiac disease. We present an overview of cardiovascular physiology in pregnancy and cardiac risks associated with pregnancy. We go on to present the available evidence regarding contraceptive safety for women with cardiac disease. Cardiac conditions are presented according to a hybrid pregnancy risk stratification schema. We conclude with a discussion of challenges and models of contraceptive care for women with cardiac disease and suggestions for future areas of research.

Reproductive Counseling Experiences of Women with Cardiac Disease

In light of the complexity of pregnancy and contraceptive management of women with cardiac disease, appropriate contraceptive counseling for these women is extremely important. Gaps exist in the reproductive health care of women with cardiac disease. Reid et al. conducted a survey of 16–20-year-olds with moderate-to-complex congenital heart disease and found that 14 % of adolescents (16–18-year-olds) and 48 % of young adults (19–20-year-olds) had been sexually active in the past 3 months. 36 % of sexually active young adults engaged in risky sexual behavior including having two or more sexual partners in the past 3 months and using drugs or alcohol at least sometimes before sex [5].

An assessment of adults with congenital heart disease found that 23 % had concerns about contraception and 28 % had concerns about pregnancy. Furthermore, 22 % had unanswered questions regarding contraception and 36 % had unanswered questions regarding pregnancy [6]. A German survey found that 20 % of women with congenital heart disease who were contracepting were using a contraindicated method and that 28 % of sexually active women with high-risk conditions were not using contraception. Overall, 43 % of women reported not receiving contraceptive counseling and 48 % reported not receiving information regarding pregnancy-related risks attributed to their condition [7].

These gaps in reproductive health counseling highlight the need to develop counseling approaches for this population. The American College of Obstetricians and Gynecologists (ACOG) recommends an initial gynecology visit for adolescents between 13 and 15 years of age [8]. The early initiation of a relationship with a women's health provider is especially important for girls and young women with cardiac disease to introduce concepts such as safe contraception, pregnancy risks, and how to optimize prepregnancy health. While the clinician should be aware of the potential to overwhelm adolescents with reproductive health information, it is important to initiate these discussions prior to the onset of sexual activity. Ensuring a positive relationship between the patient and her women's health provider requires a good patient-clinician rapport, which is usually developed gradually and over time.

Hemodynamic Changes Associated with Pregnancy and Cardiovascular Implications

Pregnancy results in major cardiovascular adaptations, which can precipitate significant morbidity and mortality in women with cardiovascular disease. Cardiac output increases by as much as 50 % due to increased blood volume (increased preload), increased stroke volume, increased heart rate, and decreased peripheral resistance (decreased afterload). The increase in plasma volume exceeds the increase in hemoglobin, resulting in the "physiologic anemia" of pregnancy. Increased blood volume can be problematic for women with left ventricular dysfunction. Maternal heart rate typically increases and is responsible for maintaining cardiac output later in pregnancy.

Tachycardia may increase the risk of arrhythmia and impair ventricular filling, which can be challenging for women with obstructive lesions such as mitral stenosis [9]. Left ventricular ejection fraction increases a small amount [10]. Left ventricular end-diastolic blood pressure remains normal, and systemic vascular resistance (SVR) decreases [11]. Systolic blood pressure (BP) begins to decrease at 7 weeks' gestation, nadirs mid-pregnancy, and gradually returns to or exceeds pre-pregnancy levels at the end of pregnancy.

Labor and delivery result in additional increases in cardiac output requirements. Uterine contractions can transfer 300–500 mL volume into the general circulation, increasing preload. Pain and anxiety increase sympathetic tone leading to elevations of heart rate (HR) and blood pressure. Maternal pushing efforts further increase cardiac output. Immediately postpartum, cardiac output continues to rise due to autotransfusion of blood from the uterus coupled with improved venous return from relief of inferior vena cava compression [12, 13]. This autotransfusion can exacerbate volume overload in women at risk of right or left heart failure. Postpartum, hemodynamic changes rapidly return to baseline with the substantial normalization within 2 weeks [12].

Pregnancy is a hypercoagulable state resulting in the increasing propensity for thromboembolic complications. This may be especially important for women predisposed to thrombosis such as women with a history of mitral stenosis, prosthetic valves, or congenital heart disease [14–16]. Alterations in glucose metabolism and cholesterol levels secondary to hormonal shifts may increase the risk of ischemic events [17, 18]. Physiologic changes in pregnancy can affect the bioavailability of cardiovascular drugs, and potential teratogenicity may lead to conflicting maternal-fetal risk-benefit ratios.

Schema for Risk Stratification

Cardiac conditions are presented throughout this chapter according to a hybrid risk stratification schema. Several larger prospective studies identify maternal cardiac risk factors in pregnancy.

Table 2.1 New York Heart Association Functional Classification

Functional class	Symptoms
I	No limitations of physical activity.
II	Mild limitations of physical activity. Ordinary activity results in dyspnea, fatigue, and palpitations.
III	Marked limitations of physical activity. No symptoms at rest but less than ordinary activity results in dyspnea, fatigue, and palpitations.
IV	Unable to carry out physical activity without symptoms. Dyspnea, fatigue, palpitations at rest.

Siu and colleagues prospectively followed 562 women with cardiovascular disease through 599 pregnancies (CARPREG study) to identify risk factors associated with adverse outcomes. Major risk factors for adverse pregnancy outcomes included a history of prior cardiac event (heart failure, transient ischemic attack/cerebrovascular accident prior to pregnancy, or arrhythmia); New York Heart Association (NYHA) functional class III or IV at baseline (Table 2.1) or cyanosis; history of left heart obstruction (aortic stenosis, mitral stenosis, or left ventricular outflow tract obstruction); and reduced systemic ventricular function (ejection fraction≤40 %) [19]. Similar approaches have been utilized in other studies with additional risk factors identified including the presence of a mechanical valve prosthesis, moderate-to-severe valvular regurgitation, cyanotic congenital heart disease, use of cardiac medications prior to pregnancy, and smoking history [2, 15, 20–23].

In order to help guide clinicians in appropriate counseling and management of contraception for women with heart disease, a multidisciplinary group of cardiologists, maternal-fetal medicine obstetricians, family planning physicians, and obstetric anesthesiologists convened in Britain to form a working group on pregnancy and contraception for women with heart disease [24]. The aim of this working group was to adapt the World Health Organization's (WHO) Medical Eligibility Criteria for Contraceptive Use to incorporate specific cardiovascular conditions not previously addressed. In addition, using the same classification scheme, the

Table 2.2 Classification of maternal cardiovascular risk

Risk category	Risk of pregnancy
I	No detectable increase in maternal mortality and no or mild increase in morbidity
II	Small increased risk of maternal mortality or moderate increase in morbidity
III	Significant increased risk in maternal mortality or severe morbidity. Expert counseling required.
IV	Extremely high risk of maternal mortality or severe morbidity. Pregnancy contraindicated. If occurs termination should be discussed. If pregnancy continues care as in category III.

Adapted from Heart, Thorne S, MacGregor A, Nelson-Piercy C, 92, 1520–5, 2006, with permission from BMJ Publishing Group Ltd

working group also rated each cardiac condition by pregnancy risk. In their 2006 published report, this working group classified individual cardiac conditions as category I to IV for both pregnancy and contraceptive use (Table 2.2) [25]. Women with category I conditions have low pregnancy risk. In contrast, women with conditions rated category III are at high risk of pregnancy complications, and those who are category IV should be advised against pregnancy [24]. Our approach in this chapter incorporates this published schema in order to organize the presentation of cardiac conditions, and to give guidance to clinicians so that they may best counsel cardiac patients about their particular relative risk of pregnancy and contraceptive use.

General Considerations Regarding Contraception in Women with Heart Disease

We consider several primary concerns for contraceptive safety in women with cardiac disease: thrombogenic alterations, the potential for fluid retention, blood pressure changes, pro-arrhythmic effects, potential changes in glucose metabolism and lipid profiles, bleeding on warfarin, bacteremia/endocarditis risk, and vasovagal reactions. Additionally, contraceptive counseling for women with cardiac disease must weigh potential contraceptive safety concerns with the risks of unintended pregnancy and differences in method efficacy. Combined hormonal contraception (CHC) has several adverse cardiac effects. Most importantly, the estrogen component alters the coagulation profile by increasing hepatic production of pro-coagulation factors (factors VII, VIII, and X), and decreasing production of fibrinolytic factors (tissue plasminogen activator and anti-plasmin). These changes result in increased rates of thromboembolic complications [26, 27]. Possible fluid retention resulting from the estrogen component of CHC may also influence contraceptive risk for women with cardiovascular disease [28]. Finally, CHC should be avoided in women with severe hypertension and in those with significant liver disease which may coexist in women with cardiac disease [29]. Progestin-only contraceptive methods are not associated with increased risk of thrombotic events and are considered safe in most women with cardiac disease.

In postmenopausal women on hormone therapy, estrogen has been demonstrated to prolong the QT interval. Progestins have been associated with a decrease in the QT interval and the combination of estrogen plus progestin has been found to have no effect. However, no studies specifically evaluate the impact of contraceptive hormones on QT intervals and arrhythmias [30, 31]. Contraceptive hormones have been found to alter lipid profiles and have inconsistent effects on glucose tolerance and diabetes mellitus [31]. Therefore, contraceptive recommendations with regard to pro-arrhythmic, lipid, and glucose considerations are primarily based on expert opinions.

Women with cardiac disease are sometimes anticoagulated with warfarin; oral anticoagulation poses unique considerations to contraceptive use. First, it should be noted that both estrogens and progestins might have the potential to interfere with warfarin metabolism [32–34]. For this reason, the international normalized ratio (INR) in women concurrently on warfarin therapy and any hormonal contraception should be closely monitored. Second, depot medroxyprogesterone acetate (DMPA) use in anticoagulated women carries with it a theoretical risk for hematoma formation at the intramuscular (IM) injection site [35]. To our knowledge, no studies have been published on the safety of intramuscular DMPA injections in anticoagulated women that specifically look at the concern for bleeding at the injection site. However, a prospective series followed 13 women on chronic anticoagulation with a history of bleeding complications from ruptured corpus lutea who had subsequently been started on DMPA for ovarian suppression. After monitoring these women for a mean of 40 months, the authors reported that there were no recurrent ovarian bleeding events. The authors did not indicate that there had been any DMPA injection site bleeding issues in their paper [36]. Several prospective studies comparing the safety of IM to subcutaneous (SC) injections of influenza vaccine in anticoagulated patients have shown no significant difference in risk of hematoma formation [37–40]. Although data showing an association between IM-administered DMPA injections and hematoma formation among anticoagulated women is lacking, we nonetheless recognize the theoretical risk. Therefore, while the use of DMPA in anticoagulated women has both contraceptive and ovarian suppression benefits, these women should be counseled regarding the possibility of intramuscular hematoma formation. As with all agents, which could affect anticoagulation levels in patients on warfarin, the INR should be followed when this method is utilized.

Data on the safety of subdermal implants in anticoagulated women are also lacking. We can, however, extrapolate from the studies evaluating safety of SC injections among warfarin users, and conclude that this procedure is safe. Moreover, unlike deep hematoma formation that may occur with IM injections, superficial hematomas are easy to detect and to monitor. Thus, although we recognize the potential for bleeding at insertion site, we assert that subdermal contraceptive implants are a preferable contraceptive method to DMPA in anticoagulated women.

Finally, anticoagulated women are at risk for heavy menstrual bleeding, and may benefit from the use of contraceptive methods that reduce menstrual flow or induce amenorrhea. A theoretical concern with intrauterine devices (IUD) for women with cardiac disease is the possible increased risk of endocarditis in high-risk women (see section "Valvular Heart Disease"). However, prophylactic antibiotics prior to IUD insertion are no longer recommended for the prevention of infectious endocarditis [41]. Another consideration for women with certain complex cardiac conditions is the potential for serious complications (cardiovascular collapse) in the event of a vasovagal reaction, which occurs in a minority of IUD insertions, especially in nulligravid or nulliparous women [35].

These considerations inform the Centers for Disease Control and Prevention's (CDC) contraceptive recommendations for women with certain cardiac conditions in the US Medical Eligibility Criteria for Contraceptive Use (USMEC) [29]. Additionally, the working group on pregnancy and contraception for women with cardiac disease, as described previously, provides a risk classification system specifically for contraception for women with cardiac disease [24]. This group adapted and expanded on the World Health Organization's contraceptive risk classification system and used the same four-tiered risk stratification (1 = no restriction, 2 = advantages generally outweigh theoretical or proven risk, 3 = theoretical or proven risk generally outweighs advantages, and 4 = unacceptable method). Throughout the text, we refer to the CDC contraceptive recommendations as the USMEC and the interdisciplinary working group's recommendations as the Working Group. We include tables of cardiac conditions grouped by pregnancy risk with each condition's primary contraceptive concerns and available contraceptive risk categories from the USMEC and/or the Working Group.

Low-Risk Conditions

Small Shunts

Simple and fully repaired cardiac shunts include atrial septal defects (ASD), ventricular septal defects (VSD), patent ducti arteriosis (PDA) and patent foramen ovales (PFO). Together, atrial and ventricular septal defects account for just over

Table 2.3 Contraception for low pregnancy risk conditions

Condition	CHC	POP	Injection	Implant	LNG-IUD	Cu-IUD	1⁰ contraceptive concerns
Small Shunts							• Thrombogenic
ASD	**1/3**[a]	**1**	**1**	**1**	**1**	**1**	
VSD	**1/2**[a]	**1**	**1**	**1**	**1**	**1**	
PDA	**1/2**[a]	**1**	**1**	**1**	**1**	**1**	
PFO	**2/4**[b]	**1**	**1**	**1**	**1**	**1**	
Mitral valve prolapse without significant insufficiency	**1**/2	1	1	1	1	1	• Thrombogenic
Mild pulmonary stenosis	**1**/2	1	1	1	1	1	• Thrombogenic
Isolated PVCs and PACs	**1**	**1**	**1**	**1**	**1**	**1**	• Arrhythmic • Thrombogenic

CHC Combined hormonal contraception, *POP* Progestin-only pills, *LNG-IUD* Levonorgestrel intrauterine device, *Cu-IUD* Copper intrauterine device
Bold = Working Group
Red = USMEC
Underlined = Working Group and USMEC
[a]Repaired without sequelae vs. non-repaired
[b]Incidental vs. symptomatic

one-third of all cases of congenital heart disease among adults [24, 42–45]. These defects are classified by their size and anatomic location. When small, they are asymptomatic and pose little risk to a pregnant woman [24].

To our knowledge, no prospective studies exist evaluating the safety of combined hormonal contraception (CHC), which includes the combined pill, patch, or ring, in women with small cardiac shunts. Women with repaired simple cardiac shunts and no residual disease do not carry a risk of clot formation and are, therefore, appropriate for all forms of contraception (Table 2.3) [24]. Atrial septal defects can result in right-to-left shunting following a valsalva maneuver with a theoretical increased risk of paradoxical thromboembolism and stroke [24]. CHCs are considered by the Working Group to be category 3 for women with unrepaired ASDs [24]. Progestin-only contraceptive methods (pills, injection, implant, IUD) and the copper IUD are considered safe in women with these lesions [35]. Ventricular septal defects without complications, repaired and unrepaired, do not carry the same risk of paradoxical embolism. Therefore, all contraceptive methods are considered broadly safe to use with this lesion [24, 35].

Patent ductus arteriosus (PDA) occurs when the fetal ductus arteriosus fails to spontaneously close after birth. Patients with PDAs account for approximately 10–18 % of congenital heart disease and are usually asymptomatic when the degree of shunting is small [46]. All patients with a PDA carry a risk of bacterial endarteritis/endocarditis. As for women with a VSD, shunt flow with a small PDA is left to right since pulmonary vascular resistance is less than systemic vascular resistance. Consequently, there is not an associated risk of paradoxical embolism [47]. Women with small unrepaired or repaired PDAs without complications (e.g., residual lesion, congestive heart failure, endarteritis, presence of ductal aneurysm, pulmonary hypertension) may therefore safely use all forms of contraception, including IUDs [35].

A patent foramen ovale (PFO) results from failure of the fetal septum primum to fuse with the septum secundum after birth. Autopsy studies suggest that PFO may be present in up to 25–35 % of adults [48]. Flow across a PFO is functional and dependent on relative pressure differences between the left and right atria. Therefore, a PFO is undetectable on physical exam and found only when there has been a clinical event or when echocardiographic screen is performed for another reason. Several case–control studies of cryptogenic strokes have shown an increased incidence of PFO in comparison with the general population, suggesting that a paradoxical embolism may play a role in the pathophysiology [49–51]. However, two community-based studies of asymptomatic patients with incidentally identified PFOs failed to find that PFOs were independently associated with increased risk of a cerebrovascular event [52, 53].

The Working Group recommends that women in whom the PFO was discovered following a clinical event (stroke or transient ischemic attack) should avoid CHC [35]. However, CHC is considered permissible in asymptomatic women with incidental PFOs. Screening for PFO prior to initiation of CHC is not recommended [35]. Progestin-only contraceptive methods and both types of IUDs are safe to use in women with PFOs [35].

Mitral valve prolapse (MVP) occurs when there is the abnormal displacement of mitral leaflets into the left atrium during systole. Mitral valve prolapse affects between 2 and 3 % of the population, and is more common in females [54–56]. Many patients are asymptomatic with normal life expectancy and without significant morbidity. Some women with mitral regurgitation develop the need for surgical intervention, arrhythmias, endocarditis, or thromboembolic complications [57]. The best predictor of cardiovascular complications in pregnancy is the degree of associated mitral regurgitation. Mitral valve prolapse without significant mitral insufficiency tends to be well tolerated in pregnancy [24, 58, 59]. Several studies suggest an association between MVP and stroke; however, to date, this association remains unclear [56, 60–62].

The Working Group suggests that women with MVP with minimal or no mitral regurgitation may safely use CHC [24]. Of note, the USMEC considers CHC in women with uncomplicated valvular heart disease to be a category 2 due to low thrombotic risk [25, 29]. The USMEC category 2 rating does not distinguish between the different types of uncomplicated valvular disease. The Working Group, however, specifically delineates MVP without significant regurgitation as low risk for thrombotic events, and therefore rates CHCs for women with this condition as category 1. Both rating systems consider progestin-only methods and both IUDs to be category 1 for these women [25, 29, 35].

Mild Pulmonic Stenosis

Pulmonic stenosis (PS) occurs when there is an obstruction of blood flow from the right ventricle (RV) to the pulmonary artery. Mild pulmonic stenosis is defined as a peak gradient less than 36 mmHg [63]. This condition occurs in 1 in 2,000 live births, accounting for approximately 8 % of congenital heart disease [64]. While PS is usually an isolated lesion, it can be associated with other congenital heart defects, most commonly septal defects. Pulmonic stenosis is often a correctible condition resulting in an increasing number of people living with long-term sequelae such as pulmonary regurgitation, restenosis, and arrhythmias [65]. However, pregnancy is well tolerated in women with mild-to-moderate PS, both in individuals with native valves as well as those who have undergone surgical correction [24, 65–67]. As in MVP, the Working Group considers mild PS low thrombotic risk and rates CHC as category 1, while the USMEC does not distinguish mild PS from other forms of uncomplicated valvular heart disease and considers this group in general to be a category 2 (see Table 2.3) [24, 25, 29]. Women with mild PS may safely use progestin-only contraception and both IUDs (category 1) [35, 66].

Isolated Premature Atrial Contractions and Premature Ventricular Contractions

Premature atrial contractions (PACs) and premature ventricular contractions (PVCs) are common findings in patients with and without significant cardiovascular disease. The presence and type of underlying structural heart disease determine the prognosis and need for further evaluation and therapy intervention. The exact prevalence of these conditions is unknown as the estimates differ depending on the study and mode of detection. One study followed 50 young, healthy women with 24-h Holter monitors and found a 64 % prevalence of PACs and a 54 % prevalence of PVCs [68]. They are also frequently seen in pregnant women with palpitations, where they are associated with benign outcomes. These conditions are considered low risk in pregnancy [24, 69, 70]. No specific recommendations on contraceptive use in women with isolated PVCs and PACs exist. However, given high prevalence in the general population we can extrapolate that all methods of contraception are appropriate in the absence of underlying structural heart disease [24].

Moderate-Risk Conditions

Repaired Tetralogy of Fallot

Tetralogy of Fallot (TOF) is the most common form of cyanotic congenital heart disease after 1 year of age. The defect results from deviation of the outlet septum, which leads to a large VSD, overriding aorta, and outflow obstruction of the RV infundibulum, pulmonary valve, or supravalvular level, with subsequent right ventricular hypertrophy [71]. Improvements in surgical repair have enabled more women affected by TOF to survive into their reproductive years [72]. Following repair, long-term complications are related to the degree of residual RV outflow tract obstruction and pulmonic stenosis or regurgitation. Residual disease can lead to RV dilatation and failure or need for valve replacement [63]. Long-term risks include endocarditis, atrial and ventricular arrhythmias, heart block, and sudden cardiac death [63]. Pregnancy in women with TOF is increasingly common, and, often, well tolerated (category 2) [73, 74]. Surgical correction is associated with improved maternal and fetal outcomes, and, when possible, repair is indicated prior to pregnancy [15, 44, 75].

In the absence of right-to-left shunt, CHC and progestin-only methods can be used safely in women with repaired TOF (Table 2.4) [35]. Intrauterine devices are excellent forms of contraception in women with this condition, and have been used safely following cardiac surgery [76, 77]. Although the Working Group rated the LNG-IUD category 1, the group rated the copper IUD category 2 in women with repaired TOF out of concern for the theoretical increased risk of endocarditis (see discussion on IUDs in section "Valvular Heart Disease"). The USMEC does not address this condition separately.

Arrhythmias

Arrhythmia is a broad term used to describe any cardiac rhythm other than normal sinus. This includes isolated premature atrial and ventricular contractions (discussed in section "Low-Risk Conditions"), bradyarrhythmias such as heart block, and tachycardias, which include supraventricular tachycardia, atrial flutter and fibrillation, and ventricular tachycardia or fibrillation. Pregnancy risk depends on the degree of associated symptoms such as syncope or dizziness, underlying structural heart disease, and thromboembolic risk.

The Working Group considers CHC broadly usable in women with most arrhythmias. In most cases, progestin-only contraceptives and IUDs are considered safe in these women [35]. Atrial fibrillation (A-fib) and atrial flutter (A-flutter) pose exceptions, as they are prothrombotic. Therefore, women with these arrhythmias should avoid estrogen-containing methods (i.e., CHC) [35]. Long-term anticoagulation is common among women with A-fib and A-flutter. Although it does confer some protection, anticoagulation therapy does not entirely block estrogen's thrombotic effect [24]. CHC should be used with caution in anticoagulated women with A-fib or A-flutter, and is contraindicated if anticoagulation is stopped [35]. Contraceptive injections should also be used with caution in anticoagulated women due to concern for injection site hematomas and the potential interaction with warfarin as described above.

Table 2.4 Contraception for moderate pregnancy risk conditions

Condition	CHC	POP	Injection	Implant	LNG-IUD	Cu-IUD	1⁰ contraceptive concerns
Repaired Tetralogy of Fallot	**1**	**1**	**1**	**1**	**1**	**2**	• Endocarditis • Thrombogenic
Arrhythmias Atrial Fibrillation/flutter Other	 **4/3**[a] **2**	 **1** **1**	 **1/3**[a] **1/3**[a]	 **1** **1**	 **1** **1**	 --	• Thrombogenic
Mild LV dysfunction	**2**/4	**1**	**1**	**1**	**1**/2	2	• Fluid retention • Hypertension • Thrombogenic
Hypertrophic cardiomyopathy	**2/3/4**[b]	**1**	**1**	**1**	**1**	--	• Arrhythmic • Endocarditis • Thrombogenic
Moderate native valve disease	2/4[c]	1	1	1	1/**2**	*1*	• Endocarditis • Thrombogenic
Mild aortic root disease Marfan without dilatation Bicuspid aortic valve with aortic root <4.5 cm Repaired coarctation	 **2** **1** **1/3**[d]	 **1** **1** **1**	 **1** **1** **1**	 **1** **1** **1**	 **1** **1** **1**	 --	• Hypertension

CHC Combined hormonal contraception, *POP* Progestin-only pills, *LNG-IUD* Levonorgestrel intrauterine device, *Cu-IUD* Copper intrauterine device

Bold = Working Group

Red = USMEC

Underlined = Working Group and USMEC

[a]Not warfarin vs. on warfarin

[b]Isolated lesion (2) vs. with associated sequelae (3 vs. 4)

[c]Uncomplicated vs. complicated

[d]Uncomplicated vs. with hypertension or aneurysm

Although the contraceptive implant is safe and effective in women with A-fib and A-flutter, case reports suggest that in anticoagulated women the INR should be closely monitored for potential interaction between warfarin and etonogestrel [24, 34]. There are no specific recommendations for the use of the copper IUD in women with arrhythmias. However, the levonorgestrel intrauterine device (LNG-IUD) has been used safely in women on warfarin and may be more appropriate than the copper IUD in anticoagulated women due to its beneficial effects on uterine bleeding profiles [77–80]. We found no reports of interactions between warfarin and the LNG-IUD.

Mild Left Ventricular Dysfunction

Mild left ventricular dysfunction (LVD) is defined as a diminished left ventricular ejection fraction of 40–50 % [81]. LVD results from multiple etiologies, including valvular heart disease, ischemic heart disease, congenital heart disease, primary cardiac muscle problems, and metabolic abnormalities [82]. Pregnancy in women with mild LVD is classified as category 2–3, depending on the underlying etiology and patient's overall cardiac reserve [24].

While the contraceptive guidelines do not specifically address the risks for women with mild LVD, we have extrapolated the risk categories from those assigned to women with peripartum cardiomyopathy with long-term, mild cardiac impairment. CHC use in women with LVD poses the risk of complications associated with hypertension, fluid retention, and thrombosis. With regard to peripartum cardiomyopathy, the Working Group accords less risk than does the USMEC for CHC use in these women (2 vs. 4, respectively) [25, 29]. As there are no prospective data regarding the risk of CHC in women in peripartum cardiomyopathy, these recommendations are based on expert opinion, which may vary. Decisions regarding the use of CHC in women with a history of peripartum cardiomyopathy should depend on symptomatology. Progestin-only contraceptive methods, on the other hand, do not carry the same cardiovascular risk, and are appropriate for women with mild LVD (category 1) [35]. Both IUDs are considered safe and appropriate options for women with this cardiac condition [35].

Hypertrophic Cardiomyopathy

Hypertrophic cardiomyopathy (HCM) is the most common genetic cardiac disease with a prevalence of about 1:500 in the general population [83]. Cardiac risks of pregnancy include diastolic heart failure due to a hypertrophied noncompliant ventricle or outflow tract obstruction, heart failure due to associated mitral regurgitation, and risk of arrhythmias (atrial fibrillation and sudden cardiac death secondary to ventricular arrhythmia). Children of parents with hypertrophic cardiomyopathy also have an inheritance risk of 50 % as the disease is autosomal dominant [44, 84]. Women with hypertrophic cardiomyopathy are typically considered pregnancy category 2 or 3 (moderate risk). Mortality with pregnancy is low except with advanced disease [85]. The 2011 American College of Cardiology Foundation/American Heart Association guidelines for management suggest that in the setting of advanced heart failure, pregnancy is associated with excess morbidity and mortality and should be avoided [84]. However, in most other women with asymptomatic HCM or with symptoms adequately controlled with medical therapy, pregnancy is reasonable [44, 84]. For any woman of childbearing age with HCM, genetic and preconceptual counseling is mandatory.

The Working Group classifies CHC as risk category 2 for women with isolated HCM lacking other high-risk cardiac conditions. However, the risk of CHC use in women with hypertrophic cardiomyopathy with additional sequelae, or with other high-risk cardiac conditions, is generally upgraded according to the condition or the symptoms [24].

Contraceptive concerns with CHC are related to potential long-term sequelae of HCM including thrombogenic risk, arrhythmias, and potential for endocarditis. Progestin-only contraceptive methods and the LNG-IUD are safe and appropriate for women with HCM (category 1) [24]. Although the safety of the copper IUD is not specifically addressed in the classification systems, we can infer that these devices are appropriate for women with this condition.

Valvular Heart Disease

Valvular heart disease can be secondary to congenital or acquired abnormalities and is classified as either stenotic (such as mitral stenosis and aortic stenosis) or regurgitant (such as mitral regurgitation and aortic regurgitation). In the European registry of heart disease in pregnancy, mitral stenosis (MS) and mitral regurgitation (MR) comprised the most common lesions (63 %), while aortic disease occurred in 23 % [23]. In the USA and Europe, aortic stenosis (AS) in reproductive-aged women is most frequently congenital as rheumatic disease is increasingly rare in developed countries [86]. The severity of valvular heart disease is defined according to the (1) degree of valvular dysfunction and/or (2) associated clinical sequelae. Pregnancy risk in women with valvular heart disease depends on the severity of the lesion. Women with mild or moderate disease do well in pregnancy; severe disease, however, is less well tolerated [44, 57, 73, 87]. For the purpose of this chapter, we define disease severity accordingly:

- Mitral stenosis: mild or moderate: >2.0 cm^2, severe: <2.0 cm^2, or symptomatic [57]
- Aortic stenosis: mild or moderate: >1.0 cm^2, severe: <1.0 cm^2, or symptomatic [57]

Thrombotic risk for women with valvular disease depends on the type of lesion and its severity. The USMEC and the Working Group consider CHC "broadly useable" in women with uncomplicated disease (category 2) [25, 29, 35]. The USMEC defines uncomplicated valvular heart disease as valvular disease without other coexisting sequelae such as atrial fibrillation, pulmonary hypertension, or previous endocarditis [29]. Women who choose a CHC should be aware of the potential, albeit low, for thromboembolic events [25, 29, 35]. Progestin-only forms of contraception are considered safe in women with valvular disease—both the USMEC and the Working Group rate these methods category 1, with the exception that the Working Group rates the LNG-IUD category 2 [25, 29, 35].

IUDs were previously thought to pose a significant risk of bacteremia-associated endocarditis in women with valvular disease, especially at the time of insertion or removal. The actual risk of IUD-associated infective endocarditis is unclear. One study evaluated blood cultures in 40 women with cardiac disease who received copper IUDs [88]. Although cultures were collected after antibiotic prophylaxis, all cultures were sterile and the investigators failed to detect any cases of endocarditis [88]. The Working Group considers the risk of IUD-associated endocarditis to be higher than does the USMEC and recommends antibiotic prophylaxis. The USMEC considers the risk of endocarditis to be minor, and categorizes both IUDs as category 1, while the Working Group rates the LNG-IUD category 2 for uncomplicated valvular disease [35]. It should be noted that the Working Group guidelines were published in 2006, prior to the most recent American Heart Association guidelines for endocarditis prophylaxis, which do not recommend antibiotics prior to IUD insertion [41]. We concur with these newer recommendations.

Mild Aortic Root Diseases (Marfan Without Dilation, Ehlers Danlos, and Repaired Coarctation)

Marfan Syndrome

Marfan syndrome (MFS) is an autosomal dominant disorder of the connective tissue. It is one of the most common inherited connective tissue disorders with an estimated incidence of 2–3 per 10,000 [89]. Marfan syndrome poses a significant risk to pregnancy. Women without aortic root dilation carry a small risk of aortic dissection, and this risk increases with increasing aortic root dilation [44, 73, 90–94]. The Working Group classifies MFS as pregnancy risk category 2–3 in women without significant dilation and as category 4 in those with aortic roots >4 cm diameter [35]. Women with MFS may safely use most forms of contraception. The Working Group rates CHC as risk category 2 for women with MFS without aortic root dilatation [24]. MFS with complications is addressed separately under high-risk lesions. The USMEC does not separately address MFS. All progestin-only contraceptive methods and both the copper IUD and the LNG-IUD are safe and excellent contraceptive methods for women with MFS (category 1) [35].

Ehlers-Danlos Syndrome and Other Connective Tissue Disorders

Ehlers-Danlos syndrome (EDS) refers to a group of genetic connective tissue disorders. These disorders have an overall frequency of 1 in 5,000 [95]. Pregnancy is usually well tolerated in women with EDS, although serious maternal complications have been reported mostly in women with type IV (vascular) EDS [96, 97]. Complications include aortic dissection, ruptured bowel, and uterine rupture [98, 99]. Because no specific contraceptive recommendations exist for this condition, we can extrapolate from recommendations for use in MFS and conclude that CHC is considered category 2 in women without aortic root dilation and category 3 in those with dilation. Progestin-only contraceptives and both IUDs should be considered safe in these women [35].

Repaired Aortic Coarctation

Coarctation of the aorta is characterized as the narrowing of the aortic lumen, usually distal to the left subclavian artery, resulting in hypertension in the arms [46]. Aortic coarctation accounts for 4–6 % of congenital heart disease [100]. Surgical repair of aortic coarctation in childhood is associated with over 80 % 25-year survival and when possible should be performed prior to pregnancy [44, 46]. Pregnancy in women with repaired aortic coarctation is usually well tolerated (pregnancy risk category 2) but can be associated with increased risk of gestational hypertension, preeclampsia, and aortic dissection [42, 44, 101].

Contraceptive options in women with repaired aortic coarctation are varied. In women with an isolated repaired lesion who are otherwise asymptomatic, CHC is considered by the Working Group to be category 1 [35]. In those with known aneurysm or persistent hypertension, the risk of CHC is increased to category 3 due to hypertensive concerns [35]. All progestin-only methods including the LNG-IUD as well as the copper IUD are safe in women with repaired aortic coarctation (category 1) [35]. In women who are considering any form of surgical correction prior to achieving pregnancy, CHC would be less ideal due to the additive thrombotic risk of surgery. Moreover, women should be clearly informed about their individual pregnancy risks in the postoperative period following coarctation repair. For this reason, the contraceptive provider and cardiologists should work together to ensure that the most effective and appropriate form of contraception is arranged.

High-Risk Pregnancy Conditions

Ischemic Cardiovascular Disease/ Myocardial Infarction

While ischemic heart disease has historically been considered a rare disease among reproductive-aged women, its burden is increasing. The estimated prevalence of coronary heart disease and acute myocardial infarction (MI) is estimated to be 0.6 % in women between the ages of 20 and 39 years, with an estimated 5,000 myocardial infarcts and deaths per year in women aged 35–45 years [102]. It is likely that ischemic heart disease will be an increasingly common problem among women of reproductive age as a result of the increasing prevalence of obesity, diabetes, hypertension, sedentary lifestyle, and trend toward older maternal age [103, 104].

Acute myocardial infarction in pregnancy is a rare but deadly condition with an estimated mortality rate of 5–10 % [44, 105]. Data on pregnancy risk in women with a history of MI are lacking. Risk of pregnancy in women with a history of coronary disease depends in part on the etiology but also on overall left ventricular function and risk for additional ischemia. In the setting of significant LV dysfunction or New York Heart Association (NYHA) class III or IV symptoms, pregnancy risk is considered category IV [24].

Ischemic heart disease is considered a contraindication to CHC due to concerns for hypertension, hyperlipidemia, impaired glucose metabolism, and thrombosis and should be avoided [24, 25, 29]. Concern exists about the hypoestrogenic effect and the reduction in HDL that can occur with long-term use of the injectable progestin-only method, DMPA. For this reason, the USMEC rates DMPA as category 3 in these women. POPs, the LNG-IUD, and the contraceptive implant are considered by the USMEC to be category 2 for initiation and category 3 for continuation (Table 2.5). However, the Working Group rates all progestin-only methods category 1 [25, 29, 35]. It should be noted that the risks of pregnancy should weigh heavily into the contraceptive decision making of women with this condition. Although the copper IUD is the ideal option for women with ischemic heart disease, if for any reason this method is not an option, another LARC method should be encouraged.

Mechanical Prosthetic Valve

Prosthetic heart valves (PHV) are commonly placed in children and women of childbearing age for congenital and acquired valvular disease,

Table 2.5 Contraception for high pregnancy risk conditions

Condition	CHC	POP	Injection	Implant	LNG-IUD	Cu-IUD	1^0 contraceptive concerns
Myocardial Infarction	4	1/2/3[a]	1/3	1/2/3[a]	1/2/3[a]	1	• Glucose metabolism • Hypertension • Lipid metabolism • Thrombogenic
Mechanical prosthetic valve	3/4[b]	1	1/3[c]	1	3	4	• Bleeding on anticoagulation • Endocardits • Thrombogenic
Complex CHD							• Thrombogenic • Arrhythmia • Bleeding on anticoagulation • Vasovagal
Cyanotic heart disease without pulmonary hypertension	4	1	2/3[c]	1	2	3	
Fontan circulation	4	1	3	1	3/4[d]	4	
Aortic root dilation (>4 cm)	3	1	1	1	1	--	• Hypertension
Peripartum cardiomyopathy							• Arrhythmia • Endocarditis • Fluid retention • Thrombogenic
Normal/mild impairment	2/3/[e]	1	1	1	1/2	2	
Moderate or severe impairment	4	1/2	1/2	1/2	1/2	2	

CHC Combined hormonal contraception, *POP* Progestin-only pills, *LNG-IUD* Levonorgestrel intrauterine device, *Cu-IUD* Copper intrauterine device
Bold = Working Group
Red = USMEC
Underlined = Working Group and USMEC
[a]Initiation vs. continuation for USMEC
[b]Bi-leaflet mechanical valve on warfarin vs. Bjork-Shiley or Starr-Edwards valves on warfarin
[c]Not on warfarin vs. on warfarin
[d]3 if no other method appropriate and risk of pregnancy outweighs vasovagal risk of insertion
[e]<6 months vs. ≥6 months for USMEC

though the exact prevalence is unclear [106]. These valves pose unique challenges to pregnant women, including the risk of thromboembolism, prosthetic valvular degeneration, heart failure, pregnancy loss, and bleeding as a result of anti-coagulation [106–108]. Although women of childbearing age are more likely to have newer, less thrombogenic valves, pregnancy-related thromboembolic risk remains high [109]. Thrombotic risk is highest with older valves and when the valve is in the mitral rather than the aortic position. Pregnancy in women with a mechanical valve is considered risk category 3 [24].

Unfortunately, contraceptive options in women with PHV are limited. Combined hormonal contraceptives should be used with caution (category 3), or are contraindicated (category 4), depending on the type of valve, due to the thrombotic risk [24, 25, 29]. Women with PHV are frequently anticoagulated. Given the potential for alteration in warfarin metabolism with either estrogen or progestin, frequent INR monitoring should be performed in women using a hormonal method [24, 32–34]. Progestin-only methods are safe in women with PHV and the contraceptive implant is a better option than DMPA or POPs due to its superior effectiveness and the theoretical concern for hematoma formation at the DMPA injection site in anticoagulated women.

One prospective cohort study followed 20 anticoagulated women who had undergone cardiac valve replacement and subsequently received the LNG-IUD [77]. Compared to the control group, women with the IUD had significantly less menstrual blood loss and higher hemoglobin levels. The two groups did not differ in coagulation parameters and there were no cases of infective endocarditis. Although this study is small, it supports the assertion that the LNG-IUD can safely be used in women with mechanical valve replacement and especially in those women on anticoagulation. It should be noted that women in both groups received antibiotic prophylaxis for insertion, although current guidelines do not recommend prophylaxis [77]. Although the LNG-IUD is rated category 3 by the Working Group, modifications in risk assessment and recommendations regarding prophylactic antibiotic use for IUD insertion in women with cardiac disease have been subsequently updated and are likely not reflected in the Working Group's publication, as discussed above.

Complex Congenital Heart Disease

Complex CHD encompasses a variety of congenital disorders, many of which have a cyanotic component in which there is communication between the systemic and pulmonary circulation. Fontan-type circulation, in which the systemic venous circulation is surgically connected to the pulmonary artery in cases of a univentricular heart, also falls under this category [110]. The prevalence of complex CHD in the year 2000 was estimated to be 1.5 in 1,000 people, though this number varies depending on the study and the specific inclusion criteria [100, 111]. Improvements in management of CHD have led to more individuals with complex lesions reaching adulthood [112]. Pregnancy in women with Fontan-type circulation is considered by the Working Group to be high risk or contraindicated (category 3 or 4) [35, 44]. Pregnant women with this condition have a limited ability to increase their cardiac output, which can lead to heart failure. They are also prone to arrhythmias and thromboembolic events [42, 44, 73].

Given the serious pregnancy complications associated with these conditions, highly effective contraception is advised. The contraceptive implant is safe and is the optimal form of reversible contraception in these women [35, 113]. Intrauterine devices are not recommended for women with Fontan circulation due to the risk of cardiovascular collapse if they were to experience a vasovagal reaction, which occurs in approximately 2 % of women at the time of IUD insertion, especially if nulligravid or nulliparous [114]. Paracervical blocks and spinal anesthesia may reduce the risk of vagal response, but should only be used in situations in which no other appropriate contraceptive options are available and the risk of pregnancy outweighs the insertion risk [35]. Depot medroxyprogesterone acetate injection should be used with caution in women with cyanotic heart disease and in women with Fontan circulation who are anticoagulated as discussed above [35]. Progestin-only pills, while considered safe, are a poor option for women with complex CHD due to their high typical-use failure rates. CHC should be avoided in women with cyanotic heart disease and Fontan circulation because these conditions are associated with pulmonary artery thrombosis and pulmonary emboli [35, 113].

Aortic Root Dilatation (>4 cm)

Aortic root dilatation of >4 cm is considered a high-risk pregnancy condition due to risk for dissection [44]. With regard to CHC, the Working Group classifies aortic root dilatation >4 cm associated with MFS as category 3 in contrast to the category 2 rating for lesions <4 cm. This upgrade in CHC risk categorization is due to hypertension-related risk of aortic dissection with larger lesions due to concerns for worsening hypertension with these medications. Contraceptive risk for progestin-only methods and IUDs remains low, consistent with mild aortic root diseases (category 1) [35].

Peripartum Cardiomyopathy

Peripartum cardiomyopathy (PPCM) is a diagnosis of exclusion and is defined as the onset of left ventricular dysfunction and heart failure occurring within the last month of pregnancy or 5 months postpartum [115]. This condition is associated with significant maternal morbidity and mortality [76]. Recent estimates of maternal mortality among women with PPCM range from 7 to 15 % [116, 117]. The need for a heart transplant among women with this condition is estimated to be 6 % [116]. The epidemiology of PPCM varies by race, ethnicity, and geography, likely reflecting genetic and diagnostic variations. Recent US data report 3.6–4.8 cases per 10,000 live births [118, 119]. The safety of a subsequent pregnancy in women with a history of PPCM is largely related to interim recovery of left ventricular function [120, 121].

A systematic review by Tepper et al., which forms the basis for the recommendations used in the USMEC, failed to find studies regarding contraceptive safety for women with PPCM. Contraceptive recommendations in the USMEC are, therefore, based on concerns for risk of venous thrombotic events, fluid retention, arrhythmias, and endocarditis [28]. Fett and Murphy documented the contraceptive use of 100 women with PPCM in Haiti. Although they did not identify any contraception-related complications, only 62 women used contraception: 10 tubal sterilization, 11 5-year levonorgestrel implant, 29 DMPA, 3 combined oral contraceptives, and 9 barrier methods [122]. The USMEC categorizes contraceptive safety with PPCM according to (1) New York Heart Association classification and (2) time since delivery of either less than 6 months or 6 months or more, while the Working Group categorizes safety only according to cardiac impairment. Notable differences between the two categorizations include that the Working Group rates CHC for women with normal cardiac function to be category 2, while the USMEC categorizes it as a 3 or a 4 depending on the time since delivery. Though the Working Group does not provide a rating for CHC in women with impaired cardiac function due to PPCM, they do rate CHC use category 4 in women with severe left ventricular dysfunction. The Working Group rates all progestin-only methods category 1 for women with a history of peripartum cardiomyopathy, regardless of cardiac impairment. In contrast, the USMEC categorizes progestin-only pills, injection, or implants category 1 for women with normal to mildly impaired cardiac function and category 2 for women with moderate-to-severe impairment. The USMEC also rates the LNG-IUD category 2 for all women with PPCM, regardless of cardiac function [29, 35]. Of note, the copper IUD is considered category 2 by the USMEC and the Working Group does not comment on the use of this device in this population.

Pregnancy Contraindicated

NYHA Class III or IV Symptoms

The New York Heart Association (NYHA) functional classification system is commonly used to classify cardiac patients according to the severity of their symptoms [123]. Patients are rated on a scale of I to IV based on their degree of physical limitations attributable to their heart disease. Advanced NYHA functional class (class III or IV) is a strong predictor of adverse cardiac outcomes in pregnancy; pregnancy is considered contraindicated in women with NYHA III-IV [21, 44, 73, 101].

Because the NYHA classification system describes an individual's functional status rather than her underlying cardiac condition, no general guidelines regarding appropriate contraceptive methods can be made for women with advanced NYHA class. It is imperative, however, for these women to be well informed of their pregnancy risk, and effective contraception appropriately tailored to her underlying condition should be a top medical priority.

Severe Pulmonary Hypertension

Pulmonary hypertension (PH) is defined as the elevation in peak pulmonary systolic pressure exceeding 30 mmHg. The etiology of PH varies,

Table 2.6 Contraception for conditions in which pregnancy is contraindicated

Condition	CHC	POP	Injection	Implant	LNG-IUD	Cu-IUD	1⁰ contraceptive concerns
NYHA Class III or IV symptoms related to underlying disease							• Depends on underlying etiology
Severe Pulmonary Hypertension (including Eisenmenger syndrome)	**4**	**1/4**[a]	**1/3**[b]	**1**[c]	**3/4**[d]	**4**	• Bleeding • Hypertension • Thrombogenic • Vasovagal
Significant LV dysfunction	**4**	**1**	**1**	**1**	**1**	--	• Arrhythmia • Fluid retention • Hypertension • Thrombogenic
Severe aortic or mitral stenosis (adapted from mild valvular disease)	**2/4**[e]	1	1/3[b]	1	1/2	1/3	• Arrhythmia • Endocarditis • Thrombogenic

CHC Combined hormonal contraception, *POP* Progestin-only pills, *LNG-IUD* Levonorgestrel intrauterine device, *Cu-IUD* Copper intrauterine device
Bold = Working Group
Red = USMEC
Underlined = Working Group and USMEC
[a]Not on bosentan vs. on bosentan
[b]Not on warfarin vs. on warfarin
[c]Recommend using back-up contraception if on bosentan
[d]3 if no other method appropriate and risk of pregnancy outweighs vasovagal risk of insertion
[e]Without or with sequelae

and can be classified as primary (idiopathic) or secondary [124]. Idiopathic PH is rare with an estimated prevalence of 6.6 per one million individuals. Secondary PH can arise from congenital heart disease, collagen vascular disease, left heart failure or valvular disease, chronic thromboembolic disease, pulmonary disease, HIV, portal hypertension, and various drugs [125, 126]. A classic example of secondary PH is Eisenmenger syndrome, in which a left-to-right shunt causes increased flow through the pulmonary vasculature and results in pulmonary hypertension. Among individuals with CHD who do not undergo surgical correction, approximately one-third will develop PH [127]. Pulmonary hypertension from any cause is exceedingly dangerous in pregnancy. Maternal mortality in women with PH had been estimated to be as high as 50 %, although more recent studies report mortality risk around 33 % [42, 44]. Pregnancy in women with PH is associated with arrhythmias, heart failure, and endocarditis [42]. Death occurs as a result of pulmonary hypertensive crises, pulmonary thrombosis, and right heart failure [44].

Women with pulmonary hypertension should be advised against pregnancy and the option for pregnancy termination should be discussed with women who do become pregnant. Contraceptive options for women with PH are limited (Table 2.6). CHC is contraindicated in women with PH due to thrombotic and hypertensive risks [35]. Bosentan, an endothelial receptor antagonist used to treat many types of PH, interacts with ethinyl estradiol and several progestins, including etonogestrel, the active component of the contraceptive implant, and norethindrone, which is used in the progestin-only pill available in the USA. While the Working Group does not specifically upgrade the risk category for the contraceptive implant in women on bosentan therapy, it does recommend that a backup method be used along with the implant due to concern for compromised effectiveness [35]. The Working Group considers the standard POP to be category 4 in women with PH on bosentan therapy due to drug-drug interaction [35]. Depot medroxyprogesterone acetate does not interact with bosentan and therefore is theoretically safe and effective for women on this treatment. However, women with PH are often anticoagulated with warfarin, and the theoretical risks of DMPA use in women on warfarin, as previously discussed, also apply [35]. Although levonorgestrel, the progestin component of the LNG-IUD, does not interact with bosentan, intrauterine devices are not recommended in women with pulmonary hypertension due to the potential fatal effects of a vasovagal reaction [35]. However, the Working Group recognizes that when no other suitable method is available, the LNG-IUD may be considered in women with this condition [35].

Significant LV Dysfunction

The risk of pregnancy increases as ventricular function worsens. Significant systemic ventricular dysfunction (NYHA III-IV or EF<30 %) is considered a pregnancy category 4 condition [35]. In one large study of pregnancy outcomes in women with heart disease, a left ventricular ejection fraction <40 % was found to be an independent risk factor for cardiac events in pregnancy [101]. Women with significant LV dysfunction carry the same contraceptive considerations as those with mild dysfunction; however the contraceptive risks may be higher. The increased relative risk of pregnancy in these women should factor into their contraceptive counseling and decision making. The more effective LARC methods are therefore most appropriate for women with severe LV dysfunction.

Severe or Complicated Aortic or Mitral Stenosis

As previously noted, complicated valvular heart disease is defined as coexisting atrial fibrillation, pulmonary hypertension, or previous endocarditis [29]. Pregnancy in women with complicated or severe (as defined above) aortic or mitral stenosis is considered contraindicated [44]. Maternal pregnancy risks include increased rate of hospitalization, pulmonary edema, heart failure, arrhythmias especially atrial fibrillation with the associated thromboembolic risk, and the need for subsequent valvular repair [44, 87, 113, 128].

In women with severe or complicated valvular disease, the risks of CHC outweigh the benefits, and these women should be advised to use a non-estrogen-containing contraceptive method [25, 29]. While no categorization exists for severe lesions, the risk of estrogen-containing contraception associated with the downstream effects of these lesions—A-fib/A-flutter, heart failure, or mechanical valves—is considered category 4 [35]. The USMEC rates all progestin-only methods category 1 in women with severe MS [35]. While the Working Group considers IUD insertion and removal to increase endocarditis risk in women with severe valvular disease, the USMEC considers both IUDs to be safe (category 1) for women with severe MS [29, 35]. The Working Group rates the LNG-IUD category 2–3 depending on the perceived risk of endocarditis. While to our knowledge there are no published studies showing an increased risk of infective endocarditis with the copper over the LNG-IUD, there remains a theoretical distinction: the LNG-IUD creates a cervical mucus barrier similar to that seen in pregnancy, which is thought to provide protection against uterine entry of pathogens. For this reason, the Working Group grades the copper IUD as risk category 3 and the LNG-IUD category 2 for women with complicated valvular disease [35].

Contraceptive Counseling Opportunities for Women with Cardiac Disease

Women with cardiac disease have reported the value of collaborative contraceptive counseling with both obstetrician-gynecologists and cardiologists. Joint counseling prevents women from going back and forth between providers, and from receiving conflicting information regarding contraceptive safety [129]. Rogers et al. developed a monthly contraceptive clinic for adults with congenital heart disease, which was jointly run by a cardiologist and a family planning (FP) physician [130]. Women presenting to the clinic have an initial cardiology consultation. For women who desire contraception, the cardiologist and FP physician meet to review the cardiac diagnosis, medications, contraceptive contraindications, and maternal and fetal risks of unplanned pregnancy. Patients then meet with the FP doctor to discuss sexual history and contraceptive methods at which point the patient receives a prescription for contraception or is scheduled for a follow-up visit to receive a long-term method. Upon conclusion of the clinic visit, a letter is sent to the patient's primary care provider summarizing the consultation [130].

A collaborative model of care can result in improved contraceptive knowledge and increased utilization of appropriate contraception among cardiac patients [130]. However, the quality of contraceptive counseling for women with cardiac disease is dependent on the quality of evidence regarding the safety and efficacy of contraceptive methods for these women. In reviewing the existing literature, we found few prospective studies to inform contraceptive recommendations for women with cardiac disease. This is an important area for future research and becomes increasingly important with the rise of both acquired and congenital cardiac disease.

References

1. Leary PJ, Leary SE, Stout KK, Schwartz SM, Easterling TR. Maternal, perinatal, and postneonatal outcomes in women with chronic heart disease in Washington State. Obstet Gynecol. 2012;120: 1283–90.
2. Berg CJ, Mackay AP, Qin C, Callaghan WM. Overview of maternal morbidity during hospitalization for labor and delivery in the United States: 1993–1997 and 2001–2005. Obstet Gynecol. 2009; 113:1075–81.
3. Small MJ, James AH, Kershaw T, Thames B, Gunatilake R, Brown H. Near-miss maternal mortality: cardiac dysfunction as the principal cause of obstetric intensive care unit admissions. Obstet Gynecol. 2012;119:250–5.
4. Pijuan-Domenech A, Baro-Marine F, Rojas-Torrijos M, Dos-Subira L, Pedrosa-Del Moral V, Subirana-Domenech MT, et al. Usefulness of progesterone-only components for contraception in patients with congenital heart disease. Am J Cardiol. 2013;112: 590–3.
5. Reid GJ, Siu SC, McCrindle BW, Irvine MJ, Webb GD. Sexual behavior and reproductive concerns among adolescents and young adults with congenital heart disease. Int J Cardiol. 2008;125:332–8.
6. Simko LC, McGinnis KA, Schembri J. Educational needs of adults with congenital heart disease. J Cardiovasc Nurs. 2006;21:85–94.
7. Vigl M, Kaemmerer M, Seifert-Klauss V, Niggemeyer E, Nagdyman N, Trigas V, et al. Contraception in women with congenital heart disease. Am J Cardiol. 2010;06:1317–21.
8. ACOG. Committee opinion no. 460: the initial reproductive health visit. Obstet Gynecol. 2010; 116:240–3.
9. Silversides CK, Harris L, Haberer K, Sermer M, Colman JM, Siu SC. Recurrence rates of arrhythmias during pregnancy in women with previous tachyarrhythmia and impact on fetal and neonatal outcomes. Am J Cardiol. 2006;97:1206–12.
10. Ouzounian JG, Elkayam U. Physiologic changes during normal pregnancy and delivery. Cardiol Clin. 2012;30:317–29.
11. Bamfo JE, Kametas NA, Nicolaides KH, Chambers JB. Reference ranges for tissue Doppler measures of maternal systolic and diastolic left ventricular function. Ultrasound Obstet Gynecol. 2007;29:414–20.
12. Robson SC, Hunter S, Moore M, Dunlop W. Haemodynamic changes during the puerperium: a Doppler and M-mode echocardiographic study. Br J Obstet Gynaecol. 1987;94:1028–39.
13. Robson SC, Dunlop W, Hunter S. Haemodynamic changes during the early puerperium. Br Med J (Clin Res Ed). 1987;294:1065.
14. Hameed A, Akhter MW, Bitar F, Khan SA, Sarma R, Goodwin TM, et al. Left atrial thrombosis in

pregnant women with mitral stenosis and sinus rhythm. Am J Obstet Gynecol. 2005;193:501–4.
15. Drenthen W, Pieper PG, Roos-Hesselink JW, van Lottum WA, Voors AA, Mulder BJ, et al. Outcome of pregnancy in women with congenital heart disease: a literature review. J Am Coll Cardiol. 2007; 49:2303–11.
16. Elkayam U, Singh H, Irani A, Akhter MW. Anticoagulation in pregnant women with prosthetic heart valves. J Cardiovasc Pharmacol Ther. 2004; 9:107–15.
17. Lippi G, Albiero A, Montagnana M, Salvagno GL, Scevarolli S, Franchi M, et al. Lipid and lipoprotein profile in physiological pregnancy. Clin Lab. 2007; 53:173–7.
18. Roth A, Elkayam U. Acute myocardial infarction associated with pregnancy. J Am Coll Cardiol. 2008; 52:171–80.
19. Tzemos N, Silversides CK, Colman JM, Therrien J, Webb GD, Mason J, et al. Late cardiac outcomes after pregnancy in women with congenital aortic stenosis. Am Heart J. 2009;157:474–80.
20. Yap SC, Roos-Hesselink JW, Hoendermis ES, Budts W, Vliegen HW, Mulder BJ, et al. Outcome of implantable cardioverter defibrillators in adults with congenital heart disease: a multi-centre study. Eur Heart J. 2007;28:1854–61.
21. Khairy P, Ouyang DW, Fernandes SM, Lee-Parritz A, Economy KE, Landzberg MJ. Pregnancy outcomes in women with congenital heart disease. Circulation. 2006;113:517–24.
22. Drenthen W, Boersma E, Balci A, Moons P, Roos-Hesselink JW, Mulder BJ, et al. Predictors of pregnancy complications in women with congenital heart disease. Eur Heart J. 2010;31:2124–32.
23. Roos-Hesselink JW, Ruys TP, Stein JI, Thilen U, Webb GD, Niwa K, et al. Outcome of pregnancy in patients with structural or ischaemic heart disease: results of a registry of the European Society of Cardiology. Eur Heart J. 2013;34:657–65.
24. Thorne S, MacGregor A, Nelson-Piercy C. Risks of contraception and pregnancy in heart disease. Heart. 2006;92:1520–5.
25. World Health Organization. Medical eligibility criteria for contraceptive use. Geneva, Switzerland: World Health Organization; 2009.
26. Peragallo Urrutia R, Coeytaux RR, McBroom AJ, Gierisch JM, Havrilesky LJ, Moorman PG, et al. Risk of acute thromboembolic events with oral contraceptive use: a systematic review and meta-analysis. Obstet Gynecol. 2013;122:380–9.
27. Hatcher RA. Contraceptive technology. 20th rev. ed. New York, NY: Ardent Media; 2011.
28. Tepper NK, Paulen ME, Marchbanks PA, Curtis KM. Safety of contraceptive use among women with peripartum cardiomyopathy: a systematic review. Contraception. 2010;82:95–101.
29. Centers for Disease Control. U.S. medical eligibility criteria for contraceptive use, 2010. Atlanta, GA: Centers for Disease Control; 2010.
30. Sedlak T, Bairey Merz CN, Shufelt C, Gregory KD, Hamilton MA. Contraception in patients with heart failure. Circulation. 2012;126:1396–400.
31. Shufelt CL, Bairey Merz CN. Contraceptive hormone use and cardiovascular disease. J Am Coll Cardiol. 2009;53:221–31.
32. de Teresa E, Vera A, Ortigosa J, Pulpon LA, Arus AP, de Artaza M. Interaction between anticoagulants and contraceptives: an unsuspected finding. Br Med J. 1979;2:1260–1.
33. Ellison J, Thomson AJ, Greer IA, Walker ID. Drug points: apparent interaction between warfarin and levonorgestrel used for emergency contraception. BMJ. 2000;321:1382.
34. Zingone MM, Guirguis AB, Airee A, Cobb D. Probable drug interaction between warfarin and hormonal contraceptives. Ann Pharmacother. 2009; 43:2096–102.
35. Thorne S, Nelson-Piercy C, MacGregor A, Gibbs S, Crowhurst J, Panay N, et al. Pregnancy and contraception in heart disease and pulmonary arterial hypertension. J Fam Plann Reprod Health Care. 2006;32(2):75–81.
36. Sonmezer M, Atabekoglu C, Cengiz B, Dokmeci F, Cengiz SD. Depot-medroxyprogesterone acetate in anticoagulated patients with previous hemorrhagic corpus luteum. Eur J Contracept Reprod Health Care. 2005;10:9–14.
37. Delafuente JC, Davis JA, Meuleman JR, Jones RA. Influenza vaccination and warfarin anticoagulation: a comparison of subcutaneous and intramuscular routes of administration in elderly men. Pharmacotherapy. 1998;18:631–6.
38. Raj G, Kumar R, McKinney WP. Safety of intramuscular influenza immunization among patients receiving long-term warfarin anticoagulation therapy. Arch Intern Med. 1995;155:1529–31.
39. Iorio A, Basileo M, Marcucci M, Guercini F, Camilloni B, Paccamiccio E, et al. Influenza vaccination and vitamin K antagonist treatment: a placebo-controlled, randomized, double-blind crossover study. Arch Intern Med. 2010;170:609–16.
40. Casajuana J, Iglesias B, Fabregas M, Fina F, Valles JA, Aragones R, et al. Safety of intramuscular influenza vaccine in patients receiving oral anticoagulation therapy: a single blinded multi-centre randomized controlled clinical trial. BMC Blood Disord. 2008;8:1.
41. Wilson W, Taubert KA, Gewitz M, Lockhart PB, Baddour LM, Levison M, et al. Prevention of infective endocarditis: guidelines from the American Heart Association: a guideline from the American Heart Association Rheumatic Fever, Endocarditis, and Kawasaki Disease Committee, Council on Cardiovascular Disease in the Young, and the Council on Clinical Cardiology, Council on Cardiovascular Surgery and Anesthesia, and the Quality of Care and Outcomes Research Interdisciplinary Working Group. Circulation. 2007; 116:1736–54.

42. Uebing A, Steer PJ, Yentis SM, Gatzoulis MA. Pregnancy and congenital heart disease. BMJ. 2006;332:401–6.
43. Yap SC, Drenthen W, Pieper PG, Moons P, Mulder BJ, Vliegen HW, et al. Pregnancy outcome in women with repaired versus unrepaired isolated ventricular septal defect. BJOG. 2010;117:683–9.
44. Regitz-Zagrosek V, Blomstrom Lundqvist C, Borghi C, Cifkova R, Ferreira R, Foidart JM, et al. ESC Guidelines on the management of cardiovascular diseases during pregnancy: the Task Force on the Management of Cardiovascular Diseases during Pregnancy of the European Society of Cardiology (ESC). Eur Heart J. 2011;32(24):3147–97.
45. Yap SC, Drenthen W, Meijboom FJ, Moons P, Mulder BJ, Vliegen HW, et al. Comparison of pregnancy outcomes in women with repaired versus unrepaired atrial septal defect. BJOG. 2009;116: 1593–601.
46. Brickner ME, Hillis LD, Lange RA. Congenital heart disease in adults. First of two parts. N Engl J Med. 2000;342:256–63.
47. Schneider DJ, Moore JW. Patent ductus arteriosus. Circulation. 2006;114:1873–82.
48. Hagen PT, Scholz DG, Edwards WD. Incidence and size of patent foramen ovale during the first 10 decades of life: an autopsy study of 965 normal hearts. Mayo Clin Proc. 1984;59:17–20.
49. Cabanes L, Mas JL, Cohen A, Amarenco P, Cabanes PA, Oubary P, et al. Atrial septal aneurysm and patent foramen ovale as risk factors for cryptogenic stroke in patients less than 55 years of age. A study using transesophageal echocardiography. Stroke. 1993;24:1865–73.
50. Lechat P, Mas JL, Lascault G, Loron P, Theard M, Klimczac M, et al. Prevalence of patent foramen ovale in patients with stroke. N Engl J Med. 1988; 318:1148–52.
51. Pearson AC, Nagelhout D, Castello R, Gomez CR, Labovitz AJ. Atrial septal aneurysm and stroke: a transesophageal echocardiographic study. J Am Coll Cardiol. 1991;18:1223–9.
52. Di Tullio MR, Sacco RL, Sciacca RR, Jin Z, Homma S. Patent foramen ovale and the risk of ischemic stroke in a multiethnic population. J Am Coll Cardiol. 2007;49:797–802.
53. Meissner I, Khandheria BK, Heit JA, Petty GW, Sheps SG, Schwartz GL, et al. Patent foramen ovale: innocent or guilty? Evidence from a prospective population-based study. J Am Coll Cardiol. 2006;47: 440–5.
54. Freed LA, Levy D, Levine RA, Larson MG, Evans JC, Fuller DL, et al. Prevalence and clinical outcome of mitral-valve prolapse. N Engl J Med. 1999; 341:1–7.
55. Theal M, Sleik K, Anand S, Yi Q, Yusuf S, Lonn E. Prevalence of mitral valve prolapse in ethnic groups. Can J Cardiol. 2004;20:511–5.
56. Avierinos JF, Gersh BJ, Melton 3rd LJ, Bailey KR, Shub C, Nishimura RA, et al. Natural history of asymptomatic mitral valve prolapse in the community. Circulation. 2002;106:1355–61.
57. Bonow RO, Carabello BA, Chatterjee K, De Leon Jr AC, Faxon DP, Freed MD, et al. Focused update incorporated into the ACC/AHA 2006 guidelines for the management of patients with valvular heart disease: a report of the American College of Cardiology/American Heart Association Task Force on Practice Guidelines (Writing Committee to Revise the 1998 Guidelines for the Management of Patients With Valvular Heart Disease): endorsed by the Society of Cardiovascular Anesthesiologists, Society for Cardiovascular Angiography and Interventions, and Society of Thoracic Surgeons. Circulation. 2008; 118:e523–661.
58. Chia YT, Yeoh SC, Lim MC, Viegas OA, Ratnam SS. Pregnancy outcome and mitral valve prolapse. Asia Oceania J Obstet Gynaecol. 1994;20:383–8.
59. Tang LC, Chan SY, Wong VC, Ma HK. Pregnancy in patients with mitral valve prolapse. Int J Gynaecol Obstet. 1985;23:217–21.
60. Kostuk WJ, Boughner DR, Barnett HJ, Silver MD. Strokes: a complication of mitral-leaflet prolapse? Lancet. 1977;2:313–6.
61. Hirsowitz GS, Saffer D. Hemiplegia and the billowing mitral leaflet syndrome. J Neurol Neurosurg Psychiatry. 1978;41:381–3.
62. Elam MB, Viar MJ, Ratts TE, Chesney CM. Mitral valve prolapse in women with oral contraceptive-related cerebrovascular insufficiency. Associated persistent hypercoagulable state. Arch Intern Med. 1986;146:73–7.
63. Baumgartner H, Bonhoeffer P, De Groot NM, de Haan F, Deanfield JE, Galie N, et al. Task Force on the Management of Grown-up Congenital Heart Disease of the European Society of Cardiology (ESC); Association for European Paediatric Cardiology (AEPC); ESC Committee for Practice Guidelines (CPG). ESC Guidelines for the management of grown-up congenital heart disease (new version 2010). Eur Heart J. 2010;31:2915–57.
64. van der Linde D, Konings EE, Slager MA, Witsenburg M, Helbing WA, Takkenberg JJ, et al. Birth prevalence of congenital heart disease worldwide: a systematic review and meta-analysis. J Am Coll Cardiol. 2011;58:2241–7.
65. Cuypers JA, Witsenburg M, van der Linde D, Roos-Hesselink JW. Pulmonary stenosis: update on diagnosis and therapeutic options. Heart. 2013;99:339–47.
66. Wald RM, Sermer M, Colman JM. Pregnancy and contraception in young women with congenital heart disease: general considerations. Paediatr Child Health. 2011;16:e25–9.
67. Reimold SC, Rutherford JD. Clinical practice. Valvular heart disease in pregnancy. N Engl J Med. 2003;349:52–9.

68. Sobotka PA, Mayer JH, Bauernfeind RA, Kanakis Jr C, Rosen KM. Arrhythmias documented by 24-hour continuous ambulatory electrocardiographic monitoring in young women without apparent heart disease. Am Heart J. 1981;101:753–9.
69. Shotan A, Ostrzega E, Mehra A, Johnson JV, Elkayam U. Incidence of arrhythmias in normal pregnancy and relation to palpitations, dizziness, and syncope. Am J Cardiol. 1997;79:1061–4.
70. Cruz MO, Hibbard JU, Alexander T, Briller J. Ambulatory arrhythmia monitoring in pregnant patients with palpitations. Am J Perinatol. 2013;30:53–8.
71. Hoffman JI. Incidence of congenital heart disease: I. Postnatal incidence. Pediatr Cardiol. 1995;16:103–13.
72. Hokanson JS, Moller JH. Adults with tetralogy of Fallot: long-term follow-up. Cardiol Rev. 1999;7:149–55.
73. Thorne SA. Pregnancy in heart disease. Heart. 2004;90:450–6.
74. Veldtman GR, Connolly HM, Grogan M, Ammash NM, Warnes CA. Outcomes of pregnancy in women with tetralogy of Fallot. J Am Coll Cardiol. 2004;44:174–80.
75. Kaur H, Suri V, Aggarwal N, Chopra S, Vijayvergiya R, Talwar KK. Pregnancy in patients with tetralogy of fallot: outcome and management. World J Pediatr Congenit Heart Surg. 2010;1:170–4.
76. Abdalla MY, el Din Mostafa E. Contraception after heart surgery. Contraception. 1992;45:73–80.
77. Kilic S, Yuksel B, Doganay M, Bardakci H, Akinsu F, Uzunlar O, et al. The effect of levonorgestrel-releasing intrauterine device on menorrhagia in women taking anticoagulant medication after cardiac valve replacement. Contraception. 2009;80:152–7.
78. Culwell KR, Curtis KM. Use of contraceptive methods by women with current venous thrombosis on anticoagulant therapy: a systematic review. Contraception. 2009;80:337–45.
79. Pisoni CN, Cuadrado MJ, Khamashta MA, Hunt BJ. Treatment of menorrhagia associated with oral anticoagulation: efficacy and safety of the levonorgestrel releasing intrauterine device (Mirena coil). Lupus. 2006;15:877–80.
80. Kadir RA, Chi C. Levonorgestrel intrauterine system: bleeding disorders and anticoagulant therapy. Contraception. 2007;75:S123–9.
81. Wang TJ, Levy D, Benjamin EJ, Vasan RS. The epidemiology of "asymptomatic" left ventricular systolic dysfunction: implications for screening. Ann Intern Med. 2003;138:907–16.
82. Yancy CW, Jessup M, Bozkurt B, Butler J, Casey Jr DE, Drazner MH, et al. 2013 ACCF/AHA guideline for the management of heart failure: a report of the American College of Cardiology Foundation/American Heart Association Task Force on Practice Guidelines. Circulation. 2013;128(16):e240–327.
83. Maron BJ, Gardin JM, Flack JM, Gidding SS, Kurosaki TT, Bild DE. Prevalence of hypertrophic cardiomyopathy in a general population of young adults: echocardiographic analysis of 4111 subjects in the CARDIA Study. Coronary artery risk development in (young) adults. Circulation. 1995;92:785–9.
84. Gersh BJ, Maron BJ, Bonow RO, Dearani JA, Fifer MA, Link MS, et al. American College of Cardiology Foundation/American Heart Association Task Force on Practice. 2011 ACCF/AHA guideline for the diagnosis and treatment of hypertrophic cardiomyopathy: a report of the American College of Cardiology Foundation/American Heart Association Task Force on Practice Guidelines. Developed in collaboration with the American Association for Thoracic Surgery, American Society of Echocardiography, American Society of Nuclear Cardiology, Heart Failure Society of America, Heart Rhythm Society, Society for Cardiovascular Angiography and Interventions, and Society of Thoracic Surgeons. J Am Coll Cardiol. 2011;58:e212–60.
85. Autore C, Conte MR, Piccininno M, Bernabo P, Bonfiglio G, Bruzzi P, et al. Risk associated with pregnancy in hypertrophic cardiomyopathy. J Am Coll Cardiol. 2002;40:1864–9.
86. Vahanian A, Alfieri O, Andreotti F, Antunes MJ, Baron-Esquivias G, Baumgartner H, et al. [Guidelines on the management of valvular heart disease (version). The Joint Task Force on the Management of Valvular Heart Disease of the European Society of Cardiology (ESC) and the European Association for Cardio-Thoracic Surgery (EACTS)]. G Ital Cardiol (Rome). 2013;14:167–214.
87. Hameed A, Karaalp IS, Tummala PP, Wani OR, Canetti M, Akhter MW, et al. The effect of valvular heart disease on maternal and fetal outcome of pregnancy. J Am Coll Cardiol. 2001;37:893–9.
88. Suri V, Aggarwal N, Kaur R, Chaudhary N, Ray P, Grover A. Safety of intrauterine contraceptive device (copper T 200 B) in women with cardiac disease. Contraception. 2008;78:315–8.
89. Judge DP, Dietz HC. Marfan's syndrome. Lancet. 2005;366:1965–76.
90. Lalchandani S, Wingfield M. Pregnancy in women with Marfan's Syndrome. Eur J Obstet Gynecol Reprod Biol. 2003;110:125–30.
91. Rahman J, Rahman FZ, Rahman W, al-Suleiman SA, Rahman MS. Obstetric and gynecologic complications in women with Marfan syndrome. J Reprod Med. 2003;48:723–8.
92. Volach V, Elami A, Gilon D, Pollak A, Ginosar Y, Ezra Y. Pregnancy in Marfan syndrome after aortic root replacement: a case report and review of the literature. Congenit Heart Dis. 2006;1:184–8.
93. Pyeritz RE. Maternal and fetal complications of pregnancy in the Marfan syndrome. Am J Med. 1981;71:784–90.
94. Lind J, Wallenburg HC. The Marfan syndrome and pregnancy: a retrospective study in a Dutch

population. Eur J Obstet Gynecol Reprod Biol. 2001;98:28–35.
95. Beighton P, De Paepe A, Steinmann B, Tsipouras P, Wenstrup RJ. Ehlers-Danlos syndromes: revised nosology, Villefranche, Ehlers-Danlos National Foundation (USA) and Ehlers-Danlos Support Group (UK). Am J Med Genet. 1998;77:31–7.
96. Lind J, Wallenburg HC. Pregnancy and the Ehlers-Danlos syndrome: a retrospective study in a Dutch population. Acta Obstet Gynecol Scand. 2002;81: 293–300.
97. Volkov N, Nisenblat V, Ohel G, Gonen R. Ehlers-Danlos syndrome: insights on obstetric aspects. Obstet Gynecol Surv. 2007;62:51–7.
98. Peaceman AM, Cruikshank DP. Ehlers-Danlos syndrome and pregnancy: association of type IV disease with maternal death. Obstet Gynecol. 1987;69: 428–31.
99. Rudd NL, Nimrod C, Holbrook KA, Byers PH. Pregnancy complications in type IV Ehlers-Danlos Syndrome. Lancet. 1983;1:50–3.
100. Hoffman JI, Kaplan S. The incidence of congenital heart disease. J Am Coll Cardiol. 2002;39: 1890–900.
101. Siu SC, Sermer M, Colman JM, Alvarez AN, Mercier LA, Morton BC, et al. Prospective multicenter study of pregnancy outcomes in women with heart disease. Circulation. 2001;104:515–21.
102. Go AS, Mozaffarian D, Roger VL, Benjamin EJ, Berry JD, Borden WB, et al. American Heart Association Statistics, and S. Stroke Statistics. Heart disease and stroke statistics—2013 update: a report from the American Heart Association. Circulation. 2013;127:e6–245.
103. Lloyd-Jones D, Adams RJ, Brown TM, Carnethon M, Dai S, De Simone G, et al. Executive summary: heart disease and stroke statistics—2010 update: a report from the American Heart Association. Circulation. 2010;121:948–54.
104. Yang Q, Cogswell ME, Flanders WD, Hong Y, Zhang Z, Loustalot F, et al. Trends in cardiovascular health metrics and associations with all-cause and CVD mortality among US adults. JAMA. 2012; 307:1273–83.
105. James AH, Jamison MG, Biswas MS, Brancazio LR, Swamy GK, Myers ER. Acute myocardial infarction in pregnancy: a United States population-based study. Circulation. 2006;113:1564–71.
106. Elkayam U, Bitar F. Valvular heart disease and pregnancy: part II: prosthetic valves. J Am Coll Cardiol. 2005;46:403–10.
107. Sadler L, McCowan L, White H, Stewart A, Bracken M, North R. Pregnancy outcomes and cardiac complications in women with mechanical, bioprosthetic and homograft valves. BJOG. 2000;107:245–53.
108. Chan WS, Anand S, Ginsberg JS. Anticoagulation of pregnant women with mechanical heart valves: a systematic review of the literature. Arch Intern Med. 2000;160:191–6.
109. North RA, Sadler L, Stewart AW, McCowan LM, Kerr AR, White HD. Long-term survival and valve-related complications in young women with cardiac valve replacements. Circulation. 1999;99:2669–76.
110. Gewillig M. The Fontan circulation. Heart. 2005;91:839–46.
111. Warnes CA, Liberthson R, Danielson GK, Dore A, Harris L, Hoffman JI, Somerville J, et al. Task force 1: the changing profile of congenital heart disease in adult life. J Am Coll Cardiol. 2001;37:1170–5.
112. D'Alto M, Mahadevan VS. Pulmonary arterial hypertension associated with congenital heart disease. Eur Respir Rev. 2012;21:328–37.
113. Silversides CK, Colman JM, Sermer M, Siu SC. Cardiac risk in pregnant women with rheumatic mitral stenosis. Am J Cardiol. 2003;91:1382–5.
114. Farmer M, Webb A. Intrauterine device insertion-related complications: can they be predicted? J Fam Plann Reprod Health Care. 2003;29:227–31.
115. Demakis JG, Rahimtoola SH. Peripartum cardiomyopathy. Circulation. 1971;44:964–8.
116. Goland S, Modi K, Bitar F, Janmohamed M, Mirocha JM, Czer LS, et al. Clinical profile and predictors of complications in peripartum cardiomyopathy. J Card Fail. 2009;15:645–50.
117. Modi KA, Illum S, Jariatul K, Caldito G, Reddy PC. Poor outcome of indigent patients with peripartum cardiomyopathy in the United States. Am J Obstet Gynecol. 2009;201:171 e1–5.
118. Gunderson EP, Croen LA, Chiang V, Yoshida CK, Walton D, Go AS. Epidemiology of peripartum cardiomyopathy: incidence, predictors, and outcomes. Obstet Gynecol. 2011;118:583–91.
119. Harper MA, Meyer RE, Berg CJ. Peripartum cardiomyopathy: population-based birth prevalence and 7-year mortality. Obstet Gynecol. 2012;120:1013–9.
120. Pearson GD, Veille JC, Rahimtoola S, Hsia J, Oakley CM, Hosenpud JD, et al. Peripartum cardiomyopathy: National Heart, Lung, and Blood Institute and Office of Rare Diseases (National Institutes of Health) workshop recommendations and review. JAMA. 2000;283:1183–8.
121. Blauwet LA, Cooper LT. Diagnosis and management of peripartum cardiomyopathy. Heart. 2011; 97:1970–81.
122. Fett JD, Murphy JG. Prevention and control of Peripartum cardiomyopathy in Haiti. Prev Control. 2005;1:305–7.
123. New York Heart Association. Criteria Committee and New York Heart Association. Nomenclature and criteria for diagnosis of diseases of the heart and great vessels. 8th ed. Boston: Little, Brown; 1979.
124. Simonneau G, Robbins IM, Beghetti M, Channick RN, Delcroix M, Denton CP, et al. Updated clinical classification of pulmonary hypertension. J Am Coll Cardiol. 2009;54:S43–54.
125. Ling Y, Johnson MK, Kiely DG, Condliffe R, Elliot CA, Gibbs JS, et al. Changing demographics, epidemiology, and survival of incident pulmonary arterial

hypertension: results from the pulmonary hypertension registry of the United Kingdom and Ireland. Am J Respir Crit Care Med. 2012;186:790–6.
126. McLaughlin VV, Archer SL, Badesch DB, Barst RJ, Farber HW, Lindner JR, et al. AHA 2009 expert consensus document on pulmonary hypertension: a report of the American College of Cardiology Foundation Task Force on Expert Consensus Documents and the American Heart Association: developed in collaboration with the American College of Chest Physicians, American Thoracic Society, Inc., and the Pulmonary Hypertension Association. Circulation. 2009;119:2250–94.
127. Friedman WF. Proceedings of National Heart, Lung, and Blood Institute pediatric cardiology workshop: pulmonary hypertension. Pediatr Res. 1986;20: 811–24.
128. Akhter N, Rahman F, Salman M, Anam K, Begum N, Naher S, et al. Valvular heart disease in pregnancy: maternal and fetal outcome. Mymensingh Med J. 2011;20:436–40.
129. Chor J, Oswald L, Briller J, Cowett A, Peacock N, Harwood B. Reproductive health experiences of women with cardiovascular disease. Contraception. 2012;86:464–9.
130. Rogers P, Mansour D, Mattinson A, O'Sullivan JJ. A collaborative clinic between contraception and sexual health services and an adult congenital heart disease clinic. J Fam Plann Reprod Health Care. 2007;33:17–21.

Contraception Use in Women with Hypertension

3

Jennifer Corbelli and Eleanor Bimla Schwarz

Introduction

Hypertension is among the most common conditions that affect women of reproductive age. National data show that 32 % of adult women meet criteria for hypertension [1], defined as blood pressures over 140/90 [2], as do 8 % of women ages 20–44. Although rates of optimal blood pressure control are similar among US men and women [3], nationally patients ages 18–39 with hypertension are less likely to be well controlled than those over 40 [4]. Certain groups of young women face even greater risk for hypertension, specifically, women who are obese, non-Hispanic black, or have diabetes or chronic kidney disease. In addition, the prevalence of hypertension increases as women age. When women of reproductive age are treated for hypertension, they most commonly receive diuretics, beta-blockers, and angiotensin-converting enzyme (ACE) inhibitors [5], medications that have all been labeled by the US Food and Drug Administration (FDA) as potentially contraindicated in pregnancy [6]. For this, among other, reasons, hypertension among younger women is often undertreated: only half of women of reproductive age with hypertension are prescribed antihypertensive therapy [5]. Thus, many women of reproductive age may be unaware of their hypertension and have uncontrolled hypertension, which places them at risk for multiple cardiovascular and pregnancy complications.

Although the risks of hypertension have been well established for decades, very little data exist on risks specific to women of reproductive age beyond the serious complications associated with hypertensive disorders of pregnancy [7]. With time, patients with hypertension develop complications, including end-stage renal disease and cardiovascular disease such as stroke, myocardial infarction (MI), congestive heart failure, and ventricular arrhythmias [8]. Patients who are diagnosed with hypertension at a young age and are effectively treated can delay the onset of this end-organ damage, and potentially avoid such complications entirely.

Hypertension and Pregnancy

To optimally meet the needs of women of reproductive age affected by hypertension, clinicians need to understand the ways in which hypertension affects pregnancy outcomes. Clinicians must also develop a framework for understanding the ways in which hypertension may affect the risks of using certain contraceptives. The impact of

J. Corbelli, M.D., M.S. (✉)
Division of General Internal Medicine, University of Pittsburgh Medical Center, Pittsburgh, PA, USA
e-mail: corbellija@upmc.edu

E.B. Schwarz, M.D., M.S.
Women's Health Services Research Unit, Center for Research on Health Care, University of Pittsburgh, Pittsburgh, PA, USA
e-mail: Schwarzeb@upmc.edu

R.H. Allen and C.A. Cwiak (eds.), *Contraception for the Medically Challenging Patient*,
DOI 10.1007/978-1-4939-1233-9_3, © Springer Science+Business Media New York 2014

Table 3.1 Risks of adverse events associated with hypertension in pregnancy

	Placental abruption (%)	Preterm birth (%)	Small for gestational age (%)	Preeclampsia (%)
Mild hypertension (variable treatment across studies, 10–50 %)	0.7–1.4	12–35	8–16	10–25
Severe hypertension (all subjects treated)	5–10	62–70	31–40	~50

hypertension on pregnancy is significant and multifaceted. This is true of both women with preexisting hypertension and women with gestational hypertension (defined as a blood pressure >140/90 that develops after 20 weeks gestation). Gestational hypertension may unmask early cardiovascular risk: approximately 15 % of women who develop gestational hypertension will go on to develop chronic hypertension [9]. Gestational hypertension has therefore been defined by the American Heart Association as a major risk factor for the subsequent development of cardiovascular disease [10]. Thus, when assessing overall cardiovascular risk, clinicians should ask all women about any prior pregnancies and pregnancy complications.

The normal physiology of pregnancy results in a decrease in blood pressure, with the nadir typically in the second trimester. This decrease is primarily due to decreases in systemic vascular resistance, mediated by increased endothelial nitric oxide and prostacyclin production. Therefore, women with mild preexisting hypertension may no longer require medication during pregnancy (although blood pressure may again reach pre-pregnancy levels by the third trimester). One of the most serious sequelae of hypertension in pregnancy is preeclampsia, defined by hypertension and proteinuria. Women with preexisting hypertension are at significantly increased risk for preeclampsia as compared to normotensive women [11]. Approximately 50 % of women with severe hypertension (defined as >160/100) will develop preeclampsia, as compared to between 10 and 25 % of women with mild hypertension (140–159/90–99) [12]. The mechanism for this relationship relates to factors released into the maternal bloodstream when the placenta becomes ischemic due to hypertension. Widespread endothelial dysfunction ensues, leading to worsening hypertension, generalized and/or pulmonary edema due to capillary leak, proteinuria, acute kidney injury, and hepatic ischemia. Women with preeclampsia are at significantly increased risk for the development of both chronic hypertension and cardiovascular disease in the future [13].

Other well-established pregnancy-related complications of hypertension share a common etiology of placental hypoperfusion. Some of these complications include placental abruption, small for gestational age infants, and preterm birth. Table 3.1 summarizes these risks, with data drawn from four large observational studies [12].

The extent to which treatment of hypertension in pregnancy prevents development of these complications is less clear. Although the data listed in Table 3.1 suggest that women with mild hypertension are at risk for complications, this does not prove that treatment decreases these risks. Importantly, blood pressure targets in pregnant women are significantly higher than in nonpregnant women. While nonpregnant women, including those who desire pregnancy, should be treated to a goal blood pressure of no higher than 140/90, the risks of treatment of pregnant women with mild hypertension may outweigh the benefits. Relative placental hypoperfusion can result from treating blood pressure in pregnant women even to levels that are otherwise considered normal. A meta-analysis of 46 randomized controlled trials showed no difference with treatment versus placebo in risks of preeclampsia, fetal mortality, preterm birth, small for gestational age infants, or placental abruption in women with mild hypertension (defined as <170/110 for the meta-analysis).

However, treatment did show a significantly decreased risk of progression to severe hypertension, with a number needed to treat between 8 and 13 [14]. Data also suggest that treatment of maternal hypertension may be harmful: in meta-analysis even a 10 mmHg decrease in maternal mean arterial pressure was associated with a 176 g (6 oz) decrease in birth weight. These results were consistent for all medications and all durations of treatment, and were observed in women treated for both mild and severe hypertension [15].

Although it is clear that all women in pregnancy with severe hypertension should be treated, in pregnant women with mild hypertension, decisions on the risks and benefits of treatment should be made on an individual basis. At a minimum, all women should be closely monitored for progression to severe hypertension. Antihypertensives should generally be avoided in young women with stable, mild hypertension, as the best data available do not show a significantly decreased risk of pregnancy complications with treatment. When treatment is indicated during pregnancy, methyldopa (class B) and labetalol (class C) are the drugs of choice [16]. Decades of data support the safety of these two agents. Long-acting calcium channel blockers (primarily nifedipine) are considered second-line, primarily due to a paucity of data [17]. Clonidine has also been shown to have outcomes similar to methyldopa [18]. While hydralazine is commonly used in the inpatient setting, it has been shown to carry increased risk of maternal hypotension and placental abruption [19], and therefore should be a third-line agent for outpatient hypertension treatment. Finally, ACE inhibitors and angiotensin receptor blockers (ARBs) should be strictly avoided during pregnancy, due to risk of oligohydramnios and other congenital abnormalities.

Combined Hormonal Contraceptives

Although it is imperative for providers who care for women of reproductive age to be able to recognize and manage the effects of hypertension on pregnancy, the high prevalence of hypertension among women desiring contraception also compels providers to learn to optimally navigate this common clinical scenario. Many forms of contraception directly impact blood pressure. Among the most notable and perhaps most notorious are estrogen-containing contraceptives. The link between estrogen-containing contraceptives, or combined hormonal contraceptives (CHC) and hypertension was first established in 1967: 11 women developed hypertension after starting combined hormonal pills, all of whom resumed normotension after the medication was discontinued. Women were also found to have elevations in renin substrates [20]. It has since been recognized that estrogen both stimulates production of angiotensinogen from the liver and increases activation of the renin-angiotensin system [21]. Although the estrogen doses (up to 200 μg ethinyl estradiol) used in early pill formulations were much higher than current CHCs, the wealth of data that has resulted since the landmark 1967 publication has repeatedly demonstrated a clear causal link between hypertension and CHC.

Much of the data available on the impact of estrogen on hypertension comes from studies of CHCs, which like all hormonal contraceptives contain progestins. CHCs have been shown, on average, to increase systolic and diastolic blood pressure by 8 and 6 mmHg, respectively [22]. Although this may seem to be a fairly mild increase, it may have an adverse clinical impact. Indeed, even normotensive women on combined oral contraceptives (COCs) have been shown to have higher blood pressures and increased urinary aldosterone excretion compared to controls not taking COCs [23]. In studies controlling for age, longer duration of COC use has also been shown to increase hypertension risk as compared to shorter durations, and women taking COCs have a small increased risk for both moderate and severe hypertension [24]. Longitudinal observational data from the Nurse's Health Study (NHS) have shown that the risk of hypertension among women taking COCs increases with age, body mass index, and duration of use [25]. Furthermore, NHS data show that women with a past history of COC use have a small but significantly increased

Table 3.2 Hypertension among never, past, and current users of OCs[a]

Hypertension	OC use Never	Past	Current
Cases, *n*	211	1193	163
Person-years[b]	35,333	167,236	28,437
Age-adjusted RR	1.0 (Referent)	1.1 (0.9–1.2)	1.5 (1.2–1.8)
Age- and BMI-adjusted RR[c]	1.0 (Referent)	1.2 (1.0–1.4)	1.8 (1.5–2.3)
Age-adjusted RR after adjustment for baseline BP[e]	1.0 (Referent)	1.2 (1.0–1.4)	1.7 (1.3–2.1)
Multivariate RR after adjustment for baseline BP[e]	1.0 (Referent)	1.2 (1.0–1.5)	1.9 (1.6–2.4)

Values in parentheses are 95 % CIs

BP blood pressure, *RR* relative risk, *BMI* body mass index

[a]Reprinted with permission from Chasan-Taber L, Willett WC, Manson JE, Spiegelman D, Hunter DJ, Curhan G, et al. Prospective study of oral contraceptives and hypertension among women in the United States. Circulation. 1996 Aug 1;94(3):483–9

[b]Person-years of exposure among the entire cohort

[c]After controlling for 5-year age categories and ten categories of BMI

[d]Multivariate model includes age (years) (25–29, 30–34, 35–39, 40–44, 45–49), BMI (deciles), cigarette smoking (cigarettes/day) (never, past, 1–14, 15–24, 25–34, 35+), family history of hypertension (no, yes), parity (number of pregnancies) (nulliparous, 1–2, 3–4, 5+), physical activity (quintiles), alcohol (g/day) (none, 0.1 to <1.5, 1.5 to <5.0, 5.0 to <15.0, 15+), and ethnicity (white, black, Hispanic, Asian, or unknown)

[e]Systolic BP (mmHg) (unknown, <105, 105–114, 115–124, 125–134, 135–144, 145–154, 155–164, 165–174, 175+) and diastolic BP (mmHg) (unknown, <65, 65–74, 75–84, 85–89, 90–94, 95–104, 105+)

Table 3.3 Number of cardiovascular events per million woman-years, ages 30–34

	Myocardial infarction	Ischemic stroke
Normotensive non-COC user	1.7	9.8
Normotensive COC user	4.2	24.6
Hypertensive non-COC user	10.2	39.3
Hypertensive COC user	25.5	98.4

risk of hypertension compared to women who never used COCs, after adjustment for age and baseline blood pressure (Table 3.2). This finding begs the question of whether COCs unmask hypertension in women who were prone to its development in later life.

Although the degree of blood pressure increase associated with COCs is not dramatic, data show a clear link between COCs use in women with hypertension and subsequent myocardial infarction. Estrogens are well known to be pro-thrombotic. Unfortunately, little data exist to define the absolute risk of cardiovascular events in women of reproductive age; rather, the majority of existing literature provide relative risks. Yet, data do exist to demonstrate that although the absolute risk of these events is low, it increases with both hypertension and COC use (Table 3.3) [26].

Early data showed that among women who use COCs, those with hypertension had nearly fourfold increased risk of myocardial infarction as compared to normotensive women [27]. Subsequent investigations showed even more concerning findings, specifically a 17-fold higher risk of MI in COC users with hypertension versus COC users without [28]. A 2006 systematic review showed that in a review of available data, the relative risk of MI among COC users with hypertension was approximately 12, as compared to nonusers with hypertension [29]. This analysis also examined the association between MI risk and whether blood pressure was measured prior to initiating COCs. The risk for MI was higher among women who had not had their blood pressure measured prior to COC initiation (OR range 2.76–9.47, 95 % CI range 1.36–24.1), as compared to women who had (OR range 1.07–3.48, 95 % CI range 0.66–8.70). These results suggest that blood pressure assessment prior to initiation of estrogen-containing contraception may mitigate MI risk among women with hypertension, particularly if estrogen-containing methods are avoided by hypertensive women.

In addition to myocardial infarction risk, data demonstrate a link between CHC use and both stroke and peripheral arterial disease (PAD) in women with hypertension. A study of 152 women ages 18–49 with PAD confirmed by angiography found an odds ratio for PAD of 8.8 (95 % CI 3.9–19.8) among hypertensive COC users, compared with normotensive COC users [30]. Although PAD is rare among women of reproductive age, these results are further evidence of the adverse impact of COCs on the endothelium of hypertensive women. As compared to the data available on PAD and COC use, the data on stroke risk are more abundant. Importantly, a dose–response relationship has been shown. Women (all-comers) using 50 μg of ethinyl estradiol were found to have an OR for stroke of 4.5 (95 % CI 2.6–7.7), as compared to women on 30–40 μg COCs (OR 1.6, 95 % CI 1.3–2.0), women on 20 μg COCs (OR 1.7, 95 % CI 1.0–3.1), and women on the progestin-only pill (OR 1.0, 95 % CI 0.3–3.0) [31]. Further evidence exists to demonstrate this dose-dependent relationship. Among users (all-comers) of COCs containing <50 μg ethinyl estradiol (EE), compared with women who had never used COCs, the odds ratio for ischemic stroke was 0.66 (95 % CI 0.29–1.47). Among prior COC users the odds ratio was 1.09 (95 % CI, 0.54–2.21). These data show that for women using COCs containing <50 μg of EE, no increased stroke risk was seen, even in analyses for women age 35 and older or those with untreated hypertension [32]. These results reinforce the reasons for which COCs with 50 μg of EE are now usually avoided.

In an international study of developed countries, the odds ratio for ischemic stroke among COC users with hypertension compared to those without hypertension was found to be 10.7 (95 % CI 2.04–56.6) and 2.71 (95 % CI 1.47–4.99), respectively [33]. Similarly, one systematic review found that most studies examining the risk of ischemic stroke among hypertensive COC users reported risks 1.5–2 times higher than those of normotensive COC users. As with data on myocardial infarction, COC users who had not had their blood pressure checked had a higher risk (1.7- to 2.5-fold increase) of ischemic stroke than COC users who had, although this increased risk was not observed for hemorrhagic stroke [29]. These data for stroke in COC users with hypertension are concerning, despite the existence of some conflicting data. Specifically, at least one study has found a higher stroke risk among hypertensive non-COC users than hypertensive women taking COCs [34]. Additionally, a similarly conducted meta-analysis found that COC users with hypertension did not have a higher stroke than COC users without hypertension [35]. Both systematic reviews included studies from the 1960s forward; therefore, it is unlikely that disparate inclusion of older studies using higher EE doses can explain the differences in these findings.

Overall, despite some data to the contrary, the available evidence suggests a probable increased risk of ischemic stroke among hypertensive women who use COCs, and likely all estrogen-containing contraceptives. Although data suggest a clear increased risk for myocardial infarction in women with hypertension who use COCs, and a possible increased risk of ischemic stroke, it is important to recognize that the prevalence of these conditions in women of reproductive age is very low. Based on a meta-analysis of overall myocardial infarction and stroke risk in women on estrogen-containing contraception, it is estimated that 10,000 women would need to be treated with a pill containing 20 μg EE for 1 year to cause two cardiovascular events (MI or thrombotic stroke) [36]. The exact extent to which this baseline risk changes in women with hypertension is unclear, although we might expect an increase in risk.

Among women with hypertension on COCs, those who discontinued use had a mean decrease in systolic blood pressure of 15 mmHg versus a decrease of 2.8 mmHg in women who continued use. Mean decreases in diastolic blood pressure for women who discontinued compared to those who did not were 10.4 mmHg and 2.2 mmHg, respectively [24]. These results are surprising in light of the above results which showed an average increase in systolic and diastolic blood pressure of 8 and 6 mmHg. However, the latter data were in all-comers, and it is probable than women with baseline hypertension experience a greater increase in blood pressure with COC initiation versus normotensive women. Overall, these data suggest that clinicians can reassure women who are hypertensive while using COCs that blood pressure is likely to significantly decrease once the pills are discontinued.

For those women who desire CHCs over other forms of contraception, it is critical to weigh these risks against the risks of the pregnancy complications associated with hypertension. When CHCs are chosen, the best choice is the lowest-dose EE possible. Data exist to support this EE dose-dependent relationship and risk of adverse outcome: for the same progestin, relative risk for both stroke and myocardial infarction tends to increase as EE dose increases from 20 to 30–40 μg [37]. The US Centers for Disease Control and Prevention's Medical Eligibility Criteria for Contraceptive Use (USMEC) defines CHCs as category 4 (method poses an unacceptable health risk) for women with blood pressures >160/100, and category 3 (method usually is not recommended unless other more appropriate methods are not available or acceptable) for women with blood pressures 140–159/90–99 or women with adequately treated hypertension [38] (see Table 3.3). It is likely that CHCs are considered category 3 in women with well-controlled hypertension because of the known risks in women with hypertension as a whole. Citing evidence (much of which is summarized previously) on the increased risk of cardiovascular events in women with hypertension using CHCs, the USMEC concludes that for women with blood pressure <160/100 for whom CHCs are the contraceptive of choice, it is reasonable to initiate CHCs with very close follow-up. However, non-estrogen-containing options, as discussed in the following section, offer superior safety for these women and should be encouraged by all providers.

Data on the effects of other estrogen-containing contraceptive options on blood pressure, specifically the patch and the ring, are minimal as compared to data available on combined oral contraceptives. Systemic EE levels achieved with the ring are approximately 50 % that achieved with COCs [39]. EE levels achieved with the patch have been shown to be higher than with COCs [40]. Therefore, although direct evidence does not exist, USMEC recommendations do not make a distinction between use of the patch or ring compared to COCs in women with hypertension. Available evidence shows that in all-comers, the contraceptive ring significantly increases stroke risk, although no significant MI risk was seen with either the patch or ring [37].

Progestin-Only Contraceptives

Given the multiple risks of CHC in women with hypertension, an understanding of the impact of progestins on blood pressure is important. Progesterone is a known vasodilator [41], and progestins do not have the pro-thrombotic effects of estrogen. Data exist to show that the progestin-only pill (POP) offers a superior safety profile to CHCs, with respect to both MI and stroke. Specifically, women (all-comers) taking the POP have been shown to be at no increased risk of MI or thrombotic stroke as compared to contraception nonusers [34, 37]. Although relative little data exist on the impact of POP on cardiovascular risk in women with hypertension, there are data to shed light on the potential association between the POP and development of hypertension. A 2004 literature review identified three prospective studies evaluating this relationship [42]. In one study of Black normotensive women under age 35 taking the POP, no overall increase in systolic blood pressure was observed and diastolic blood pressures were decreased [43]. Other studies again showed no increase in blood pressure over 2 years of follow-up [44, 45].

There is only one known study examining the risk of cardiovascular events associated with the POP in women with hypertension specifically. A 1998 case–control study done by the World Health Organization (WHO) showed an increased risk of all cardiovascular events among women with hypertension whether they were using POP (OR 6.78, 95 % CI 2.82–16.3) or not (OR 5.87,95 % CI 5.12–6.73) [46] compared to women without hypertension. As the difference in effect size is small, and the confidence intervals overlap, the CDC's US Selected Practice Recommendations do not recommend blood pressure measurement prior to initiation of the POP [38]. The POP is rated as category 1 (no restrictions) in women with adequately controlled or mild hypertension, and category 2 (advantages generally outweigh theoretical or proven risks) in women with blood pressures >160/100.

Although again limited, some additional data shed light on the relationship between other forms of progestin-only contraceptives and blood pressure. For example, depot medroxyprogesterone acetate (DMPA) has been shown to be safe in women with cardiovascular contraindications to estrogen [47]. Per the USMEC, blood pressure measurement is not necessary prior to initiation of DMPA, although DMPA is rated category 3 in women with blood pressures >160/110 and as category 2 in women with adequately controlled or mild hypertension. The reasons for the category 3 rating in women with severe hypertension are based primarily on the same 1998 WHO case–control study discussed previously (the only study cited in these guidelines), which showed an increased risk of all cardiovascular events among women with hypertension whether they used DMPA (OR 7.16, 95 % CI 1.32–38.7) or not (OR 5.87,95 % CI 5.12–6.73) compared to women without hypertension [46]. As these confidence intervals overlap considerably, it is unclear why DMPA is rated as category 3 for women with severe hypertension, when the POP is rated as category 2. In the absence of data demonstrating a true increase in risk of cardiovascular events, both DMPA and the progestin-only pill should be considered safe methods of contraception for women with hypertension. The only caveat with DMPA is that it cannot be immediately discontinued if adverse effects arise.

There are several other considerations regarding the impact of different progestins on hypertension. One such consideration is the role of the progestin, drospirenone. Drospirenone has a known anti-mineralocorticoid effect, and therefore it is biologically plausible that it may cause a decrease in blood pressure. Although limited data exist on the impact of drospirenone on blood pressure in women of reproductive age, when used in combination with estradiol, it has been shown to lower blood pressure in postmenopausal women with mild hypertension [48, 49]. One recent study examined the effects of drospirenone combined with 30 μg EE on 24-h ambulatory blood pressure and heart rate in normotensive women of reproductive age. Results showed no impact on blood pressure and a small but significant increase in heart rate [50]. Importantly, as discussed in Chap. 12, COCs containing drospirenone have been associated in multiple studies with a relatively increased risk of venous thromboembolism as compared to COCs containing other progestins, particularly levonorgestrel [51, 52]. The prospective EURAS study, however, has not found such an association [53]. Additionally, no progestin-only pill containing drospirenone exists, and therefore any woman taking drospirenone is at risk for the effects of COCs on blood pressure. Therefore, despite drospirenone's potential to decrease blood pressure, COCs containing drospirenone should not be preferentially used in women who are hypertensive or otherwise poor candidates for COCs.

Intrauterine Devices and Implants

No discussion of contraception should neglect consideration of highly effective reversible contraception, specifically intrauterine devices (IUDs) containing either copper (ParaGard, Teva, Israel) or levonorgestrel (LNG-IUD, Mirena, Sklya, Bayer Healthcare Pharmaceuticals, Wayne, NJ, USA), and the subdermal etonogestrel implant (Nexplanon, Merck, Whitehouse Station, NJ, USA). Given the evidence discussed above which show that progestin-only pills do not increase risk of hypertension, there is no biologic plausibility to suggest a risk associated with these methods. Unfortunately, no studies have explicitly documented the impact of these methods on blood pressure. USMEC guidelines give

Table 3.4 Summary: US medical eligibility criteria for contraceptive use in women with hypertension

Blood pressure	CHC	POP	DMPA	Implant	LNG-IUD	Copper IUD
Adequately controlled	3	1	2	1	1	1
140–159/90–99	3	1	2	1	1	1
≥160/100	4	2	3	2	2	1

CHC combined hormonal contraception, *POP* progestin-only pill, *DMPA* depot medroxyprogesterone acetate, *LNG-IUD* levonorgestrel intrauterine device, *Copper IUD* copper intrauterine device

both the implant and the LNG-IUD the same rating as the progestin-only pill: category 1 for women with adequately controlled and mild hypertension, and category 2 for women with severe hypertension (>160/110) although no studies to support this caution are cited. The copper IUD is category 1 for women with any degree of hypertension. Given the excellent efficacy, safety, and tolerability of IUDs and implants, clinicians should offer these highly effective reversible contraceptives as first-line options for women with any degree of hypertension. Table 3.4 summarizes USMEC guidelines for contraception in women with hypertension.

Patient Assessment and Counseling

In light of the many considerations required before initiation of contraception in women with hypertension, optimal patient assessment is key to both minimizing risks and optimizing opportunities for patient counseling. Patient assessment will differ depending on the type of contraceptive desired. Several systematic reviews have demonstrated that women who do not have their blood pressure measured prior to initiation of CHCs are at significantly higher risk for myocardial infarction and ischemic stroke as compared to women whose blood pressure was measured [29, 54]. For these reasons, blood pressure measurement is recommended for all women prior to initiation of CHC and, if blood pressure is severely elevated, an alternate contraceptive option should be chosen. Systematic review of the literature has not identified any studies which have demonstrated that blood pressure assessment prior to initiation of progestin-only methods changes outcomes [54]. Despite the lack of the direct data, existing evidence demonstrates no increased risk of incident hypertension among women using progestin-only contraceptives. For these reasons, among women choosing progestin-only methods including DMPA and implants, it is not necessary to assess blood pressure prior to initiation [38].

When blood pressure assessment prior to contraception initiation is necessary, proper technique and approach is important. Many women will require a large cuff: the bladder inside the cuff should encircle 80 % of an adult's arm. When in doubt, opt for the larger cuff. Use of a poorly fitting cuff will skew measurement results, with small cuffs producing inaccurately high readings. Providers should not make the diagnosis of hypertension based on one blood pressure reading alone. Rather, patients should be seen in close follow-up to have blood pressure repeated once at a minimum, and ideally twice to rule in the diagnosis. Whenever measuring blood pressure, the patient should be sitting in a quiet environment for at least 5 min. Her arm should be rested on a table or other support, such that the midpoint of the upper arm is at the same level as the heart. Providers should be aware of the many factors that can impact office blood pressure measurement, including caffeine, smoking, pain, anxiety, and errors in technique. "White coat" hypertension, in which blood pressure transiently increases due to the stress associated with medical evaluation but is otherwise normal, is also a phenomenon well documented in the literature [55]. Nevertheless, it is important to recognize that patients whose hypertension is seen only on clinical evaluation but not in ambulatory settings still have increased atherosclerotic risk compared to patients without white coat hypertension [56].

An elevated blood pressure should not delay or prevent initiation of contraception. The importance of this point cannot be underestimated: the adverse health effects, both cardiovascular and otherwise, of an unwanted pregnancy are both more common and serious. In all instances, an elevated blood pressure will inform the need for follow-up and a discussion of whether antihypertensive medication should be initiated. In the event that a CHC is preferred by the patient and her blood pressure is found to be >160/100, an alternative contraceptive should be encouraged. If a patient declines all other options, an individual assessment of the risks and benefits of CHC initiation as well as shared patient–provider decision making are key to considering initiation of a CHC in a woman using an antihypertensive. If this approach is chosen, blood pressure should be reassessed within 1 week. If blood pressure at follow-up is in the mild hypertensive or normal range, long-term use of CHCs in combination with antihypertensive medication is reasonable. Importantly, when initiating contraception in women with hypertension, providers should capitalize on opportunities to counsel and intervene on other risk factors for cardiovascular disease, such as smoking, diabetes, salt intake, and obesity, which are common challenges for hypertensive patients.

Little data exist to guide specific follow-up after initiation of contraception in women with hypertension. Ideally, women with hypertension who are started on a CHC should be prescribed a blood pressure cuff and instructed to record measurements and call their provider if they see readings >140/90. In settings where either cuffs are not available or it is not feasible for patients to self-monitor blood pressure, initiation of contraception should not be delayed or deferred. Women with hypertension should be scheduled for a visit for blood pressure measurement 1–2 weeks after CHC initiation. No additional follow-up, other than what would normally be recommended for hypertensive patients, is necessary after initiation of progestin-only methods and IUDs.

Despite clear evidence for the risk of hypertension after CHC initiation, a systematic review of the literature found that only a small percentage of women developed incident hypertension in up to 2 years of follow-up after starting a CHC. Furthermore, even in studies in which the mean blood pressure was higher in the CHC group than in the placebo group, the mean blood pressures among CHC users largely remained well below levels consistent with a diagnosis of hypertension [57]. Although it is reasonable to check blood pressure in routine follow-up of all women using CHC, these data should reassure providers that no specific blood pressure monitoring is necessary after initiation of a CHC by women who are normotensive at baseline.

No known medication interactions exist between any contraceptive method and antihypertensive agents. The major considerations for medication effects in women of reproductive age with hypertension involve pregnancy and breastfeeding. Agents of choice are discussed previously in this chapter. Although there are important medication interactions that can occur with contraceptive agents as discussed in Chap. 20, providers can be reassured that no interactions with agents used to treat hypertension have been identified.

Pulmonary Arterial Hypertension

A detailed discussion of pulmonary arterial hypertension (PAH) is beyond the scope of this chapter (see Chap. 2). Although pulmonary hypertension is much less common than systemic hypertension, PAH disproportionately impacts reproductive-aged women more than men [58]. The gender differences in the prevalence of this disease are thought to be largely driven by hormonal factors (specifically the effects of altered estrogen metabolism on pulmonary circulation) [59], and therefore a basic understanding of the impact of contraceptive agents on this disease is imperative for any provider who cares for women.

Medical therapy for pulmonary arterial hypertension should be managed by a pulmonologist with expertise in this disease process. Yet, primary care providers play a crucial role in counseling affected women regarding contraception and pregnancy. Unfortunately, pregnancy is often a time when PAH presents, in part, due to the increased stroke volume, cardiac output, and hypercoagulability associated with pregnancy. Even with treatment, maternal mortality is as high 33–50 % [60, 61], with the majority of these tragic fatalities occurring within 35 days of delivery [62]. For these reasons, pregnancy in women with PAH of any cause is classified by the WHO as contraindicated [60].

Given the very high maternal mortality with PAH, safe effective contraception use for women in this patient population is paramount. However, data are very limited and existing guidelines have largely been generated by expert consensus. Neither the CDC nor the WHO MEC specifically discusses pulmonary hypertension. However, as both CHC and PAH increase risk of pulmonary embolism, CHC should be avoided by women with PAH. IUDs and the subdermal implant are first-line agents for any woman with high risk of pregnancy related morbidity or mortality. However, before placing an IUD for a woman with PAH, providers should consider that up to 2 % of women will experience a vasovagal response at the time of IUD placement, especially nulliparous women. As a vagal response for a woman with PAH poses a risk of cardiac collapse, IUD placement should be performed in a carefully monitored setting. The etonogestrel implant may therefore be the preferred contraceptive option for women with PAH. However, when PAH is treated with bosentan (a teratogenic drug commonly used to treat PAH) this medication causes known induction of cytochrome p450, which may reduce the efficacy of the implant as well as POPs [63]. DMPA, due to its relatively higher dose, is thought to remain effective despite cytochrome-inducing agents such as bosentan, and offers another safe alternative. Emergency contraception, which contains no estrogen, is thought to be safe for all women, including those with PAH or cardiac disease of any kind.

Research Gaps

As noted throughout this chapter, many important research gaps exist with respect to contraception use in women either with or at risk of hypertension. One significant gap is that much of what is known about the cardiovascular effects of various contraceptive agents derives from studies in normotensive women. Data are also fairly limited regarding use of the patch and ring. However, given the associated risks seen in these studies as well as the USMEC ratings of 3 and 4 for CHC options in women with varying degrees of hypertension, it is unlikely that additional prospective research in this population will become available. There is also no evidence available regarding the LNG-IUD, the copper IUD, or subdermal implant. The field would benefit from further data on progestin-only methods in women with hypertension. Currently there is only one study examining this relationship, and it does not include the LNG-IUD or subdermal implant. Existing data show the potential for a small increase in cardiovascular risks associated with POP or depot medroxyprogesterone acetate use by hypertensive women. However, these data are far from definitive. Further data on the safety of these methods could potentially change USMEC ratings, especially for progestin-only methods in women with severe hypertension who face significant risk of adverse pregnancy outcomes.

In summary, most women will have no adverse effects from any type of contraception, whether or not they have hypertension. Highly effective reversible contraception such as the contraceptive implant and intrauterine devices are more effective than oral and injectable contraceptives. For this reason, as well as for their favorable safety profiles, they should be recommended as first-line for contraception to women with hypertension. Progestin-only contraceptives and the copper intrauterine device can be used safely in women with hypertension, even if blood pressure is poorly controlled. Blood pressure assessment is not necessary prior to use of these methods. In most cases, the risks and harms associated with an unplanned pregnancy will be greater than any risks associated with contraception for a woman with hypertension; thus, when a combined hormonal method is a woman's preferred contraceptive, use of such a method may be clinically indicated with clear documentation of extended discussion of the risks versus potential benefits of such an approach. Women with known hypertension or risk factors for it should have their blood pressure measured prior to initiation of CHC. These women should also be seen in follow-up to screen for development of worsening hypertension. In general, CHC should be avoided (category 4) in women with blood pressures >160/100. Because of data demonstrating a dose-dependent risk of cardiovascular events in women using contraceptives containing ethinyl estradiol, when these methods are selected, doses ≤35 μg are universally preferred.

References

1. Centers for Disease Control and Prevention. Vital signs: prevalence, treatment, and control of hypertension – United States, 1999–2002 and 2005–2008. MMWR. 2011;60(4):103–8. PubMed PMID: 21293325.
2. Chobanian AV, Bakris GL, Black HR, Cushman WC, Green LA, Izzo Jr JL, et al. The seventh report of the Joint National Committee on Prevention, Detection, Evaluation, and Treatment of High Blood Pressure: the JNC 7 report. JAMA. 2003;289(19):2560–72. PubMed PMID: 12748199.
3. Ong KL, Tso AW, Lam KS, Cheung BM. Gender difference in blood pressure control and cardiovascular risk factors in Americans with diagnosed hypertension. Hypertension. 2008;51(4):1142–8. PubMed PMID: 18259031.
4. Egan BM, Zhao YM, Axon RN. US trends in prevalence, awareness, treatment, and control of hypertension, 1988–2008. JAMA. 2010;303(20): 2043–50. PubMed PMID: WOS:000278018200028. English.
5. Bateman BT, Shaw KM, Kuklina EV, Callaghan WM, Seely EW, Hernandez-Diaz S. Hypertension in women of reproductive age in the United States: NHANES 1999–2008. PLoS One. 2012;7(4):e36171. PubMed PMID: 22558371. Pubmed Central PMCID: 3340351.
6. Schwarz EB, Postlethwaite DA, Hung YY, Armstrong MA. Documentation of contraception and pregnancy when prescribing potentially teratogenic medications for reproductive-age women. Ann Intern Med. 2007;147(6):370–6. PubMed PMID: 17876020. Pubmed Central PMCID: 2941151.
7. American College of Obstetricians and Gynecologists Task Force on Hypertension in Pregnancy. Report of the American College of Obstetricians and Gynecologists' Task Force on Hypertension in Pregnancy. Obstet Gynecol. 2013;122(5):1122–31. PubMed PMID: 24150027.
8. Hsu CY, McCulloch CE, Darbinian J, Go AS, Iribarren C. Elevated blood pressure and risk of end-stage renal disease in subjects without baseline kidney disease. Arch Intern Med. 2005;165(8):923–8. PubMed PMID: 15851645.
9. Reiter L, Brown MA, Whitworth JA. Hypertension in pregnancy: the incidence of underlying renal disease and essential hypertension. Am J Kidney Dis. 1994;24(6):883–7. PubMed PMID: 7985664.
10. Mosca L, Benjamin EJ, Berra K, Bezanson JL, Dolor RJ, Lloyd-Jones DM, et al. Effectiveness-based guidelines for the prevention of cardiovascular disease in women – 2011 update: a guideline from the American Heart Association. J Am Coll Cardiol. 2011;57(12):1404–23. PubMed PMID: 21388771. Pubmed Central PMCID: 3124072.
11. Chappell LC, Enye S, Seed P, Briley AL, Poston L, Shennan AH. Adverse perinatal outcomes and risk factors for preeclampsia in women with chronic hypertension: a prospective study. Hypertension. 2008;51(4):1002–9. PubMed PMID: 18259010.
12. Sibai BM. Chronic hypertension in pregnancy. Obstet Gynecol. 2002;100(2):369–77. PubMed PMID: 12151166.
13. Bellamy L, Casas JP, Hingorani AD, Williams DJ. Pre-eclampsia and risk of cardiovascular disease and cancer in later life: systematic review and meta-analysis. BMJ (Clin Res Ed). 2007;335(7627):974. PubMed PMID: 17975258. Pubmed Central PMCID: 2072042.
14. Abalos E, Duley L, Steyn DW, Henderson-Smart DJ. Antihypertensive drug therapy for mild to moderate hypertension during pregnancy. Cochrane Database Syst Rev. 2007;1, CD002252. PubMed PMID: 17253478.
15. von Dadelszen P, Ornstein MP, Bull SB, Logan AG, Koren G, Magee LA. Fall in mean arterial pressure and fetal growth restriction in pregnancy hypertension: a meta-analysis. Lancet. 2000;355(9198):87–92. PubMed PMID: 10675164.
16. Seely EW, Ecker J. Clinical practice. Chronic hypertension in pregnancy. N Engl J Med. 2011;365(5):439–46. PubMed PMID: 21812673.
17. Aleksandrov NA, Fraser W, Audibert F. Diagnosis, management, and evaluation of hypertensive disorders of pregnancy. J Obstet Gynaecol Can. 2008;30(11):1000. Author reply – 1. PubMed PMID: 19126280.
18. Horvath JS, Phippard A, Korda A, Henderson-Smart DJ, Child A, Tiller DJ. Clonidine hydrochloride – a safe and effective antihypertensive agent in pregnancy. Obstet Gynecol. 1985;66(5):634–8. PubMed PMID: 3903581.
19. Magee LA, Cham C, Waterman EJ, Ohlsson A, von Dadelszen P. Hydralazine for treatment of severe hypertension in pregnancy: meta-analysis. BMJ (Clin Res Ed). 2003;327(7421):955–60. PubMed PMID: 14576246. Pubmed Central PMCID: 259162.
20. Laragh JH, Sealey JE, Ledingha JG, Newton MA. Oral contraceptives – renin aldosterone and high blood pressure. JAMA. 1967;201(12):918. PubMed PMID: WOS:A19679882400003. English.

21. August P. Hypertension in women. Adv Chronic Kidney D. 2013;20(5):396–401. PubMed PMID: WOS:000324445200005. English.
22. Cardoso F, Polonia J, Santos A, Silva-Carvalho J, Ferreira-de-Almeida J. Low-dose oral contraceptives and 24-hour ambulatory blood pressure. Int J Gynecol Obstet. 1997;59(3):237–43. PubMed PMID: WOS:000071653600008. English.
23. Heintz B, Schmauder C, Witte K, Breuer I, Baltzer K, Sieberth HG, et al. Blood pressure rhythm and endocrine functions in normotensive women on oral contraceptives. J Hypertens. 1996;14(3):333–9. PubMed PMID: WOS:A1996UJ80600010. English.
24. Lubianca JN, Faccin CS, Fuchs FD. Oral contraceptives: a risk factor for uncontrolled blood pressure among hypertensive women. Contraception. 2003;67(1): 19–24. PubMed PMID: WOS:000180496200004. English.
25. Chasan-Taber L, Willett WC, Manson JE, Spiegelman D, Hunter DJ, Curhan G, et al. Prospective study of oral contraceptives and hypertension among women in the United States. Circulation. 1996;94(3):483–9. PubMed PMID: WOS:A1996UZ05100038. English.
26. Farley TM, Collins J, Schlesselman JJ. Hormonal contraception and risk of cardiovascular disease. An international perspective. Contraception. 1998;57(3):211–30. PubMed PMID: 9617537.
27. Croft P, Hannaford PC. Risk-factors for acute myocardial-infarction in women – evidence from the Royal College of General Practitioners Oral Contraception Study. BMJ. 1989;298(6667):165–8. PubMed PMID: WOS:A1989R926400028. English.
28. Poulter NR, Chang CL, Farley TMM, Kelaghan J, Meirlk O, Marmot MG, et al. Acute myocardial infarction and combined oral contraceptives: results of an international multicentre case–control study. Lancet. 1997;349(9060):1202–9. PubMed PMID: WOS:A1997WW71700009. English.
29. Curtis KM, Mohllajee AP, Martins SL, Peterson HB. Combined oral contraceptive use among women with hypertension: a systematic review. Contraception. 2006;73(2):179–88. PubMed PMID: WOS:000235252500008. English.
30. Van Den Bosch MAAJ, Kemmeren JM, Tanis BC, Mali WPTM, Helmerhorst FM, Rosendaal FR, et al. The RATIO study: oral contraceptives and the risk of peripheral arterial disease in young women. J Thromb Haemost. 2003;1(3):439–44. PubMed PMID: WOS:000183061900011. English.
31. Lidegaard O, Kreiner S. Contraceptives and cerebral thrombosis: a five-year national case–control study. Contraception. 2002;65(3):197–205. PubMed PMID: WOS:000174908400002. English.
32. Schwartz SM, Petitti DB, Siscovick DS, Longstreth WT, Sidney S, Raghunathan TE, et al. Stroke and use of low-dose oral contraceptives in young women – a pooled analysis of two US studies. Stroke. 1998;29(11):2277–84. PubMed PMID: WOS:000076754100006. English.
33. WHO. Ischaemic stroke and combined oral contraceptives: results of an international, multicentre, case–control study WHO collaborative study of cardiovascular disease and steroid hormone contraception. Lancet. 1996;348(9026):498–505. PubMed PMID: 8757151.
34. Heinemann LA, Lewis MA, Spitzer WO, Thorogood M, Guggenmoos-Holzmann I, Bruppacher R. Thromboembolic stroke in young women. A European case–control study on oral contraceptives. Transnational research group on oral contraceptives and the health of young women. Contraception. 1998;57(1):29–37. PubMed PMID: 9554248.
35. Gillum LA, Mamidipudi SK, Johnston SC. Ischemic stroke risk with oral contraceptives: a meta-analysis. JAMA. 2000;284(1):72–8. PubMed PMID: 10872016.
36. Petitti DB. Hormonal contraceptives and arterial thrombosis – not risk-free but safe enough. N Engl J Med. 2012;366(24):2316–8. PubMed PMID: 22694003.
37. Lidegaard O, Lokkegaard E, Jensen A, Skovlund CW, Keiding N. Thrombotic stroke and myocardial infarction with hormonal contraception. N Engl J Med. 2012;366(24):2257–66. PubMed PMID: 22693997.
38. Division of Reproductive Health NCfCDP, Health Promotion CfDC, Prevention. U.S. selected practice recommendations for contraceptive use, 2013: adapted from the World Health Organization selected practice recommendations for contraceptive use, 2nd edn. MMWR. 2013;62(RR-05):1–60. PubMed PMID: 23784109.
39. Timmer CJ, Mulders TM. Pharmacokinetics of etonogestrel and ethinylestradiol released from a combined contraceptive vaginal ring. Clin Pharmacokinet. 2000;39(3):233–42. PubMed PMID: 11020137.
40. Devineni D, Skee D, Vaccaro N, Massarella J, Janssens L, LaGuardia KD, et al. Pharmacokinetics and pharmacodynamics of a transdermal contraceptive patch and an oral contraceptive. J Clin Pharmacol. 2007;47(4):497–509. PubMed PMID: 17389559.
41. Minshall RD, Pavcnik D, Browne DL, Hermsmeyer K. Nongenomic vasodilator action of progesterone on primate coronary arteries. J Appl Physiol (1985). 2002;92(2):701–8. PubMed PMID: 11796684.
42. Hussain SF. Progestogen-only pills and high blood pressure: is there an association? A literature review. Contraception. 2004;69(2):89–97. PubMed PMID: 14759612.
43. Hall WD, Douglas MB, Blumenstein BA, Hatcher RA. Blood pressure and oral progestational agents. A prospective study of 119 black women. Am J Obstet Gynecol. 1980;136(3):344–8.
44. Spellacy WN, Birk SA. The effect of intrauterine devices, oral contraceptives, estrogens, and progestogens on blood pressure. Am J Obstet Gynecol. 1972;112(7):912–9. PubMed PMID: 4114467.
45. Wilson ES, Cruickshank J, McMaster M, Weir RJ. A prospective controlled study of the effect on blood pressure of contraceptive preparations containing different types and dosages of progestogen. Br J Obstet Gynecol. 1984;91(12):1254–60. PubMed PMID: 6440589.

46. WHO. Cardiovascular disease and use of oral and injectable progestogen-only contraceptives and combined injectable contraceptives. Results of an international, multicenter, case–control study. World Health Organization collaborative study of cardiovascular disease and steroid hormone contraception. Contraception. 1998;57(5):315–24. PubMed PMID: 9673838.
47. Frederiksen MC. Depot medroxyprogesterone acetate contraception in women with medical problems. J Reprod Med. 1996;41(5 Suppl):414–8. PubMed PMID: 8725704.
48. White WB, Pitt B, Preston RA, Hanes V. Antihypertensive effects of drospirenone with 17beta-estradiol, a novel hormone treatment in postmenopausal women with stage 1 hypertension. Circulation. 2005;112(13):1979–84. PubMed PMID: 16186434.
49. Oelkers W, Foidart JM, Dombrovicz N, Welter A, Heithecker R. Effects of a new oral contraceptive containing an antimineralocorticoid progestogen, drospirenone, on the renin-aldosterone system, body weight, blood pressure, glucose tolerance, and lipid metabolism. J Clin Endocrinol Metab. 1995;80(6):1816–21. PubMed PMID: 7775629.
50. Cagnacci A, Ferrari S, Napolitano A, Piacenti I, Arangino S, Volpe A. Combined oral contraceptive containing drospirenone does not modify 24-h ambulatory blood pressure but increases heart rate in healthy young women: prospective study. Contraception. 2013;88(3):413–7. PubMed PMID: 23312932.
51. Stegeman BH, de Bastos M, Rosendaal FR, van HylckamaVlieg A, Helmerhorst FM, Stijnen T, et al. Different combined oral contraceptives and the risk of venous thrombosis: systematic review and network meta-analysis. BMJ (Clin Res Ed). 2013;347:f5298. PubMed PMID: 24030561. Pubmed Central PMCID: 3771677.
52. Lidegaard O, Nielsen LH, Skovlund CW, Skjeldestad FE, Lokkegaard E. Risk of venous thromboembolism from use of oral contraceptives containing different progestogens and oestrogen doses: Danish cohort study, 2001–9. BMJ (Clin Res Ed). 2011;343:d6423. PubMed PMID: 22027398. Pubmed Central PMCID: 3202015.
53. Dinger JC, Heinemann LA, Kuhl-Habich D. The safety of a drospirenone-containing oral contraceptive: final results from the European Active Surveillance Study on oral contraceptives based on 142,475 women-years of observation. Contraception. 2007;75(5):344–54. PubMed PMID: 17434015.
54. Tepper NK, Curtis KM, Steenland MW, Marchbanks PA. Blood pressure measurement prior to initiating hormonal contraception: a systematic review. Contraception. 2013;87(5):631–8. PubMed PMID: 23063336.
55. Reeves RA. The rational clinical examination. Does this patient have hypertension? How to measure blood pressure. JAMA. 1995;273(15):1211–8.
56. Muldoon MF, Nazzaro P, Sutton-Tyrrell K, Manuck SB. White-coat hypertension and carotid artery atherosclerosis: a matching study. Arch Intern Med. 2000;160(10):1507–12. PubMed PMID: 10826466.
57. Steenland MW, Zapata LB, Brahmi D, Marchbanks PA, Curtis KM. Appropriate follow up to detect potential adverse events after initiation of select contraceptive methods: a systematic review. Contraception. 2013;87(5):611–24. PubMed PMID: 23177264.
58. Shapiro S, Traiger GL, Turner M, McGoon MD, Wason P, Barst RJ. Sex differences in the diagnosis, treatment, and outcome of patients with pulmonary arterial hypertension enrolled in the registry to evaluate early and long-term pulmonary arterial hypertension disease management. Chest. 2012;141(2):363–73. PubMed PMID: 21757572.
59. Pugh ME, Hemnes AR. Pulmonary hypertension in women. Expert Rev Cardiovasc Ther. 2010;8(11):1549–58. PubMed PMID: 21090930. Pubmed Central PMCID: 3077035.
60. Thorne S, Nelson-Piercy C, MacGregor A, Gibbs S, Crowhurst J, Panay N, et al. Pregnancy and contraception in heart disease and pulmonary arterial hypertension. J Fam Plann Reprod Health Care. 2006;32(2):75–81. PubMed PMID: 16824295.
61. European Society of G, Association for European Paediatric C, German Society for Gender M, Regitz-Zagrosek V, Blomstrom Lundqvist C, Borghi C, et al. ESC guidelines on the management of cardiovascular diseases during pregnancy: the Task Force on the Management of Cardiovascular Diseases During Pregnancy of the European Society of Cardiology (ESC). Eur Heart J. 2011;32(24):3147–97. PubMed PMID: 21873418.
62. Weiss BM, Zemp L, Seifert B, Hess OM. Outcome of pulmonary vascular disease in pregnancy: a systematic overview from 1978 through 1996. J Am Coll Cardiol. 1998;31(7):1650–7. PubMed PMID: 9626847.
63. Venitz J, Zack J, Gillies H, Allard M, Regnault J, Dufton C. Clinical pharmacokinetics and drug–drug interactions of endothelin receptor antagonists in pulmonary arterial hypertension. J Clin Pharmacol. 2012;52(12):1784–805. PubMed PMID: 22205719.

Contraception and Diabetes

4

Meredith Macrae Warden, Jody Steinauer, and Elizabeth Harleman

Epidemiology of Diabetes in the United States

Diabetes is a common condition in the United States. In 2010, almost 26 million people, or 8.3 % of the US population, had diabetes, 12.6 million of whom were women [2]. The incidence of diabetes in US women is increasing, from 4.5 per 1,000 in 1997 to 7.5 per 1,000 in 2011 (Fig. 4.1) [3]. Among those less than age 20, a recent estimate from 2010 showed that 215,000 people have diabetes. Between 2005 and 2008, 35 % of US adults were diagnosed with prediabetes (fasting glucose of 100–125 mg/dL), a condition that carries an increased risk of not only diabetes, but also heart disease and stroke. Prediabetes is also increasing in US women, with recent data suggesting that between 2002 and 2010, the prevalence of prediabetes among women increased by 8 % [4]. Both prediabetes and diabetes are also increasing among US adolescents [5]. The increase of both prediabetes and diabetes in the United States is likely at least in part due to increasing obesity.

The increasing prevalence of diabetes is of concern given that diabetes increases the risk of a number of medical complications, as well as negatively impacting overall life expectancy [6]. Microvascular complications of both type 1 and type 2 diabetes include nephropathy, neuropathy, and retinopathy [7]. Nephropathy is characterized by albuminuria, typically urinary albumin excretion of 30–300 mg/day. Interestingly, the degree of albuminuria is not necessarily associated with the severity of nephropathy. Diabetic nephropathy is the most common cause of dialysis in the United States [8]. Nephropathy and diabetic retinopathy often coexist within patients. Diabetic retinopathy is one of the leading causes of vision loss, and is typically diagnosed on a retinal exam. Diabetic neuropathy is a clinical diagnosis, based on a neurological exam, and is characterized by symmetrical sensory polyneuropathy. The progression of diabetic neuropathy correlates directly with hyperglycemia, and is a major source of pain in patients with diabetes. Diabetes also dramatically increases the risk of cardiovascular disease, including coronary artery disease, stroke, and peripheral vascular disease [6]. It is these macrovascular complications that often contribute to mortality in diabetic patients.

M.M. Warden, M.D., M.P.H. (✉)
Department of Obstetrics, Gynecology and Reproductive Sciences, San Francisco General Hospital, University of California, San Francisco, San Francisco, CA, USA
e-mail: wardenm@obgyn.ucsf.edu

J. Steinauer, M.D., M.A.S.
Department of Obstetrics, Gynecology and Reproductive Sciences, San Francisco General Hospital, San Francisco, CA, USA
e-mail: steinauerj@obgyn.ucsf.edu

E. Harleman, M.D.
Department of Internal Medicine, San Francisco General Hospital, University of California, San Francisco, San Francisco, CA, USA
e-mail: eharleman@medsfgh.ucsf.edu

R.H. Allen and C.A. Cwiak (eds.), *Contraception for the Medically Challenging Patient*,
DOI 10.1007/978-1-4939-1233-9_4, © Springer Science+Business Media New York 2014

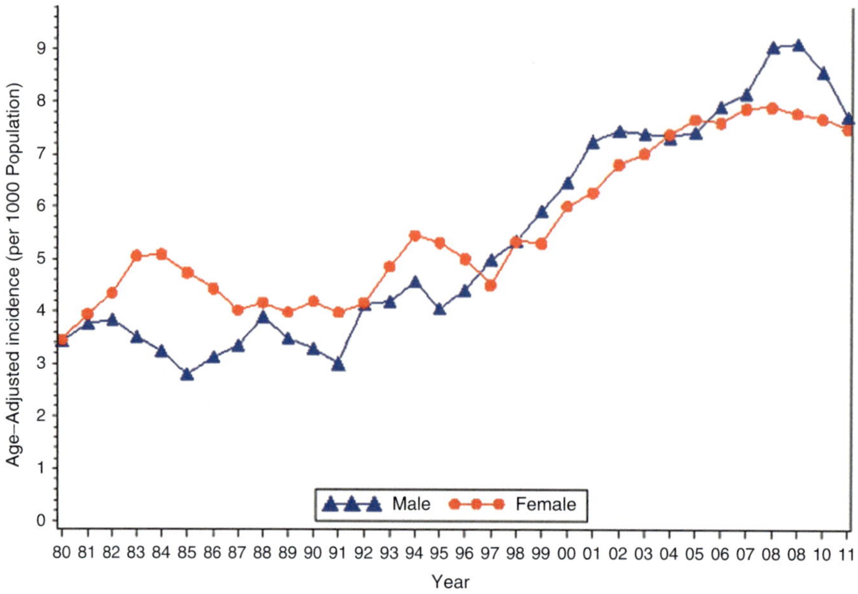

Fig. 4.1 Age-adjusted incidence of diagnosed diabetes per 1,000 population aged 18–79 years, by sex, United States, 1980–2011

Major trials examining the effect of treatment of diabetes and its associated comorbidities, hypertension and hyperlipidemia, consistently show that while glycemic control may limit the progression of microvascular complications, control of blood pressure and lipids has the most potent effect on mortality [9–11].

Preexisting diabetes in women who become pregnant is also a major cause of both maternal and fetal morbidity. Poorly controlled diabetes increases the risk of spontaneous abortion as well as the risk of major congenital malformations [12]. Pregnant patients often have significant insulin resistance, necessitating dose increases of medications as well as much closer blood glucose monitoring. Preexisting diabetes also increases the risk of preeclampsia and cesarean delivery [13]. Metabolic imprinting of the fetus is thought to contribute to the increased risk of obesity, insulin resistance, diabetes, and cardiovascular disease in the offspring of diabetic mothers [14, 15].

Preexisting end organ disease often worsens in pregnant diabetic women. The increased glomerular filtration rate associated with the physiologic expansion of blood volume in pregnancy tends to worsen preexisting renal and retinal disease. Worsening renal disease, particularly nephrotic conditions, is associated with an increased risk of pregnancy complications including preeclampsia and preterm delivery [16]. Evidence from small case series suggests that for women with moderate renal insufficiency, up to 30 % may experience an irreversible decline in renal function [17], and a small proportion of patients without preexisting renal disease may experience a permanent decline in renal function. A recent meta-analysis showed that women with preexisting renal impairment were more likely to develop hypertensive disorders of pregnancy than women without renal disease (12 % vs. 2 %), and there was an increased but nonsignificant trend in maternal mortality (4 % vs. 1 %) [18]. Diabetic nephropathy also increases the risk of preterm birth secondary to worsening maternal disease, fetal growth restriction, and perinatal mortality.

Gestational diabetes, which affects 2–10 % of pregnancies, also carries an increased risk of both maternal and fetal complications [2]. It is a known risk factor for macrosomia, which can increase the risk of operative vaginal delivery, cesarean section, and brachial plexus injury in the infant [19]. It has also been associated with preeclampsia in pregnancy. Gestational diabetes substantially increases the risk that a woman will subsequently develop type 2 diabetes, with up to a third having impaired glucose tolerance or overt diabetes at postpartum follow-up, and up to 50 % developing type 2 diabetes in the 10 years following pregnancy [20]. As such, the population of women with a history of gestational diabetes mellitus (GDM) represents a uniquely well-defined cohort of patients at risk for development of a chronic disease with lifelong implications. Since each subsequent pregnancy is associated with a period of worsening metabolic control, potential end organ damage, and for many women, a permanent increase in body weight, assisting women with a history of GDM in accessing effective contraception can be one of the most important preventive steps a physician can take.

Pathophysiology, Diagnosis, and Treatment of Diabetes Mellitus

Diabetes mellitus is characterized by abnormal glucose metabolism. There are two main types of diabetes. Type 1, which develops due to autoimmune destruction of the pancreatic islet cells, most commonly affects younger patients who may have a normal body mass index (BMI). Patients with type 1 diabetes generally have modest but essential exogenous insulin requirements. They are at risk for diabetic ketoacidosis, a ketotic state that can have disastrous consequences if untreated. Much more common is type 2 diabetes, which is caused by relative peripheral insulin resistance. Though type 2 diabetes classically affects older, overweight patients, it can also develop in normal weight patients, and is becoming increasingly common in children and adolescents due in part to the epidemic of obesity. Type 2 diabetes outside of pregnancy may be treated with diet and exercise alone, or a variety of medications, both oral and injectable, can be added to improve glycemic control if needed. The landscape of therapies for type 2 diabetes has changed significantly over the past 10 years, with a number of new drugs becoming available. Nevertheless, type 2 diabetes, like type 1, is usually a lifelong chronic disease that must be managed in close partnership with the individual patient.

Table 4.1 Diagnosis of diabetes mellitus and prediabetes

Diagnosis of diabetes mellitus: (only one required for diagnosis)	Fasting blood glucose ≥126 mg/dL
	HbA1C ≥6.5 %
	Random blood glucose ≥200 mg/dL in persons with symptoms of hyperglycemia or hyperglycemic crisis
	2-h 75 g OGTT ≥200 mg/dL
Diagnosis of prediabetes: (only one required for diagnosis)	Fasting blood glucose 100–125 mg/dL
	HbA1C 5.7–6.4 %
	2-h 75 g OGTT of 140–199 mg/dL

OGTT oral glucose tolerance test

Since 1997, the diagnosis of type 2 diabetes (formerly known as adult-onset diabetes) has been based on two confirmed fasting plasma glucose levels of 126 mg/dL or greater (Table 4.1) [21]. Alternatively, a random plasma glucose of at least 200 mg/dL is also diagnostic of type 2 diabetes (T2DM) in patients with symptoms of hyperglycemia such as polyuria, polydipsia, and polyphagia. Glycated hemoglobin (HbA1C) is now internationally standardized, and since 2009, a HbA1C of ≥6.5 % is also diagnostic of T2DM. Given their more complex and costly nature, oral glucose tolerance tests are rarely used outside of pregnancy, the postpartum period, and in research settings to identify individuals with diabetes and gestational diabetes. The preference for their use in pregnant and postpartum women is due to both historical norms and the greater sensitivity of the oral glucose tolerance test, which performs better than the fasting glucose or HgBA1C at identifying women with impaired glucose tolerance in the postpartum period.

Impaired fasting glucose is now recognized as a prediabetic state, and is defined as a fasting glucose of 100–125 mg/dL (see Table 4.1). Having impaired fasting glucose is associated with a 5–10 % annual risk of developing type 2 diabetes, which is 5–10 times that of people with normal fasting glucose. Prediabetic HbA1C levels are defined as 5.7–6.4 %.

Contraceptive Practices of Women with Diabetes in the United States

There is an unmet need for contraception among women with diabetes in the United States. Given the well-documented increased risk of both maternal and fetal morbidity due to diabetes in pregnancy, use of effective contraception to enable optimal pregnancy planning is essential in women with diabetes. However, women with diabetes are more likely to not use contraception than either overweight or obese women [22]. Several studies have also demonstrated that women with diabetes are less likely to receive contraceptive counseling, prescriptions for birth control, or contraceptive services [23–26]. One study suggested that a third of adolescents with diabetes perceived that contraceptive options were very limited because of their diabetes, and 43 % believed that all birth control methods are less effective in women with diabetes [26]. Women with diabetes are also less likely to use highly effective reversible methods of contraception, but are more likely to undergo sterilization, highlighting the lack of appropriate contraceptive counseling among women with diabetes who have not yet completed childbearing [23, 25].

Physiologic Changes of Contraception on Glycemic Control in Nondiabetic Women

Levonorgestrel IUD

There are scant data evaluating the effect of the levonorgestrel (LNG) IUD on glycemic control. One study that compared 31 women randomized to either the copper IUD, the LNG-IUD, or LNG-containing combined oral contraceptives (COCs) found no significant differences over 3 months in fasting glucose or insulin concentrations [27]. A prospective population-based study of the Northern Finland Birth Cohort compared insulin and glucose measures at 31 years of age in users of nonhormonal contraception, combined oral contraceptives (COCs), and the LNG-IUD [28]. In their adjusted analysis, the metabolic parameters of LNG-IUD users were similar to nonhormonal users, but COC users were more likely to have insulin resistance despite having lower BMIs. This finding may reflect prescribing practice or other factors in the COC users, as these results are inconsistent with the larger body of literature on insulin resistance in COC users (see below).

Contraceptive Implant

The data that exist on carbohydrate metabolism in women using the levonorgestrel implant (Norplant), which is no longer available in the United States, is inconsistent, but overall suggests minimal impact on insulin resistance or glucose metabolism, though there may be at least initially a decrease in insulin sensitivity [29]. The studies that assessed glucose metabolism beyond 6 months did not tend to show significant effects on insulin sensitivity or glucose levels.

A two-rod system of 140 mg of LNG (Jadelle) is available outside of the United States, and is approved for use up to 5 years. Studies have assessed OGTTs in healthy women for up to 5 years post-insertion which found that although there were statistically significant increases in 1-h glucose levels up to three years (between 139 and 142 mg/dL), these slight increases were mild and not progressive, and returned to normal by the fourth and fifth years post-insertion [29]. Fasting and 2-h glucose levels were not statistically significantly different from baseline at any time point.

As with the levonorgestrel IUD, few studies have assessed the effect of the etonogestrel (ENG) implant (Implanon, Nexplanon, Merck, Whitehouse Station, NJ, USA) on carbohydrate metabolism. One non-randomized prospective study of 46 Brazilian women using either the ENG implant or the copper IUD followed OGTT and HbA1C at baseline, 6 and 12 months [30]. Though fasting insulin was slightly higher in the implant group at 6 months, it was not statistically different from the IUD users, and there was no difference at 12 months. There were no differences in fasting glucose, 2-h OGTT glucose levels, or HbA1C levels at 6 or 12 months. Biswas et al. compared 80 women randomized to the 6-rod levonorgestrel implant or the ENG implant, and followed them for 2 years [31]. Area under the curve (AUC) for both insulin and glucose, OGTTs, mean fasting insulin, and HbA1C levels was statistically higher than baseline in both groups at 24 months, but all of these values were still within normal limits for healthy women. A study of 70 women using the ENG implant did not find any differences between baseline and 3-year fasting glucose levels [32]. Overall, these studies suggest minimal impact of the etonogestrel implant on glucose metabolism, though as with other methods, studies involving women who may be at risk for diabetes or obese women are lacking.

Injectable Contraception

Glycemic control in injectable contraception has been studied with inconsistent results [33]. One trial randomized 40 women to either injectable 150 mg DMPA or 200 mg norethisterone enanthate and followed them for 1 year [34]. The DMPA group had higher mean fasting glucose levels, fasting serum insulin, and mean glucose 2-h responses, but no difference in insulin 2-h responses. More recently, Berenson et al. followed over 700 women using either DMPA, CHCs, or nonhormonal contraception for 3 years and found that DMPA users had a small increase in serum glucose levels that remained stable after 18 months [33]. DMPA users also had slightly greater insulin levels compared to CHC users, suggesting that DMPA may worsen peripheral sensitivity to insulin, predisposing patients to the development of type 2 diabetes. Of note, the increases were not clinically significant for any of the DMPA studies.

Combined Hormonal Contraception

The impact of CHC on glycemic control has been studied extensively in women without diabetes. Comparing desogestrel- vs. LNG-containing COC, meta-analyses showed that the desogestrel group had higher mean fasting glucose at 6 months that resolved by 12 months compared to the LNG-containing COC, but individual studies showed inconsistencies [34]. Other COC comparisons between formulations with gestodene, drospirenone, and norethindrone showed no significant differences in glucose or insulin measures. Studies of extended cycle formulations are limited, but have shown no significant differences in glycemic metabolism [34]. Similarly, the etonogestrel-containing vaginal ring has not been associated with any changes in carbohydrate metabolism when compared to either COCs or LNG implants. One small study of the contraceptive patch in Thai women showed no changes in mean fasting glucose in patch users compared to baseline over 3 months [35].

Physiologic Changes of Contraception on Glycemic Control in Nondiabetic Obese Women

More recently, studies assessing carbohydrate metabolism in obese and non-obese women have been published. A recent small study comparing eight women using nonhormonal contraception to eight etonogestrel implant users and to nine LNG-IUD users over 6 months, all with BMI of 30 or greater, showed that fasting glucose was significantly increased in both LNG and ENG users compared to nonhormonal users, with an average of 92.6, 101, and 86.6 mg/dL, respectively, at 6 months [36]. These differences reflected minimal if any clinical significance, did not seem to increase between 3 and 6 months, and were not associated with differences in insulin levels between the groups. Also interestingly, within groups, the insulin sensitivity decreased over 6 months in the ENG and LNG users compared to the nonhormonal users, but there was no statistically significant mean difference between the groups. Another study compared the metabolic effects of DMPA in a predominantly Latina population of 10 obese (BMI of 30 kg/m^2 or greater) vs. 5 normal weight women (BMI 18.5–24.9 kg/m^2) over 7 months [37]. In this study, a measure of insulin resistance was increased in the obese women on DMPA compared to the normal weight women. Though the long-term clinical significance of this biochemical finding is unclear, it suggests the need for future study to better define and quantify the risk of progression to T2DM, particularly in obese women using injectable contraceptives.

In summary, some evidence suggests that hormonal contraception may change carbohydrate metabolism but not in clinically meaningful ways, particularly for IUDs and CHC. Other evidence shows that hormonal contraception has no effect. These studies are limited by small numbers of participants, and the variation in duration of follow-up and outcome measures. The emerging data on whether carbohydrate metabolism is truly affected, and whether it is affected in a more clinically meaningful way in obese women, warrants further study.

Contraception in Women with Diabetes Mellitus

The literature on contraceptives in women with diabetes is less robust than that of women without diabetes. Just as studies in nondiabetic women tend to exclude women with obesity and prediabetes, studies in diabetic women frequently exclude women with complications from diabetes. In this section, we will review the literature on various contraceptive methods in women with diabetes, with close examination of the severity or classification of diabetes in study participants.

Intrauterine Device

One randomized controlled trial by Rogovskaya et al. compared the LNG-IUD to the copper IUD in women with type 1 diabetes [38]. This study randomized a total of 62 women to either the copper IUD or the LNG-IUD, and women were followed for 12 months with metabolic measures at baseline, 6 weeks, 6 months, and 12 months. The copper IUD is a nonhormonal method of contraception and therefore would not be expected to alter carbohydrate metabolism, and is a MEC category 1 for all types of diabetes. All participants were seen by a diabetologist, an ophthalmologist, and a gynecologist. As this study was designed to evaluate the effects of the LNG-IUD on women with well-controlled type 1 diabetes, only women with "normal" glucose and HbA1C levels, and without evidence of "retinopathy or nephropathy" (also not defined), were included. The average duration of diabetes was 6–7 years for both groups. There were no significant differences in fasting glucose levels, HbA1C levels, or insulin requirements between LNG-IUD users compared to copper IUD users at any time point. There were statistically significant increases in HbA1C levels from 5.5 to 5.6 % at baseline to 6.3 % in both groups over the 12-month study period, but these increases occurred in both groups nondifferentially.

Grigoryan et al. assessed carbohydrate and lipid metabolism in perimenopausal women with diabetes using different combinations of COCs, the copper IUD, and the LNG-IUD [39]. This study followed women ages 39–50 with type 1 and type 2 DM for 12 months. The study excluded women with proliferative retinopathy, nephropathy, or macrovascular complications. The average duration of diabetes for the T1 diabetics was 14.3 years, and for T2 diabetics it was 5.3 years. One hundred and three women were randomized to one of five treatment groups, with age-matched controls who were using no contraception. The treatment groups included three COC groups, a copper IUD group, and an LNG-IUD group. This study showed no significant differences in HbA1C levels between any of the groups at 12 months, and no differences in insulin requirements for either IUD group compared to controls at 12 months.

These two randomized controlled trials by Rogovskaya and Grigoryan, one of which included older women with diabetes who may be at increased risk of metabolic complications from hormonal contraception, provide evidence that the LNG-IUD does not affect carbohydrate metabolism measures in women with diabetes. Thus, the MEC category 2 for the LNG-IUD in women with diabetes is overly cautious, and could be reduced to a category 1.

Etonogestrel Implant

No randomized studies have been conducted assessing the effect of the contraceptive progestin-only implant on carbohydrate metabolism in diabetic users. One prospective study of 23 diabetic women using the etonogestrel implant measured carbohydrate and lipid metabolic markers over 24 months [40]. There were no significant changes in weight, HbA1C, or insulin requirements over the study period. And though total high density lipoprotein (HDL) cholesterol did decrease over time (from a baseline mean of 62 to 57 mg/dL), there was also a decrease in total cholesterol (209–193 mg/dL) and low density lipoprotein (LDL) (125–119 mg/dL) levels.

Injectable Contraception

There have been no randomized controlled trials of DMPA in women with diabetes. A single prospective study of 80 type 1 and 2 diabetics compared carbohydrate and lipid measurements over 9 months in women using patient-selected methods of contraception (DMPA, the 6 rod levonorgestrel implant or a low-dose COC, compared to copper IUD controls) [41]. Women with retinopathy, nephropathy, uncontrolled diabetes (HbA1C over 8 %), hypertension, or liver disease were excluded. Participants choosing the implant were more likely to be older and have higher parity than those choosing the IUD; otherwise, participants had similar study characteristics at baseline. There was no increase in fasting blood glucose (FBG) or insulin requirements for the implant users, but in the DMPA users, FBG increased significantly from a baseline mean of 102.7 to 112.9 mg/dL. Also in injectable users, HDL significantly decreased over the study period from 44.6 at baseline to 34.4 mg/dL, but otherwise there was no change in any other measured parameters in this group. There was a statistically significant increase in percent change of fasting glucose in each of the groups (implant, COCs, and DMPA) when compared to the IUD group, but no significant changes of insulin or oral hypoglycemic requirements occurred in any of the groups.

To our knowledge this single study is the only one to assess the effects of DMPA use on metabolic parameters in diabetic women. High-quality studies evaluating the effect of DMPA on women with diabetes are needed to determine whether the benefits of this highly effective contraceptive outweigh any possible impairment of glucose metabolism in women with diabetes.

Combined Oral Contraceptives and Progestin-Only Pills

Several studies have evaluated the impact of oral contraceptives on metabolic parameters in women with diabetes, three of which are randomized controlled trials. Two of the studies were in women with T1DM, but one included both T2DM and T1DM [42]. The Grigoryan study reviewed previously randomized women to either the LNG-IUD, the copper IUD, or one of three formulations of COCs: 20 mcg ethinyl estradiol (EE) + 150 mcg desogestrel (DSG), 30 mcg EE + 150 mcg DSG, or 30 mcg EE + 75 mcg DSG [39]. Overall, there were no clinically significant changes in fasting glucose or HbA1C levels in any of the COC groups compared to the copper IUD, but there was a statistically significant within-group increase of 21 % in insulin requirements among the 30EE/DSG participants at 12 months. There were otherwise favorable changes in lipid metabolism, including an increase in HDL levels and a decrease in triglyceride levels in one of the COC groups.

Similarly, a study which randomized women to four different COC preparations or one progestin-only pill (POP) in T1 diabetics found no changes in HbA1C levels, fasting glucose, or insulin requirements in any of the groups at 6 months [43]. HDL levels were significantly lower in one of the COC formulations, but triglycerides and VLDL were lower in other groups.

Another study which randomized diabetic women to either the progestin-only lynestrenol (LYN) 0.5 mg pill or the combined 50 mcg EE plus 2.5 mg LYN pill found that with the progestin only formulation, there were no changes in insulin requirements at 6 months [44]. The COC users had a statistically significant, but minor, increase in insulin requirements but no change in fasting blood glucose measurements. The LYN-only group had significant reductions in triglycerides and total cholesterol.

These data are limited by small numbers of participants, variations in outcomes and duration of follow-up, as well as the overall lack of quality randomized controlled trials. However, overall any negative effect of COCs or POPs on carbohydrate and lipid metabolism appears to be minimal if at all present.

Contraceptive Patch/Ring

No randomized trials have been conducted in women with diabetes using the contraceptive patch or ring. One study of 25 women with T1DM using the contraceptive ENG ring compared to 20 age-matched controls with T1DM using no contraception and to 20 nondiabetic women using the ring for 6 months [45]. Of note, the average age of the women in this study was 40.3 years. There were no significant changes in insulin requirements, HbA1C levels, or lipid measures in women using the ring.

Another study evaluated the effect of continuous contraceptive ring use on carbohydrate metabolism in 109 women with T1DM [46]. In this study women were assigned to using the contraceptive ring in the routine 21/7 day regimen, 42/7 regimen, 84/7 or 357/7 regimen. They were compared with 22 age-matched controls with T1DM using no contraception. There were no changes in HbA1C levels or insulin requirements over 24 months. Neither of these studies provided comparative analyses between ring users and controls.

We were unable to identify any studies evaluating the patch in women with diabetes. Overall, the literature on the patch and ring suffers from the same limitations as the COC literature; but there appears to be a minimal effect of any CHC method on carbohydrate metabolism.

Contraception in Women with a History of Gestational Diabetes

Gestational diabetes mellitus (GDM) affects 2–10 % of pregnant women [2, 47]. As many as one-third of healthy women who develop GDM have impaired glucose tolerance or diabetes at their postpartum visit [20]. Women who have had GDM have a 35–60 % chance of developing type 2 diabetes in the 10–20 years following their pregnancies [2]. In fact, a recent study of nearly 600 Latina women in southern California found that of women with a history of GDM, 9 % had diabetes diagnosed at the first postpartum visit and of those followed for 2 years an additional 19 % were diagnosed [48]. In all women, provision of postpartum contraception is critical to support planned birth spacing and avoid unintended pregnancy, but in women with GDM it is especially critical. Completing additional pregnancies after diagnosis of GDM increases the risk of development of type 2 diabetes [49]. And as described earlier, conceiving without tight control of diabetes increases risk of malformations.

There has been concern that hormonal contraceptive use in women with GDM may increase the likelihood of development of type 2 diabetes. Observational studies have examined whether hormonal contraception alters glucose metabolism in otherwise healthy women with a history of GDM. Current evidence suggests that today's formulations of low-dose combined hormonal contraceptives and progestin-only methods, including the pill, injection, implant, and IUD, are safe in women with a history of GDM.

Combined Oral Contraceptives

Postpartum use of low-dose COCs is safe in otherwise healthy women with a history of GDM and does not appear to alter glucose metabolism, weight, serum lipids, or blood pressure [50]. A retrospective cohort study of women with GDM, of whom 443 used nonhormonal contraceptives and 383 used COCs, found that the incidence of type 2 diabetes was 9 and 10 % for women using nonhormonal contraception and COCs, respectively, over up to 7.5 years of follow-up [51]. Thus, their data support the lack of association between COCs and postpartum development of diabetes in women with a history of GDM.

Progestin-Only Oral Contraceptives

The literature about postpartum use of progestin-only methods, specifically the progestin pill and DMPA, is conflicting. The study by Kjos et al., described previously, included 78 women who desired oral contraceptives but planned to breastfeed and were therefore prescribed progestin-only pills (POPs) until the end of breastfeeding [51]. Among them, the incidence of type 2 diabetes in the same time period was 26 %, higher than in either the nonhormonal or combined contraception arms. However, compared with women using COCs who did not breastfeed, those who breastfed and thus used POPs had higher baseline parity, BMI, cholesterol levels, and higher weight gain in pregnancy, all of which are risk factors for diabetes. In proportional hazards regression analysis controlling for insulin treatment during the index pregnancy, glucose AUC at the baseline OGTT, weight change, and completion of an additional pregnancy during follow-up, use of POPs was associated with increased risk of development of type 2 diabetes (adjusted RR, 2.87; 95 % CI, 1.57–5.27). The other variables that differed at baseline, when included in the analysis, did not affect the hazard ratios. However, this observational study is limited by the inability to control for all potential confounders, as well as the fact that every woman in the POP arm was breastfeeding. A retrospective cohort study of 572 women, of whom 189 were followed for up to 2 years beyond their first postpartum visit and contributed contraception data, found that ever or constant use of progestin oral contraception was not associated with worsening of glucose tolerance compared with combined contraception or nonhormonal contraception [48].

Injectable Contraception

There is concern that DMPA might alter glucose metabolism or increase risk of subsequent development of diabetes in women with a history of GDM. A prospective cohort study of 526 women who chose either DMPA ($n=96$) or low-dose COCs ($n=430$) found an annual DM incidence of 19 % in the DMPA group and 12 % in the COC group. Women who chose DMPA had higher BMI and more family members with diabetes, and had lower HDL and TGs compared with women who chose COCs. While the unadjusted model found an association between DMPA and diabetes diagnosis, the multivariate model adjusting for the variables different at baseline found no association (1.18; 95 % CI 0.67–2.28, $p=0.57$) and adjustment for weight gain during follow-up decreased the association further (1.07; 0.61–1.89; $p=0.81$) [52]. The retrospective cohort study of 189 women [48] who had been followed beyond the first postpartum visit and contributed contraception information also estimated the incidence of worsening glucose tolerance, defined as a change in one category level—from normal to prediabetes, or prediabetes to diabetes (based on category definitions established by the American Diabetes Association in 2007, see Table 4.1)—in DMPA users. They found that women who used DMPA constantly since delivery had no worsening, but women who had used it at least once in the first postpartum year were more likely to have moved to a worse glucose category during follow-up (43 % vs. 23 %). Given the discrepancy between ever use and constant use and that they were unable to control for confounders (but noted that the baseline BMI did not differ by method choice), we do not conclude from this study that DMPA increases risk of diabetes.

Also, given that the previous study found no association in adjusted analyses, there is no strong evidence to support the idea that DMPA increases risk.

Other Methods

We were unable to identify any studies of the ring, patch, or implant, but based on the evidence provided above for similar methods we believe that these should not increase development of type 2 diabetes in women with a history of GDM.

Application of Available Evidence to CDC Medical Eligibility Criteria

In 1996, the WHO first published the Medical Eligibility Criteria for Contraceptive Use (MEC) to provide evidence-based guidance for health care professionals on the safety of contraceptive methods in women with various medical conditions. The CDC has modified the WHO's MEC for the US population and provides specific guidance on the safety of the use of contraception in women with diabetes and gestational diabetes (Table 4.2). A category 1 indicates that there are no restrictions for use of that method. Category 2 indicates that benefits to using the method generally outweigh theoretical or proven risks of using the method. Category 3 indicates that theoretical or proven risks generally outweigh the benefits of using the method. Finally, a category 4 indicates that using the method carries an unacceptable health risk, and that the method should not be used. The 3/4 category has a clarification which states that the category should be assessed according to the severity of the condition. In this section we will review the specific evidence on subcategories of the CDC's MEC section on diabetes.

Women with evidence of microvascular disease (retinopathy, nephropathy, or neuropathy) are listed as category 3/4 for combined hormonal contraceptives (pill, patch, ring), category 3 for injectables, but are otherwise category 2 for the progestin-only pill, implant, and the IUDs. Similarly, any vascular disease or having diabetes of a duration longer than 20 years is also a category 3/4 for combined hormonal contraceptives, category 3 for injectables, but category 2 for all other hormonal methods of contraception. As discussed previously, the copper IUD is a category 1 for any woman with diabetes or history of GDM.

Radberg et al. is the only study to evaluate the effect of a 50 mcg EE-containing COC, a POP, or the copper IUD in diabetic women fitting in any of the MEC subcategories [44]. The average duration of diabetes was 10.3 years in the POP group, 10.8 in the CHC group, and 13.3 in the IUD group. Given the published standard deviation, only in the IUD group could a participant have had diabetes for greater than 20 years. Three to four patients in each group may have had some element of nephropathy, retinopathy, or concurrent hypertension in this study. None of the POP patients had any significant effects on their glycemic control, and though the COC group had slightly increased insulin requirements they were overall small and not associated with a change in fasting glucose measures in that group. Only one other study included women whose average duration of disease was 22.1 years, and that study found no negative effects of glycemic control in diabetic women using the contraceptive ring [45].

One study performed a sub-analysis of diabetic women under good glycemic control (HbA1c less than 7 %) compared to women with poor control (HbA1c 7–9 % or greater) and found that COCs did not change lipid profile in diabetics with good control but when looking at women with poor control, COC users experienced increases in LDL and triglycerides of up to 4.2 and 31 % by 12 months compared to baseline [39]. The participants taking COCs with poor control also had statistically significant elevations in total cholesterol by 2.5 %, an increase in LDL, and a decrease in HDL at 12 months. A similar analysis comparing carbohydrate metabolism in women with good versus poor glycemic control was not reported in this study.

Table 4.2 CDC medical eligibility criteria for diabetes mellitus

Condition	Sub-condition	Combined pill, patch, ring	Progestin-only pill	Injection	Implant	LNG-IUD	Copper-IUD
Diabetes mellitus (DM)	(a) History of gestational DM only	1	1	1	1	1	1
	(b) Nonvascular disease						
	1. Non-insulin dependent	2	2	2	2	2	1
	2. Insulin dependent[b]	2	2	2	2	2	1
	(c) Nephropathy/retinopathy/neuropathy[b]	3/4[a]	2	3	2	2	1
	(d) Other vascular disease or diabetes of 20 years' duration[b]	3/4[a]	2	3	2	2	1

I initiation of contraceptive method, *C* continuation of contraceptive method, *NA* not applicable, *LNG* levonorgestrel

[a]Please see the complete guidance for a clarification to this classification: www.cdc.gov/reproductive health/unintendedpregnancy/USMEC.htm

[b]Condition that exposes a woman to increased risk as a result of unintended pregnancy

There is a considerable lack of evidence on women with complications of diabetes and on women with suboptimal glycemic control to guide our recommendations for contraceptive use in this population. Given the known increased cardiovascular and renal risks for women with complicated diabetes, the 3/4 category discouraging use of combined hormonal contraception in these patients seems reasonable. Additionally, clinicians should consider the presence of other cardiovascular risk factors in a diabetic patient, such as obesity, smoking, etc., when determining if CHC may be appropriate for use in their diabetic patients. We would caution, however, that the risks of diabetes in pregnancy are so substantial that benefits of CHC in this population may outweigh risks if other methods are not available or acceptable to patients with micro- or macrovascular complications of diabetes.

We have extremely limited data to suggest that injectable contraception adversely impacts glycemic control in women with diabetes. Additionally, it is important to consider concerns that DMPA may be associated with weight gain in at least some populations of users, which could further exacerbate diabetic control. We would maintain that effective contraception is of vital importance as the risks of pregnancy in women with complicated diabetes likely outweigh the possible risks of deterioration of disease. Thus, the current MEC category 3 recommendation is conservative, and we feel that perhaps a category 2 would be more appropriate, unless patients experience significant weight gain with DMPA, in which case, another method would be recommended.

Regarding contraception use in women with a history of GDM, we interpret the current Level 2 evidence (i.e., based on observational studies) as supporting use of nonhormonal contraception, COCS, POPs, and DMPA in women with a history of GDM. This recommendation is supported by the CDC's U.S. Medical Eligibility Criteria, which list all methods of contraception as category 1 in women with a history of GDM. We would not recommend against progestin-only contraceptive use in these women, whether breastfeeding or not. However, the one note of caution is that DMPA has been associated with increased weight gain in postpartum women with a history of GDM [50, 52]. When controlling for weight gain, the association with DMPA and DM disappears, but weight gain is an independent risk factor for development of DM. However, if a woman desires DMPA as the only method she will use, we believe that the risk of unintended pregnancy and its deleterious effect on diabetes risk outweighs potential risk from weight gain. Finally, it is critical for all women with GDM to obtain postpartum glucose testing and close follow-up because of a high risk of development of diabetes regardless of their use of contraception.

References

1. Narayan KM, Boyle JP, Thompson TJ, Sorensen SW, Williamson DF. Lifetime risk for diabetes mellitus in the United States. JAMA. 2003;290(14):1884–90. PubMed PMID: 14532317.
2. Centers for Disease Control and Prevention. National diabetes fact sheet: national estimates and general information on diabetes and prediabetes in the United States, 2011. Atlanta, GA: U.S. Department of Health and Human Services, Centers for Disease Control and Prevention; 2011.
3. Centers for Disease Control and Prevention. Age-Adjusted Incidence of Diagnosed Diabetes per 1,000 Population Aged 18–79 Years, by Sex, United States, 1980–2011 [October 13, 2013]. http://www.cdc.gov/diabetes/statistics/incidence/fig4.htm.
4. Bullard KM, Saydah SH, Imperatore G, Cowie CC, Gregg EW, Geiss LS, et al. Secular changes in U.S. Prediabetes prevalence defined by hemoglobin A1c and fasting plasma glucose: National Health and Nutrition Examination Surveys, 1999–2010. Diabetes Care. 2013;36(8):2286–93.
5. May AL, Kuklina EV, Yoon PW. Prevalence of cardiovascular disease risk factors among US adolescents, 1999–2008. Pediatrics. 2012;129(6):1035–41. PubMed PMID: 22614778.
6. Wang CC, Reusch JE. Diabetes and cardiovascular disease: changing the focus from glycemic control to improving long-term survival. Am J Cardiol. 2012;110(9 Suppl):58B–68. PubMed PMID: 23062569. Pubmed Central PMCID: 3480668.
7. Hemmingsen B, Lund SS, Gluud C, Vaag A, Almdal T, Hemmingsen C, et al. Targeting intensive glycaemic control versus targeting conventional glycaemic control for type 2 diabetes mellitus. Cochrane Database Syst Rev. 2011;6, CD008143. PubMed PMID: 21678374.
8. Centers for Disease Control and Prevention. Incidence of end-stage renal disease attributed to diabetes among persons diagnosed with diabetes—United

States and Puerto Rico, 1996–2007. Atlanta, GA: U.S. Department of Health and Human Services, Centers for Disease Control and Prevention; 2010.

9. Intensive blood-glucose control with sulphonylureas or insulin compared with conventional treatment and risk of complications in patients with type 2 diabetes (UKPDS 33). UK Prospective Diabetes Study (UKPDS) Group. Lancet. 1998;352(9131):837–53. PubMed PMID: 9742976.
10. Action to Control Cardiovascular Risk in Diabetes Study G, Gerstein HC, Miller ME, Byington RP, Goff Jr DC, Bigger JT, et al. Effects of intensive glucose lowering in type 2 diabetes. N Engl J Med. 2008;358(24):2545–59. PubMed PMID: 18539917.
11. Group AC, Patel A, MacMahon S, Chalmers J, Neal B, Billot L, et al. Intensive blood glucose control and vascular outcomes in patients with type 2 diabetes. N Engl J Med. 2008;358(24):2560–72. PubMed PMID: 18539916.
12. Gabbe SG, Graves CR. Management of diabetes mellitus complicating pregnancy. Obstet Gynecol. 2003;102(4):857–68. PubMed PMID: 14551019.
13. Persson M, Norman M, Hanson U. Obstetric and perinatal outcomes in type 1 diabetic pregnancies: a large, population-based study. Diabetes Care. 2009;32(11):2005–9. PubMed PMID: 19675195. Pubmed Central PMCID: 2768194.
14. Hunter WA, Cundy T, Rabone D, Hofman PL, Harris M, Regan F, et al. Insulin sensitivity in the offspring of women with type 1 and type 2 diabetes. Diabetes Care. 2004;27(5):1148–52. PubMed PMID: 15111536.
15. Sobngwi E, Boudou P, Mauvais-Jarvis F, Leblanc H, Velho G, Vexiau P, et al. Effect of a diabetic environment in utero on predisposition to type 2 diabetes. Lancet. 2003;361(9372):1861–5. PubMed PMID: 12788573.
16. Sibai BM, Caritis S, Hauth J, Lindheimer M, VanDorsten JP, MacPherson C, et al. Risks of preeclampsia and adverse neonatal outcomes among women with pregestational diabetes mellitus. National Institute of Child Health and Human Development Network of Maternal-Fetal Medicine Units. Am J Obstet Gynecol. 2000;182(2):364–9. PubMed PMID: 10694338.
17. Podymow T, August P, Akbari A. Management of renal disease in pregnancy. Obstet Gynecol Clin N Am. 2010;37(2):195–210. PubMed PMID: 20685548.
18. Nevis IF, Reitsma A, Dominic A, McDonald S, Thabane L, Akl EA, et al. Pregnancy outcomes in women with chronic kidney disease: a systematic review. Clin J Am Soc Nephrol. 2011;6(11):2587–98. PubMed PMID: 21940842. Pubmed Central PMCID: 3359575.
19. WendLand EM, Torloni MR, Falavigna M, Trujillo J, Dode MA, Campos MA, et al. Gestational diabetes and pregnancy outcomes—a systematic review of the World Health Organization (WHO) and the International Association of Diabetes in Pregnancy Study Groups (IADPSG) diagnostic criteria. BMC Pregnancy Childbirth. 2012;12:23. PubMed PMID: 22462760. Pubmed Central PMCID: 3352245.
20. England LJ, Dietz PM, Njoroge T, Callaghan WM, Bruce C, Buus RM, et al. Preventing type 2 diabetes: public health implications for women with a history of gestational diabetes mellitus. Am J Obstet Gynecol. 2009;200(4):365e1–8. PubMed PMID: 18691691.
21. Inzucchi SE. Clinical practice. Diagnosis of diabetes. N Engl J Med. 2012;367(6):542–50. PubMed PMID: 22873534.
22. Chuang CH, Chase GA, Bensyl DM, Weisman CS. Contraceptive use by diabetic and obese women. Womens Health Issues. 2005;15(4):167–73. PubMed PMID: 16051107.
23. Schwarz EB, Postlethwaite D, Hung YY, Lantzman E, Armstrong MA, Horberg MA. Provision of contraceptive services to women with diabetes mellitus. J Gen Intern Med. 2012;27(2):196–201. PubMed PMID: 21922154. Pubmed Central PMCID: 3270235.
24. Vahratian A, Barber JS, Lawrence JM, Kim C. Family-planning practices among women with diabetes and overweight and obese women in the 2002 National Survey For Family Growth. Diabetes Care. 2009;32(6):1026–31. PubMed PMID: 19279299. Pubmed Central PMCID: 2681041.
25. Shawe J, Smith P, Stephenson J. Use of contraception by women with type 1 or type 2 diabetes mellitus: 'it's funny that nobody really spoke to me about it'. Eur J Contracept Reprod Health Care. 2011;16(5):350–8. PubMed PMID: 21777049.
26. Schwarz EB, Sobota M, Charron-Prochownik D. Perceived access to contraception among adolescents with diabetes: barriers to preventing pregnancy complications. Diabetes Educ. 2010;36(3):489–94. PubMed PMID: 20332282.
27. Pakarinen P, Lahteenmaki P, Rutanen EM. The effect of intrauterine and oral levonorgestrel administration on serum concentrations of sex hormone-binding globulin, insulin and insulin-like growth factor binding protein-1. Acta Obstet Gynecol Scand. 1999;78(5):423–8. PubMed PMID: 10326889.
28. Morin-Papunen L, Martikainen H, McCarthy MI, Franks S, Sovio U, Hartikainen AL, et al. Comparison of metabolic and inflammatory outcomes in women who used oral contraceptives and the levonorgestrel-releasing intrauterine device in a general population. Am J Obstet Gynecol. 2008;199(5):529e1–e10. PubMed PMID: 18533124.
29. Dorflinger LJ. Metabolic effects of implantable steroid contraceptives for women. Contraception. 2002;65(1):47–62. PubMed PMID: 11861055.
30. Oderich CL, Wender MC, Lubianca JN, Santos LM, de Mello GC. Impact of etonogestrel-releasing implant and copper intrauterine device on carbohydrate metabolism: a comparative study. Contraception. 2012;85(2):173–6. PubMed PMID: 22067787.
31. Biswas A, Viegas OA, Coeling Bennink HJ, Korver T, Ratnam SS. Implanon contraceptive implants: effects on carbohydrate metabolism. Contraception. 2001;63(3):137–41. PubMed PMID: 11368985.

32. Inal MM, Yildirim Y, Ertopcu K, Avci ME, Ozelmas I, Tinar S. Effect of the subdermal contraceptive etonogestrel implant (implanon) on biochemical and hormonal parameters (three years follow-up). Eur J Contracept Reprod Health Care. 2008;13(3):238–42. PubMed PMID: 18609340.
33. Berenson AB, van den Berg P, Williams KJ, Rahman M. Effect of injectable and oral contraceptives on glucose and insulin levels. Obstet Gynecol. 2011;117(1):41–7. PubMed PMID: 21173642. Pubmed Central PMCID: 3079533.
34. Lopez LM, Grimes DA, Schulz KF. Steroidal contraceptives: effect on carbohydrate metabolism in women without diabetes mellitus. Cochrane Database Syst Rev. 2012;4, CD006133. PubMed PMID: 22513937.
35. Kiriwat O, Petyim S. The effects of transdermal contraception on lipid profiles, carbohydrate metabolism and coagulogram in Thai women. Gynecol Endocrinol. 2010;26(5):361–5. PubMed PMID: 20050766.
36. Bender NM, Segall-Gutierrez P, Najera SO, Stanczyk FZ, Montoro M, Mishell Jr DR. Effects of progestin-only long-acting contraception on metabolic markers in obese women. Contraception. 2013;88(3):418–25. PubMed PMID: 23410714.
37. Segall-Gutierrez P, Xiang AH, Watanabe RM, Trigo E, Stanczyk FZ, Liu X, et al. Deterioration in cardiometabolic risk markers in obese women during depot medroxyprogesterone acetate use. Contraception. 2012;85(1):36–41. PubMed PMID: 22067800.
38. Rogovskaya S, Rivera R, Grimes DA, Chen PL, Pierre-Louis B, Prilepskaya V, et al. Effect of a levonorgestrel intrauterine system on women with type 1 diabetes: a randomized trial. Obstet Gynecol. 2005;105(4):811–5. PubMed PMID: 15802410.
39. Grigoryan OR, Grodnitskaya EE, Andreeva EN, Shestakova MV, Melnichenko GA, Dedov II. Contraception in perimenopausal women with diabetes mellitus. Gynecol Endocrinol. 2006;22(4):198–206. PubMed PMID: 16723306.
40. Vicente L, Mendonca D, Dingle M, Duarte R, Boavida JM. Etonogestrel implant in women with diabetes mellitus. Eur J Contracept Reprod Health Care. 2008;13(4):387–95. PubMed PMID: 19117254.
41. Diab KM, Zaki MM. Contraception in diabetic women: comparative metabolic study of Norplant, depot medroxyprogesterone acetate, low dose oral contraceptive pill and CuT380A. J Obstet Gynaecol Res. 2000;26(1):17–26. PubMed PMID: 10761326.
42. Visser J, Snel M, Van Vliet HA. Hormonal versus non-hormonal contraceptives in women with diabetes mellitus type 1 and 2. Cochrane Database Syst Rev. 2013;3, CD003990. PubMed PMID: 23543528.
43. Skouby SO, Molsted-Pedersen L, Kuhl C, Bennet P. Oral contraceptives in diabetic women: metabolic effects of four compounds with different estrogen/progestogen profiles. Fertil Steril. 1986;46(5):858–64. PubMed PMID: 3781003.
44. Radberg, Gustafson A, Skryten A, Karlsson K. Oral contraception in diabetic women. Diabetes control, serum and high density lipoprotein lipids during low-dose progestogen, combined oestrogen/progestogen and non-hormonal contraception. Acta Endocrinol (Copenh). 1981;98(2):246–51.
45. Grigoryan OR, Grodnitskaya EE, Andreeva EN, Chebotnikova TV, Melnichenko GA. Use of the NuvaRing hormone-releasing system in late reproductive-age women with type 1 diabetes mellitus. Gynecol Endocrinol. 2008;24(2):99–104. PubMed PMID: 18210334.
46. Grodnitskaya EE, Grigoryan OR, Klinyshkova EV, Andreeva EN, Melnichenko GA, Dedov II. Effect on carbohydrate metabolism and analysis of acceptability (menstrual cycle control) of extended regimens of the vaginally inserted hormone-releasing system 'NuvaRing' as compared with the standard 21/7 regime in reproductive-age women with type 1 diabetes mellitus. Gynecol Endocrinol. 2010;26(9):663–8. PubMed PMID: 20334583.
47. Perritt JB, Burke A, JamshidLi R, Wang J, Fox M. Contraception counseling, pregnancy intention and contraception use in women with medical problems: an analysis of data from the Maryland Pregnancy Risk Assessment Monitoring System (PRAMS). Contraception. 2013;88(2):263–8. PubMed PMID: 23245354.
48. Nelson AL, Le MH, Musherraf Z, Vanberckelaer A. Intermediate-term glucose tolerance in women with a history of gestational diabetes: natural history and potential associations with breastfeeding and contraception. Am J Obstet Gynecol. 2008;198(6):699 e1–7. discussion e7–8. PubMed PMID: 18439553.
49. Kjos SL, Peters RK, Xiang A, Schaefer U, Buchanan TA. Hormonal choices after gestational diabetes. Subsequent pregnancy, contraception, and hormone replacement. Diabetes Care. 1998;Suppl 2:B50–7. PubMed PMID: 9704227.
50. Xiang AH, Kawakubo M, Buchanan TA, Kjos SL. A longitudinal study of lipids and blood pressure in relation to method of contraception in Latino women with prior gestational diabetes mellitus. Diabetes Care. 2007;30(8):1952–8. PubMed PMID: 17519432.
51. Kjos SL, Peters RK, Xiang A, Thomas D, Schaefer U, Buchanan TA. Contraception and the risk of type 2 diabetes mellitus in Latina women with prior gestational diabetes mellitus. JAMA. 1998;280(6):533–8. PubMed PMID: 9707143.
52. Xiang AH, Kawakubo M, Kjos SL, Buchanan TA. Long-acting injectable progestin contraception and risk of type 2 diabetes in Latino women with prior gestational diabetes mellitus. Diabetes Care. 2006;29(3):613–7. PubMed PMID: 16505515.

Contraception for Women with Mental Health Conditions

5

Kelli Stidham Hall, Julia R. Steinberg, and Sheila M. Marcus

Part I: Contraception and Common Mental Health Conditions

Scope of Common Mental Health Conditions Among Reproductive-Aged Women

Depressive and anxiety disorders are among the leading causes of disability in the USA and worldwide [1–8]. In the USA, women are 55 % more likely to experience a depressive disorder during their lifetime compared to men [8]. Approximately 20 % of women ages 18 years and older will experience a depressive disorder in their lifetime; 8.6 % will experience one each year [8]. Anxiety disorders are also common, with lifetime and 12-month prevalence rates estimated at 36 % and 23 %, respectively [8]. Depression and anxiety are frequently comorbid with one another and with other mental health disorders, including substance abuse and eating disorders. US nationally representative data show that of people with a depressive disorder in the past year, approximately 60 % also had an anxiety disorder and nearly 9 % had a substance use disorder [9]. Prevalence rates of depressive and anxiety disorders among new generations of adolescent and young women appear to be increasing in recent years [10–12].

Despite a clear need for women's mental health care, mental health service utilization in the USA is low [13, 14]. Depression and anxiety disorders often go undetected and untreated among reproductive-aged women [15–21]. Sixty-three percent of adults who have depression do not talk to a professional in the first year of having the disorder [22]. In recent years, less than half of pregnant and nonpregnant US women with a major depressive episode received a mental health diagnosis or treatment [17, 19, 21]. A population-based study of over 70,000 nonpregnant women found that half of women meeting criteria for depression did not receive a diagnosis or treatment, even though more than 70 % had contact with a health provider in the last year [17]. Black and Hispanic women are even less likely to receive a mental health diagnosis and treatment than White women [17, 23, 24]. These same groups of women disproportionately experience high unintended pregnancy rates [25].

K.S. Hall, Ph.D., M.S. (✉)
Department of Obstetrics and Gynecology, Institute for Social Research, University of Michigan, Ann Arbor, MI, USA
e-mail: hkelli@umich.edu

J.R. Steinberg, Ph.D., M.A.
Department of Psychiatry, University of California, San Francisco, San Francisco, CA, USA
e-mail: Julia.Steinberg@ucsf.edu

S.M. Marcus, M.D.
Department of Psychiatry, University of Michigan, Ann Arbor, MI, USA
e-mail: smmarcus@med.umich.edu

R.H. Allen and C.A. Cwiak (eds.), *Contraception for the Medically Challenging Patient*,
DOI 10.1007/978-1-4939-1233-9_5, © Springer Science+Business Media New York 2014

Certain social circumstances such as poverty, unemployment, and having less education are associated with experiencing common mental health conditions [10, 26–28]. Other risk factors for depression and anxiety include having a personal or family history of a mental health disorder, having other chronic medical illnesses such as cancer, stroke, or HIV/AIDs, and having adverse life experiences, including physical and sexual violence or trauma [1–4]. Some of these same characteristics, such as having less education or experiencing physical and sexual violence, also increase women's risk of contraceptive non- or misuse [29–31], suggesting similar groups of women are vulnerable to mental health disorders and unintended pregnancy. In the pages that follow, we discuss more direct evidence that connects mental health disorders, contraception, and unintended pregnancy.

Relationships Between Reproductive Health and Depression and Anxiety

Research has examined the interplay between depressive or anxiety disorders and reproductive health [32–49]. Some studies have found depression and anxiety are precursors to a variety of negative reproductive outcomes, including maternal and infant morbidity, obstetrical complications, preterm labor, stillbirth, and low birth weight [32, 34, 35]. In addition, women with depression and anxiety appear to be at greater risk of experiencing an unintended pregnancy, and those pregnancies may be more likely to end in induced abortion, compared to women without depression and anxiety [38–40, 42, 43]. Depression and anxiety before pregnancy also consistently predict depression and anxiety after pregnancy [41, 42, 44, 45]. On the other hand, studies have also found that reproductive health influences subsequent mental health outcomes. For instance, women who carry their unintended pregnancies to term are at risk for antepartum and postpartum depression [44–50]. Some groups of women, including poor, underinsured, undereducated, and minority women, disproportionately experience adverse mental *and* reproductive health outcomes due to common risk factors, including limited health knowledge, access to medical resources, and social support [10–12, 17, 23, 25–28, 44, 48, 50, 51].

Effects of Contraception on Mental Health

While the causes of depression and anxiety are not fully understood, deficiencies in neurotransmitters (serotonin, norepinephrine, dopamine, GABA, and peptides) that impact mood have been implicated in clinical studies of depression and anxiety [1–4]. Genetic predisposition and psychosocial stressors appear to be important precursors to neurotransmitter deficiencies and contribute to these disorders [4]. Soon after the combined oral contraceptive pill (COC) was made available in 1960, researchers hypothesized that synthetic estrogens and progestins in COCs could potentially interact with mood-related neurotransmitters [52–55]. Articles published in the 1970s and 1980s suggested that the large steroid dosages in COCs (e.g., Enovid: 5 mg norethynodrel, 75 mcg mestranol) could interfere with serotonin, noradrenaline, tryptophan (an amino acid precursor to serotonin), and vitamin and endocrine metabolism [52–55]. Estrogen was thought to reduce noradrenaline and serotonin in the hypothalamus, resulting in pyridoxine deficiency [52, 53, 55]; progestins were thought to cause cerebral monoamine oxidase activity, triggering enzymatic breakdown of neurotransmitters [54].

However, given the significantly lower steroid dosages in modern hormonal contraceptives, these mechanistic theories appear to no longer be relevant. While few (if any) recent clinical trials have used brain imaging and hormonal bioassays to clarify these relationships, a notable newer body of scientific evidence suggests that the steroidal activity of modern methods does not have a clinically relevant physiological impact on women's mood or mood-related neuroendocrine functioning [56–73]. In a comprehensive review, Robinson et al. analyzed seven studies examining COC pharmacological properties and mood-related side effects [56]. The researchers found no evidence for an association between the intrinsic biochemical mechanisms of COCs and mood effects reported by COC users. In the Medical Eligibility Criteria for Contraceptive Use report published in 2010, the US Centers for Disease Control and Prevention concluded there are no contraindications to hormonal contraception for women with depression, basing their recommendation on evidence that does not support a causal relationship [57]. Prospective clinical placebo-controlled and population-based cohort studies have reported similar or even lower rates of depression or mood symptoms between women who use COCs and those who do not [58–65]. The best scientific evidence to date suggests that modern COC formulations do not cause depression or mood symptoms among the women that use them, and in fact, COCs may improve depression and mood symptoms for some women.

Clinical research studies have examined whether mental health symptoms increase among women initiating other hormonal contraceptive methods, including the depot medroxyprogesterone acetate (DMPA) contraceptive injectable (e.g., Depo-Provera, Pfizer Inc., New York NY, USA), transdermal patch (e.g., Ortho-Evra patch, Ortho-McNeil Pharmaceutical Inc., Raritan, NJ, USA), vaginal ring (e.g., NuvaRing, Merck, Whitehouse Station, NJ, USA), and long-acting reversible contraceptive methods (LARC) such as the subdermal implant (e.g., Implanon, Nexplanon), levonorgestrel-releasing intrauterine device (IUD, e.g., Mirena, Bayer Healthcare Pharmaceuticals, Wayne, NJ, USA), and copper-containing IUD (e.g., ParaGard, Teva, Israel) [56–73]. Collectively, these studies have found no adverse effects of these methods on depression, anxiety, or mood [56–73].

Effects of Mental Health on Contraceptive Use

Compared to the large literature investigating the mental health effects of contraception, less research has focused on the extent to which mental health influences contraceptive behaviors. Even though, as detailed above, the literature does not support a causal relationship between contraception and negative mental health outcomes, perceived mood symptoms continue to be a primary reason why women report not using, misusing, or discontinuing hormonal contraceptives [74–77]. COC discontinuation rates from perceived mood symptoms have ranged from 14 to 21 % [74–77]. Some research has suggested that women with depression, anxiety, and related stress symptoms are more likely to perceive negative mood symptoms than those without those symptoms [77]. Yet, how depression and anxiety may influence perceived contraceptive side effects and use has not been well studied. It may be that neuroendocrine pathology amplifies physical symptomatology attributed to COCs. However, this hypothesis has not been studied.

Alternatively, cognitive processes related to "perceptions" of physical symptoms, rather than pathophysiological processes themselves, may be altered in COC users with mental health conditions. A study by Rubino-Watkins et al. found that COC users with psychological stress had higher self-reported negative cognitive patterns and emotions over time than stressed OC nonusers, and greater negative affect was attributed to more daily stressors among OC users versus nonusers [78]. Other researchers have found that higher levels of somatization (recurrent and frequently changing physical symptoms which cannot be explained by any known medical condition) and hypochondriasis (excessive worry about illness and the belief that one has an undiagnosed physical disease) are associated with higher rates of reported side effects among those using both active and placebo medications [79, 80]. Because depressed individuals are attuned to negative cues in their environment [81, 82], depressed women may internalize negative information about hormonal contraceptives (e.g., side effects and risks), which could preclude initiation or continuation. With anxiety, excessive worry could potentially contribute to irrational concerns about contraceptive safety or side effects, leading to misuse and discontinuation, though this has not been examined.

Depression and anxiety may also affect cognitive and behavioral processes related to use of contraception, including risk assessment, planning, and social learning, as well as perceptions of benefits and threats of contraception and perceived susceptibility to pregnancy [83–87]. Decreased motivation and desire for self-care, which may accompany depression [88, 89], could impact women's abilities to use certain methods, like daily COCs. Anxiety symptoms also have the potential to interfere with contraceptive decision-making processes [90], leading women to make suboptimal contraceptive choices.

To our knowledge, no research studies have investigated these hypotheses directly, but scientific evidence indirectly supports a link between mental health and family planning. Some recent studies have shown that women with elevated depressive, anxiety, and stress symptoms have higher rates of risky sexual behaviors (e.g., increased numbers of sexual partners, earlier sexual debut) and contraceptive nonuse, misuse, discontinuation, and use of less effective methods, compared to women without elevated mental health symptoms [18, 66, 73, 91–99]. These findings have been most widely noted for condoms and COCs but have also been demonstrated for the DMPA injectable, IUDs, and implants [66, 69, 73].

Some emerging research also suggests that depression and anxiety may affect contraceptive method selection and use differently depending upon the health setting or social context of the woman. Garbers et al. found that among 2,476 urban women presenting to a health department clinic, those who screened positive for depression had 45 % higher odds of selecting condoms (compared to more effective methods) and 39 % lower odds of selecting hormonal methods (compared to less effective methods) at their routine clinic visit compared to women without depressive symptoms [94]. Similar findings have been noted among clinical and population-based samples of nonpregnant women [18, 95–97]. On the other hand, a study of abortion patients initiating contraception immediately following their abortion found that those with higher mental distress symptoms before their abortion had increased odds of leaving their visit with more effective methods including IUDs and implants compared to women without distress [99]. While reasons for these differences in associations between mental health and contraceptive method selection are not fully clear and may be partially attributed to different measurement approaches, it is possible that women with depression who have already experienced an unintended pregnancy are motivated to avoid a subsequent pregnancy due to their mental health concerns and stressful life circumstances. Research is warranted to clarify the role of mental health in women's contraceptive decision-making and behavior across different life circumstances and health care contexts.

Clinical Assessment: Mental Health and Contraception

Common mental health disorders frequently go undiagnosed among reproductive-aged women, and yet underlying symptoms and the disorders themselves can impact women's perceived and actual family planning needs [17, 18, 21, 94–97, 99]. A lack of detection and diagnosis of depression and anxiety among women points to the potential role that depression and anxiety screening and management may play in reproductive health contexts. In obstetrical settings, health providers may see women with postpartum depression who need assistance choosing a contraceptive method that is effective in preventing rapid repeat pregnancy and also safe for breastfeeding. Women presenting for abortion care may need education on contraceptive methods that will effectively prevent another unintended pregnancy, in addition to counseling on strategies and resources to cope with their stressful life experience. Women presenting for sexually transmitted infection (STI) treatment require counseling on dual method use and safe sex and may also need an evaluation of mental distress related to the STI diagnosis. These are just a few examples of clinical encounters in which family planning and mental health issues may interact. Symptoms of depression and anxiety can take many different forms, and signs may not be obvious to the provider or patient [100–105]. The following discussion highlights aspects of the clinical encounter relevant to mental health and contraception.

First, depression and anxiety may impact patient-provider communication and interaction in important ways [100–105]. A careful review of the past medical history will identify any personal or family risk factors for new, recurring, or chronic mental health conditions. For undiagnosed conditions, disclosure of mental health symptoms may be difficult for patients due to perceived stigma, as well as women's lack of awareness and insight into their own mental health status [100–105]. Health providers should routinely engage their patients in a discussion about overall health, including psychological well-being, and its impact on sexual and reproductive health. Employing patience, empathy, and a nonjudgmental tone can help patients feel more comfortable discussing their mental health issues [100–105]. Directive, confrontational questions should be avoided. Mental health concerns can be introduced with a simple educational statement such as, "Did you know that a fifth of women will experience depression in their lifetimes? Because depression is so common, I like to check in with all my patients about their own mental health." This approach can alert patients to the provider's concern but also normalize the experience. Reflective listening, use of open-ended questions, and careful patient observation can help providers pick up subtle cues of an underlying mental health condition [100–105]. A clinical presentation of a sad voice, anxious expressions, or lethargic posture would raise suspicions of a mental health issue. Providers should also reflect on their own feelings, emotions, and mood during and after the clinical encounter and be attuned to transference (i.e., feeling down, sad, or upset after seeing a patient with depression or anxiety) [100, 101]. Finally, women with diagnosed or undiagnosed mental health conditions commonly present with multiple, vague complaints, nonspecific symptoms or pain-related syndromes. In women's health contexts, complaints may include nonspecific vulva, pelvic, vaginal, coital, or menstrual-related pain, headaches, or gastrointestinal disturbances [105]. Cues such as these should alert the provider to an underlying mental health condition requiring further evaluation.

Second, use of standardized mental health screening instruments may be an effective, efficient method to screen patients for common mental health conditions and identify those who may need follow-up psychiatric care [106–113]. Commonly used, evidence-based depression and anxiety screens are presented in Tables 5.1 and 5.2. In busy clinical settings, use of an abbreviated tool, such as the Patient Health Questionnaire (PHQ), is ideal. Such screening instruments can be seamlessly included in electronic medical record charting and should be used routinely and systematically, for instance with all well-woman exams or new patients.

Third, clinical diagnosis of a mental health disorder is ideally made by a trained mental health care professional, such as a psychiatrist or clinical psychologist [4, 100–104, 106]. However, when standardized diagnostic criteria are followed, common mental health disorders like depression and anxiety may be diagnosed in non-specialty health care settings including family practice and reproductive health. While a structured psychiatric interview, such as the Composite International Diagnostic Interview or the Structured Clinical Interview for Diagnostic and Statistical Manual of Mental Disorders (DSM), is the gold standard [4, 10–104, 106, 121], use of self-report instruments may be more feasible in settings where large volumes of patients are seen and time per patient is limited.

Differential diagnoses of reproductive-aged women presenting with new onset mental health symptoms should be evaluated [100, 102–105]. Chronic diseases such as hypothyroidism, diabetes mellitus, anemia, cancer, and multiple sclerosis, which are not uncommon among reproductive-aged women, can cause mood-related symptoms that may mimic depression or anxiety [100, 102–105]. Women with acute stress or grief may exhibit transient or chronic mood symptoms, as well as reproductive symptoms like irregular menses. Women with anorexia nervosa or bulimia nervosa may similarly experience co-occurring depression or anxiety and amenorrhea or irregular menses. Finally, medica-

Table 5.1 Screening instruments for depression

Measure name and citation	How/where to obtain measure	Description	Sample items
1. Center for Epidemiological Study of Depression Scale (CES-D) [109, 114]	Radloff LS. The CES-D Scale: A self-report depression scale for research in the general population. Applied Psych Measur 1977; 1(3):385–401	20-item measure, also 10-item available; rate items from 0 = rarely or none of the time to 3 = most or all of the time	During past week… 1. I was bothered by things that usually don't bother me 2. I felt that everything I did was an effort 3. I talked less than usual
2. The Primary Care Evaluation of Mental Disorders (Prime-MD) Depression subscale [111, 115]	Spitzer RL, Kroenke K, Williams JBW, and the Patient Health Questionnaire Primary Care Study Group. Validation and utility of a self-report version of PRIME-MD: The PHQ Primary Care Study. JAMA 1999; 282 (18): 1737–1744.	9-item measure; rate items from 0 = not at all to 3 = nearly every day; also available as a 2-item measure	Over the last 2 weeks how often have you… 1. Had little interest or pleasure in doing things 2. Been feeling down, depressed, or hopeless 3. Had trouble concentrating on things such as reading the newspaper or watching television
3. Beck Depression Inventory-Revised (also known as II) [116]	Available from Pearson for a fee	21 groups of statements and choose one of each group	Pick the one state of each group that best describes how you have been feeling during the past 2 weeks, including today Group 1 I do not feel sad I feel sad much of the time I am sad all the time I am so sad or unhappy that I can't stand it
4. Depression Anxiety Stress Scales (DASS)—depression subscale [117]	Lovibond PF, Lovibond SH. The structure of negative emotional states: Comparison of the Depression Anxiety Stress Scales (DASS) with The Beck Depression and Anxiety Inventories. Behav Res Ther. 1995;33(3): 335–343 Order scoring manual from: http://www2.psy.unsw.edu.au/Groups/Dass/order.htm	A 42-item measure, where 14 items measure depression, 14 measure anxiety, and 14 measure stress; a 2-item version is also available—7 items for each measure; 0 = not at all to 3 = very much or most of the time	How much has each statement applied to you over the past week? 1. I felt downhearted and blue 2. I felt that life was meaningless 3. I felt I was pretty worthless

Table 5.2 Screening instruments for anxiety

Measure name and citation	How/where to obtain measure	Description	Sample items
1. Beck Anxiety Inventory (BAI) [118, 119]	Available from Pearson for a fee	21 items rated from 0 = not at all to 3 = severely-it bothered me a lot	Rate how much bothered by each of the following: 1. Numbness or tingling 2. Terrified or afraid 3. Fear of losing control
2. The Primary Care Evaluation of Mental Disorders (Prime-MD) Anxiety subscale [115]	Spitzer RL, Kroenke K, Williams JBW, and the Patient Health Questionnaire Primary Care Study Group. Validation and utility of a self-report version of PRIME-MD: The PHQ Primary Care Study. JAMA 1999; 282 (18): 1737–1744	5 items with the first item being the main item and all the rest following from that rated as Yes or No	1. In the last 4 weeks, have you had an anxiety attack—suddenly feeling fear or panic? 2. Has this ever happened before? 3. Do these attacks bother you a lot or are you worried about having another attack?
3. Spielberger state and trait anxiety [120]	For a fee, available at: http://www.mindgarden.com/products/staisad.htm#ms	20 items for trait and 20 for state anxiety rated with 0 = almost never to 3 = almost always	State: Rate how true about self 1. I am tense 2. I am worried 3. I feel calm Trait: 1. I worry too much over something that really doesn't matter 2. I am content; I am a steady person
4. Depression Anxiety Stress Scales (DASS)—anxiety subscale [117]	Lovibond PF, Lovibond SH. The structure of negative emotional states: Comparison of the Depression Anxiety Stress Scales (DASS) with The Beck Depression and Anxiety Inventories. Behav Res Ther. 1995;33(3): 335–343 Order scoring manual from: http://www2.psy.unsw.edu.au/Groups/Dass/order.htm	A 42-item measure, where 14 items measure depression, 14 measure anxiety, and 14 measure stress; a 21-item version is also available—7 items for each measure	How much has each statement applied to you over the past week? 0 = not at all to 3 = very much or most of the time 1. I was aware of the action of my heart in the absence of physical exertion (e.g., sense of heart rate increase, heart missing a beat) 2. I was aware of dryness of my mouth 3. I was worried about situations in which I might panic or make a fool of myself

tions such as beta blockers or calcium channel blockers, glucocorticoids, and GnRH analogues (e.g., Lupron) can cause mood changes [100, 102–105]. Therefore, reproductive health providers should be able to screen for depression and anxiety, differentiate subclinical symptomatology from a diagnosable disorder, rule out differential diagnoses, and provide or refer for further mental health evaluation and treatment when indicated.

Contraceptive Management for Women with Common Mental Health Conditions

Eligibility and Drug Interaction Considerations

Women with depression and anxiety are generally good candidates for all contraceptive methods. In most cases, contraceptive method selection should not be limited by the mental health diagnosis or treatment but rather should occur through shared decision-making between patient and provider based upon individual health circumstances, contraceptive preferences, and family planning needs. The CDC Medical Eligibility Criteria for Contraceptive Use lists depression as Category 1 for eligibility, stating that there are no restrictions for use of hormonal contraception for women with depression and related disorders [57]. Drug interactions between modern pharmacologic antidepressant agents and hormonal contraception are relatively rare. The most widely used antidepressants include selective serotonin reuptake inhibitors (SSRIs, such as fluoxetine, citalopram, escitalopram, and sertraline) and more recently serotonin norepinephrine reuptake inhibitors (SNRIs, such as venlafaxine and duloxetine) [100, 102–105]. The best available scientific evidence suggests SSRIs and SNRIs do not interact with hepatic metabolism of synthetic steroids in COCs [122–125]. Women on SSRIs and SNRIs should be offered the full range of contraceptive methods.

Older generation antidepressant agents such as tricyclics (TCAs, such as amitriptyline or nortriptyline) and monoamine oxidase inhibitors (MAOIs, such as phenelzine and tranylcypromine), which are still used in treatment-refractive chronic depression, are highly interactive with other foods and drugs [100–105]. TCAs and MAOIs may interact with contraceptive steroid metabolism in the liver, potentially leading to decreased contraceptive efficacy; reduced hepatic metabolism can also lead to antidepressant side effects or toxicity [125]. In addition, while the scientific evidence is inconsistent, St. John's wort (hypericum perforatum), an alternative over-the-counter antidepressant therapy, may also induce the cytochrome P450 system and subsequently reduce contraceptive steroid availability, by 13–15 % one study found [126, 127]. Thus, women who require more intensive psychiatric treatment with TCAs, MAOIs, or those using St. John's wort are not ideal candidates for COCs or other systemic hormonal contraceptives. Other locally acting hormonal contraceptive methods, such as the levonorgestrel-releasing IUD, as well as nonhormonal methods like the copper-containing IUD, appear to be safe for women on TCAs, MAOIs, and St. John's wort [128] (see Chap. 20 for more details).

Many women with depression and anxiety are treated with non-pharmacologic therapies including cognitive behavioral therapy, interpersonal psychotherapy, and adjunct therapies like exercise, sleep, and healthy diet [100–105, 129–131]. These treatments should not interfere with contraception or preclude use of any methods. Providers can encourage women to participate in these treatment modalities since the principles and self-care techniques learned (e.g., problem-solving and coping skills) may also benefit women's reproductive health decision-making and behaviors.

Contraceptive Method Considerations

We present an overview of contraceptive method options and considerations for women with specific mental health issues in Table 5.3. In most cases, the full range of contraceptive methods is safe and suitable for women with depression and anxiety. Potential contraceptive adherence issues, however, may be an important factor for selection of the most appropriate method [132–138].

Table 5.3 Effective contraceptive method options for specific mental health considerations

Mental health considerations	Effective contraceptive method options				
	Long-acting reversible contraceptives (LARC) (copper-containing intrauterine device (IUD), levonorgestrel IUD, subdermal implants)	Progestin-only contraceptives (Depot medroxyprogesterone acetate injectable (DMPA), progestin-only pills (POP))	Other combined hormonal contraceptives (vaginal ring, transdermal patch)	Combined oral contraceptives (COCs)	Condoms
1. Adherence concerns	Highly effective and reversible with low user maintenance; should be considered first line	DMPA acceptable option; POPs not optimal because vulnerable to missed or late pill dosages	Less ideal than LARC and DMPA because requires monthly (ring) or weekly (patch) replacement, but acceptable; counseling on appropriate use and regular assessment for adherence necessary; emergency contraceptive provision as backup	Not optimal; requires counseling and education on appropriate use and frequent assessment of daily adherence and missed pills; emergency contraceptive provision as backup	Dual use of condoms plus another more effective method should be routinely encouraged to prevent sexually transmitted infections; not an optimal option for primary contraceptive method in most cases due to higher typical use failure rates than other effective methods, adherence concerns considerable user effort, and necessary partner cooperation; acceptable when all other effective options are not feasible
2. Mood side effect concerns	Copper-containing IUD optimal option for women who prefer not to take hormones, other LARC methods also acceptable; no evidence to support LARC causes mood symptoms	Acceptable; no evidence to support DMPA or POPs cause mood symptoms	Acceptable; no evidence to support ring or patch causes mood symptoms; assess regularly for adherence issues	No evidence to support COCs cause mood symptoms; may consider lower dosage and monophasic formulations, extended cycle regimens or continuous dosing; assess regularly for adherence issues	
3. Menstrual irregularity concerns	Copper-containing IUD optimal option for women who prefer regular menses; other LARC methods also acceptable; irregular bleeding patterns possible	Acceptable; irregular bleeding patterns possible with DMPA; irregular bleeding may occur with missed dosages of POPs	Acceptable	Optimal option for menstrual control; may be optimal option for women who prefer to be in "regular" control of using contraception	

(continued)

Table 5.3 (continued)

Mental health considerations	Effective contraceptive method options				
	Long-acting reversible contraceptives (LARC) (copper-containing intrauterine device (IUD), levonorgestrel IUD, subdermal implants)	Progestin-only contraceptives (Depot medroxyprogesterone acetate injectable (DMPA), progestin-only pills (POP))	Other combined hormonal contraceptives (vaginal ring, transdermal patch)	Combined oral contraceptives (COCs)	Condoms
4. Postpartum depression and breast feeding	Acceptable	Acceptable	CDC MEC category 3 for women <1 month postpartum due to VTE risk	CDC MEC category 3 for women <1 month postpartum due to VTE risk	
5. Perimenopausal depression	Acceptable	Acceptable	Acceptable; assess for contraindications to estrogen	Optimal option; has therapeutic benefit for perimenopausal symptoms; assess for contraindications to estrogen	
6. Premenstrual dysphoric disorder (PMDD)	Acceptable	Acceptable	Acceptable	Drospirenone-containing COCs have FDA approval for PMDD	
7. Medical comorbidities including cardiovascular risks, age >35 years and a smoker, and other estrogen contraindications	Acceptable	DMPA acceptable; may monitor for weight gain, truncal fat deposit, and peripheral glucose intolerance	CDC MEC categories 3–4; contraindicated due to increased risk of MI, stroke, and VTE	CDC MEC categories 3–4; contraindicated due to increased risk of MI, stroke, and VTE	
8. Taking modern antidepressants including SSRIs or SNRIs	Acceptable	Acceptable	Acceptable	Acceptable	
9. Taking older generation antidepressants including TCAs, MAOIs, or St. John's wort	IUDs acceptable; subdermal implant not recommended due to potential drug interactions	DMPA acceptable; POPs not recommended due to potential drug interactions	Not recommended due to potential drug interactions	Not recommended due to potential drug interactions	

10. Taking mood stabilizers and/or antiepileptics	IUDs acceptable; subdermal implant not recommended due to potential drug interactions	DMPA acceptable; POPs not recommended due to potential drug interactions	Not recommended due to potential drug interactions	Not optimal due to potential drug interactions; monitor psychiatric drug levels, adjust dosages as necessary if other methods not feasible
11. Taking atypical antipsychotics	Acceptable	Acceptable	Acceptable	Acceptable; may have therapeutic benefit for hyperprolactinemia
12. Intimate partner violence	May be optimal option due to inconspicuous nature and infrequent health service visit requirements	DMPA optimal option due to inconspicuous nature but requires more frequent health service visits	Not optimal option for women with unsupportive partner due to conspicuous nature	Not optimal option for women with unsupportive partner due to conspicuous nature
13. Impaired decision-making capacity	Ethical considerations due to long-term nature and informed consent for medical procedures, although reversible	DMPA optimal option given less invasive highly effective and reversible	Not optimal since requires intact cognitive functioning	Not optimal since requires intact cognitive functioning

LARC long-acting reversible contraception, *IUD* intrauterine device, *DMPA* depot medroxyprogesterone acetate, *POPs* progestin-only pills, *COCs* combined oral contraceptives, *TCAs* tricyclic antidepressants, *MAOIs* monoamine oxidase inhibitors, *CDC MEC* Center for Disease Control and Prevention Medical Eligibility Criteria for Contraceptive Use 2010, *VTE* venous thromboembolism, *SSRI* selective serotonin reuptake inhibitors, *SNRI* serotonin norepinephrine reuptake inhibitors

As mentioned earlier, women with depression and anxiety have more perceived contraceptive side effects and may misuse and discontinue methods at higher rates than women without these mental health conditions, with the greatest body of evidence available for user-dependent methods including condoms and COCs [18, 66, 73, 93–99]. Women with depression or anxiety may find it difficult to remember or find the energy to take a COC every day or may be too distracted, worried, or emotional to encourage their partner to apply a condom at every intercourse. LARC methods, including IUDs and the subdermal implant, require little user burden, have less worry and hassle, and offer the greatest contraceptive efficacy, making them ideal options for women with mental health conditions who wish to avoid an unintended pregnancy [128, 135, 136]. These "fit and forget" methods are also cost effective, which may be beneficial to women who have long-term financial concerns. On the other hand, not all women prefer long-acting methods. Women with depression or anxiety may prefer to be in regular control of using their method or may worry about menstrual irregularity. In this case, the vaginal ring, transdermal patch, or COCs are alternative options.

For providers who are initiating COCs or managing women with mental health conditions who have difficulty finding a satisfactory COC, several considerations may be useful. First, research has suggested that women's experiences with perceived side effects are similar across different types of COCs [139], even though more than 90 different formulations are used by women in the USA alone [128, 136, 137, 140]. Thus, health providers can counsel their patients that most women do well with any COC. Second, a dose–response relationship with COCs and side effects was noted in the 1970s and 1980s, when contraceptive steroid dosages were significantly higher [128]. While modern formulations generally have low steroid dosages, providers may choose formulations with lower dosages (i.e., 20 mcg versus >20 mcg) in an attempt to minimize their patients' risk of mood side effects [141]. On the other hand, lower dosage COCs are associated with other side effects like irregular bleeding, as well as vulnerable efficacy levels with missed pills [128, 141]. Providers should help women balance concerns about side effects and adherence. Second, in regard to the type of progestin, second-generation levonorgestrel- and norgestrel-containing COCs are the most widely used and are not known to contribute to mental health symptoms [140, 142, 143]. Newer fourth-generation drospirenone-containing COCs (e.g., Yaz, 3 mg drospirenone and 20 mcg ethinyl estradiol) are approved by the Food and Drug Administration (FDA) for treatment of mood symptoms occurring with premenstrual dysphoric disorder (PMDD) and may also be an option for women with depression and anxiety disorders [128]. Third, women's experiences with mood symptoms can be worse during certain periods of the menstrual cycle, for instance during ovulation or menses, due to variable circulating estrogen levels. Theoretically, monophasic formulations, which offer a steady dose (versus multiphasic formulations), could better stabilize hormone levels to minimize the risk of mood symptoms [144]. Women who report mood symptoms during their placebo weeks (i.e., estrogen withdrawal) may benefit from COCs with extended cycle regimens (e.g., 24/4) or continuous dosing (i.e., skipping inactive pills), which would reduce or eliminate the estrogen withdrawal period [128, 145]. While a dearth of scientific evidence exists to support these strategies, they may be clinically useful for COC management of women with mood concerns.

Additional contraceptive method considerations may be specific to the mental health disorder itself. For instance, postpartum and perimenopausal depression, which affect approximately 10–20 % of women, have similar diagnostic criteria to major depressive disorder except onset occurs following pregnancy or during perimenopause, respectively [4, 45–48]. Explicit conversations about contraception are needed during these periods since postpartum and perimenopausal women may not be aware of their risks for unintended pregnancy. Mental health treatment options for postpartum depression (psychotherapy and SSRIs are the first lines of defense) should not interfere with modern contraceptive methods [33–39]. Postpartum women who are breastfeeding generally should not be initiated on estrogen-containing contraceptives due to possible reduction in breast milk production and VTE risk, and progestin-only methods including the levonorgestrel-releasing IUD, subdermal implant, DMPA injectable, or progestin-only pills can be used instead [57, 128]. Perimenopausal women may be ideal candidates for COCs, the patch, or ring, which can help stabilize hormonal fluctuations and control mood, menstrual, and hot flash symptoms while also preventing pregnancy [146–152]. Perimenopausal women should be evaluated for cardiovascular risks, tobacco use, and other contraindications to estrogen use prior to initiation and throughout treatment [57].

Education and Counseling

Education and counseling is a critical component of contraceptive initiation and management for women with mental health conditions [105, 125]. The scope of counseling needs among women with depression and anxiety may be broad and counseling should ultimately be tailored to individual patient's specific needs and circumstances. Several key education and counseling considerations may be universally applicable: (1) accurate contraceptive information emphasizing method effectiveness, (2) mental health assessment, and (3) ongoing discussions about intimate partner violence.

Research has shown that women's knowledge of contraception, including use, effectiveness, benefits, risks, and side effects of different contraceptive methods, is consistently low [153–160]. Women with mental health conditions may benefit from repeated and specific information on user-related method effectiveness rates. If a patient presenting for contraceptive initiation understands that her likelihood of becoming pregnant depends upon her ability to remember to take her pill every day and she is motivated to initiate or switch methods, then she may be more inclined to choose a highly effective method like an IUD that does not require daily diligence. Providers should encourage and support depressed women in taking action to select the most appropriate contraceptive method. Providers should also assess for and counsel on concurrent treatment adherence issues among patients who are taking antidepressants and contraception [133, 134]. If a patient reports that she is missing dosages or has stopped taking her antidepressant, this may alert the provider to contraceptive misuse or discontinuation. Counseling should focus on ways to improve accuracy and consistency of medication use in the context of her daily life, such as setting a cell phone reminder or taking pills when she brushes her teeth before bedtime [128]. Contraceptive counseling should also dispel myths and misperceptions of side effects and reinforce the benefits of modern methods for pregnancy prevention and non-contraceptive effects (e.g., improved mood and acne, protection from ovarian and uterine cancer) [154, 160]. Finally, women with depression and anxiety should be counseled on sexual risk behaviors and condom use given an increased risk for sexually transmitted infections [89–93].

Women who present for contraception with underlying mental health conditions (newly detected or previously diagnosed) may benefit from education on the prevalence, signs, and symptoms, and treatment options for depression, anxiety, and related disorders [105, 147, 149]. Helping a patient to understand that her mental health is as important as her reproductive health and that the two are interrelated may facilitate honesty, trust, and communication. Evidence-based counseling techniques like motivational interviewing can be used to focus attention on specific behaviors that may need to change (e.g., frequent missed pills, condom nonuse), to evoke motivation for change by increasing confidence and readiness, and to plan practical steps to improve contraceptive behaviors [105, 147, 149, 155]. Providers should also assess for other dimensions of patients' lives that impact their mental and reproductive health, for example, financial considerations, social support, and coping resources. Having readily available education and resource materials for local social work counselors, psychology or psychiatric services, and insurance or medication assistance programs can help patients address their mental health needs and potential life stressors which may be implicated in their mental health. Promoting mental health may ultimately promote positive family planning outcomes.

Contraceptive counseling should also include a discussion of intimate partner violence, which may be a contributing factor to depression and anxiety and which has serious implications for women's reproductive autonomy and health. More than one in three women are estimated to experience some form of intimate partner violence—either rape, physical violence, or stalking by a sexual partner—in their lifetime [161–164]. Rates of mood and anxiety disorders are higher among women who have experienced violence compared to those who have not [42]. Women in violent relationships may experience reproductive coercion, birth control sabotage, intentional exposure to sexually transmitted infections, unintended pregnancy, and lack of control over their pregnancy outcomes, access to health services, and use of contraception [31, 161]. While most research has focused on the mental health effects of intimate partner violence, women with mental health disorders may be particularly susceptible to being victims of intimate partner violence or reproductive coercion [163]. Routine screening for intimate partner violence with simple questions such as "Has your partner ever hit, slapped, kicked, bitten, pushed, choked, shoved or physically hurt you?" can identify patients who may have special contraceptive considerations [161, 162]. Providers can assist patients in selecting methods that maximize contraceptive control and minimize the likelihood of exacerbating partner resistance or violence. The DMPA injectable is an effective, inconspicuous contraceptive method that is controlled by the woman. IUDs or the subdermal implant may offer other subtle, highly effective options that require less frequent health service visits. Overall, the individual situation and specific mental health and intimate partner violence concerns should be taken into account during contraceptive decision-making and management.

Part II: Contraception and Other Serious Mental Illnesses

While psychotic disorders like schizophrenia, bipolar disorder, and borderline personality disorder are less common than depression and anxiety disorders [164, 165], these other serious mental illnesses (SMI) have important implications for women's reproductive health [165–170]. Women with other SMI may experience cognitive impairments, impulsivity, self-destructive behaviors, poor judgment, and co-occurring substance use that can affect family planning decision-making and contraceptive behaviors [125, 165–174]. Women with severe depression and anxiety may also exhibit similar symptoms. Women with SMI experience higher rates of non-adherence to contraceptives, unintended pregnancy, sexually transmitted infections, and nonconsensual and transactional sex than the general population of women [125, 166–181]. Unintended pregnancy for women with SMI, especially those taking teratogenic mood stabilizers, can have adverse physical, psychological, and social consequences for women and their offspring [166, 167, 169]. Thus, helping women with SMI prevent unintended pregnancy is a clinical priority. Health providers who care for with women with SMI may avoid contraceptive care due to insufficient knowledge and training, negative countertransference with regard to patients' sexuality, incorrect assumptions about sexual activity, perceptions of contraception as secondary to psychiatric care, and concerns about ethical issues [125, 170–173, 182–185]. In this section, we offer strategies for contraceptive counseling and management for women with SMI.

Contraceptive Counseling Considerations for Other Serious Mental Illnesses

Some research on schizophrenia and bipolar disorder has found that some women with psychotic disorders lack basic knowledge of sexuality and reproduction, have misperceptions about contraception, and are concerned about access to contraceptive methods [125, 166–171, 175]. Thus, reproductive health education for women with SMI may need to be extensive. Contraceptive counseling should occur within a larger discussion of sexuality, reproductive health promotion, risk reduction and disease prevention, pregnancy intentions and readiness for pregnancy (emphasizing the value of stable social conditions and interpersonal relationships), and individual contraceptive expectations and preferences [125, 169]. Contraceptive information presented should be accurate, simple, clear, and provided at a time when patients are most receptive [125]. For instance, acutely psychotic patients are unlikely to have adequate attention and organization to assimilate contraceptive information [125, 171]. Counseling should be supplemented with simple written educational materials. Information on contraceptive methods should emphasize method-specific effectiveness rates, many of which are highly dependent upon correct use [128, 135, 154]. Effective use of some methods, like condoms, rely upon partner cooperation and support, and because women with SMI may have difficulties negotiating contraceptive use before or during sex, it is important for providers to engage partners in contraceptive counseling and education sessions when possible [170].

Contraceptive Method Considerations for Serious Mental Illness

The majority of women with SMI are eligible for the wide range of available contraceptive methods. In most cases, LARC methods, including the levonorgestrel-releasing and copper-containing IUDs and subdermal implant, should be considered as first line methods for women with SMI who wish to avoid an unintended pregnancy. LARC methods are highly effective, have few adherence issues, and do not contain estrogen, which eliminates cardiovascular risk concerns for women with chronic medical morbidities like diabetes, obesity, breast cancer, or hypertension, and women over 35 years of age who smoke. These are all health conditions which may co-occur with SMI and are CDC MEC contraindications to combined hormonal method use [57, 128, 135, 136, 171, 176]. Other progestin-only methods, including the DMPA injectable and progestin-only pills (POPs), are alterative options for women who do not wish to use LARC methods but have contraindications to estrogen. Monitoring for weight gain, truncal fat deposit, and peripheral glucose intolerance in the case of DMPA, especially among women using neuroleptics, may be useful since these potential side effects are of concern in the context of other medical morbidities [186–188]. Additionally, POPs require a relatively strict daily regimen for effectiveness (must be taken within a 3 h time frame daily) and are associated with irregular bleeding profiles, especially with missed or late dosages [128]. Barrier methods like condoms and diaphragms should be considered lower priority options for primary contraception for women with SMI given the amount of user involvement that is necessary [128, 135, 136].

For women with SMI who are eligible for estrogen-containing contraceptives and who do not want or have access to LARC, combined hormonal methods, including the vaginal ring, transdermal patch, and COCs, are reasonable options [128, 135, 136]. The effectiveness of these methods relies heavily on correct use. Health providers should work with women with SMI to optimize contraceptive choice based on co-occurring medical conditions, individual preferences, and the likelihood of method success. In all cases, dual method use (i.e., condoms plus another effective contraceptive) should be encouraged for HIV/STI prevention and unintended pregnancy protection [166, 167, 171, 175, 177–182]. Finally, because sexual intercourse is often unplanned (among all women but especially among those with SMI), emergency contraception is a necessary back up and is safe [171].

Contraceptive and Drug Interaction Considerations for Serious Mental Illness

Hyperprolactinemia and suppression of the hypothalamic–pituitary–gonadal axis is commonly experienced among women with schizophrenia on atypical antipsychotics (risperidone > aripiprazole > ziprasidone), which can lead to menstrual irregularities, amenorrhoea, sexual dysfunction, infertility issues, and galactorrhoea [189, 190]. Women taking atypical antipsychotics may believe they are not at risk for pregnancy because of menstrual irregularities or they may believe that their antipsychotic medication offers contraceptive protection, both of which are not accurate [189, 190]. Women who continue taking atypical antipsychotics with hyperprolactinemia should receive estradiol supplementation for neuroendocrine regulation, and some research has shown that estrogen may modulate and improve the expression of psychotic symptoms [189–194]. Thus, COCs may offer therapeutic effects for women on older atypical antipsychotics. However, frequent assessment of COC adherence and counseling on condom use would be essential. Women taking newer antipsychotics are less likely to experience elevated prolactin, so use of COCs for therapeutic purposes is less of a concern [189, 190, 194].

Women with schizophrenia and bipolar disorder may be treated with mood stabilizers, including antiepileptic medications including lamotrigine, carbamazepine, and topiramate. Many of these medications can induce cytochrome P450 3A4 causing enhanced hepatic metabolism of contraceptive steroids and potentially decreased contraceptive efficacy [125, 171, 176, 187, 188, 195–201]. Contraceptive steroids can also decrease levels of antiepileptics, such as valproate and lamotrigine, rendering them less effective [201–204]. Antipsychotic medications, including clozapine and chlorpromazine, are also metabolized by the liver, and contraceptive steroids can cause a significant increase in antipsychotic medication levels resulting in severe side effects such as hypotension, sedation, and tremor [202–204]. Providers should monitor psychiatric drug levels and adjust dosages as needed for hormonal contraceptive users [200–204] (see Chap. 8 for more information).

For women with SMI and drug interaction concerns, the local action of the IUDs, or the high dose of the DMPA injectable, offers effective alternative contraceptive options [128]. The injectable requires more effort on the part of the user (i.e., injections required every 3 months) compared to IUDs [128, 135]. Research that has compared these methods among women with SMI has found higher continuation rates for IUDs than for DMPA, with no differences in psychiatric complication and hospitalization rates between methods [176–185].

Ethical Considerations for Contraception in Serious Mental Illness

One of the most important and controversial but understudied topics in regard to contraception for women with SMI is how to best assess, promote, and protect women's reproductive autonomy. SMIs are often accompanied by deficits in reality testing that can negatively impact their decision-making capabilities. This may present an ethical dilemma for health providers who wish to help protect their patients from unintended pregnancy and avoid contraceptive coercion [172, 173]. Routine mental status exams of women with acute or chronic SMI symptoms are required during all phases of contraceptive care. Women should be able to consent to contraception—specifically, attend to, absorb, retain, and recall information disclosed in contraceptive counseling sessions, appreciate the information and its significance for their lives, evaluate the consequences, express both cognitive and evaluative understanding, and communicate a decision based upon that understanding [172, 173]. Thus, the first goal of contraceptive management among patients with chronic and variable impaired autonomy and reality testing is to restore decision-making capacities. In most cases, treatment of the underlying SMI can improve functioning, which will enhance understanding of contraceptive information and the ability to apply it to family planning decision-making and behavior [172, 173]. Providers have an ethical responsibility to help patients with SMI understand the implications of unintended pregnancy and should assist in weighing the risks of pregnancy with individual reproductive values (which may be dynamic). As opposed to sterilization, LARC methods are highly effective and reversible [128]. However, these methods require provider-controlled insertion and removal procedures, which may present a dilemma for informed consent. Other long-acting methods like the DMPA injectable are less invasive but also effective and reversible [128]. When possible, spouses, partners, or family members should be engaged in contraceptive counseling and management for patients with SMI since they can provide insight into reproductive values and treatment preferences [170, 172, 173]. Providers should be aware of any undue pressure from family or signs of intimate partner violence, and patients should always be provided with ample opportunities to discuss contraception in private [172, 173].

Conclusion

Depression, anxiety, and related disorders are common among reproductive-aged women and have significant implications for women's risk of unintended pregnancy. While other serious mental illnesses like schizophrenia and bipolar disorders are less common, these conditions can have especially adverse consequences for the health and well-being of women and their offspring. There has been a lack of attention to mental health in family planning settings, and significant research gaps prevent an in-depth understanding of the most effective approaches for contraceptive management among women with mental health conditions. From the best available scientific evidence, however, we have offered several take-home messages.

First, modern contraceptives do not appear to *cause* clinically significant mood symptoms or mental health conditions. The impact of hormonal contraceptives on perceived mood symptoms among women with preexisting mental health disorders warrants additional scientific investigation. Second, potential neuroendocrine, cognitive, and behavioral pathways may link mental health conditions with contraceptive decision-making and behaviors and place women at risk of unintended pregnancy. Additional research is needed to better understand these mechanisms. Third, contraceptive education and counseling is essential for women with mental health conditions who wish to avoid an unintended pregnancy. Special attention should be given to method effectiveness and adherence issues. Fourth, modern contraceptive methods are generally safe for women with mental health conditions and should be made available. Selection of an appropriate method should occur through shared decision-making. LARC methods offer strong options for women with mental health conditions since they are highly effective, are reversible, and have little user-burden. Fifth, while drug interactions with modern antidepressant and contraceptive therapies are rare, hormonal contraceptives and older antidepressant agents and some antipsychotics and mood stabilizers can interact. Similarly, chronic comorbid diseases, which commonly co-occur with mental health conditions and that may preclude estrogen use, should be taken into account. Finally, attention to ethical issues around reproductive autonomy and contraceptive decision-making, especially for women with SMI who have significant cognitive impairments, is essential. Treatment of the underlying mental health condition can restore cognitive functioning to improve contraceptive decision-making capacities.

Overall, while additional scientific research can improve our understanding of the role of mental health in contraception (and vice versa), health providers should prioritize contraceptive counseling and management for women with mental health conditions who wish to avoid unintended pregnancy. An integrated approach is needed to address interrelated mental and reproductive health issues, ultimately to improve the health and well-being of women, their families, and society [205].

References

1. U.S. Department of Health and Human Services' Office on Women's Health; Substance Abuse and Mental Health Services Administration. Action Steps for Improving Women's Mental Health. 2009. Author.
2. U.S. Department of Health and Human Services. Mental Health. Healthy People 2020. http://www.healthypeople.gov/2020/LHI/mentalHealth.aspx. Accessed 27 Sept 2013.
3. World Health Organization. The World Health Report 2001, Mental Health: New Understanding, New Hope. 2001. Geneva, Switzerland: World Health Organization; 2001.
4. American Psychiatric Association. Diagnostic and statistical manual of mental disorders, 4th edition, text revised. Washington, DC: American Psychiatric Association; 2000.
5. Gore FM, Bloem PJN, Patton GC, Ferguson J, Joseph V, Coffey C, et al. Global burden of disease in young people aged 10–24 years: a systematic analysis. Lancet. 2011;377:2093–102.
6. WHO. The global burden of disease: 2004 update 2008. Geneva, Switzerland: WHO; 2008.
7. Kessler RC. Epidemiology of women and depression. J Affect Disord. 2003;74(1):5–13.
8. Harvard Medical School. National Comorbidity Survey. 2009. http://www.hcp.med.harvard.edu/ncs/index.php. Accessed 27 Sept 2013.
9. Kessler RC, Berglund P, Demler O, Jin R, Koretz D, Merikangas KR, et al. The epidemiology of major depressive disorder: results from the National Comorbidity Survey Replication (NCS-R). JAMA. 2003;289(23):3095–105.
10. Twenge JM, Gentile B, DeWall N, Ma D, Lacefield K, Schurtz DR. Birth cohort increases in psychopathology among young Americans, 1938–2007: a cross-temporal meta-analysis of the MMPI. Clin Psychol Rev. 2010;30(2):145–54.
11. Cross-National Collaborative Group. The changing rate of major depression. Cross-national comparisons. JAMA. 1992;268(21):3098–105.
12. Compton WM, Conway KP, Stinson FS, Grant BF. Changes in the prevalence of major depression and substance use disorders in the United States between 1991–1992 and 2001–2002. Am J Psychiatry. 2006;163(12):2141–7.
13. National Institute of Mental Health [internet]. Use of mental health services and treatment among adults. http://www.nimh.nih.gov/statistics/3USE_MT_ADULT.shtml. Accessed 24 Oct 2012.
14. National Institute of Mental Health [internet]. Use of mental health services and treatment among children. http://www.nimh.nih.gov/statistics/1NHANES.shtml. Accessed 24 Oct 2012.
15. Barrio L, Burt V. Depression in pregnancy: strategies for primary care management. Dealing with underdiagnosed and undertreated problem. Wom Health Prim Care. 2000;3:490.
16. Miranda J, Chung JY, Green BL, Krupnick J, Siddique J, Revicki DA, Belin T. Treating depression in predominantly low-income young minority women: a randomized controlled trial. JAMA. 2003;290:57–65.
17. Farr SL, Dietz PM, Williams JR, Gibbs FA, Tregear S. Depression screening and treatment among nonpregnant women of reproductive age in the United States, 1990–2010. Prev Chron Dis. 2011;8:A122.
18. Li-Ching L, Casanueva CE, Martin SL. Depression among female family planning patients: prevalence, risk factors and use of mental health services. J Womens Health. 2005;14:225–32.
19. Ko JY, Farr SL, Dietz PM, Robbins CL. Depression and treatment among US pregnant and non-pregnant women of reproductive age, 2005–2009. J Womens Health. 2012;21:830–6.
20. Dennis CL, Ross LE, Grigoriadis S. Psychosocial and psychological interventions for treating antenatal depression. Cochrane Database Syst Rev. 2007;3. Art. No.: CD006309. DOI: 10.1002/14651858.CD006309.pub2.
21. Farr SL, Bitsko RH, Hayes DK, Dietz PM. Mental health and access to services among US women of reproductive aged. Am J Obstet Gynecol. 2010; 203:e1–9.
22. Wang PS, Lane M, Olfson M, Pincus HA, Wells KB, Kessler RC. Twelve month use of mental health services in the United States. Arch Gen Psychiatry. 2005;62:629–40.
23. Carrington CH. Clinical depression in African American women: diagnosis, treatment and research. J Clin Psychol. 2006;62:779–91.
24. Das AK, Ofson M, McCurtis HL, Weissman MM. Depression in African Americans: breaking barriers to detection and treatment. J Fam Pract. 2006;55:30–9.
25. Finer LB, Henshaw SK. Disparities in rates of unintended pregnancy in the United States, 1994 and 2001. Perspect Sex Reprod Health. 2006;38:90–6.
26. American Psychological Association [internet]. Women and depression. http://www.apa.org/about/gr/issues/women/depression.aspx. Accessed 24 Oct 2012.
27. Mcleod JD, Kessler RC. Socioeconomic status differences in vulnerability to undesired life events. J Health Soc Behav. 1990;31:162–72.
28. U.S. Department of Health and Human Services. Mental Health: Culture, Race, and Ethnicity: A Supplement to Mental Health: A Report of the Surgeon General. Rockville, MD: US Dept of Health and Human Services, Public Health Service, Office of the Surgeon General; 2001.
29. Frost JJ, Singh S, Finer LB. Factors associated with contraceptive use and nonuse, United States, 2004. Perspect Sex Reprod Health. 2007;39(1):48–55.
30. Gee RE, Mitra N, Wan F, Chavkin DE, Long JA. Power over parity: intimate partner violence and issues of fertility control. Am J Obstet Gynecol. 2009;201(148):e1–7.

31. Miller E, Decker MR, McCauley HL, Tancredi DJ, Levenson RR, Waldman J, et al. Pregnancy coercion, intimate partner violence and unintended pregnancy. Contraception. 2010;81(4):316–22.
32. Grote NK, Bridge JA, Gavin AR, Melville JL, Iyengar S, Katon WJ. A meta-analysis of depression during pregnancy and the risk of pre-term birth, low birth weight and intrauterine growth restriction. Arch Gen Psychiatry. 2010;67:1012–24.
33. Flynn HA, Walton MA, Chermack ST, Cunningham RM, Marcus SM. Brief detection and co-occurrence of violence, depression and alcohol risk in prenatal care settings. Arch Womens Ment Health. 2007;10:155–61.
34. Alder J, Fink N, Bitzer J, Hosli I, Holzgreve W. Depression and anxiety during pregnancy: a risk factor the obstetric, fetal and neonatal outcome? A critical review of the literature. J Matern Fetal Neonatal Med. 2007;20:189–209.
35. Kelly RH, Russo J, Holt V, Danielsen BH, Zatzick DF, Walker E, et al. Psychiatric and substance use disorders as risk factors for low birth weight and preterm delivery. Obstet Gynecol. 2002;100:297–304.
36. Vesga-Lopez O, Blanco C, Keyes K, Olfson M, Grant BF, Hasin DS. Psychiatric disorders in pregnant and postpartum women in the United States. Arch Gen Psychiatry. 2008;65:805–15.
37. Williams KE, Marsh WK, Rasgon NL. Mood disorders and fertility in women: a critical review of the literature and implications for future research. Hum Reprod Update. 2007;13:607–16.
38. Bennett IM, Culhane JF, McColuum KF, Elo IT. Unintended rapid repeat pregnancy and low education status: any role for depression and contraceptive use? Obstet Gynecol. 2006;194:749–54.
39. Steinberg JR, Trussell J, Hall KS, Guthrie K. Fatal flaws in a recent meta-analysis on abortion and mental health. Contraception. 2012;86(5):4307.
40. Takahashi S, Tsuchiya KJ, Matsumoto K, Suzuki K, Mori N, Takei N. Psychosocial determinants of mistimed and unwanted pregnancy: the Hamamatsu Birth Cohort Study. Matern Child Health J. 2012; 16(5):947–55.
41. Steinberg JR, Becker D, Henderson JT. Does the outcome of a first pregnancy predict depression, suicidal ideation, or lower self-esteem? Data from the National Comorbidity Survey. Am J Orthopsychiatry. 2011;81(2):193–201.
42. Steinberg JR, Finer LB. Examining the association of abortion history and current mental health: a reanalysis of the National Comorbidity Survey using a common-risk-factors model. Soc Sci Med. 2011;72:72–82.
43. Kessler RC, Berglund PA, Foster CL, Saunders WB, Stang PE. Walters EE Social consequences of psychiatric disorders. II: Teenage parenthood. Am J Psychiatry. 1997;154(10):1405–11.
44. Lancaster CA, Gold KJ, Flynn HA, Yoo H, Marcus SM, Davis MM. Risk factors for depressive symptoms during pregnancy: a systematic review. Am J Obstet Gynecol. 2010;205(3):5–14.
45. Gavin NI, Gaynes BN, Lohr KN, Meltzer-Brody S, Gartlehner G, Swinson T. Perinatal depression: a systematic review of prevalence and incidence. Obstet Gynecol. 2005;106(5):1071–83.
46. Marcus S, Flynn H, Blow F, Barry K. Depressive symptoms among pregnant women screening in obstetrics settings. J Womens Health. 2003;12(4):373–80.
47. Milgrom J, Gemmill AW, Bilszta JL, Hayes B, Barnett B, Brooks J, et al. Antenatal risk factors for postnatal depression: a large prospective study. J Affect Disord. 2008;108(1–2):147–57.
48. Beck CT. Predictors of postpartum depression: an update. Nurs Res. 2001;50(5):278–85.
49. Marcus SM, Flynn HA, Young E, Ghaziuddin N, Mudd S. Recurrent depression in women through the lifespan. In: Riba M, Oldham J, editors. American psychiatric press review of psychiatry. Washington, DC: American Psychiatric Press, Inc.; 2001. p. 19–50.
50. Silverman JG, Raj A, Mucci LA, Hathaway JE. Dating violence against adolescent girls and associated substance use, unhealthy weight control, sexual risk behavior, pregnancy, and suicidality. JAMA. 2001;286:572–9.
51. Wittchen H, Zhao S, Kessler RC, Eaton WW. DSM-III-R generalized anxiety disorder in the National Comorbidity Survey. Arch Gen Psychiatry. 1994;51: 355–64.
52. Moller SE. Effect of oral contraceptives on tryptophan and tyrosine availability: evidence for a possible contribution to mental depression. Neuropsychobiology. 1981;7:192–200.
53. Parry BL, Rush AJ. Oral contraceptives and depressive symptomatology: biologic mechanisms. Compr Psychiatry. 1979;20:347–58.
54. Sheenan DV, Sheenan KH. Psychiatric aspects of oral contraceptive use. Psychiatr Ann. 1976;6:500–8.
55. Winston F. Oral contraceptives, pyridoxine and depression. Am J Psychiatry. 1973;130:1217–21.
56. Robinson SA, Dowell M, Pedulla D, McCauley L. Do the emotional side-effects of hormonal contraceptives come from pharmacologic or psychological mechanisms? Med Hypotheses. 2004;63:268–73.
57. CDC. U.S. Medical eligibility criteria for contraceptive use, 2010. MMWR. 2010;59.
58. Vessey MP, McPherson K, Lawless M, Yeates D. Oral contraception and serious psychiatric illness: absence of an association. Br J Psychiatry. 1985;146:45–9.
59. Duke JM, Sibbritt DW, Young AF. Is there an association between the use of oral contraception and depressive symptoms in young Australian women? Contraception. 2007;75:27–31.
60. Walker A, Bancroft J. Relationship between premenstrual symptoms and oral contraceptive use: a controlled study. Psychosom Med. 1990;52:86–96.
61. O'Connell K, Davis AR, Kerns J. Oral contraceptives: side effects and depression in adolescent girls. Contraception. 2007;75:299–304.
62. Deijen JB, Duyn KJ, Jansen WA, Klittsie JW. Use of a monophasic low-dose oral contraceptive in relation to mental functioning. Contraception. 1992;46:359–67.

63. Almagor M, Ben-Porath MS. Mood changes during the menstrual cycle and their relation to the use of oral contraceptives. J Psychosom Res. 1991;35:721–8.
64. Sanders SA, Graham CA, Bass JL, Bancroft J. A prospective study of the effects of oral contraceptives on sexuality and wellbeing and their relationship to discontinuation. Contraception. 2001;64:51–8.
65. Segebladh B, Borgstrom A, Odlind V, Bixo M, Sundstrom-Poromaa I. Prevalence of psychiatric disorders and premenstrual dysphoric symptoms in patients with experience of adverse mood during treatment with combined oral contraceptives. Contraception. 2009;79:50–5.
66. Westhoff C, Truman C, Kalmuss D, Cushman L, Davidson A, Rulin M, et al. Depressive symptoms and depo-provera. Contraception. 1998;57:237–40.
67. Gupta N, O'Brien R, Jacobsen LJ, Davis A, Zuckerman A, Supran S, et al. Mood changes in adolescents using depo-medroxyprogesterone acetate for contraception. J Pediatr Adolesc Gynecol. 2001;14:71–6.
68. Tsai S. Effect of depot medroxyprogesterone acetate on postpartum depression. Contraception. 2010;82:174–7.
69. Westhoff C, Truman C, Kalmuss D, Cushman L, Rulin M, Heartwell S, et al. Depressive symptoms and Norplant contraceptive implants. Contraception. 1998;57(4):241–5.
70. Lopez LM, Grimes DA, Gallo MF, Schulz KF. Skin patch and vaginal ring versus combined oral contraceptives for contraception. Cochrane Database Syst Rev. 2010;17(3)pub3.
71. Sucato GS, Land SR, Murray PJ, Cecchini R, Gold MA. Adolescents experiences using the contraceptive patch versus pills. J Pediatr Adolesc Gynecol. 2011;24:197–203.
72. Mansour D, Korver T, Marintcheva-Petrova M, Fraser IS. The effects of Implanon on menstrual bleeding patterns. Eur J Contracept Reprod Health Care. 2008;13:13–28.
73. Elovainio M, Teperi J, Aalto AM, Grenman S, Kivelä A, Kujansuu E, et al. Depressive symptoms as a predictor of discontinuation of treatment of menorrhagia by levoenorgesterol releasing intrauterine system. Int J Behav Med. 2007;14:70–5.
74. Westhoff C, Heartwell S, Edwards S, Zieman M, Stuart G, Cwiak C, et al. Oral contraceptive discontinuation: do side effects matter? Am J Obstet Gynecol. 2007;196:412e1–7.
75. Rosenberg MJ, Waugh MS, Long S. Unintended pregnancies and use, misuse and discontinuation of oral contraceptives. J Reprod Med. 1995;40:355–60.
76. Stenchever MA, Herbst AL, Droegemueller W, Mishell D, editors. Comprehensive gynecology. St. Louis: Elsevier Health Sciences; 2001.
77. Hall K, Reame N, O'Connell K, Rickert V, Weshoff C. Influence of depressed mood and psychological stress symptoms on perceived oral contraceptive side effects and discontinuation in young minority women. Contraception. 2012;86:518–25.
78. Rubino-Watkins MF, Doster JA, Franks S, Kelly KS, Sonnier BL, Goven AJ, et al. Oral contraceptive use: implications for cognitive and emotional functioning. J Nerv Ment Dis. 1999;187:275–80.
79. Barsky AJ, Saintfort R, Rogers MP, Borus JF. Nonspecific medication side effects and the Nocebo phenomenon. JAMA. 2002;287:22–7.
80. Katon W, Lin E, Von Korff M, Russo J, Lipscomb P, Bush T. Somatization: a spectrum of severity. Am J Psychiatry. 1991;148:34–40.
81. Mathews A, MacLeod C. Cognitive vulnerability to emotional disorders. Annu Rev Clin Psychol. 2005; 1:167–95.
82. Beck AT. Cognitive models of depression. J Cognit Psychother. 1987;1(1):5–37.
83. Maner JK, Schmidt NB. The role of risk avoidance in anxiety. Behav Ther. 2006;37(2):181–9.
84. Yuen KSL, Lee TMC. Could mood state affect risk-taking decisions? J Affect Disord. 2003;75(1):11–8.
85. Ruscher S, de Wit R, Mazimanian D. Psychiatric patients' attitudes about medication and factors affecting noncompliance. Psychiatr Serv. 1997;48:82–5.
86. Patel MS, David AS. Medication adherence: predictive factors and enhancement strategies. Psychiatry. 2004;3:41–4.
87. Calev A. Assessment of neuropsychological functions in psychotic disorders. Washington, DC: American Psychiatric Press; 1999.
88. Alvy LM, McKirnan DJ, Mansergh G, Koblin B, Colfax GN, Flores SA, et al. Project MIX Study Group. Depression is associated with sexual risk among men who have sex with men, but is mediated by cognitive escape and self-efficacy. AIDS Behav. 2011;15(6):1171–9.
89. Clery-Melin ML, Schmidt L, Lafargue G, Baup N, Fossati P, Pessiglione M. Why don't you try harder? An investigation of effort production in major depression. PLoS One. 2011;6(7):e23178. 1–8.
90. Hartley CA, Phelps EA. Anxiety and decision-making. Biol Psychiatr. 2012;72(2):113–8.
91. Lehrer JA, Shrier LA, Gortmaker S, Buka S. Depressive symptoms as longitudinal predictors of sexual risk behaviors among US middle and high school students. Pediatrics. 2006;118:189–200.
92. Shrier LA, Harris SK, Sternberg M, Beardslee WR. Associations of depression, self-esteem, and substance use with sexual risk among adolescents. Prev Med. 2001;33(3):179–89.
93. Chen YW, Stiffman AR, Cheng LC, Dore P. Mental health, social environment and sexual risk behaviors of adolescent service users: a gender comparison. J Child Fam Stud. 1997;6:9–25.
94. Garbers S, Correa N, Tobier N, Blust S, Chiasson MA. Associations between symptoms of depression and contraceptive method choices among low-income women at urban reproductive health centers. Matern Child Health J. 2010;14:102–9.
95. Hall K, Moreau C, Trussell J, Barber J. Role of young women's depression and stress symptoms in

their weekly use and nonuse of contraceptive methods. J Adolesc Health. 2013;53(2):241–8.
96. Hall K, Moreau C, Trussell J, Barber J. Young women's consistency of contraceptive use—do depression and stress matter? Contraception. 2013;88(5):641–9.
97. Brooks TL, Harris SK, Thrall JS. Woods ER Association of adolescent risk behaviors with mental health symptoms in high school students. J Adolesc Health. 2002;31:240–6.
98. Zink TM, Shireman TI, Ho M, Buchanan T. High-risk teen compliance with prescription contraception: an analysis of Ohio medicaid claims. J Pediatr Adolesc Gynecol. 2002;15:15–21.
99. Steinberg JR, Tschann JM, Henderson JT, Drey EA, Steinauer JE, Harper CC. Psychological distress and post-abortion contraceptive choice at an urban clinic. Contraception. 2013;88:717–24.
100. Mann JJ. The medical management of depression. N Engl J Med. 2005;353:1819–34.
101. Roter DL, Frankel RM, Hall JA, Sluyter D. The expression of emotion through nonverbal behavior in medical visits. Mechanisms and outcomes. J Gen Intern Med. 2006;21:s28–34.
102. Hackley B, Sharma C, Kedzior A, Sreenivasan S. Managing mental health conditions in primary care settings. J Midwifery Womens Health. 2010; 55(1):9–19.
103. National Institute for Health and Clinical Excellence Clinical guidelines CG90, TMAP Guidelines, The MacArthur Initiative on Depression and Primary Care. 2009.
104. University of Michigan Depression Center Toolkit [internet]. http://depressiontoolkit.org/treatmentoptions/Psychotherapy/dbt.asp. Accessed 20 Dec 2012.
105. ARHP's Clinical Advisory Committee for The Reproductive Health Implications of Depression [internet]. 2011. http://www.arhp.org/core. Accessed 1 Feb 2013.
106. American Psychological Association [internet]. Assessment tools. http://www.apa.org/pi/about/publications/caregivers/practice settings/assessment/tools/index.aspx. Accessed 1 Feb 2013.
107. Bohannon RW, Maljanian R, Goethe J. Screening for depression in clinical practice: reliability and validity of a five-item subset of the CES-depression. Percept Mot Skills. 2003;97:855–61.
108. Cohen S, Kamarck T, Mermelstein R. A global measure of perceived stress. J Health Soc Behav. 1993;24:385–96.
109. Radloff LS. The CES-D scale: a self-report depression scale for research in the general population. Appl Psychol Meas. 1977;1:385–401.
110. Ewing JA. Detecting alcoholism. The CAGE questionnaire. JAMA. 1984;12(14):1905–7.
111. Kroenke K, Spitzer RL, Williams JB. The patient health questionnaire-2: validity of a two-item depression screener. Med Care. 2003;41:1284–92.
112. Cotton MA, Ball C, Robinson P. Four simple questions can help screen for eating disorders. J Gen Intern Med. 2003;18:53–6.
113. McDowell AK, Lineberry TW, Bostwick JM. Practical suicide-risk management for the busy primary care physician. Mayo Clin Proc. 2011;86: 792–800.
114. Andresen EM, Malmgren JA, Carter WB, Patrick DL. Screening for depression in well older adults: evaluation of a short form of the CES-D (Center for Epidemiologic Studies Depression Scale). Am J Prev Med. 1994;10(2):77–84.
115. Spitzer RL, Kroenke K, Williams JBW, Patient Health Questionnaire Primary Care Study Group. Validation and utility of a self-report version of PRIME-MD: the PHQ primary care study. JAMA. 1999;282(18):1737–44.
116. Richter P, Werner J, Heerlein A, Kraus A, Sauer H. On the validity of the beck depression inventory: a review. Psychopathology. 1998;31(3):160–8.
117. Lovibond PF, Lovibond SH. The structure of negative emotional states: comparison of the depression anxiety stress scales (DASS) with the beck depression and anxiety inventories. Behav Res Ther. 1995;33(3):335–43.
118. Fydrich T, Dowdall D, Chambless DL. Reliability and validity of the beck anxiety inventory. J Anxiety Dis. 1992;6(1):55–61.
119. Beck AT, Steer RA. Manual for the beck anxiety inventory. San Antonio, TX: Psychological Corporation; 1990.
120. Spielberger CD, Gorsuch RL, Lushene R, Vagg PR, Jacobs GA. State-trait anxiety inventory for adults: manual, test booklet and scoring key 1983. Palo Alto, CA: Consulting Psychologist Press, Inc.; 1983.
121. Higgins ES. A review of unrecognized mental illness in primary care prevalence, natural history and efforts to change the course. Arch Fam Med. 1994;3:908–17.
122. Koke SC, Brown EB, Miner CM. Safety and efficacy of fluoxetine in patients who receive oral contraceptive therapy. Am J Obstet Gynecol. 2002;187:551–5.
123. D'Arcy PF. Drug interactions with oral contraceptives. Drug Intell Clin Pharm. 1986;20:353 62.
124. Anderson IM, Edwards JG. Guidelines for choice of selective serotonin reuptake inhibitor in depressive illness. Adv Psychiatr Treat. 2001;7:170–80.
125. Buckley P, editor. Sexuality and serious mental illness. Netherlands: Harwood Academic Publishers; 2013.
126. Will-Shahab L, Bauer S, Kunter U, Roots I, Brattstrom A. St John's wort extract (Ze 117) does not alter the pharmacokinetics of a low dose oral contraceptive. Eur J Clin Pharmacol. 2009;65:287–94.
127. Murphy PA, Kern SE, Stanczyk FZ, Westhoff CL. Interaction of St. John's wort with oral contraceptives; effects on the pharmacokinetics of norethindrone and ethinyl estradiol, ovarian activity and breakthrough bleeding. Contraception. 2005;71: 402–8.
128. Hatcher RA, Trussell J, Stewart F, et al. Contraceptive technology. 20 (Revised)th ed. New York, NY: Ardent Media; 2004.

129. Hunot VM, Caldwell D, Jones DP, Furukawa TA, Lewis G, Churchhill R. Cognitive behavioural therapies versus treatment as usual for depression. Cochrane Database Syst Rev. 2010; DOI: 10.1002/14651858.CD008699.
130. Hunot V, Churchill R, Teixeira V, Silva de Lima M. Psychological therapies for generalised anxiety disorder. Cochrane Data Syst Rev. 2007;1, Art. No.: CD001848. DOI:10.1002/14651858
131. Churchill R, Davies P, Caldwell D, Moore THM, Jones H, Lewis G, Hunot V. Interpersonal, cognitive analytic and other integrative therapies versus treatment as usual for depression. Cochrane Database Syst Rev. 2010;9, Art. No.: CD008703. DOI:10.1002/14651858.CD008703.
132. Hall KS, Reame N, O'Connell K, Westhoff C. Studying the use of oral contraception: a review of measurement approaches. J Womens Health. 2010;19:2203–10.
133. DiMatteo MR, Lepper HS, Croghan TW. Depression is a risk factor for noncompliance with medical treatment: meta-analysis of the effects of anxiety and depression on patient adherence. Arch Intern Med. 2000;160:2101–7.
134. Osterberg L, Blascke T. Adherence to medication. N Engl J Med. 2005;353:487–97.
135. World Health Organization (WHO) Department of Reproductive Health and Research, Johns Hopkins Bloomberg School of Public Health/Center for Communication Programs (CCP). Knowledge for health project. Family planning: a global handbook for providers (2011 update). Baltimore, MD; Geneva, Switzerland: CCP and WHO; 2011.
136. Trussell J, Vaughn B. Contraceptive failure, method-related discontinuation and resumption of use: results from the 1995 NSFG. Fam Plann Perspect. 1999;31:64–72. 93.
137. Mosher WD, Jones J. Use of contraception in the United States: 1982–2008. Vital Health Stat. 2010;23:1–43.
138. Kost K, Singh S, Vaughan B, Trussell J, Bankole A. Estimates of contraceptive failure from the 2002 National Survey of Family Growth. Contraception. 2008;77:10–21.
139. Moreau C, Trussell J, Gilbert F, Bajos N, Bouyer J. Oral contraceptive tolerance: does the type of pill matter? Obstet Gynecol. 2007;109:1277–85.
140. Hall KS, Trussell J. Types of combined oral contraceptives used by US women. Contraception. 2012;86(6):659–65.
141. Gallo MF, Grimes NK, Lopez LM, Schulz KF. 20ug versus >20ug estrogen combined oral contraceptives for contraception. Cochrane Collab Rev. 2011;1. http://www.thecochranelibrary.com.
142. Maitra NN, Kulier R, Bloemenkamp K, Helmerhorst FM, Gulmezogul AM. Progestogens in combined oral contraceptives for contraception. Cochrane Collab Rev. 2011;3. http://www.thecochranelibrary.com.
143. Lawrie TA, Helmerhorst FM, Maitra NN, Kulier R, Bloemenkamp K, Gulmezoglu AM. Types of progestogens in combined oral contraception: effectiveness and side-effects Cochrane Collab Rev. 2011;5. http://www.thecochranelibrary.com.
144. Van Vliet HAAM, Grimes DA, Lopez LM, Schulz KF, Helmerhorst FM. Triphasic versus monophasic oral contraceptives for contraception. Cochrane Collab Rev. 2011;12. http://www.thecochranelibrary.com.
145. Edelman A, Gallo MF, Jensen JT, Nichols MD, Grimes DA. Continuous or extended cycle vs. cyclic use of combined hormonal contraceptives for contraception. Cochrane Collab Rev. 2011;8. http://www.thecochranelibrary.com.
146. Ward RK, Zamorski MA. Benefits and risks of psychiatric medication during pregnancy. Am Fan Physician. 2002;66:629–36.
147. Flynn HA, O'Mahen HA, Massey L, Marcus S. The impact of a brief obstetrics clinic-based intervention on treatment use for perinatal depression. J Womens Health. 2006;15:1195–204.
148. Marcus SM, Barry KL, Flynn HA, Tandon R, Greden JF. Treatment guidelines for depression in pregnancy. Int J Gynecol Obstet. 2001;72:61–70.
149. O'Mahen HA, Himle JA, Fedock G, Henshaw E, Flynn HA. A pilot randomized controlled trial of cognitive behavioral therapy for perinatal depression adapted for women with low incomes. Depress Anxiety. 2013;30(7):679–87.
150. Freeman EW, Samuel MD, Lin H, Nelson DB. Associations of hormones and menopausal status with depressed mood in women with no history of depression. Arch Gen Psychiatry. 2006;63(4): 375–82.
151. Parry BL. Optimal management of perimenopausal depression. Int J Womens Health. 2010;2:143–51.
152. Steinberg EM, Rubinow DR, Bartko JJ, Fortinsky PM, Haq N, Thompson K, et al. A cross-sectional evaluation of perimenopausal depression. J Clin Psychiatry. 2008;69(6):973–80.
153. Frost JJ, Lindberg LD, Finer LB. Young adults' contraceptive knowledge, norms and attitudes: associations with risk of unintended pregnancy. Perspect Sex Reprod Health. 2012;44(2):107–16.
154. Hall KS, Castano P, Stone P, Westhoff C. Measuring oral contraceptive knowledge: a review of research findings and limitations. Patient Educ Couns. 2010;81:388–94.
155. Akers AY, Gold MA, Borrero S, Santucci A, Schwarz EB. Structured contraceptive counseling—a randomized controlled trial. J Womens Health. 2010; 19:1163–70.
156. Hall K. The health belief model can guide modern contraceptive research. J Midwifery Womens Health. 2011;57:74–81.
157. Lopez LM, Tolley EE, Grimes DA, Mario CM. Theory-based strategies for improving contraceptive use: a systematic review. Contraception. 2009;79:411–7.
158. Tessler SL, Peipert JF. Perceptions of contraceptive effectiveness and health effects of oral contraception. Womens Health Issues. 1997;7:400–6.

159. Rickert VI, Berenson AB, Williamson AJ, Wiemann CM. Immediate recall of oral contraceptive instructions: implications for providers. Am J Obstet Gynecol. 1999;180:1399–406.
160. Grimes DA, Schulz KF. Nonspecific side effects of oral contraceptives: nocebo or noise? Contraception. 2011;83(1):5–9.
161. ACOG. Intimate partner violence. Committee Opinion No. 518. American College of Obstetricians and Gynecologists. Obstet Gynecol. 2012;119:412–7.
162. Black MC, Basile KC, Breidig MJ, Smith SG, Walters ML, Merrick MT, et al. The National Intimate Partner and Sexual Violence Survey (NISVS): 2010 summary report. Atlanta (GA): National Center for Injury Prevention and Control, Centers for Disease Control and Prevention; 2011.
163. Lehrer JA, Buka B, Gortmaker S, Shrier LA. Depressive symptomatology as a predictor of exposure to intimate partner violence among US female adolescents and young adults. Arch Pediatr Adolesc Med. 2006;160(3):270–6.
164. National Alliance on Mental Illness [internet]. About mental illness. http://www.nami.org/template.cfm?section=about_mental_illness. Accessed 2 June 2013
165. National Institute of Mental Health [internet]. Prevalence of serious mental illness among U.S. Adults by age, sex and race. http://www.nimh.nih.gov/statistics/SMI_AASR.shtml. Accessed 20 Aug 2013.
166. Matevosyan NR. Reproductive health in women with serious mental illnesses: a review. Sex Disabil. 2009;27:109–18.
167. Miller LJ. Sexuality, reproduction, and family planning in women with schizophrenia. Schizopr Bull. 1997;23(4):623–35.
168. Miller LJ, Finnerty M. Family planning knowledge, attitudes and practices in women with schizophrenic spectrum disorders. J Psychosom Obstet Gynaecol. 1998;19:210–7.
169. Krumm S, Killan R, Becker T. Mentally ill women's subjective views on social context of desire for children. A qualitative approach. Psychiatr Prax. 2011;38(1):23–30.
170. Guedes TG, Moura ERF, Almeida PC. Particularities of family planning in women with mental disorders. Rev Lat Am Enfermagem. 2009;17(5):639–44.
171. Seeman MV, Ross R. Prescribing contraceptives for women with schizophrenia. J Psychiatr Pract. 2011; 17:258–69.
172. McCullough LB, Coverdale J, Bayer T, Chernenak FA. Ethically justified guidelines for family planning interventions to prevent pregnancy in female patients with chronic mental illness. Am J Obstet Gynecol. 1992;167:19–25.
173. Coverdale JH, Bayer TL, McCullough LB, Chervenak FA. Respecting the autonomy of chronic mentally ill women in decisions about contraception. Hosp Community Psychiatry. 1993;44(7):671–4.
174. Magalhaes PVS, Kapczinkski F, Kauer-Sant'Anna M. Use of contraceptive methods among women treated for bipolar disorder. Arch Womens Ment Health. 2009;12:183–5.
175. Lang DL, Sales JM, Salazar LR, DiClemente RJ, Crosby RA, Brown LK, et al. Determinants of multimethod contraceptive use in a sample of adolescent women diagnosed with psychological disorders. Infect Dis Obstet Gynecol. 2000;2011:1–8.
176. Berenson AB, Asem H, Tan A, Wilkinson GS. Continuation rates and complications of intrauterine contraception in women diagnosed with bipolar disorder. Obstet Gynecol. 2011;118(6):1331–6.
177. Whitmore EA, Mikulich SK, Ehlers KM, Crowley TJ. One-year outcome of adolescent females referred for conduct disorder and substance abuse/dependence. Drug Alcohol Depend. 2000;59(2):131–41.
178. Smith MD. HIV risk in adolescents with severe mental illness: literature review. J Adolesc Health. 2001;29(5):320–9.
179. Auslander WF, McMillen JC, Elze D, Thompson R, Jonson-Reid M, Stiffman A. Mental health problems and sexual abuse among adolescents in foster care: relationship to HIV risk behaviors and intentions. AIDS Behav. 2002;6(4):351–9.
180. Tubman JG, Gil AG, Wagner EF, Artigues H. Patterns of sexual risk behaviors and psychiatric disorders in a community sample of young adults. J Behav Med. 2003;26(5):473–500.
181. DiClemente RJ, Ponton LE. HIV-related risk behaviors among psychiatrically hospitalized adolescents and school- based adolescents. Am J Psychiatry. 1993;150(2):324–5.
182. Haboubi NH, Lincoln N. Views of health professionals on discussing sexual issues with patients. Disabil Rehabil. 2003;25:291–6.
183. Wright ER, Wright DE, Perry BL, Foote-Ardah CE. Stigma and the sexual isolation of people with serious mental illness. Soc Prob. 2007;54:78–98.
184. Abel K, Rees S. Reproductive and sexual health of women service users: what's the fuss? Adv Psychiatr Treat. 2010;16:279–80.
185. Cropsey KL, Matthews C, Campbel S, Ivey S, Adawadkar S. Long-term, reversible contraception use among high-risk women treated in a university-based gynecology clinic: comparison between IUD and depo-provera. J Womens Health (Larchmt). 2010;19:349 53.
186. Verhaeghe J. Hormonal contraception in women with the metabolic syndrome: a narrative review. Eur J Contracept Reprod Health Care. 2010; 15:305–13.
187. Crawford P. Interactions between antiepileptic drugs and hormonal contraception. CNS Drugs. 2002;16:263–72.
188. Dutton C, Foldvary-Schaefer N. Contraception in women with epilepsy: pharmacokinetic interactions, contraceptive options, and management. Int Rev Neurobiol. 2008;83:113–34.
189. Seeman MV. Antipsychotic-induced amenorrhea. J Ment Health. 2011;20(5):484–91.
190. Richer-Rossler A, Schmid C, Bleuer S, Birkhauser M. Antipsychotics and hyperprolactinaemia: pathophysiology, clinical relevance, diagnosis and therapy. Neuropsychiatr. 2009;23(2):71–83.

191. Riecher-Rössler A. Oestrogen effects in schizophrenia and their potential therapeutic implications—review. Arch Womens Ment Health. 2002;5(3):111–8.
192. Kulkarni J, de Castella A, Fitzgerald PB, Gurvich CT, Bailey M, Bartholomeusz C, et al. Estrogen in severe mental illness: a potential new treatment approach. Arch Gen Psychiatry. 2008;65:955–60.
193. Riecher-Rössler A, de Geyter C. The forthcoming role of treatment with oestrogens in mental health. Swiss Med Wkly. 2007;137:565–72.
194. Currier GW, Simpson GM. Psychopharmacology: antipsychotic medications and fertility. Psychiatr Serv. 1998;49:175–6.
195. Gaffield ME, Culwell KR, Lee CR. The use of hormonal contraception among women taking anticonvulsant therapy. Contraception. 2011;83:16–29.
196. Spina E, Pisani F, Perucca E. Clinically significant pharmacokinetic drug interactions with carbamazepine. An update. Clin Pharmacokinet. 1996;31:198–214.
197. Herzog AG, Blum AS, Farina EL, Maestri XE, Newman J, Garcia E, et al. Valproate and lamotrigine level variation with menstrual cycle phase and oral contraceptive use. Neurology. 2009;72:911–4.
198. Wegner I, Edelbroek PM, Bulk S, Lindhout D. Lamotrigine kinetics within the menstrual cycle, after menopause, and with oral contraceptives. Neurology. 2009;73:1388–93.
199. Bialer M, Doose DR, Murthy B, Curtin C, Wang SS, Twyman RE, et al. Pharmacokinetic interactions of topiramate. Clin Pharmacokinet. 2004;43:763–80.
200. Johannessen Landmark C, Patsalos PN. Drug interactions involving the new second- and third-generation antiepileptic drugs. Expert Rev Neurother. 2010;10:119–40.
201. Reddy DS. Clinical pharmacokinetic interactions between antiepileptic drugs and hormonal contraceptives. Expert Rev Clin Pharmacol. 2010;3:183–92.
202. Gabbay V, O'Dowd MA, Mamamtavrishvili M, Asnis GM. Clozapine and oral contraceptives: a possible drug interaction. J Clin Psychopharmacol. 2002;22:621–2.
203. Brown D, Goosen TC, Chetty M, Hamman JH. Effect of oral contraceptives on the transport of chlorpromazine across the CACO-2 intestinal epithelial cell line. Eur J Pharm Biopharm. 2003;56:159–65.
204. Chetty M, Miller R. Oral contraceptives increase the plasma concentrations of chlorpromazine. Ther Drug Monit. 2001;23:556–8.
205. World Health Organization. Mental Health Aspects of Women's Reproductive Health: A global review of the literature. Geneva, Switzerland:WHO; 2009.

Contraception for Women Living with HIV

6

Lisa B. Haddad, Jessica Tarleton, Anandi N. Sheth, and Ighovwerha Ofotokun

Background on the HIV Epidemic: Globally and in the USA

Human immunodeficiency virus (HIV), the virus that causes acquired immunodeficiency syndrome (AIDS), survives via inhabiting and killing the immune cells that fight infections. The first cases of AIDS were recognized in the early 1980s in the USA, with the first published case series from the US Centers for Disease Control and Prevention (CDC) in 1981 of five homosexual men [1]. Since then, global recognition of the virus has led to great advances in our understanding of the disease, transmission, pathogenesis, prognosis, and treatment. Although there is no cure for HIV infection at this time, with the development of highly active antiretroviral therapy (HAART), individuals with HIV infection can live longer and transmission can be reduced. While the incidence of new HIV infections and HIV-related mortality continues to decline due to improvements in care and treatment, the prevalence of HIV infections globally continues to rise, and HIV infection remains a leading cause of death among women of childbearing age worldwide [2, 3].

L.B. Haddad, M.D., M.S., M.P.H. (✉)
J. Tarleton, M.D., M.P.H.
Department of Gynecology and Obstetrics, Emory University School of Medicine, Atlanta, GA, USA
e-mail: lbhadda@emory.edu; jtarlet@emory.edu

A.N. Sheth, M.D. • I. Ofotokun, M.D., M.Sc.
Division of Infectious Diseases, Department of Medicine, Emory University School of Medicine, Atlanta, GA, USA
e-mail: ansheth@emory.edu; iofotok@emory.edu

The Global Epidemic

As of 2012, an estimated 35.3 million people were living with HIV worldwide [4]. Sub-Saharan Africa contains two-thirds of the world's HIV-infected population. In this region, HIV disproportionately affects women, who make up 58 % of those infected. In the Caribbean region, with the second highest prevalence of HIV in the world, 1 in 100 people live with HIV infection [4]. It should be noted that a large proportion of the data on women with HIV infection stems from international research efforts particularly in sub-Saharan Africa. Furthermore, given immigration to the USA, it is important that health care providers, especially those who serve low-income and migrant populations, are aware of the global context of the HIV/AIDS epidemic.

United States

An estimated 1.1 million people in America are living with HIV, and nearly 1 in 5 are unaware of

R.H. Allen and C.A. Cwiak (eds.), *Contraception for the Medically Challenging Patient*, DOI 10.1007/978-1-4939-1233-9_6, © Springer Science+Business Media New York 2014

their infection [5]. Approximately 50,000 new people are additionally infected each year [5, 6]. The proportion of HIV/AIDS cases diagnosed among women in the USA has grown annually from 8 % in 1985 to an estimated 25 % in 2010. HIV disproportionately affects black women in the USA. In 2010, heterosexual transmission among black women made up one of the most common routes of new infections, with greater than 5,000 new infections transmitted in this way. Of the total number of new HIV infections among women in the USA in 2010, 64 % occurred in black women, 18 % were in white women, and 15 % were in Hispanic women. Young women ages 25–44 years accounted for the majority of new infections in women in 2010. Fortunately, among all racial groups, the rate of new infections in women has been slowly declining [7].

Why Are Women at Risk?

Due to a complex array of factors, women are particularly vulnerable to acquiring HIV. Women may not be aware of their partner's risk factors for HIV and may not be able to successfully negotiate consistent condom use or mutual monogamy with their partners. The vast majority of these new infections come from heterosexual contact with men who have risk factors that are unknown to their female partners (e.g., men who have sex with other men or inject illicit drugs) [8]. Challenges that many women face, such as domestic violence, discrimination, stigma, substance abuse, mental health disorders, and poverty, increase their HIV susceptibility. Additionally, women are more susceptible to acquiring HIV during unprotected vaginal sex than men, with even higher risk during unprotected anal sex, due to a variety of factors, including the concentration of virus in semen, delicacy of vaginal tissues, and cervical ectropion.

For women who are aware of their partner's HIV status, they often lack the ability to advocate for the use of strategies to reduce HIV transmission risk, such as condoms and male circumcision. HIV pre-exposure prophylaxis, a strategy in which antiretroviral drugs are used orally or topically by HIV-uninfected persons before potential HIV exposure, has recently shown promise in HIV prevention. The daily use of oral fixed-dose combination tablets containing tenofovir, disoproxil, fumarate, and emtricitabine is approved by the Food and Drug Administration for use among sexually active adults at risk for HIV infection. Additionally, a tenofovir-containing vaginal microbicide has shown promise for HIV prevention in at-risk women and is being explored further [9].

Unfortunately, it is estimated that in the USA almost 1 in 5 women who are HIV-infected are unaware of their status. This highlights the importance of routine HIV testing in women, as recommended by CDC guidelines, to improve women's health and prevent HIV transmission. Linking HIV-infected women into appropriate medical care, retaining them in care, and optimizing HIV therapy for affected women are crucial to maintain health, improve survival, and reduce HIV transmission in the community [10, 11]. Relative to men, women living with HIV infection in the USA have been shown to be more vulnerable with regard to health care resource utilization [12, 13], potentially due to challenges such as transportation, childcare, insurance, substance abuse, and stigma. Key health indicators such as rates of clinic visits, antiretroviral treatment adherence, virologic suppression, and mean CD4 T-cell counts are lower for the HIV-infected women of racial/ethnic minority backgrounds [14, 15]. Since many of these women are the sole providers of care for their children, illness and death ultimately threaten the stability and welfare of families in their communities. These statistics underscore the urgent need for interventions aimed at women for the prevention and effective treatment of HIV infection. Family planning clinics provide an important venue for women of reproductive age who are living with or at risk for HIV to access the health care system, and serve as a crucial step for women to receive HIV testing and for HIV-infected women to be linked into appropriate medical care.

Living with HIV: HIV Care over the Past 30 Years

Primary HIV infection is often asymptomatic and if symptoms do occur they can be nonspecific and flu-like in nature. After the primary infection, many months or years may pass before the person is diagnosed. Symptoms that may prompt evaluation include opportunistic infections, or minor skin or constitutional symptoms. Women may present at a later stage of the disease or may discover their HIV-positive status during routine prenatal testing.

The natural history of HIV infection has changed over the past few decades with the use of HAART [16]. Mortality from HIV infection has declined and opportunistic infections are becoming less common, with more than half of the deaths among individuals with HIV infection now related to conditions other than AIDS. The paradigm of care in HIV infection in the era of HAART has shifted to that of chronic disease management. Despite this, some women still are diagnosed or present to care late in their disease course with conditions related to AIDS. In caring for HIV-infected women, care providers must therefore consider their overall health in relation to chronic non-AIDS complications such as cardiovascular disease (CVD), bone disease, renal disease, liver disease, and malignancies whose prevalence are significantly high, particularly among women (relative to men) living with HIV/AIDS [17], as well as possible immune suppression if AIDS-related conditions are present.

AIDS-Related Complications

Compared to women without HIV infection, HIV-infected women are at risk for recurrent candida vulvovaginitis, recurrent or complicated pelvic inflammatory disease, persistent or recurrent bacterial vaginosis, severe and prolonged genital herpes infections, cervical dysplasia and cancer, and abnormal uterine bleeding. The presence of any of these conditions should trigger HIV testing in a woman who does not have a diagnosis of HIV, and women with HIV should be screened regularly and managed aggressively for these conditions as several of them can increase their risk of transmitting HIV to their partner (see the section "Reproductive Health Care for Women with HIV").

Rarely, AIDS-defining conditions may involve the female reproductive tract, and women with such conditions may present to a reproductive care provider. These conditions include invasive cervical cancer, pelvic or genital tract tuberculosis infection, genital tract lymphoma, or endometritis due to uncommon pathogens. Women with these conditions should be carefully evaluated for signs of systemic infection and referred to a specialist for appropriate management.

Non-AIDS Complications

Early recognition and effective management of certain non-AIDS conditions could have implications on the reproductive and contraceptive choices available to women living with HIV/AIDS. HIV infection confers a heightened risk of CVD beyond that accounted for by traditional risk factors. The risk of CVD is up to 50 % higher for HIV-infected individuals relative to the general population [18–26]; this HIV-related risk may be more pronounced in women [22]. HIV infection precipitates premature CVD at an average age of 44 years, 10–15 years earlier than in the uninfected population [27, 28]. Finally, rates and the severity of CVD complications, such as ischemic cardiomyopathy and acute myocardial infarction, are aggravated by HIV infection [29–32]. Certain risk factors for CVD, such as diabetes mellitus and hyperlipidemia, may be more common in HIV-infected women, particularly in the setting of exposure to certain antiretroviral drugs.

Chronic liver disease due to chronic viral hepatitis, alcohol use, or fatty liver disease is also one of the leading causes of hospitalization and death in HIV-infected persons [17]. Similarly, HIV-infected patients are increasingly affected by kidney disease due to either traditional risk factors, such as diabetes and hypertension, HIV itself, drug toxicities, or other comorbidities, such as hepatitis [33]. The risk of venous thromboembolism may also be higher in HIV-infected patients [34]. Additionally, osteopenia and osteoporosis are seen in up to 70 % and 15 %, respectively, of HIV-infected patients in the USA [35–37], a risk that is over six and three times that of HIV-negative persons. Consequently, fracture rates several-fold higher than the general population are being reported in persons with HIV infection [38–42]. While the risk of certain non-AIDS-defining cancers, such as anal, liver, and lung cancer, have been shown to be higher in HIV-infected patients compared to the general population, the risk of breast cancer appears to be similar between HIV-infected and HIV-uninfected women [43]. Finally, HIV-infected women may also be at particular risk for neurocognitive disease [44], depression [45], and intimate partner violence [46].

Overview of the Importance of Balanced Family Planning for Women with HIV

Fertility Intentions

Several studies have explored the impact of HIV infection on fertility decisions and pregnancy rates [47–53]. Evidence suggests that sociocultural factors play a large role in fertility decision-making and that there is a rich and complex range of factors, including HIV status and HAART use, which influence reproductive decisions [53, 54]. Previous studies in Malawi [55] and Uganda [56] suggested that desire for children was lower among HIV-infected women in comparison to their uninfected peers. Among HIV-infected women in Côte d'Ivoire and Kenya, more education [57] and marriage [58] were associated with increased contraceptive use while in Uganda previous discussions of family planning with a partner and a current marital relationship increased the likelihood of contraceptive use [59]. Among HIV-infected women, contraceptive use might change over time on HAART [60, 61], possibly due to improved health, changing desires for family size, or concerns about interactions of contraceptives and HAART [62]. Previous studies have shown that among HIV-infected women in Rwanda, despite high initial contraceptive uptake after counseling, contraceptive use declined over time [60, 61]. Although these studies noted changes in fertility intentions and contraceptive use among those with HIV infection, the role of HAART on these decisions remains unclear.

There are few studies evaluating fertility intentions among women with HIV infection in the USA. A 2001 study showed that nearly 70 % of HIV-infected women (about one quarter of whom had no children) surveyed did not desire future fertility, and 31 % said if they became pregnant, they "definitely would" have an abortion [47]. Desires and expectations for future fertility in HIV-infected women were less than HIV-negative women; however, notably with the increase in HAART use, this difference may not be as sizable.

Importance of Family Planning

Prevention of unintended pregnancy among women with HIV infection is critical to prevent the unnecessary morbidity and mortality associated with pregnancy, and to prevent vertical transmission of HIV. The World Health Organization's (WHO's) 4-Component Strategy for prevention of maternal to child transmission includes: (1) prevention of HIV infection in women, especially young women; (2) prevention of unintended pregnancies in HIV-infected women; (3) prevention of transmission from HIV-infected women to their infants; and (4) support for HIV-infected women, their infants, and their families [63].

Health Risks Among HIV-Infected Women During Pregnancy

HIV infection contributes to the global maternal mortality with an estimated 56,100 pregnancy-related deaths attributed to HIV infection in 2011 [64]. HIV-infected pregnant women are at two- to tenfold higher risk of death compared to

HIV-negative pregnant women [65–67]; thus the CDC considers HIV/AIDS a condition that is associated with increased risk of adverse health events as a result of unintended pregnancy [68]. Infectious etiologies such as tuberculosis (TB), meningitis, and pneumonia are large contributors to this increased risk; however, puerperal sepsis, largely related to cesarean section and abortion, is also a major contributor [67]. Furthermore, there is higher morbidity in pregnancy among women with HIV infection with higher risks of prematurity [69] and low birth weight [70] compared to HIV-negative women. One should note however that it is challenging to distinguish the impact of HIV infection itself from the effects of poverty, addiction, or poor generalized health on pregnancy outcomes in this population. Interestingly, HAART appears to modify this risk, reducing the incidence of maternal morbidity and mortality [71, 72]. It should be noted that a vast majority of the data on health outcomes in pregnancy have been generated from studies in low-income countries where the maternal health infrastructure may be fragile. Data from the US and other high-income countries show better outcomes, though maternal morbidity and mortality in the setting of HIV infection are compromised even in this setting [73]. In general, most women in the USA with HIV infection who choose to have a child have uncomplicated pregnancies with favorable outcomes.

Transmission of HIV to the Child: Prevention of Maternal to Child Transmission (PMTCT)

In the late 1980s and early 1990s, perinatal transmission and progression of perinatally transmitted neonatal infection was a major health concern in the pediatric population. At that time, the risk of perinatal transmission of HIV was as high as 20–30 %, and factors predicting which women were more or less likely to transmit the virus were mostly unknown. Diagnosis of infection in the first year of life was still very difficult, and it was thought that infected babies faced an imminent risk of early childhood death. In these early days of the epidemic, the CDC recommended that HIV-infected women delay or defer childbirth until more was known about the virus [8].

However, since that time, the standard of intrapartum care in the setting of HIV infection has dramatically changed globally. Most treatment guidelines now recommend HAART for women during pregnancy regardless of CD4 T-cell counts or plasma HIV-RNA PCR (viral loads) [74, 75]. Those with viral loads greater than 400 copies/mL should receive zidovudine before vaginal or cesarean delivery, those with viral loads greater than 1,000 are recommended to undergo cesarean section before the onset of labor to reduce the risk of perinatal transmission, and all infants should be referred for prophylaxis after birth. With these recommendations, the risk of perinatal HIV transmission has dropped significantly in most countries, and in the USA, it is now lower than 3 % [6]. Public health authorities in many countries including the World Health Organization (WHO), U.S. Preventive Services Task Force (USPSTF), and the CDC have since revised their reproductive policy recommendations for HIV-infected women to a policy of non-directed reproductive counseling that is supportive of the patient's reproductive desires [76].

These recommendations notwithstanding, in 2010, 390,000 children became infected with the HIV globally, 90 % of which were acquired through mother-to-child transmission (MTCT) during pregnancy, labor and delivery, or breastfeeding, and nearly all of them were born in sub-Saharan Africa [77]. Global prevention of pediatric HIV infection therefore remains a sexual and reproductive health priority and is highlighted in 4 of the 8 United Nations Millennium Development Goals—promoting gender equality and empowering women, reducing child mortality, improving maternal health, and combating HIV/AIDS, malaria, and other diseases [78].

Transmission of HIV to the Partner

An additional issue of public health importance is that several studies have suggested that the risk of acquiring HIV or transmitting HIV to an uninfected partner may be higher during pregnancy [79, 80]. Although not all studies have supported this finding [81], this only adds to the imperative of effectively preventing unintended pregnancy as a HIV prevention effort. Condom use promotion and effective use of antiretroviral therapy is paramount to the prevention of transmission. In addition, as previously mentioned, the daily oral fixed-dose combination tablet containing tenofovir, disoproxil, fumarate, and emtricitabine is approved for use for HIV prevention among sexually active adults at risk for HIV infection and serves as an additional prevention tool for certain individuals.

Contraceptive Care: Setting and Counseling

Integration of Family Planning and HIV Care

In regions of the USA and globally with a high prevalence of HIV and sexually transmitted infections (STI) in heterosexual populations, target audiences for HIV/STI and family planning services overlap broadly and can benefit from, and in fact prefer, joint services [82–87]. Barriers to integration have roots in historical, philosophical, and structural differences in the areas of family planning and HIV prevention [88], which has resulted in disjointed services in many regions. Clinic staff often view family planning and HIV prevention as mutually independent services and are not trained to administer them together [89]. Service delivery in family planning clinics tends to be an instructive and fact-giving approach, while HIV-testing service delivery is often a client-centered, counseling approach [90]. Dual-method use is not widely promoted; family planning programs often emphasize condom use rather than dual-method use despite the high failure rate of condoms for prevention of pregnancy [88]. Given the importance of dual-method use, it is therefore encouraged that HIV prevention and family planning programs provide integrated services mutually reinforcing HIV prevention and family planning goals [84, 88, 91].

Barriers to Contraceptive Use

Common factors influencing nonuse of contraception are lack of female decision-making power [62], poor economic resources [92], low quality care of family planning services, and desire for large families. The influence of HIV infection and HAART on these factors is poorly understood. Fear of side effects from contraception may be amplified among HIV-infected individuals who are often sensitive to their health status [62].

Fertility-Based Contraceptive Counseling

As with all women, it is important to develop a reproductive health plan that allows them to decide whether and when to have children. For women with HIV infection, it is especially important to consider the status of their disease in this counseling. As noted, when HIV infection is well controlled, the risks of maternal complications and transmission potential to the infant are significantly reduced. It is also important to recognize that HIV infection is not in itself a reason to assume that a woman does not desire to have children or to encourage women to not have children. One recent study among women attending an HIV clinic in Atlanta reported that the most common form of contraception was a tubal ligation, but many of these women regretted this decision and desired future fertility [93]. This same study reported that only about half of the women who were sexually active had discussed their contraceptive plans with their provider within the past year. This observation highlights the fact that although many women with HIV infection may access care, their care may not include a discussion of their fertility intentions or contraceptive needs.

For a woman who desires fertility, it is important to counsel her or refer her to a practitioner who can counsel her regarding optimization of her HIV status, potential health risks of pregnancy, the risk of transmission to her child, choice of antiretroviral medications that are safer to use during pregnancy, and methods to conceive that will reduce exposure and transmission to an HIV-negative partner. Women with HIV can successfully have a healthy pregnancy and, with correct use of effective antiretroviral therapy, have a very low risk of transmission of HIV to the child. While outside the scope of this chapter, this topic is extremely important for the health of the mother and her child and is the subject of US Department of Health and Human Services (DHHS) guidelines [76].

Reproductive Health Care for Women with HIV

As encounters for contraception are frequently combined with encounters for general and/or gynecologic wellness, a few practical considerations should be kept in mind when providing gynecologic care for women with HIV. Beyond the increased health risks associated with HIV infection discussed previously, women with HIV may be at greater risk of STIs, more frequent outbreaks from herpes simplex virus (HSV) and condyloma, vaginitis with candida and bacterial vaginosis, irregular menses, and early menopause. Furthermore, HPV-related vulvar, vaginal, and cervical dysplasias may occur more commonly among HIV-infected women, who have higher rates of HPV persistence and progression to cancer. Based on these increased risks, when providing reproductive health care the following are recommended.

Screening for STIs

The CDC recommends yearly screening for syphilis, gonorrhea, and chlamydia in women with HIV [94]. Although the prevalence of these infections tends to be the same as the prevalence in HIV-negative women, co-infection with STIs other than HIV can increase the transmission of HIV. Diagnosis and treatment of syphilis, trichomonas, gonorrhea, and chlamydial infections are the same as in HIV-negative women. Pelvic inflammatory disease may be more severe or complicated in HIV-infected women, but management does not differ overall from HIV-negative women [95].

HIV-infected women are more likely to suffer from recurrent HSV outbreaks that are extremely painful and may take longer to resolve. Some women require suppressive therapy to reduce the frequency of outbreaks. Because there is evidence that HIV transmission may be increased among women with genital HSV even without active lesions and that the treatment of HSV can reduce plasma and genital HIV viral load [96–98], some providers support suppressive therapy for HIV-infected women with HSV seropositivity. This is not a universal recommendation, however, as the most recent clinical trials have not shown a reduction in HIV or HSV transmission risk [99, 100]. Active and suppressive treatment of HSV for women with HIV infection typically requires higher doses and longer durations of appropriate antiviral agents. Current recommendations are available from the CDC (http://www.cdc.gov/std/treatment/2010/genital-ulcers.htm#hsv). Importantly, if women fail to respond to treatment, a viral culture should be obtained with sensitivity testing done for evaluation of resistant infections. Similar to HSV, chancroid (ulcers that occur following infection with *H. ducreyi*) requires close monitoring and typically longer therapy for resolution among HIV-infected women and should be treated per CDC guidelines.

Cervical Dysplasia and Cervical Cancer Screening

Current cervical cancer screening recommendations for HIV-infected women call for screening twice in the first year after diagnosis of HIV infection and then annually if the first two test results are normal. Although the incidence of cervical dysplasia is increased in women with HIV, women who undergo the recommended screening for and treatment of cervical dysplasia are not at increased risk of cervical cancer [95]. The role of HPV testing in the screening of HIV-infected women for cervical dysplasia has not been established but is likely to be the subject of future guidelines.

Vulvar, Vaginal, and Rectal Dysplasia, and Cancer

Although there are no well-established guidelines for screening for vulvar or vaginal dysplasia, a careful vulvar and vaginal examination should be done whenever a pelvic examination is performed. HIV-infected women should, therefore, undergo a pelvic examination annually at a minimum, based on cervical cancer screening guidelines. There are no guidelines for rectal pap smears among HIV-infected women; thus at this time a comprehensive evaluation of risk factors and symptoms in combination with an annual external examination at the time of a pelvic examination is recommended. Clinical manifestations of vulvar intraepithelial neoplasia (VIN) and vaginal intraepithelial neoplasia (VAIN) in HIV-infected women are similar as for women without HIV infection. Approximately 50 % of women with VIN are asymptomatic. In symptomatic women, the most common complaint is vulvar pruritus; other presentations include perineal pain or burning, dysuria, a visible lesion, or a palpable abnormality.

Human Papillomavirus (HPV) Vaccination

Efficacy of HPV vaccination in HIV-infected women is currently unknown and studies addressing this question are in progress [101, 102]. Many believe that, similar to the general population, HPV vaccination would offer some benefit to women with HIV infection, and since it is not contraindicated with immunosuppression, is recommended by some guidelines for HIV-infected males and females ages 13–26 years [75]. Both quadrivalent (for HPV types 6, 11, 16, 18) and bivalent (for HPV types 16 and 18) formulations are available, but the quadrivalent vaccine offers the additional potential benefit of prevention of anogenital warts associated with HPV types 6 and 11, which can be extensive in immunosuppressed patients.

Vulvovaginal Candidiasis (VVC) and Bacterial Vaginosis (BV)

The incidence of VVC is higher among HIV-infected women compared to uninfected women and correlates to the severity of immunodeficiency. Further, these infections may recur frequently especially among women with poorly controlled HIV infection. Treatment for VVC should not differ for HIV-infected women from that of uninfected women with the added importance of optimizing their HIV control [94, 103]. Recurrent infections, defined as four or more episodes each year, should be treated as complicated infections and treated with prolonged therapy. Women with CD4 counts less than 200 may have more persistent BV infections than those with well-controlled HIV. Similar to VVC, the treatment for BV in HIV positive women is the same as in uninfected women [94, 95].

Menstrual Problems

Evaluation of abnormal uterine bleeding among HIV-infected women should follow the same principles as among uninfected women. Evaluation should include the same endocrinologic evaluations (such as thyroid stimulating hormone [TSH] and prolactin levels), infection evaluation (such as gonorrhea and Chlamydia testing), imaging studies, and endometrial biopsy when indicated. Treatment to improve bleeding should consider the future fertility goals and expectations of the patient in terms of desired bleeding pattern.

Menopause

Menopause may occur earlier in HIV-positive women than HIV-negative women for reasons that remain poorly understood. Early menopause and the associated hypoestrogenemia may further heighten CVD and fragility bone disease risks for women living with HIV/AIDS [104]. As with HIV-negative women, hormone therapy may be considered for management of bothersome symptoms. Little has been studied about the interaction of hormone therapy with antiretroviral medications. A transdermal route may avoid first-pass metabolism and decrease drug interactions [105].

Starting a Birth Control Method

Taking a History

Prior to starting a contraceptive method for any woman, clinicians should obtain a directed history. This will include a medical history, contraceptive history, psychosocial and sexual history, as well as an assessment of her beliefs, possible misconceptions and fears, and her expectations with regard to use of contraception.

For women with HIV, specific history questions should include the following:

1 Do you have any medical problems? Do you have high blood pressure or diabetes? Do you get frequent headaches or migraines? Have you ever had a blood clot? Do you have active liver disease? Have you ever had cancer? Do you smoke?

Medical conditions or behaviors that limit the use of certain contraceptives need to be assessed among all women, including women with HIV. Other medical comorbidities such as hypertension, diabetes, breast cancer, or vascular disease will be important to consider when choosing a contraceptive method. Important potential contraindications will be present from conditions that may impact their vascular risk and increase their risk of blood clots including stroke associated with combined hormonal contraception. For example, it is important to probe about headaches to determine if a patient has migraines with aura that would be a contraindication to combined hormonal contraceptive methods. Some chronic medical conditions may impact women with HIV infection more commonly than those who do not have HIV infection. For example, liver diseases occur more frequently among HIV-infected women and are considered contraindicated with some contraceptives (see Chap. 18). After attaining a thorough history, referring to the CDC Medical Eligibility Criteria for Contraceptive Use (MEC) will be helpful in considering if any current medical comorbidities will limit the use of a specific contraceptive method [106].

2. What Medications Are You Currently Taking?

There are several specific medications that have drug interactions with different contraceptives. To review potential medication contraindications, the use of checklists for this purpose is encouraged as often asking directly without probing questions may overlook important issues to consider. Antiretroviral medications that are important to consider are certain protease inhibitors such as ritonavir and other pharmacologic boosters such as cobicistat that interact with the cytochrome p450 pathway and may impact the efficacy of both the contraceptive and antiretroviral drug. Antibiotics and antifungal medications are generally safe to use with any of the contraceptive methods. As new medications are developed and integrated into clinical care, it is important to evaluate for potential interactions prior to initiation. For details regarding drug interactions, including those with antibiotics and antifungals, see Chap. 20. Drug interactions with antiretroviral drugs and contraceptives are reviewed later in this chapter.

3. Have You Had Tuberculosis (TB) or Are You Currently Taking Medication for TB?

Tuberculosis is more common among HIV-infected individuals due to their immunosuppression. Although uncommon in the USA, pelvic TB is one of the rare conditions where an intrauterine device (IUD) is not recommended. Per the CDC MEC, pelvic TB is considered a category 4 (method should not be used) for initiation of an IUD and a category 3 (risks usually outweigh benefits) for continuation of an IUD [106]. Thus in most cases, IUDs should not be placed and should be removed for women with pelvic TB. History of successfully treated pelvic TB, however, should not preclude IUD use.

Rifampin and rifabutin, which are commonly used for treatment of TB, are considered a category 3 for combined hormonal contraceptives, progestin-only pills, and contraceptive implants due to drug–drug interactions. For details regarding drug interactions, see Chap. 20.

4. Have You Recently Been Ill? Were You Recently Started on HAART? What Is Your Most Recent CD4 Count?

Accessing the individuals' current HIV status is important before initiating a contraceptive method. HIV is not a contraindication for initiating any contraceptive, but caution should be exercised in placing an IUD in a woman with late-stage AIDS who is not receiving antiretroviral medications. Although IUD use over time is not associated with an increase in pelvic infections and may actually reduce the risk of pelvic infections, there is a slightly increased risk in pelvic infection over the first few weeks after placement. In women with AIDS who are severely immunocompromised with low CD4 T-cell counts or an active opportunistic infection, it may be prudent to delay an IUD placement until active opportunistic infections are controlled and/or immune status is improved with HAART (risks for these individuals typically outweigh the benefits in a CDC category 3 recommendation). Of note, these women are still at risk for pregnancy, and it is particularly important to protect from unplanned pregnancy given the increased risk of poor maternal and fetal outcomes. For these women, initiating an effective contraceptive immediately while concurrently stabilizing their HIV infection is a priority. Once their HIV is controlled with HAART, an IUD may be placed and may remain without increased risk of pelvic infection even if clinical status declines.

5. What Have You Used Before? What Have You Been Told? What Are You Looking for with a Contraceptive Method?

Many women have had prior experience with different birth control methods. This experience may impact their willingness to use a method, both favorably and unfavorably. Added on to their prior experience, many women have been told that they cannot use specific methods of contraception. The information that they have received may not always be accurate. It is therefore important to start out discussing what their knowledge and perceptions are regarding contraception as this will direct your discussion and may impact contraceptive selection and continuation.

Lastly, what are their expectations with their contraceptive? Are they looking for something that is easy to use or something that makes their periods lighter? Choice of contraceptive should be directed toward addressing the patients' specific goals. For example, women who are seeking to continue to have regular predictable cycles should consider combined hormonal contraceptives or the copper IUD. A discussion additionally should focus on the tiers of contraceptive efficacy. For example, tubal ligation, IUDs, and implants are the most effective methods to prevent pregnancy. For women desiring a highly effective long-term option, long-acting reversible contraceptives (LARCs) methods should be encouraged.

Choosing a Method

In choosing a contraceptive, you must work with the patient to identify her key goals, review the information, and help her find a method that will be best for her. Having HIV itself is not a contraindication to the use of any contraceptive method (Table 6.1); however, there are some issues to consider with each method.

For the most part, LARCs are ideal first choice methods to consider for this population given their superior effectiveness and safety profile for most women. LARC methods are user independent, meaning they do not require action by the patient to maintain effectiveness, such as the need to take pills daily or injections every 3 months. These methods are extremely safe with low risk of complications from use and are easily reversible with rapid return of fertility should the woman desire pregnancy. Furthermore, although the initial investment is high, LARCs are the most cost-effective methods for use over time as there is no additional cost accrued for the duration of contraceptive use until replaced. Further, these methods can be safely placed immediately postpartum and postabortion.

Levonorgestrel IUD (Mirena)

This LARC method is an ideal choice for many women with HIV, given that it is in the highest tier

Table 6.1 US medical eligibility criteria for contraceptive use for HIV [68]

Condition	Sub-condition	Combined pill, patch, ring	Progestin-only pill	Injection	Implant	LNG-IUD I	LNG-IUD C	Copper IUD I	Copper IUD C
HIV	High risk	1	1	1	1	2	2	2	2
	HIV infected (see also "Drug Interactions" section and Chap. 20)	1	1	1	1	2	2	2	2
	AIDS (see "Drug Interactions" section and Chap. 20)	1	1	1	1	3	2[a]	3	2[a]
	Clinically well on therapy					2	2	2	2

1 = Use without restrictions; 2 = Advantages generally outweigh the risks; 3 = Risks usually outweigh the advantages; 4 = Unacceptable health risks (method not to be used) [107]
[a]Clarification for continuation of IUD: IUD users with AIDS should be closely monitored for pelvic infection

for effectiveness, with protection from pregnancy for 5 years with some evidence of off-label efficacy for up to 7 years [108], high continuation rates, and an excellent safety and tolerability profile. Typical use and perfect use pregnancy rates with use of the levonorgestrel IUD (LNG-IUD) are equivalent since it is a user independent method, with 0.2 unplanned pregnancies per 100 women in the first year of use [109, 110]. As mentioned above, if a woman is clinically unstable with late-stage AIDS and/or active opportunistic infections, placement may need to be delayed. However, once placed, it is an ideal method for continued use irrespective of clinical status. Further, there is some evidence to suggest that the LNG-IUD may reduce the risk of pelvic inflammatory disease (PID) as its mechanism of action is to thicken the cervical mucus, providing a barrier to semen and ascending infections [111]. Additional benefits include less bleeding, which would reduce transmission risk with the handling of infectious sanitary products. Further, the LNG-IUD offers protection of the endometrium that is important for women with anovulatory cycles or other risk factors for endometrial cancer. That said, women must know prior to placement that their bleeding pattern will change, they may have irregular bleeding, lighter menses, or no bleeding. Placement of an IUD is easily accomplished during a clinic visit with mild patient discomfort of short duration. Patient counseling should focus on initial irregular bleeding with the LNG-IUD that typically improves with continued use over the first 3–6 months. Women who are at high risk for HIV are likely at high risk for other pelvic infections as well. Keep in mind that a diagnosis of cervicitis or PID in a woman with an IUD does *not* necessitate removal of the IUD and women should be encouraged to keep it in place unless PID persists or worsens despite appropriate treatment.

Copper IUD (Paragard)

Another LARC method that should be considered among the best methods for women with HIV infection is the copper IUD. With exceptional protection from pregnancy lasting for 10 years with some evidence supporting efficacy for up to 12 years [112, 113], the copper IUD can be safely placed in most women with very few restrictions. Unintended pregnancy rates with copper IUD use are low with 0.6 and 0.8 pregnancies per 100 women in the first year of use for perfect and typical use, respectively [110]. This is an ideal method for women who desire to see a regular cycle every month and who are willing to tolerate potential increases in bleeding or cramping during their cycles. There are few contraindications to placement; similar to the LNG-IUD, as long as a woman is clinically stable with regard to her HIV, the IUD can safely be placed.

Contraceptive Implants

The contraceptive implant is a LARC method similarly ideal for HIV-infected women with few exceptions that would limit its safe initiation and use. Nexplanon (Merck, Whitehouse Station, NJ, USA), an etonogestrel implant, is a single rod device that once placed can last for up to 3 years. Other implants that are not currently available in the USA but are widely used in Africa include the levonorgestrel implants Jadelle and Sino-implant, which each last for 4–5 years with high typical and perfect use effectiveness (0.05 unintended pregnancies per 100 women in the first year of use for both typical and perfect use [110]). There have been case reports of increased pregnancy rates when etonogestrel implants are used in patients taking the antiretroviral drug efavirenz, a non-nucleotide reverse transcriptase inhibitor, but data are limited to make conclusive recommendations regarding the use of the implant for women on efavirenz [114] (see the section "Drug Interactions with Antiretroviral Regimens").

Injectable Contraceptives

Depo-medroxyprogesterone acetate (DMPA) is marketed as Depo-Provera (Pfizer Inc., New York NY, USA) in the USA. Other progestin-only contraceptive injections are available in other countries. DMPA is highly convenient, requiring injections only every 3 months. With perfect use, defined as receiving an intramuscular injection every 11–13 weeks, there is a 0.2 % pregnancy rate in the first year, but a 6 % pregnancy rate with typical use [110] The most common reason for discontinuing the method is changes in bleeding pattern, but discontinuation rates are much lower among women who are adequately counseled on the possibility of irregular or heavy bleeding, or cessation of menstrual bleeding. DMPA may remain equally effective up to 15 weeks after the injection, which allows for some forgiveness in the "three month" rule [115]. However, this comes hand in hand with the disadvantage that return to fertility after discontinuation may be 9–10 months after the last injection. DMPA may cause increased weight gain in comparison to other hormonal contraceptive methods (see Chap. 10).

DMPA and other injectable progestins are widely available and affordable around the world, but some studies in high-risk populations outside the USA have raised concerns about the possibility that DMPA increases transmissibility of HIV from HIV-infected women to their uninfected partners, and increases susceptibility of HIV-negative women to the virus. However, the US Medical Eligibility Criteria continue to recommend DMPA as a "category 1," indicating that the method can be used without restrictions, although with a clarification statement that describes the inconclusive nature of the evidence and instruction to recommend condoms for prevention of HIV in these populations [107]. This topic is discussed further in the section "Controversies and Research Gaps."

Combined Hormonal Contraceptives

Combined hormonal contraceptives containing both progestin and estrogen to achieve their contraceptive benefit can be delivered via pills (many brands marketed in the USA), the transdermal patch (only available as Ortho Evra [Ortho-McNeil Pharmaceutical Inc., Raritan, NJ, USA] in the USA), and hormone-eluting vaginal ring (NuvaRing, Merck, Whitehouse Station, NJ, USA). Oral contraceptives are still the most popular hormonal contraceptive method in the USA. These methods have the benefits of being private and patient-controlled, and not requiring active involvement of medical providers after the initial prescription is given. They can be used in a cyclic way that simulates a natural monthly menstrual cycle for women who prefer that. On the other hand, they can also be used in a continuous manner to suppress menses when that is desired. With perfect use, combined contraceptive methods have a 0.3 % failure rate but a 9 % typical use pregnancy rate in the first year of use [110]. While combined contraceptive methods are recommended as safe in women with HIV or those at high risk of HIV (designated a "category 1" denoting a method that can be used without restriction in the CDC MEC), they may be contraindicated or used with caution in women who are using certain antiretroviral drugs (see the section "Drug Interactions with Antiretroviral Regimens"). As in HIV-negative women, estrogen-containing contraceptives are contraindicated in women with a history of venous thromboembolism (VTE), hypercoagulability, cardiovascular disease, migraine with aura, or smoking over the age of 35, due to increased risk of VTE or stroke in these women. Therefore, it is important to refer to the CDC MEC for guidance on contraceptive method selection for all women with complex medical conditions [106].

Progestin-Only Pills

Progestin-only pills (POPs) formulated in the USA contain 0.35 mg norethindrone. They carry the same rate of unintended pregnancy as combined contraceptives, 0.3 % with perfect use and 9 % with typical use [110]. Patients must be counseled that they should take the pill at the same time each day to provide effective contraception as the therapeutic level of each pill lasts only 25 h. The ideal candidate for this contraceptive is one who is highly reliable and has a regular daily schedule. Unlike estrogen-containing contraceptives, progestin-only pills are not contraindicated in women at risk for hypercoagulability. However, like combined contraceptives, progestin-only pills may alter and may be altered when combined with certain antiretroviral drugs (see the section "Drug Interactions with Antiretroviral Regimens").

Male and Female Condoms

Traditional male condoms have a typical use failure rate of 18 % [110], and thus are not a highly reliable single choice for contraception. However, no contraceptive method other than condoms can prevent the transmission of HIV or STIs. The simultaneous use of highly effective contraception and condom use, termed dual protection, should be strongly encouraged in women with HIV and those women at high risk of acquiring HIV in order to avoid STI transmission and acquisition. Although not many high-quality studies comparing male to female condoms exist, available evidence suggests that female condoms prevent STIs including HIV as well as male condoms [116, 117]. Every contraceptive method should be presented in conjunction with condoms as a dual preventative strategy. In discussing condom use, a discussion of both the male and female condom is essential, reviewing strategies to increase use in the context of the individual's sexual relationships, how to obtain and how to use these types of condoms correctly.

Spermicides

Spermicides are frequently used with other barrier methods of contraception such as condoms, sponges, and diaphragms. When used alone, perfect use has an 18 % failure rate, and typical use a 29 % failure rate [109]. Nonoxynol-9 is the most common active ingredient in spermicides in the USA. Besides having a high failure rate, it also may cause irritation and epithelial erosions of the vagina with repeated use. This may increase the opportunity for HIV transmission. In one study of high-risk women, those who used nonoxynol-9 more than three times a day had increased rates of HIV transmission [118]. For this reason, spermicides are labeled as a "4" in the CDC MEC—method is not to be used due to unacceptable health risks—in women with HIV and women at high risk for acquiring HIV [106].

Microbicides

Studies are currently ongoing to test vaginal microbicides that can help prevent HIV in high-risk populations. While the spermicide nonoxynol-9 is effective in vitro at killing HIV virions, as previously mentioned, in vivo it was associated with a higher risk of HIV transmission, likely due to disruption in the vaginal mucosa [118]. Clinical trials involving a topical gel containing the antiretroviral drug tenofovir have shown some promise in reducing the risk of HIV transmission. Other exciting technologies in development are microbicide-eluting vaginal rings, which eventually may be able to be combined with contraceptive methods to prevent both pregnancy and HIV in a single system. At this time, no effective microbicide is commercially available [119].

Lactational Amenorrhea

For HIV-infected mothers, recommendations in the USA are to bottle-feed infants to reduce the risk of postnatal HIV transmission via breast milk. This recommendation is different in developing countries where clean water, milk, or formula availability may limit adequate and safe nutrition for the baby. HIV transmission risk from breast milk can vary based upon maternal viral load, antiretroviral medications, and exclusivity of feeding. However, in countries where supplemental access to enriched formula is available, it is currently believed that the risks of breastfeeding in terms of HIV transmission to the child outweigh the potential benefits to the mother and the baby.

Cervical Cap or Diaphragm

Cervical caps and diaphragms are barrier contraceptives that are not commonly used. These methods have low levels of typical use effectiveness [110] and studies have shown that they do not reduce the risk of HIV transmission [120].

Emergency Contraceptives

Currently available emergency contraceptives include both the emergency contraceptive pills and the copper IUD. For pills, there are currently two drugs available for use, levonorgestrel-based regimens and ulipristal acetate. Ulipristal is more effective than levonorgestrel-based emergency contraceptives from 4 to 5 days after unprotected intercourse [121], and neither is recommended as reliable pregnancy prevention more than 5 days after unprotected intercourse. There is little data on the influence of HAART regimens on the effectiveness of these drug regimens; however there is some suggestion that the effectiveness will be reduced when taken with drugs that impact cytochrome p450 (see the section "Drug Interactions with Antiretroviral Regimens"). That said, as an "emergency" regimen, it is a last effort to reduce the risk of pregnancy when more effective contraceptive methods were not employed or a condom slipped or broke. For women using condoms as a primary birth control method, information about emergency contraception is imperative. Although some formulations are available over the counter, a prescription may be most affordable for certain patients and should be provided when appropriate. As the copper IUD is the most effective form of emergency contraceptive, it avoids all potential challenges associated with drug interactions, and offers long-term protection from pregnancy, this is an ideal method to promote in the setting when emergency contraception is needed.

Continuation of Contraception

For many contraceptive methods, anticipatory guidance can help avoid discontinuation of contraception. Many studies show that counseling on changes in bleeding patterns anticipated by contraceptive methods, such as progestin-only methods, helps reduce discontinuation of these methods. Many women will be reassured that although progestin-only methods cause irregular bleeding, for most women, the overall quantity of bleeding will be reduced and may completely stop after 1 year of use. Frequent visits when initiating a new method of contraception can help alleviate concerns. Women with HIV may also have frequent changes in their health status—e.g., changes in HAART regimens or development of liver disease—that may necessitate frequent reevaluation of the appropriateness of their contraceptive plan.

Drug Interactions with Antiretroviral Regimens

Antiretroviral drugs may affect the level of steroid hormones in the blood and vice versa, owing to shared metabolic pathways utilizing hepatic cytochrome P450 [68, 75, 76]. This could potentially change the effectiveness and/or safety of either the contraceptive method or the antiretroviral drug. Several antiretroviral drugs (ARVs) have interactions with combined oral contraceptives that either decrease or increase blood levels of ethinyl estradiol or the progestin component, which could potentially decrease contraceptive effectiveness or increase estrogen- or progestin-related adverse effects, respectively. In particular, ritonavir-boosted protease inhibitors may substantially decrease the bioavailable steroid hormone [122, 123] in combined oral contraceptives, which may lead to contraceptive failure. The use of oral contraceptives, both combined and progestin-only, in women on ritonavir-boosted protease inhibitors is considered a category 3 per the CDC MEC [68], meaning that the risks of use typically outweigh the benefits of use. The newer pharmacologic booster cobicistat also affects the cytochrome P450 system and may result in increased progestin levels. The effects of this are not yet known and current guidelines for the USMEC do not specify specific guidelines to avoid these combined regimens. However, whenever possible, alternative contraceptives should be considered. Neither DMPA nor LNG-IUDs have been demonstrated to significantly interact with antiretroviral regimens [124]. The action of the copper IUD is independent of drug metabolism mechanisms and carries no theoretical or actual interactions with antiretroviral therapy.

No interactions have been reported between nucleoside reverse transcription inhibitor (NRTI) drugs and contraceptives. The clinical significance of smaller alterations in hormonal bioavailability from non-nucleoside reverse transcription inhibitor (NNRTI) drugs is unclear. The NIH Guidelines for Antiretroviral Use recommend the use of alternative or additional contraceptive methods for the use of certain NNRTIs [125]; however the CDC MEC currently considers use of progestin-only pills, hormonal implants, and all combined hormonal methods to be a category 2, meaning that the benefits typically outweigh the risks [106]. Overall, data are relatively limited and the clinical implications of these findings are unclear. Recommendations regarding other combined hormonal contraceptive methods are based on combined oral contraceptive pill use, as very little evidence is available regarding the effects of ARVs on bioavailable hormone from transdermal patches or vaginal rings [126]. Small studies of HIV-infected women receiving DMPA while on ART showed no significant interactions between DMPA and efavirenz, nevirapine, nelfinavir, or NRTI drugs [110, 127–129].

Although the data on efavirenz and birth defects are limited, due to potential teratogenic effects, it is often not used as a first-line option in women of childbearing age. If it is used, it should be accompanied by a very reliable contraceptive plan. Unfortunately, efavirenz can lead to decreases in circulating progestins [114, 130]. For progestin-containing methods, the degree of reduction in effectiveness of these methods may vary based on the method. For example, DMPA has very high circulating levels of progestin, so small reductions in the progestin concentration will likely not impact its effectiveness. Etonogestrel implants, on the other hand, have lower circulating progestin levels such that small reductions could impact the method effectiveness. The use of efavirenz has also been associated with increased risk of failure of progestin implants in case reports [114]. However, given the limited data, the current CDC MEC [68] recommendations consider the use of efavirenz a category 2 for use. There are no data at this time regarding the use of efavirenz and levonorgestrel-containing IUDs.

A summary of recommendations regarding specific antiretroviral drugs, their effect on hormone levels, and current USMEC guidelines is given in Table 6.2. Notably, current recommendations [75] support that concerns about pharmacokinetic interactions between oral and implant hormonal contraceptives and ARVs should not

Table 6.2 Antiretroviral drugs interactions with hormonal contraception and current recommendations for use

Antiretroviral drug	Contraceptive effects	Antiretroviral effects	Drug-specific comments
NRTIs			
CDC MEC Category 1: Combined pill, patch, ring; progestin only pill; injection; implant 2: LNG-IUD; copper IUD continuation 2/3: LNG-IUD; copper IUD insertion			
All NRTIs	No known effect Tenofovir: EE ↔, NGM ↔ [131]	No known effect Tenofovir ↔ with COC [131] Zidovudine ↔ with COC/ DMPA [132]	May be used without restriction
NNRTIs			
CDC MEC Category 1: Injection 2: Combined pill, patch, ring; progestin only pill; implant; LNG-IUD and copper IUD continuation 2/3:LNG-IUD; copper IUD insertion			
Efavirenz	EE ↑ [133], EE ↔ [134], NGM ↓ [134], LNG ↓ [134], ↓ ETG (implant) possible [114]	Efavirenz ↔ with COC [133, 134]	Use alternative or additional methods
	MPA ↔ [129]		Effectiveness of emergency postcoital contraception may be diminished [123]
	No ovulations during three cycles [127, 129]	Efavirenz ↔ with DMPA [129]	No dose adjustment necessary
Etravirine	EE ↔, NET ↔ [135]	Etravirine ↑ with COC but concurrent administration generally safe and well tolerated [135]	No dosage adjustment necessary
Nevirapine	EE ↔, NET ↔ [136]		Use alternative or additional methods
	MPA: ↔ [129] No ovulations during three cycles [129]		No dosage adjustment necessary
Rilpivirine	EE ↔, NET ↔ [137]		No dosage adjustment necessary
Protease inhibitors			
CDC MEC Category (ritonavir-boosted protease inhibitors) 1: Injection 2: Implant; LNG-IUD and copper IUD continuation 2/3:LNG-IUD; copper IUD insertion 3: Combined pill, patch, ring; progestin-only pill			
CDC MEC Category (protease inhibitors without ritonavir) No comment			

Atazanavir/ritonavir	EE ↓, NGM ↑ [138]		COC should contain ≥35 μg EE. COCs containing progestins other than NET or NGM have not been studied
Darunavir/ritonavir	EE ↓, NET ↔ [139]	Darunavir ↔ [139]	Use alternative or additional method
Fosamprenavir/ritonavir	EE ↓ [140, 141], NET ↓ [141]	Amprenavir ↔, ritonavir ↑, Elevated liver transaminases [140]	Use alternative or additional method
Lopinavir/ritonavir	EE ↓, NET ↔ [142], NGM ↑ [130]		Use alternative or additional method
Tipranavir/ritonavir	EE ↓ [17], NET ↔ [143]	↑ Skin and musculoskeletal adverse events; possible drug hypersensitivity reaction [144]	Use alternative or additional method
Atazanavir	EE ↑, NET ↑ [138]		Use COC ≤30 μg EE. COCs with <25 μg EE or progestins other than NET or NGM have not been studied
Fosamprenavir	EE ↑, NET ↑ [145]	Amprenavir ↓ [145]	Use alternative method
Nelfinavir	EE ↓, NET↓ [146]		Use alternative or additional method
	MPA ↔ [129]	Nelfinavir ↔ [129]	No adjustment necessary
Integrase inhibitors CDC MEC Category No comment			
Elvitegravir/Cobicistat/tenofovir/emtricitabine	EE ↓, NGM ↑ [122]		The effects of increases in progestin are not fully known. Weigh the risks and benefits of the drug, and consider alternative contraceptive method
Raltegravir	EE ↔, NGM ↔ [147]		Safe to use
CCR5 inhibitors CDC MEC Category No comment			
Maraviroc	No clinically significant effect		Safe to use

COC combined oral contraceptive, *DMPA* depot medroxyprogesterone acetate, *ARV* antiretroviral, *NRTI* nucleoside reverse transcriptase inhibitor, *NNRTI* non-nucleoside reverse transcriptase, *EE* ethinyl estradiol, *NET* norethindrone, *NGM* norgestimate, *ETG* etonogestrel, *LNG* levonorgestrel, *IUD* intrauterine device, *MPA* medroxyprogesterone acetate, *left-right arrow* no change or change ≤30 %, *up arrow* increase >30 %, *down arrow* decrease >30 % in any contraceptive pharmacokinetic parameters prevent clinicians from prescribing hormonal contraceptives for women on ART if that is their preferred contraceptive method. If a woman chooses to use hormonal contraceptives and drug interactions with ARVs are known or potential, then additional or alternative contraceptive methods may be recommended. Particularly, consistent use of condoms to prevent transmission of HIV and protect against other sexually transmitted diseases is recommended for all HIV-infected women and their partners, regardless of contraceptive use.

Controversies and Research Gaps

Concerns Regarding Increased HIV Acquisition, Transmission, and Disease Progression

Some observational studies have raised concerns about an increased risk of acquiring HIV in HIV-negative women and shedding HIV in HIV-positive women using hormonal contraception, particularly DMPA [148, 149]. Theoretically, progestins could increase susceptibility to and acquisition of HIV by thinning the vaginal epithelium, increasing the frequency of target cells, and modulating the systemic immune system [150]. However, the available population-based studies are inconsistent, underpowered, and often flawed [151]. The literature is even weaker on a possible association between oral contraceptive pills and HIV risk. No studies have examined the association of HIV susceptibility with progestin-containing implants or intrauterine devices, hormonal patches, or hormonal rings [151]. Because of the heterogeneous outcomes and low quality of the studies available on hormonal contraception and HIV risk, both the WHO and the revised USMEC put no restrictions (category 1) on contraceptive use in women at high risk for acquiring HIV or HIV-positive women. At the same time, both MECs make strong recommendations that because of the unclear information, women with HIV or those at risk for HIV should always use condoms to prevent HIV transmission [106, 107].

Theoretical concerns together with one randomized controlled trial have also called attention to the possibility of accelerated HIV/AIDS disease progression in HIV-positive women using hormonal contraception. A study by Stringer et al. [152] randomized HIV positive postpartum women to receive copper IUD or hormonal contraception (including DMPA, combined oral contraceptives, and progestin-only pills), showing an increased risk of HIV progression to CD4 count below 200 cells/mL in the hormonal contraception users. However, this study is flawed by differential losses to follow up, high rates of switching of methods, and a substandard control group (copper IUD, for which implications on HIV progression have not been studied) [153]. Other observational studies published on hormonal contraception and HIV progression show no association [154, 155].

Conclusion: Key Points in Providing Care

- Effective contraception can reduce maternal and pediatric morbidity and mortality from unintended pregnancies complicated by HIV.
- Desires for planned pregnancy should not be overlooked in women with HIV. Addressing fertility intentions can help optimize health status before pregnancy occurs.
- Family planning and STI prevention services should be integrated whenever possible as they share common goals.
- Regular STI and cervical cancer screening are critical parts of routine reproductive health care in women with HIV. Recommendations for screening may differ from those for HIV-negative women.
- Long-acting reversible contraceptives (LARCs) are highly effective and ideal for most women with HIV.
- Spermicides should be avoided in women with HIV and women at high risk for acquiring HIV.
- Interactions exist between antiretroviral drugs and oral contraceptives that may limit contraceptive effectiveness.

- All women, especially HIV-positive women and those women at high risk of acquiring HIV, should be encouraged to use "dual protection" by combining a highly effective contraceptive with condoms during sex to maximally prevent pregnancy and STI infection.

References

1. Centers for Disease Control and Prevention (CDC). Pneumocystis pneumonia – Los Angeles. MMWR. 1981;30:250–2.
2. Ribeiro PS, Jacobsen KH, Mathers CD, Garcia-Moreno C. Priorities for women's health from the Global Burden of Disease study. Int J Gynaecol Obstet. 2008;102(1):82–90. Epub 2008/04/05.
3. World Health Organization. Women and health: today's evidence, tomorrow's agenda. Geneva: World Health Organization; 2009.
4. Joint United Nations Programme on HIV/AIDS (UNAIDS). Global report: UNAIDS report on the global AIDS epidemic; 2013.
5. Centers for Disease Control and Prevention (CDC). Monitoring selected national HIV prevention and care objectives by using HIV surveillance data – United States and 6 U.S. dependent areas – 2010. HIV Surveill Suppl Rep. 2012;17(3). Epub Jun 2012.
6. Centers for Disease Control and Prevention (CDC). Estimated HIV incidence among adults and adolescents in the United States, 2007–2010. HIV Surveill Suppl Rep. 2012;17(4). Epub Dec 2012.
7. Centers for Disease Control and Prevention (CDC). Estimated HIV incidence among adults and adolescents in the United States, 2007–2010. HIV Surveill Suppl Rep. 2012;17(4).
8. Centers for Disease Control and Prevention (CDC). Recommendations for assisting in the prevention of perinatal transmission of human T-lymphotropic virus type III/lymphadenopathy-associated virus and acquired immunodeficiency syndrome. MMWR. 1985;34(48):721–6. 31–2. Epub 1985/12/06.
9. Abdool Karim Q, Abdool Karim SS, Frohlich JA, Grobler AC, Baxter C, Mansoor LE, et al. Effectiveness and safety of tenofovir gel, an antiretroviral microbicide, for the prevention of HIV infection in women. Science. 2010;329(5996):1168–74. Epub 2010/07/21.
10. Cohen MS, Chen YQ, McCauley M, Gamble T, Hosseinipour MC, Kumarasamy N, et al. Prevention of HIV-1 infection with early antiretroviral therapy. N Engl J Med. 2011;365(6):493–505. Epub 2011/07/20.
11. Reynolds SJ, Makumbi F, Nakigozi G, Kagaayi J, Gray RH, Wawer M, et al. HIV-1 transmission among HIV-1 discordant couples before and after the introduction of antiretroviral therapy. AIDS. 2011;25(4):473–7. Epub 2010/12/17.
12. Cunningham WE, Andersen RM, Katz MH, Stein MD, Turner BJ, Crystal S, et al. The impact of competing subsistence needs and barriers on access to medical care for persons with human immunodeficiency virus receiving care in the United States. Med Care. 1999;37(12):1270–81. Epub 1999/12/22.
13. Fleishman JA, Gebo KA, Reilly ED, Conviser R, Christopher Mathews W, Todd Korthuis P, et al. Hospital and outpatient health services utilization among HIV-infected adults in care 2000–2002. Med Care. 2005;43(9 Suppl):III40–52. Epub 2005/08/24.
14. Ribaudo H, Smith K, Robbins G, Flexner C, Haubrich R, Chen Y, et al. Race differences in the efficacy of initial ART on HIV infection in randomized trials undertaken by ACTG. 18th Conference on retroviruses and opportunistic infections, Boston, MA, 27 Feb to 2 Mar 2011.
15. Murphy DA, Greenwell L, Hoffman D. Factors associated with antiretroviral adherence among HIV-infected women with children. Women Health. 2002;36(1):97–111. Epub 2002/09/07.
16. Bhaskaran K, Hamouda O, Sannes M, Boufassa F, Johnson AM, Lambert PC, et al. Changes in the risk of death after HIV seroconversion compared with mortality in the general population. JAMA. 2008;300(1):51–9. Epub 2008/07/03.
17. Weber R, Sabin CA, Friis-Moller N, Reiss P, El-Sadr WM, Kirk O, et al. Liver-related deaths in persons infected with the human immunodeficiency virus: the D:A:D study. Arch Intern Med. 2006;166(15):1632–41. Epub 2006/08/16.
18. Currier JS, Taylor A, Boyd F, Dezii CM, Kawabata H, Burtcel B, et al. Coronary heart disease in HIV-infected individuals. J Acquir Immune Defic Syndr. 2003;33(4):506–12. Epub 2003/07/19.
19. Lang S, Mary-Krause M, Cotte L, Gilquin J, Partisani M, Simon A, et al. Increased risk of myocardial infarction in HIV-infected patients in France, relative to the general population. AIDS. 2010;24(8):1228–30. Epub 2010/04/20.
20. Klein D, Hurley LB, Quesenberry Jr CP, Sidney S. Do protease inhibitors increase the risk for coronary heart disease in patients with HIV-1 infection? J Acquir Immune Defic Syndr. 2002;30(5):471–7. Epub 2002/08/03.
21. Triant VA. HIV infection and coronary heart disease: an intersection of epidemics. J Infect Dis. 2012;205 Suppl 3:S355–61. Epub 2012/05/18.
22. Triant VA, Lee H, Hadigan C, Grinspoon SK. Increased acute myocardial infarction rates and cardiovascular risk factors among patients with human immunodeficiency virus disease. J Clin Endocrinol Metab. 2007;92(7):2506–12. Epub 2007/04/26.
23. Freiberg MS, Chang CC, Kuller LH, Skanderson M, Lowy E, Kraemer KL, et al. HIV infection and the risk of acute myocardial infarction. JAMA Intern Med. 2013;173(8):614–22. Epub 2013/03/06.

24. Freiberg MS, Chang CC, Skanderson M, McGinnis K, Kuller LH, Kraemer KL, et al. The risk of incident coronary heart disease among veterans with and without HIV and hepatitis C. Circ Cardiovasc Qual Outcomes. 2011;4(4):425–32. Epub 2011/06/30.
25. Durand M, Sheehy O, Baril JG, Lelorier J, Tremblay CL. Association between HIV infection, antiretroviral therapy, and risk of acute myocardial infarction: a cohort and nested case-control study using Quebec's public health insurance database. J Acquir Immune Defic Syndr. 2011;57(3):245–53. Epub 2011/04/19.
26. Obel N, Thomsen HF, Kronborg G, Larsen CS, Hildebrandt PR, Sorensen HT, et al. Ischemic heart disease in HIV-infected and HIV-uninfected individuals: a population-based cohort study. Clin Infect Dis. 2007;44(12):1625–31. Epub 2007/05/23.
27. Boccara F, Lang S, Meuleman C, Ederhy S, Mary-Krause M, Costagliola D, et al. HIV and coronary heart disease: time for a better understanding. J Am Coll Cardiol. 2013;61(5):511–23. Epub 2013/02/02.
28. WWHOT report: WWHOTwh. 2012. http://www.who.int/gho/publications/world_health_statistics/2012/en/. Accessed 8 Aug 2013
29. Pearce D, Ani C, Espinosa-Silva Y, Clark R, Fatima K, Rahman M, et al. Comparison of in-hospital mortality from acute myocardial infarction in HIV sero-positive versus sero-negative individuals. Am J Cardiol. 2012;110(8):1078–84. Epub 2012/07/06.
30. Boccara F, Mary-Krause M, Teiger E, Lang S, Lim P, Wahbi K, et al. Acute coronary syndrome in human immunodeficiency virus-infected patients: characteristics and 1 year prognosis. Eur Heart J. 2011;32(1):41–50. Epub 2010/10/23.
31. Lorgis L, Cottenet J, Molins G, Benzenine E, Zeller M, Aube H, et al. Outcomes after acute myocardial infarction in HIV-infected patients: analysis of data from a French nationwide hospital medical information database. Circulation. 2013;127(17):1767–74. Epub 2013/04/02.
32. Klein D, Leyden WA, Xu L, Chao CR, Horberg MA, Towner WJ, et al. Contribution of immunodeficiency to CHD: cohort study of HIV+ and HIV− Kaiser permanent members. Program and abstracts of the 18th conference on retroviruses and opportunitistic infections, Boston, MA; 2011.
33. Fine DM, Atta MG. Kidney disease in the HIV-infected patient. AIDS Patient Care STDS. 2007;21(11):813–24. Epub 2008/02/05.
34. Crum-Cianflone NF, Weekes J, Bavaro M. Review: thromboses among HIV-infected patients during the highly active antiretroviral therapy era. AIDS Patient Care STDS. 2008;22(10):771–8. Epub 2008/09/12.
35. Madeddu G, Spanu A, Solinas P, Calia GM, Lovigu C, Chessa F, et al. Bone mass loss and vitamin D metabolism impairment in HIV patients receiving highly active antiretroviral therapy. Q J Nucl Med Mol Imaging. 2004;48(1):39–48. Epub 2004/06/15.
36. Vescini F, Borderi M, Buffa A, Sinicropi G, Tampellini L, Chiodo F, et al. Bone mass in HIV-infected patients: focus on the role of therapy and sex. J Acquir Immune Defic Syndr. 2003;33(3):405–7. Epub 2003/07/05.
37. Brown TT, Qaqish RB. Antiretroviral therapy and the prevalence of osteopenia and osteoporosis: a meta-analytic review. AIDS. 2006;20(17):2165–74. Epub 2006/11/07.
38. Triant VA, Brown TT, Lee H, Grinspoon SK. Fracture prevalence among human immunodeficiency virus (HIV)-infected versus non-HIV-infected patients in a large U.S. health care system. J Clin Endocrinol Metab. 2008;93(9):3499–504.
39. Young B, Dao CN, Buchacz K, Baker R, Brooks JT. Increased rates of bone fracture among HIV-infected persons in the HIV Outpatient Study (HOPS) compared with the US general population, 2000–2006. Clin Infect Dis. 2011;52(8):1061–8. Epub 2011/03/15.
40. Womack JA, Goulet JL, Gibert C, Brandt C, Chang CC, Gulanski B, et al. Increased risk of fragility fractures among HIV infected compared to uninfected male veterans. PLoS One. 2011;6(2):e17217. Epub 2011/03/02.
41. Prior J, Burdge D, Maan E, Milner R, Hankins C, Klein M, et al. Fragility fractures and bone mineral density in HIV positive women: a case-control population-based study. Osteoporos Int. 2007;18(10):1345–53. Epub 2007/08/01.
42. Guerri-Fernandez R, Vestergaard P, Carbonell C, Knobel H, Aviles FF, Castro AS, et al. HIV infection is strongly associated with hip fracture risk, independently of age, gender, and comorbidities: a population-based cohort study. J Bone Miner Res. 2013;28(6):1259–63. Epub 2013/01/31.
43. Patel P, Hanson DL, Sullivan PS, Novak RM, Moorman AC, Tong TC, et al. Incidence of types of cancer among HIV-infected persons compared with the general population in the United States, 1992–2003. Ann Intern Med. 2008;148(10):728–36. Epub 2008/05/21.
44. Maki PM, Martin-Thormeyer E. HIV, cognition and women. Neuropsychol Rev. 2009;19(2):204–14. Epub 2009/05/12.
45. Ciesla JA, Roberts JE. Meta-analysis of the relationship between HIV infection and risk for depressive disorders. Am J Psychiatry. 2001;158(5):725–30. Epub 2001/05/01.
46. Siemieniuk RA, Krentz HB, Gill MJ. Intimate partner violence and HIV: a review. Curr HIV AIDS Rep. 2013;10(4):380–9.
47. Chen JL, Philips KA, Kanouse DE, Collins RL, Miu A. Fertility desires and intentions of HIV-positive men and women. Fam Plan Perspect. 2001;33(4):144–52, 65. Epub 2001/08/11.
48. Panozzo L, Battegay M, Friedl A, Vernazza PL. High risk behaviour and fertility desires among heterosexual HIV-positive patients with a serodiscordant partner – two challenging issues. Swiss Med Wkly. 2003;133(7–8):124–7. Epub 2003/03/20.

49. Ross A, Van der Paal L, Lubega R, Mayanja BN, Shafer LA, Whitworth J. HIV-1 disease progression and fertility: the incidence of recognized pregnancy and pregnancy outcome in Uganda. AIDS. 2004;18(5):799–804. Epub 2004/04/13.
50. Sherr L, Barry N. Fatherhood and HIV-positive heterosexual men. HIV Med. 2004;5(4):258–63. Epub 2004/07/09.
51. Stephenson JM, Griffioen A. The effect of HIV diagnosis on reproductive experience. Study Group for the Medical Research Council Collaborative Study of Women with HIV. AIDS. 1996;10(14):1683–7. Epub 1996/12/01.
52. Thackway SV, Furner V, Mijch A, Cooper DA, Holland D, Martinez P, et al. Fertility and reproductive choice in women with HIV-1 infection. AIDS. 1997;11(5):663–7. Epub 1997/04/01.
53. Cooper D, Moodley J, Zweigenthal V, Bekker LG, Shah I, Myer L. Fertility intentions and reproductive health care needs of people living with HIV in Cape Town, South Africa: implications for integrating reproductive health and HIV care services. AIDS Behav. 2009;13 Suppl 1:38–46. Epub 2009/04/04.
54. Nattabi B, Li J, Thompson SC, Orach CG, Earnest J. A systematic review of factors influencing fertility desires and intentions among people living with HIV/AIDS: implications for policy and service delivery. AIDS Behav. 2009;13(5):949–68. Epub 2009/03/31.
55. Hoffman IF, Martinson FE, Powers KA, Chilongozi DA, Msiska ED, Kachipapa EI, et al. The year-long effect of HIV-positive test results on pregnancy intentions, contraceptive use, and pregnancy incidence among Malawian women. J Acquir Immune Defic Syndr. 2008;47(4):477–83. Epub 2008/01/23.
56. Heys J, Kipp W, Jhangri GS, Alibhai A, Rubaale T. Fertility desires and infection with the HIV: results from a survey in rural Uganda. AIDS. 2009;23 Suppl 1:S37–45. Epub 2010/02/02.
57. Desgrées-Du-Loû A, Msellati P, Viho I, Yao A, Yapi D, Kassi P, et al. Contraceptive use, protected sexual intercourse and incidence of pregnancies among African HIV-infected women. DITRAME ANRS 049 Project, Abidjan 1995–2000. Int J STD AIDS. 2002;13(7):462–8.
58. Balkus J, Bosire R, John-Stewart G, Mbori-Ngacha D, Schiff MA, Wamalwa D, et al. High uptake of postpartum hormonal contraception among HIV-1-seropositive women in Kenya. Sex Transm Dis. 2007;34:25–9.
59. Polis CB, Gray RH, Lutalo T, Nalugoda F, Kagaayi J, Kigozi G, et al. Trends and correlates of hormonal contraceptive use among HIV-infected women in Rakai, Uganda, 1994–2006. Contraception. 2011;83:549–55.
60. King R, Estey J, Allen S, Kegeles S, Wolf W, Valentine C, et al. A family planning intervention to reduce vertical transmission of HIV in Rwanda. AIDS. 1995;9 Suppl 1:S45–51. Epub 1995/07/01.
61. Rutenberg N, Baek C. Field experiences integrating family planning into programs to prevent mother-to-child transmission of HIV. Stud Fam Plann. 2005;36(3):235–45. Epub 2005/10/08.
62. Grabbe K, Stephenson R, Vwalika B, Ahmed Y, Vwalika C, Chomba E, et al. Knowledge, use, and concerns about contraceptive methods among serodiscordant couples in Rwanda and Zambia. J Womens Health (Larchmt). 2009;18(9):1449–56. Epub 2009/08/28.
63. Pitter C. PMTCT implementation and the importance of male involvement. Washington, DC: Elizabeth Glaser Pediatric AIDS Foundation; 2010.
64. Lozano R, Wang H, Foreman KJ, Rajaratnam JK, Naghavi M, Marcus JR, et al. Progress towards millennium development goals 4 and 5 on maternal and child mortality: an updated systematic analysis. Lancet. 2011;378(9797):1139–65. Epub 2011/09/23.
65. van Dillen J, Meguid T, van Roosmalen J. Maternal mortality audit in a hospital in Northern Namibia: the impact of HIV/AIDS. Acta Obstet Gynecol Scand. 2006;85(4):499–500. Epub 2006/04/14.
66. Wandabwa JN, Doyle P, Longo-Mbenza B, Kiondo P, Khainza B, Othieno E, et al. Human immunodeficiency virus and AIDS and other important predictors of maternal mortality in Mulago Hospital Complex Kampala Uganda. BMC Public Health. 2011;11:565. Epub 2011/07/16.
67. Moran NF, Moodley J. The effect of HIV infection on maternal health and mortality. Int J Gynaecol Obstet. 2012;119 Suppl 1:S26–9. Epub 2012/08/15.
68. Centers for Disease Control and Prevention (CDC). US medical eligibility criteria for contraceptive use. MMWR. 2010;59(RR-4):1–86.
69. Mirpuri J, Jain L. Issues of prematurity and HIV infection. Clin Perinatol. 2010;37(4):887–905, xi. Epub 2010/11/17.
70. Brocklehurst P, French R. The association between maternal HIV infection and perinatal outcome: a systematic review of the literature and meta-analysis. Br J Obstet Gynaecol. 1998;105(8):836–48. Epub 1998/09/24.
71. Kuhn L, Semrau K, Ramachandran S, Sinkala M, Scott N, Kasonde P, et al. Mortality and virologic outcomes after access to antiretroviral therapy among a cohort of HIV-infected women who received single-dose nevirapine in Lusaka, Zambia. J Acquir Immune Defic Syndr. 2009;52(1):132–6. Epub 2009/06/10.
72. Marazzi MC, Palombi L, Nielsen-Saines K, Haswell J, Zimba I, Magid NA, et al. Extended antenatal use of triple antiretroviral therapy for prevention of mother-to-child transmission of HIV-1 correlates with favorable pregnancy outcomes. AIDS. 2011;25(13):1611–8. Epub 2011/06/16.
73. Parikh L, Timofeev J, Singh J, Sullivan S, Huang CC, Landy HJ, et al. Racial disparities in maternal and neonatal outcomes in HIV-1 positive mothers. Am J Perinatol. 2013. Epub 2013/09/04.

74. World Health Organization. Use of antiretroviral drugs for treating pregnant women and preventing HIV infection in infants: Programmatic update. Geneva: World Health Organization; 2012.
75. Panel on Antiretroviral Guidelines for Adults and Adolescents. Guidelines for the use of antiretroviral agents in HIV-1-infected adults and adolescents. Contract No.: Nov 12, 2013.
76. Panel on Antiretroviral Guidelines for Adults and Adolescents. Recommendations for use of antiretroviral drugs in pregnant HIV-1-infected women for maternal health and interventions to reduce perinatal HIV transmission in the United States. 2013 [updated 7/31/12]. http://aidsinfo.nih.gov/contentfiles/lvguidelines/AdultandAdolescentGL.pdf. Accessed 14 Nov 2013.
77. UNICEF. Childinfo: monitoring the situation of children and women: statistics by area/HIV/AIDS. 2012.
78. UN. The millennium development goals report 2012. New York, NY: 2012. Contract No.: 12-24532.
79. Gray RH, Li X, Kigozi G, Serwadda D, Brahmbhatt H, Wabwire-Mangen F, et al. Increased risk of incident HIV during pregnancy in Rakai, Uganda: a prospective study. Lancet. 2005;366(9492):1182–8. Epub 2005/10/04.
80. Mugo NR, Heffron R, Donnell D, Wald A, Were EO, Rees H, et al. Increased risk of HIV-1 transmission in pregnancy: a prospective study among African HIV-1-serodiscordant couples. AIDS. 2011;25(15):1887–95. Epub 2011/07/26.
81. Morrison CS, Wang J, Van Der Pol B, Padian N, Salata RA, Richardson BA. Pregnancy and the risk of HIV-1 acquisition among women in Uganda and Zimbabwe. AIDS. 2007;21(8):1027–34. Epub 2007/04/26.
82. Stover J, editor. Reducing the costs of effective AIDS control programmes through appropriate targeting of interventions. International AIDS conference, 1996, Vancouver, Canada; 1996.
83. Peterman TA, Todd KA, Mupanduki I. Opportunities for targeting publicly funded human immunodeficiency virus counseling and testing. J Acquir Immune Defic Syndr Hum Retrovirol. 1996;12(1):69–74.
84. Sweeney C. 1 of 3 Pregnancies unwanted. Popline. 1992;14:1. Epub 1992/01/01.
85. Kell PD, Barton SE, Boag FC. Incorporating patients' views in planning services for women with HIV infection. Genitourin Med. 1992;68(4):233–4.
86. McCarthy GA, Cockell AP, Kell PD, Beevor AS, Boag FC. A women-only clinic for HIV, genitourinary medicine and substance misuse. Genitourin Med. 1992;68(6):386–9.
87. Carlin EM, Russell JM, Sibley K, Boag FC. Evaluating a designated family planning clinic within a genitourinary medicine clinic [see comments]. Genitourin Med. 1995;71(2):106–8.
88. Cates Jr W, Stone K. Family planning, sexually transmitted disease, and contraceptive choice: a literature update. Part II. Fam Plann Perspect. 1992;24(3):122–8.
89. Daley D. Reproductive health and AIDS-related services for women: how well are they integrated? Fam Plann Perspect. 1994;26(6):264–9. Epub 1994/11/01.
90. Becker J, Ureno M. How HIV has helped family planning: sexuality, the essential link. International conference on AIDS, Vancover, BC, 7–12 Jul 1996
91. Chandhok K, Sankaran S, Peters S, Mathews G, Manoharan S, Thomas S, editors. Developing comprehensive intervention programs for women in the reproductive age group. International AIDS conference, Vancouver, BC, Canada; 1996.
92. Hamid S, Stephenson R. Provider and health facility influences on contraceptive adoption in urban Pakistan. Int Fam Plan Perspect. 2006;32(2):71–8. Epub 2006/07/14.
93. Badell ML, Lathrop E, Haddad LB, Goedken P, Nguyen ML, Cwiak CA. Reproductive health care needs and desires in a cohort of HIV-positive women. Infect Dis Obstet Gynecol. 2012;2012:107878. Epub 2012/07/05.
94. Centers for Disease Control and Prevention (CDC). Sexually transmitted diseases treatment guidelines, 2010. MMWR 2010;59(RR-12). Epub 17 Dec 2010.
95. ACOG Practice Bulletin No. 117: gynecologic care for women with human immunodeficiency virus. Obstet Gynecol. 2010;116(6):1492–509. Epub 26 Nov 2010.
96. Zuckerman RA, Lucchetti A, Whittington WL, Sanchez J, Coombs RW, Zuniga R, et al. Herpes simplex virus (HSV) suppression with valacyclovir reduces rectal and blood plasma HIV-1 levels in HIV-1/HSV-2-seropositive men: a randomized, double-blind, placebo-controlled crossover trial. J Infect Dis. 2007;196(10):1500–8. Epub 2007/11/17.
97. Baeten JM, Strick LB, Lucchetti A, Whittington WL, Sanchez J, Coombs RW, et al. Herpes simplex virus (HSV)-suppressive therapy decreases plasma and genital HIV-1 levels in HSV-2/HIV-1 coinfected women: a randomized, placebo-controlled, cross-over trial. J Infect Dis. 2008;198(12):1804–8. Epub 2008/10/22.
98. Dunne EF, Whitehead S, Sternberg M, Thepamnuay S, Leelawiwat W, McNicholl JM, et al. Suppressive acyclovir therapy reduces HIV cervicovaginal shedding in HIV- and HSV-2-infected women, Chiang Rai, Thailand. J Acquir Immune Defic Syndr. 2008;49(1):77–83. Epub 2008/08/01.
99. Celum C, Wald A, Lingappa JR, Magaret AS, Wang RS, Mugo N, et al. Acyclovir and transmission of HIV-1 from persons infected with HIV-1 and HSV-2. N Engl J Med. 2010;362(5):427–39. Epub 2010/01/22.
100. Mujugira A, Magaret AS, Celum C, Baeten JM, Lingappa JR, Morrow RA, et al. Daily acyclovir to decrease herpes simplex virus type 2 (HSV-2) transmission from HSV-2/HIV-1 coinfected persons: a randomized controlled trial. J Infect Dis. 2013;208(9):1366–74. Epub 2013/08/01.

101. Kojic E, Cu-Uvin S. Safety of and immune response to the human papillomavirus (HPV) vaccine in HIV-infected women. National Library of Medicine; 2013. http://clinicaltrials.gov/ct2/show/NCT00604175. Accessed 14 Nov 2013
102. Kahn J, Squires K. Impact of an HPV vaccine in HIV-infected young women. National Library of Medicine; 2013. http://clinicaltrials.gov/ct2/show/NCT00604175. Accessed 14 Nov 2013
103. Workowski KA, Berman S. Sexually transmitted diseases treatment guidelines, 2010 MMWR recommendations and reports. MMWR. 2010;59(RR-12):1–110. Epub 2010/12/17.
104. Conde DM, Silva ET, Amaral WN, Finotti MF, Ferreira RG, Costa-Paiva L, et al. HIV, reproductive aging, and health implications in women: a literature review. Menopause. 2009;16(1):199–213. Epub 2008/09/19.
105. Kanapathipillai R, Hickey M, Giles M. Human immunodeficiency virus and menopause. Menopause. 2013;20(9):983–90. Epub 2013/03/28.
106. Centers for Disease Control. U.S. medical eligibility criteria for contraceptive use, 2010. MMWR recommendations and reports: morbidity and mortality weekly report recommendations and reports. MMWR. 2010;59(RR-4):1–86. Epub 2010/06/19.
107. CDC. Update to CDC's US medical eligibility criteria for contraceptive use, 2010: revised recommendations for the use of hormonal contraception among women at high risk for HIV infection or infected with HIV. MMWR. 2012;61(24):449–52. Epub 2012/06/22.
108. Sivin I, Stern J, Coutinho E, Mattos CE, el Mahgoub S, Diaz S, et al. Prolonged intrauterine contraception: a seven-year randomized study of the levonorgestrel 20 mcg/day (LNg 20) and the Copper T380 Ag IUDS. Contraception. 1991;44(5):473–80. Epub 1991/11/01.
109. Trussell J. Contraceptive efficacy. Arch Dermatol. 1995;131(9):1064–8. Epub 1995/09/01.
110. Hatcher RA, Trussell J, Stewart FH, Nelson AL, Cates W, Guest F, et al. Contraceptive technology, 20th rev ed. New York: Ardent Media, Inc.; 2011. xxviii, 871 p., [7] p. of plates p.
111. Toivonen J, Luukkainen T, Allonen H. Protective effect of intrauterine release of levonorgestrel on pelvic infection: three years' comparative experience of levonorgestrel- and copper-releasing intrauterine devices. Obstet Gynecol. 1991;77(2):261–4. Epub 1991/02/01.
112. Long-term reversible contraception. Twelve years of experience with the TCu380A and TCu220C. Contraception. 1997;56(6):341–52. Epub 1998/03/12.
113. Hatcher R, Trussell J, Nelson A, Cates W, Stewart F, Kowel D. Contraceptive technology. 20th ed. New York: Ardent Media; 2011.
114. Leticee N, Viard JP, Yamgnane A, Karmochkine M, Benachi A. Contraceptive failure of etonogestrel implant in patients treated with antiretrovirals including efavirenz. Contraception. 2012;85(4):425–7. Epub 2011/11/01.
115. CDC. U.S. selected practice recommendations for contraceptive use, 2013: adapted from the World Health Organization selected practice recommendations for contraceptive use, 2nd ed. MMWR Centers Dis Control. 2013;62(RR-05):1–60. Epub 2013/06/21.
116. Trussell J, Sturgen K, Strickler J, Dominik R. Comparative contraceptive efficacy of the female condom and other barrier methods. Fam Plann Perspect. 1994;26(2):66–72. Epub 1994/03/01.
117. Gallo MF, Kilbourne-Brook M, Coffey PS. A review of the effectiveness and acceptability of the female condom for dual protection. Sex Health. 2012;9(1):18–26. Epub 2012/02/22.
118. Van Damme L, Ramjee G, Alary M, Vuylsteke B, Chandeying V, Rees H, et al. Effectiveness of COL-1492, a nonoxynol-9 vaginal gel, on HIV-1 transmission in female sex workers: a randomised controlled trial. Lancet. 2002;360(9338):971–7. Epub 2002/10/18.
119. Gupta SK. Nutan. Clinical use of vaginal or rectally applied microbicides in patients suffering from HIV/AIDS. HIV. HIV AIDS (Auckl). 2013;5:295–307.
120. Padian NS, van der Straten A, Ramjee G, Chipato T, de Bruyn G, Blanchard K, et al. Diaphragm and lubricant gel for prevention of HIV acquisition in southern African women: a randomised controlled trial. Lancet. 2007;370(9583):251–61. Epub 2007/07/17.
121. Brache V, Cochon L, Deniaud M, Croxatto HB. Ulipristal acetate prevents ovulation more effectively than levonorgestrel: analysis of pooled data from three randomized trials of emergency contraception regimens. Contraception. 2013;88(5):611–8. Epub 2013/07/03.
122. German P, Wang M, Warren D, Kearney B, editors. Pharmacokinetic interaction between norgestimate/ethinyl estradiol and EVG/COBI/FTC/TDF single tablet regimen. 12th International workshop on clinical pharmacology of HIV therapy, Miami, FL, Apr 2011.
123. Carten M, Kiser J, Kwara A, Ma Whinney S, S. C-U, editors. Pharmacokinetic (PK) interactions between the hormonal emergency contraception Plan B (levonorgestrel) and efavirenz (EFV). 17th Conference on retroviruses and opportunistic infection, San Francisco, Feb 2010
124. Robinson JA, Jamshidi R, Burke AE. Contraception for the HIV-positive woman: a review of interactions between hormonal contraception and antiretroviral therapy. Infect Dis Obstet Gynecol. 2012;2012:890160. Epub 2012/08/29.
125. Adolescents PoAGfAa. Guidelines for the use of antiretroviral agents in HIV-1-infected adults and adolescents. Department of Health and Human Services; 2013. http://aidsinfo.nih.gov/contentfiles/lvguidelines/AdultandAdolescentGL.pdf. Accessed 2 Nov 2013.
126. Centers for Disease Control and Prevention (CDC). Update to CDC's US medical eligibility criteria for

contraceptive use, 2010: revised recommendations for the use of hormonal contraception among women at high risk for HIV infection or infected with HIV. MMWR. 2012;61(24):449–52. Epub 22 Jun 2012.

127. Nanda K, Amaral E, Hays M, Viscola MA, Mehta N, Bahamondes L. Pharmacokinetic interactions between depot medroxyprogesterone acetate and combination antiretroviral therapy. Fertil Steril. 2008;90(4):965–71. Epub 2007/09/21.
128. Watts DH, Park JG, Cohn SE, Yu S, Hitti J, Stek A, et al. Safety and tolerability of depot medroxyprogesterone acetate among HIV-infected women on antiretroviral therapy: ACTG A5093. Contraception. 2008;77(2):84–90. Epub 2008/01/30.
129. Cohn SE, Park JG, Watts DH, Stek A, Hitti J, Clax PA, et al. Depo-medroxyprogesterone in women on antiretroviral therapy: effective contraception and lack of clinically significant interactions. Clin Pharmacol Therapy. 2007;81(2):222–7. Epub 2006/12/29.
130. Vogler MA, Patterson K, Kamemoto L, Park JG, Watts H, Aweeka F, et al. Contraceptive efficacy of oral and transdermal hormones when co-administered with protease inhibitors in HIV-1-infected women: pharmacokinetic results of ACTG trial A5188. J Acquir Immune Defic Syndr. 2010;55(4):473–82. Epub 2010/09/16.
131. Kearney B, Isaacson E, Sayre J, Cheng A, editors. Tenofovir DF and oral contraceptives: lack of a pharmacokinetic drug interaction. 43rd Interscience conference on antimicrobial agents and chemotherapy, Chicago, IL; Washington, DC, 14–17 Sep 2003.
132. Aweeka FT, Rosenkranz SL, Segal Y, Coombs RW, Bardeguez A, Thevanayagam L, et al. The impact of sex and contraceptive therapy on the plasma and intracellular pharmacokinetics of zidovudine. AIDS. 2006;20(14):1833–41. Epub 2006/09/07.
133. Joshi A, Fiske W, Benedek I, White SJ, Joseph JL, Kornhauser DM. Lack of a pharmacokinetic interaction between efavirenz (DMP 266) and ethinyl estradiol in healthy female volunteers. 5th Conference on retroviruses and opportunistic infections, Chicago, IL, 1–5 Feb 1998.
134. Sevinsky H, Eley T, He B, et al. Effect of efavirenz on the pharmacokinetics of ethinyl estradiol and norgestimate in healthy female subjects [Abstract A958]. In: Program and abstracts of the 48th interscience conference on antimicrobial agents and chemotherapy, Washington, DC, 25–28 Oct 2008. Washington, DC: American Society for Microbiology; 2008.
135. Scholler-Gyure M, Debroye C, Aharchi F, et al. No clinically relevant effect of TMC125 on the pharmacokinetics of oral contraceptives. 8th International congress on drug therapy in HIV infection, Glasgow, 12–16 Nov 2006.
136. Mildvan D, Yarrish R, Marshak A, Hutman HW, McDonough M, Lamson M, et al. Pharmacokinetic interaction between nevirapine and ethinyl estradiol/norethindrone when administered concurrently to HIV-infected women. J Acquir Immune Defic Syndr. 2002;29(5):471–7. Epub 2002/05/01.
137. Tibotec Therapeutics Inc. Edurant [package insert]. Raritan, NJ; 2011.
138. Bristol-Meyers Squibb. Reyataz (atazanavir) package label. 2010.
139. Sekar V, Lefebvre E, Seal S. Pharmacokinetic interaction between nevirapine and ethinyl estradiol, norethindrone, and TMC114, a new protease inhibitor [Abstract A-368]. San Francisco, CA: American Society for Microbiology, 27–30 Sep 2006. Report No.; 2006
140. Glaxo Smith Kline. Prescription medicines. Lexiva (fosamprenavir calcium). 2009.
141. Glaxo Smith Kline. Study APV10020. A phase I, open label, two period, single-sequence, drug–drug interaction study comparing steady-state plasma ethinyl estradiol and norethisterone pharmacokinetics following administration of brevinor for 21 days with and without fosamprenavir 700 mg twice daily (BID) and ritonavir 100 mg (BID) for 21 days in healthy adult female subjects. 2009.
142. Abbott Laboratories. Lopinavir and ritonavir prescribing information. North Chicago, IL: Abbott Laboratories; 2009.
143. Boehringer Ingelheim Pharmaceuticals I. Aptivus [package insert]. Ridgefield, CT: Nov 2005. Report No.; 2005.
144. Food and Drug Administration. Highlights of prescribing information. Aptivus (Tipranavir) Capsules. USFDA; 2009.
145. Glaxo Wellcome Inc. Agenerase [package insert]. Research Triangle Park, NC; 2004.
146. Agouron Pharmaceuticals. Viracept (Nelfinavir mesylate) prescribing information. San Diego, CA: Agouron Pharmaceuticals; 2008.
147. Anderson MS, Hanley WD, Moreau AR, Jin B, Bieberdorf FA, Kost JT, et al. Effect of raltegravir on estradiol and norgestimate plasma pharmacokinetics following oral contraceptive administration in healthy women. Br J Clin Pharmacol. 2011;71(4):616–20. Epub 2011/03/15.
148. Baeten JM, Benki S, Chohan V, Lavreys L, McClelland RS, Mandaliya K, et al. Hormonal contraceptive use, herpes simplex virus infection, and risk of HIV-1 acquisition among Kenyan women. AIDS. 2007;21(13):1771–7. Epub 2007/08/11.
149. Heffron R, Donnell D, Rees H, Celum C, Mugo N, Were E, et al. Use of hormonal contraceptives and risk of HIV-1 transmission: a prospective cohort study. Lancet Infect Dis. 2012;12(1):19–26. Epub 2011/10/07.
150. Hel Z, Stringer E, Mestecky J. Sex steroid hormones, hormonal contraception, and the immunobiology of human immunodeficiency virus-1 infection. Endocr Rev. 2010;31(1):79–97. Epub 2009/11/12.
151. Polis CB, Curtis KM. Use of hormonal contraceptives and HIV acquisition in women: a systematic review of the epidemiological evidence. Lancet Infect Dis. 2013;13(9):797–808. Epub 2013/07/23.

152. Stringer EM, Kaseba C, Levy J, Sinkala M, Goldenberg RL, Chi BH, et al. A randomized trial of the intrauterine contraceptive device vs hormonal contraception in women who are infected with the human immunodeficiency virus. Am J Obstet Gynecol. 2007;197(2):144e1-8. Epub 2007/08/11.
153. Phillips SJ, Curtis KM, Polis CB. Effect of hormonal contraceptive methods on HIV disease progression: a systematic review. AIDS. 2013;27(5):787–94. Epub 2012/11/09.
154. Cejtin HE, Jacobson L, Springer G, Watts DH, Levine A, Greenblatt R, et al. Effect of hormonal contraceptive use on plasma HIV-1-RNA levels among HIV-infected women. AIDS. 2003;17(11):1702–4. Epub 2003/07/11.
155. Richardson BA, Otieno PA, Mbori-Ngacha D, Overbaugh J, Farquhar C, John-Stewart GC. Hormonal contraception and HIV-1 disease progression among postpartum Kenyan women. AIDS. 2007;21(6):749–53. Epub 2007/04/07.

Contraceptive Options for Women with Headache Disease

7

Deborah Bartz, M. Angela O'Neal, and Andrea G. Edlow

Introduction

Forty-three percent of women in the United States (US) are affected by migraine [1]. The prevalence of migraine increases with age: 22 % of women age 20–24 years, 28 % age 25–29 years, 33 % age 30–34 years, and as many as 37 % of women age 35–39 years are affected (Fig. 7.1) [1]. During these reproductive years, hormonal contraception is the most prevalent form of birth control used, with 43 % of contracepting US women using hormone-containing pills, patches, rings, shots, implants, or intrauterine devices [2]. Given the significant proportion of reproductive-age women affected by migraine, several clinical considerations arise when evaluating women for hormonal contraceptives. Key considerations include physician selection of appropriate candidates for initiation of hormone-containing contraceptives and decision-making about method continuation in patients complaining of headache while taking hormonal contraceptives.

It is critical for physicians prescribing hormonal contraception to distinguish among different headache types to decide when the use of estrogen-containing contraception is appropriate. In addition, headache is a frequently reported side effect while using hormonal contraception and a leading reason cited for contraceptive discontinuation [3]. Contraceptive discontinuation accounts for 20 % of the 3.5 million unplanned pregnancies in the United States annually [4]. Separate from the risk of unintended pregnancy, women who discontinue hormonal contraceptives due to headaches are unable to reap the noncontraceptive benefits of these medications, including potential relief of chronic pelvic pain and endometrial protection in anovulatory states, such as polycystic ovary syndrome.

D. Bartz, M.D., M.P.H. (✉)
Department of Obstetrics, Gynecology, and Reproductive Biology, Harvard Medical School, Brigham and Women's Hospital, Boston, MA, USA
e-mail: dbartz@partners.org

M. Angela O'Neal, M.D.
Department of Neurology, Brigham and Women's Hospital, Boston, MA, USA
e-mail: maoneal@partners.org

A.G. Edlow, M.D., M.Sc.
Division of Maternal-Fetal Medicine, Department of Obstetrics and Gynecology, Tufts Medical Center, Boston, MA, USA
e-mail: agedlow@gmail.com

Diagnosis of a Headache

Migraine Without Aura

Migraine headache is distinguished from other headaches as a benign and recurring syndrome of headache, nausea, and vomiting, without other symptoms of neurologic dysfunction (Table 7.1). According to the American Migraine

R.H. Allen and C.A. Cwiak (eds.), *Contraception for the Medically Challenging Patient*, DOI 10.1007/978-1-4939-1233-9_7, © Springer Science+Business Media New York 2014

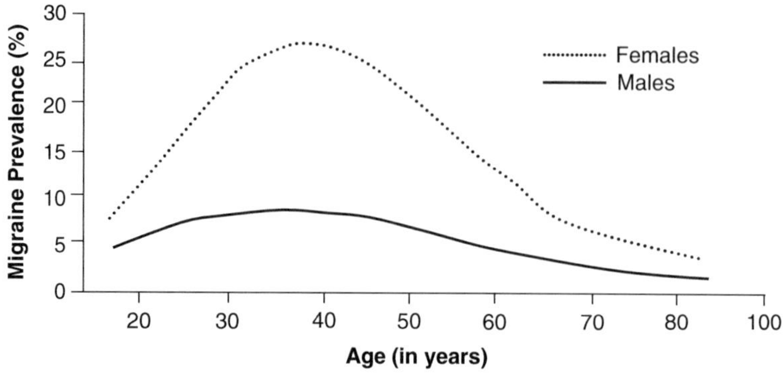

Fig. 7.1 One-year migraine prevalence by age and gender. Adapted from [5]

Table 7.1 The International Classification of Headache Disorders II (ICHD II) Diagnostic Criteria for Migraine

Without Aura
Recurring headache with at least 5 attacks fulfilling the following criteria:
Attacks last 4–72 h (untreated or unsuccessfully treated)
At least 2 of the following: – Unilateral location – Pulsating quality – Moderate or severe pain intensity – Aggravated by routine physical activity
At least 1 of the following during attack: – Nausea and/or vomiting – Photophobia and phonophobia – Not attributed to another disorder
With Aura
Must fulfill criteria for migraine listed above, and in addition, at least 2 attacks fulfilling the following criteria:
Aura consisting of at least 1 of the following, but no motor weakness: 1. Fully reversible visual symptoms including positive features (flickering lights, spots, or lines) and/or negative features (i.e., loss of vision) 2. Fully reversible sensory symptoms including positive features (i.e., pins and needles) and/or negative features (i.e., numbness) 3. Fully reversible dysphasic speech disturbance
At least two of the following other characteristics: 1. Homonymous visual symptoms and/or unilateral sensory symptoms 2. At least 1 aura symptom develops gradually over $\geq$5 min, and/or different aura symptoms occur in succession over $\geq$5 min 3. Each symptom lasts $\geq$5 and <60 min
Headache fulfilling the criteria for migraine begins during the aura or follows aura within 60 min
Not attributed to another disorder

Reprinted with permission from Headache Classification Subcommittee of the International Headache Society. The International Classification of Headache Disorders, 2nd ed. Cephalalgia. 2004;24(suppl 1):9–160

Prevalence and Prevention study, the 1-year incidence of migraine in women is about 17 %, and highest at 24 % in reproductive-age women [5]. The 1-year prevalence rate for migraine without aura (i.e., common migraine) is 11 % in women, making it the most frequent subset of migraine in women [6]. Neurologists diagnose migraines using the International Classification of Headache Disorders II (ICHD II) criteria, the official criteria of the International Headache Society (IHS) [7].

Migraine with Aura

Migraine with aura has a 1-year prevalence rate of 5 % in women [6]. Aura specifically describes a complex of neurologic symptoms that occurs just before or with the onset of migraine headache, and most often resolves completely before the onset of headache. Neurologists hypothesize that migraine aura is caused by a phenomenon called cortical spreading depression, in which changes in cellular excitability trigger waves of altered brain function [8]. Visual symptoms are the most common aura, and are a feature of 99 % of auras [9]. Other common aural symptoms include paresthesias and vertigo. According to the ICHD II criteria, migraine with aura is a recurrent disorder manifesting in attacks of reversible focal neurologic symptoms that develop gradually over 5–20 min, and last for less than 60 min (see Table 7.1). A migrainous headache, featuring throbbing and unilateral pain, follows the aura. Less commonly, the headache may lack migrainous features or be completely absent [7].

Risk of Stroke in Women with Migraines

Migraine is an independent risk factor for ischemic stroke [10–19]. However, the absolute risk of ischemic stroke is low in women of reproductive age, with reported incidence rates ranging from 5 to 11.3 per 100,000 woman-years [20, 21]. Often, a history of migraine may be the only significant risk factor for stroke in women younger than age 35 years. A history of migraine loses relevance in women over age 35, in whom more traditional atherogenic risk factors for ischemic stroke (i.e., hypertension, dyslipidemia, diabetes) dominate [17]. Although two case–control studies suggest the association between migraine and stroke may be limited to women younger than age 45 years [17, 18], a large prospective cohort study of women age ≥45 years found that active migraine with aura was associated with a significantly increased risk of major cardiovascular disease, myocardial infarction (MI), ischemic stroke, and death due to ischemic cardiovascular disease [14].

The difficulty with making a diagnosis of migrainous stroke is illustrated by the following case. Migraine and stroke share risk factors of patent foramen ovale (PFO) and are both hereditary conditions.

Case 1

A 41-year-old right-handed woman with a history of migraines and depression presents with small right parietal infarct. The patient had an episode of migraine with her usual visual symptoms of moving "puzzle pieces" followed by headache associated with nausea and vomiting, which resolved after taking Excedrin Migraine. While at the house, she started having another typical migraine. She again took Excedrin Migraine, had a cup of tea, and left the house. She remembers driving and the next thing she remembers is being at the hospital.

She had a low-velocity car accident followed by a witnessed seizure and was brought to the Emergency Department. Per report, her car rolled into another car with minimal damage. She did not fall or hit her head. En route to the hospital, she was confused. Her medications were calcium supplements and multivitamins.

Her exam was notable only for her mild confusion.

Brain MRI showed a punctate area of right parietal infarction (Fig. 7.2). Her evaluation including vascular imaging and hypercoagulable laboratories was unremarkable. Cardiac monitoring documented no arrhythmia. She had a transthoracic echocardiogram which showed a small PFO. No clots were imaged in her pelvis or lower extremities.

(continued)

(continued)

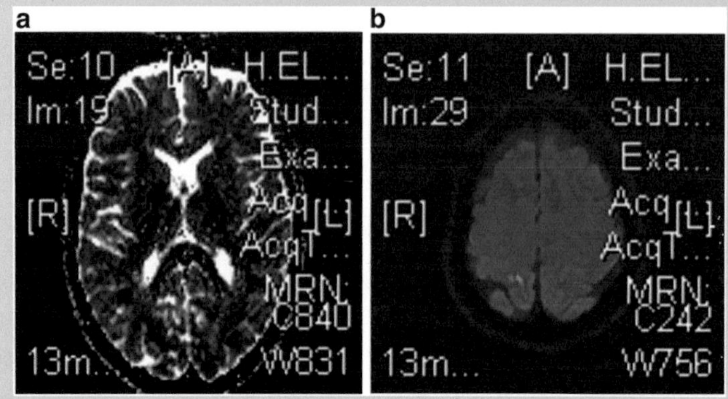

Fig. 7.2 Diffusion weighted image (DWI) (**b**) and apparent diffusion coefficient (ADC) (**a**) images showing a small right parietal infarct

Studies offer conflicting evidence with respect to risk of ischemic stroke associated with migraine without aura [11, 13, 14, 16, 22]. There is, however, a preponderance of evidence that migraine with aura is associated with a significantly elevated relative risk (RR) of ischemic stroke [11–18, 22]. A meta-analysis of 11 case–control studies and three cohort studies suggest that the RR of ischemic stroke in all migraineurs is 2.16 (95 % confidence interval [CI], 1.89–2.48); migraine with aura carried a RR of 2.27 (95 % CI, 1.61–3.19) for ischemic stroke, and migraine without aura had a RR of 1.83 (95 % CI, 1.06–3.15) of ischemic stroke [15]. The odds ratios (OR) for ischemic stroke in the setting of migraine without aura and migraine with aura are presented in Fig. 7.3.

This risk is magnified with the addition of other risk factors: age, combined oral contraceptive (COC) use, smoking, and hypertension [13]. Increased migraine frequency may be positively associated with stroke. The stroke mechanism, as in the above case, is most commonly idiopathic; vessel imaging, cardiac studies, and hypercoagulable laboratories are normal. There is no increase in atherosclerotic or cardioembolic strokes with migraine. Further, women with migraine with aura and a PFO did not have an increased stroke risk [12].

Risk of Stroke in Women Using Combined Hormonal Contraceptives (CHC)

Does Combination (Estrogen-Progestin) Hormonal Contraception Increase Stroke Risk Regardless of Migraine Status?

Combined hormonal contraceptives (CHCs) have been found to be an independent risk factor for ischemic stroke in some studies [23–27]. However, a large population-based case–control study and a pooled analysis of data from two US case–control studies found that low-dose COCs (i.e., preparations containing <50 μg of ethinyl estradiol) were not associated with an increased risk of stroke in the absence of migraine [21].

The Impact of the Ethinyl Estradiol Dose on Stroke Risk

Although evidence supports that pill formulations containing ≥50 μg of ethinyl estradiol (EE) are associated with an elevated risk of ischemic stroke compared with formulations with <50 μg, the data are not as clear regarding risk of stroke associated

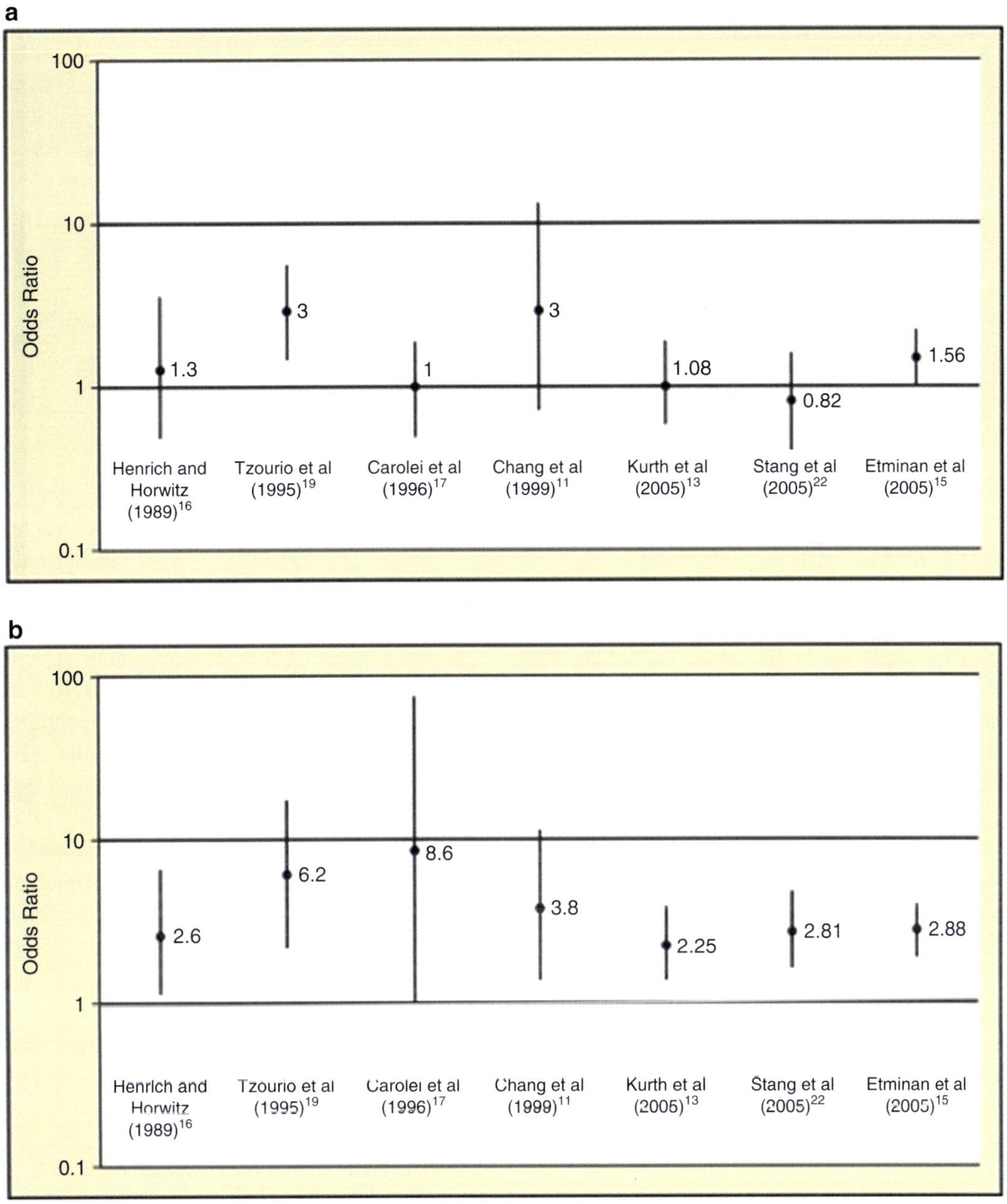

Fig. 7.3 (**a**) Migraine without aura and stroke risk. (**b**) Migraine with aura and stroke risk. Reproduced from Journal of Family Planning and Reproductive Health Care, Migraine and use of combined hormonal contraceptive: a clinical review, E. Anne MacGregor, 33, Copyright 2007, with permission from BMJ Publishing Group Ltd

with 20 μg versus 30 or 35 μg formulations. Lidegaard and colleagues reviewed data from a large, historical Danish cohort of nonpregnant women taking hormonal contraception, and assessed their 15-year risk for MI and stroke. Women, 15–49 years old, without any history of cancer or cardiovascular disease were followed and their risk for either MI or stroke was stratified according to the type and dose of CHC used (those studied included COCs stratified by estradiol dose and progestin type, transdermal patches, and a vaginal ring) [28]. The study followed

Table 7.2 USMEC Medical Eligibility for Combination Hormonal (Estrogen–Progestin) Contraceptive (CHC) Use: Women with Headache and Migraine

Category	Description	Headache/Migraine-specific recommendation
1	A condition for which there is no restriction for the use of the contraceptive method	Nonmigrainous headache
2	A condition where the advantages of using the method generally outweigh the theoretical or proven risks	Migraine without aura, age <35 years, nonsmoker
		Nonmigrainous headaches develop after initiating CHC
3	A condition where the theoretical or proven risks generally outweigh the advantages	Migraine without aura, age ≥35 years Migraines without aura develop after initiating CHC
4	A condition which represents an unacceptable health risk if the contraceptive is used	Migraines with aura, any age
		Migraines with aura develop after initiating CHC

1,626,158 women with 14,251,063 person-years of observation. A total of 3,311 thrombotic strokes and 1,725 MIs occurred. The overall risk for stroke was small, at 21.4/100,000 person-years. The study demonstrated that higher amounts of EE in the CHCs, 30–40 μg as compared with 20 μg, were associated with an increased combined risk for stroke and MI. The amount of progestin had no influence on these endpoints [28].

In the few studies that examined ischemic stroke risk associated with 20 μg EE formulations compared with 30 to 40 μg formulations, the data are conflicting. Tzourio and colleagues reported a significantly lower OR of stroke in 20 μg formulations (OR 1.7 compared with OR of 2.7 for 30–40 μg formulations) [19], whereas Lidegaard and colleagues reported a similar OR of ischemic stroke for 20 μg (OR 1.7) and for 30 to 40 μg (OR 1.6) formulations [24]. Further research with modern hormonal contraceptive methods is needed to draw conclusions regarding the impact of EE dose on stroke risk.

The Impact of Progestins on Stroke Risk

Similarly, there are conflicting data regarding whether type of progestin influences stroke risk in low-EE (<50 μg) formulations. The IHS Task Force concludes in their consensus statement that there is no difference in the ischemic stroke risk between low-EE formulations containing second-generation progestins (e.g., ethynodiol diacetate, levonorgestrel, norethisterone) versus third-generation progestins (i.e., desogestrel, gestodene, norgestimate) [20].

Although studies are limited, there is no evidence to suggest that progestin-only contraceptives increase the risk of stroke, even in women who have multiple risk factors (including age > 35 years, tobacco use, and migraines with aura). The Centers for Disease Control and Prevention (CDC) considers progestin-only pills, implants, intrauterine devices, and injectables to be category 2 for women who have migraines with aura, regardless of a woman's age, smoking status, or comorbidities [29]. There is general consensus that progestin-only contraceptives are safe for use in women who have migraine with aura, even in the presence of other risk factors for stroke [30–32].

Does Combination Hormonal Contraception (CHC) Increase Stroke Risk in Women with Migraine?

No studies have been adequately powered to directly compare stroke risk in migraineurs with aura taking CHCs with that of migraineurs without aura taking CHCs. Many studies have reported increased overall odds of stroke in migraineurs who use combination hormonal contraception, particularly among active smokers (Fig. 7.4) [11, 12, 19, 23, 33, 34]. The reported

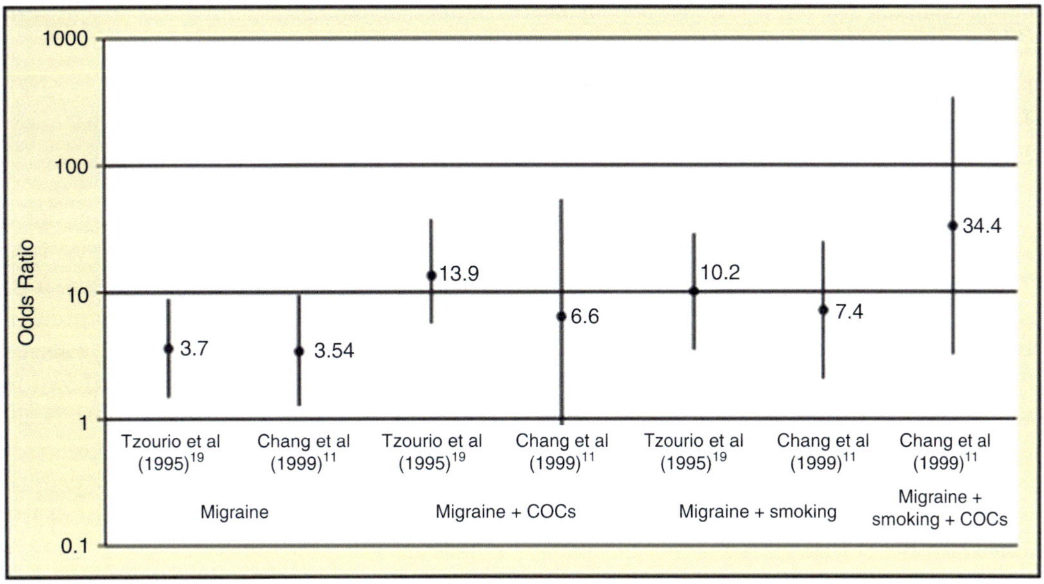

Fig. 7.4 Effect of combined oral contraceptives (COC), migraine, and smoking on stroke risk. Reproduced from Journal of Family Planning and Reproductive Health Care, Migraine and use of combined hormonal contraceptive: a clinical review, E. Anne MacGregor, 33, Copyright 2007, with permission from BMJ Publishing Group Ltd

ORs for ischemic stroke in migraineurs using CHC range from 2 to nearly 14, compared with women without migraine who are not using CHC. A recent systematic review and meta-analysis of nine studies found that the pooled RR of ischemic stroke in women age<45 years with migraine with or without aura was 3.6, and the risk of ischemic stroke was further increased to 7.2 among women currently using CHCs [35].

A case–control study by Tzourio and colleagues compared 72 women aged 18–44 years (the women were not further stratified by age) presenting with first ischemic stroke with 173 hospital-matched controls. The controls were matched for age, body mass, and educational background. They found the odds of ischemic stroke were nearly 14 times higher in migrainous women using oral contraceptives (the study did have enough power to distinguish between CHC versus progestin-only contraceptives). This increase occurred with both types of migraine, although the risk was higher with migraine with aura (odds ratio 6.2) than with migraine without aura (odds ratio 3.0). This risk persisted after controlling for age, hypertension, OC use, and smoking [19]. In a pooled analysis of data from two US case–control studies, Schwartz and colleagues studied 175 women aged 18–44 years with ischemic stroke and 1,191 controls. They found that women with a history of migraine and current low-dose COC use (<50 μg EE) had twice the odds of stroke compared with nonusers of combination contraception [33]. Chang and colleagues compared 291 women aged 20–44 years with ischemic, hemorrhagic, or unclassified arterial stroke to 736 age- and hospital-matched controls. They found that women with migraine using low-dose combination oral contraceptives (<50 μg EE) had nearly seven times the odds of ischemic stroke, and this risk increased nearly exponentially if the women were smokers (see Fig. 7.4) [11]. Another case–control study by MacClellan and colleagues examined the effect of smoking on stroke risk in migraineurs, comparing 386 women ages 15–49 years with first ischemic stroke with 614 age- and ethnicity-matched controls. This study found that migraineurs with aura who were current COC users and smokers had seven times higher odds of stroke compared with migraineurs with aura who did not smoke and did not use COCs, and 10 times higher odds of stroke compared with women without migraine who did not smoke and did not use COCs [12]. Finally, it is important to note that at least two studies found that the use of COC did not further elevate the risk of ischemic stroke in women with migraines [14, 30].

Professional Recommendations Regarding Hormone Use in Women with Migraines

Due to the preponderance of evidence that migraine with aura is associated with an elevated stroke risk compared with migraine without aura, and the assumption that this risk would be further elevated by use of CHCs, the American College of Obstetricians and Gynecologists (ACOG), the World Health Organization (WHO), and the CDC have considered migraines with aura to be an absolute contraindication to the use of combined hormonal contraception [32, 36]. The IHS Task Force on Combined Oral Contraceptives and Hormone Replacement Therapy, however, has slightly more liberal guidelines, stating, "There is a potentially increased risk of ischemic stroke in women with migraine who are using combination hormonal contraception and have additional risk factors which cannot easily be controlled, including migraine with aura. One must individually assess and evaluate these risks" [20]. Thus, use of CHC in women experiencing migraine with aura is not strictly contraindicated by the IHS. In assessing the risk of CHC or hormone therapy in patients who have migraine and migraine with aura, the IHS suggests that other independent risk factors for stroke also be assessed and taken into consideration, including age>35 years, tobacco use, dyslipidemia, family history of arterial disease age<45 years, and other relevant medical comorbidities (i.e., obesity [body mass index ≥ 30], diabetes, known vascular disease). The recommendations of the USMEC, ACOG, and the IHS Task Force regarding CHC use in women with headache and migraine are summarized in Table 7.3.

Special Considerations

Idiopathic Intracranial Hypertension (IIH)

Although migraine is the headache type most influenced by hormonal contraceptives, there are some concerns for idiopathic intracranial hypertension (IIH), formerly known as pseudotumor cerebri. The International Headache Society definition criterion for IIH is shown in Table 7.4. The incidence of IIH is approximately 21/100,000. The condition occurs four times more frequently in women, and 90 % of women with IIH are obese. The pathophysiology of IIH is unclear. The proposed mechanisms include increased intracellular fluid, excess cerebrospinal fluid (CSF) production, decreased CSF absorption, and increased cerebral venous pressure. Each of these could result in elevated intracranial pressure. The major concern for untreated IIH is visual loss due to sustained elevated intracranial pressure pressing on the optic nerves [37, 38].

There have been a number of case reports implicating COCs as causal agents in IIH. However, the current thinking is that CHCs do not play a role in the etiology of IIH. The major concern in choosing contraception for these patients is related to their obesity. For example, COCs and the combined contraceptive patch may be slightly less effective in obese individuals (see Chap. 10) [39]. In addition, obesity increases both cardiovascular risk and risk of venous thromboembolism. Therefore, a progestin-only method may be safer, though the USMEC considers the benefit from CHCs in this population greater than the risk [40].

Excessive weight gain during pregnancy will exacerbate and in some instances trigger IIH (as illustrated in the case below). Other pregnancy complications are related to obesity itself, which increases the risk of pregnancy-induced hypertension, preeclampsia, and gestational diabetes.

Table 7.3 USMEC/ACOG/IHS Task Force Recommendations Regarding Combined Hormonal Contraceptive (CHC) Use in Women with Headache and Migraine

Condition	ACOG	USMEC	IHS
Headache (nonmigrainous)	No contraindication	No contraindication	No contraindication
Migraine without Aura			
Age<35 years	No contraindication	No contraindication	Individualized assessment of risk
Age ≥35 years	Risk usually outweighs benefits	Risk usually outweighs benefits	Individualized assessment of risk, depends on number of risk factors[a]
Smokers	Risk usually outweighs benefits	Risk usually outweighs benefits	Women with migraine who smoke should stop smoking before starting CHC
Additional risk factors for ischemic stroke: hypertension, obesity, diabetes, hyperlipidemia	Risk usually outweighs benefits	Risk usually outweighs benefits	Individualized assessment of risk, depends on number of risk factors.[b] Risk factors such as hypertension and hyperlipidemia should be treated
Migraine with Aura			
Age<35 years	Risk unacceptable	Risk unacceptable	Individualized assessment of risk, depends on number of risk factors
Age ≥35 years	Risk unacceptable	Risk unacceptable	Individualized assessment of risk, depends on number of risk factors
Smokers	Risk unacceptable	Risk unacceptable	Women with migraine who smoke should stop smoking before starting CHC
Additional risk factors for ischemic stroke: hypertension, obesity, diabetes, hyperlipidemia	Risk unacceptable	Risk unacceptable	Individualized assessment of risk, depends on number of risk factors. Risk factors such as hypertension and hyperlipidemia should be treated

Abbreviations: *ACOG* American College of Obstetricians and Gynecologists, *IHS* International Headache Society, *USMEC* United States Medical Eligibility Criteria for Contraceptive Use

[a]Risk factors include age >35 years, ischemic heart disease or cardiac disease with embolic potential, diabetes mellitus, family history of arterial disease at age <45 years, hyperlipidemia, hypertension, migraine aura, obesity (body mass index >30), smoking, systemic diseases associated with stroke including sickle cell disease and connective tissue disorders.

[b]Consider non-CHC methods in women at increased risk of ischemic stroke, particularly those who have multiple risk factors

Table 7.4 Idiopathic Intracranial Hypertension (IIH) International Headache Society 2013

- Headache is usually accompanied by other signs of IIH. It remits after normalization of CSF pressure
- CSF pressure is > 250 mm
- The majority of patients have papilledema
- Other symptoms include pulsatile tinnitus, transient visual obscurations, neck or back pain, and diplopia
- Other causes of elevated ICP have been excluded

Abbreviations: *CSF* cerebrospinal fluid, *ICP* intracranial pressure

Reprinted with permission from Levin M. The International Classification of Headache Disorders, 3rd Edition (ICHD III) – Changes and Challenges. Headache: The Journal of Head and Face Pain 2013; 53: 1383–1395.

Case 2

A 22-year-old woman who is 26 weeks pregnant comes in for evaluation of headaches. She has gained 47 lb. She is currently having headaches primarily in the morning. They are worse with cough or Valsalva. She has occasional episodes of blurred vision.

New-Onset Headaches Following Initiation of Exogenous Hormones

Exogenous hormone-induced headache is defined as either new onset of headache or exacerbation of existing headache within the first 3 months of initiating hormonal therapy [7]. There is evidence that patients who have migraines with aura have four times the odds of developing worsening headaches after initiation of combination oral contraceptives compared with women who have migraines without aura [41, 42]. Exogenous hormone-induced headaches are also more common in women age>35 years and women with a family history of migraines [43]. Headache associated with CHC use typically will improve as use continues. A Scandinavian study suggests that if a headache or migraine occurs in the first cycle of combination hormonal contraceptive use, there is only a 1 in 3 risk of headache recurrence in the second cycle, and a 1 in 10 chance of headache in the third cycle [6].

Nevertheless, a recent systematic review suggests that studies on exogenous hormone-induced headache are generally of low quality, have studied older contraceptive formulations with higher EE doses that do not reflect those in current use, have failed to distinguish migraine from other headaches, and have failed to control for baseline estimates of migraine incidence or prevalence, both of which are high in women, and increase with age. The majority of studies did not include control groups of women using nonhormonal or no contraception, and so do not capture the baseline incidence of headache in reproductive-age women. The review concludes that we lack reliable evidence about the effects of hormonal contraception on headache and migraine [44]. Until better data are available, ACOG, the CDC, and the IHS Task Force recommend reevaluation or discontinuation of CHC use for women who develop escalating severity or frequency of headaches, particularly outside of the pill-free interval; new-onset migraine with aura symptoms; or nonmigrainous headaches persisting beyond 3 months of use [20, 36]. For these women, consideration should be given to a progestin-only or hormone-free method.

The effect of exogenous progestins on headache and migraine is not well understood. It has been noted that migraines may occur during episodes of uterine bleeding in women taking progestins, even if ovulation is suppressed [6, 45]. However, it is unclear whether this effect is secondary to estrogen fluctuation due to incomplete suppression of ovulation, or increased prostaglandins within the endometrium [6]. Because some progestin-only methods, such as the progestin-only pill and the levonorgestrel-IUD, may not fully suppress gonadotropins, estrogen fluctuations can occur. It has been noted that in women taking progestin-only pills, headache and migraine improve most often in those who have achieved amenorrhea [45, 46]. However, even when ovulation is completely suppressed, estrogen fluctuations have still been noted in women using progestin-only methods [47]. Third-generation progestins may be associated with fewer headaches per cycle, compared with second-generation progestins [46, 48].

Estrogen-Withdrawal Headache

In women who are not taking hormonal contraception, estrogen withdrawal during the late luteal phase is a well-recognized trigger of headache and menstrual migraines [49]. Estrogen-withdrawal headaches have also been observed in women taking CHCs as well as postmenopausal women taking estrogen-containing hormone therapy [50].

The pathophysiology triggering menstrual migraine is thought to be related to estrogen's effects on prostaglandins and the endogenous opioid pathways. Prostaglandins play a role in both neurogenic inflammation and sensitization of the central pain pathways. In addition, prostaglandins produced by the endometrium cause uterine contractions and dysmenorrhea. Studies have shown that when blood taken from women during severe dysmenorrhea episodes is autologously transfused after the pain subsides, subjects report both crampy pain and headache [51].

Estrogen also has modulatory effects on central opioid pathways involving the hypothalamic-pituitary axis. Opiate peptides cause an inhibition of the pituitary's secretion of luteinizing hormone. This response is muted in women who have menstrual migraine, suggesting altered hypothalamic opioid activity. The pituitary is the primary source of beta-endorphin, which affects pain responses and locally acts as a neurotransmitter. Levels of beta- endorphin are lower in women who suffer from menstrual migraine, suggesting that changes in central opioid pathways are linked to the onset of these headaches [52–54].

Estrogen-withdrawal headaches are defined as headaches that appear within the first 5 days of estrogen cessation, start after daily exogenous estrogen exposure for three weeks or more prior to cessation, and typically resolve within 3 days of their onset [7]. Estrogen-withdrawal headaches may also be associated with other hormone withdrawal symptoms, including breast tenderness and pelvic pain. Additional ethinyl estradiol during the perimenstrual interval can effectively reduce or prevent estrogen-withdrawal headaches [55]. Reducing the hormone-free interval to 3–4 days instead of 7 days, or eliminating the hormone-free interval entirely, has been successful in the prevention of estrogen-withdrawal headaches [42, 50, 53–56].

Menstrual Migraines

Menstrual migraines are a subset of estrogen-withdrawal headaches, typically occurring 2 days before the onset of menses and lasting through the third day of menstrual bleeding. The association of migraines with menses must occur in at least two-thirds of cycles to be classified as menstrual migraines [7]. Due to different definitions, the prevalence cited is variable. A small number of women will have menstrual migraines only, and more than 50 % of women with migraine will have menses-triggered migraines as well as migraines at other times in their cycle. This type of migraine is generally the most severe, longest, and most refractory to treatment [53].

Although menstrual migraines by definition fulfill the ICHD II criteria for migraine, they typically are not associated with an aura, even in women who experience migraine with aura at other times in their cycle [57]. Treatment of menstrual migraine depends on whether the migraine is exclusive to menstruation. If not, a prophylactic medication can be used, with consideration of increasing the dose around the time of menstruation. Before attempting hormone supplementation, nonsteroidal anti-inflammatory drugs (NSAIDs), triptans, and ergot derivatives may be attempted as initial prophylaxis and abortive therapy for women who experience menstrual migraines [58–60]. A small, randomized, placebo-controlled trial found that 550 mg naproxen twice daily for migraine prophylaxis, beginning 7 days before onset of menses and continued for 13 days, significantly decreased the frequency, severity, and duration of menstrual migraines compared with placebo [60]. Triptans have been extensively studied in treatment of menstrual migraine, and found to be superior to placebo [61]. Rizatriptan and sumatriptan have been the most well studied. A small, randomized, placebo-controlled trial found that mefenamic acid—also effective in treatment of dysmenorrhea—is superior to placeboin the treatment of menstrual migraine [62]. An NSAID/triptan combination may be another first-line therapy in women with menstrual migraines and dysmenorrhea [63]. For women whose menstrual migraines do not respond to nonhormonal therapy, supplemental EE during the late luteal phase of the menstrual cycle (day 28, 29) through cycle day 3 may reduce the severity and frequency of menstrual migraines [64].

Strategies to avoid hormone withdrawal and consequent migraine include continuous use of combination contraception or adding estrogens alone during the perimenstrual period. Use of percutaneous estradiol gel beginning 48 h prior to anticipated migraine attack and used for 7 days was found to be superior to placebo in double-blind controlled studies [54, 65–67]. A transdermal estradiol patch has also been shown to be effective in preventing menstrual migraines [64]. The minimum effective dose of estrogen in a transdermal patch has been shown to be 0.1 mg/day. Of note, patches, gels, and other hormone supplementation to prevent menstrual migraines should begin no more than 2 days before the anticipated onset of menses; starting estrogen supplementation earlier (i.e., 6 days before the first day of menses) has been associated with an increased incidence of migraine after the estrogen supplementation is withdrawn [54].

Table 7.5 Migraine preventive medications

Drug class	Generic name	Level of risk in pregnancy	CHC interaction
Beta blockers	Atenolol	D	None
	Metoprolol	C	None
	Nadolol	C	None
	Timolol	C	None
	Propranolol	C	None
Antiepileptics	Gabapentin	C	None
	Topiramate	D	At doses >200 mg/d increases metabolism of OC
	Valproate	X	None
Calcium channel blockers	Verapamil	C	None
Tricyclics	Amitriptyline	C	

Pregnancy and Migraines

Pregnancy is both a high-progesterone and a high-estrogen state in which ovulation is completely suppressed. The elevated estrogen and progesterone levels of pregnancy decline precipitously after delivery. Thus, migraine and headache symptoms might be expected to improve during pregnancy and to recur during the puerperium, if the hypothesis that menstrual migraines (which are usually migraine without aura) occur when estrogen levels decline rapidly after sustained exposure to estrogen throughout the menstrual cycle is true. There are conflicting data in this regard. The majority of available literature suggests that women typically experience improvement or no change in frequency or severity of migraines during pregnancy [68]. The percentage of women whose migraines improve in pregnancy ranges vastly in the literature, from 18 % to 86 % [69]. To date, no objective criteria have been established to determine which women are likely to have improvement of headache or migraine in pregnancy. It is a consistent finding that migraine with aura is less likely to improve in pregnancy [41, 70, 71], perhaps related to increased endothelial reactivity in these patients [60]. Findings from a large, population-based study of Norwegian women suggest that headache, both migrainous and nonmigrainous, is less prevalent in pregnancy, although this association was only true in the third trimester and in primigravidas. The decreased prevalence of headaches in pregnancy was not seen in primiparous or multiparous pregnant women [72].

Migraine Medications and Contraceptive Interactions

The medications that are used as migraine preventives include beta blockers, calcium channel blockers, and some antiepileptic drugs (AEDs). Cytochrome P450 enzyme-inducing AEDs affect hormonal contraceptive efficacy by increasing their metabolism. Topiramate is the most commonly used migraine prophylactic that can decrease both CHC and progestin-only pill and implant efficacy in this way. This effect is primarily seen in topiramate doses greater than 200 mg/day [73]. See Table 7.5 for a summary of contraceptive interaction and pregnancy classification of commonly used migraine prophylactic medications (see Chap. 20).

Conclusion

Migraine affects a little over one-third of reproductive-age women in the United States. Hormonal contraception is the most frequently used form of birth control, with up to 43 % of US women selecting a hormonal method. Evidence suggests that migraine, particularly migraine with aura, is associated with an increased risk of ischemic stroke, and that this risk may be further elevated in the setting of combined hormonal contraceptive use. There are no studies that directly compare the risk of stroke in migraineurs with and without aura using combined hormonal contraceptives. The majority of studies regarding stroke risk in women with migraine using combination hormonal contraception are retrospective case–control studies. Thus, the data are subject to recall bias and classification bias, and must be interpreted with caution.

ACOG and the CDC state that the use of CHC may be considered for women with migraine headache only if they do not experience aura, do not smoke, are otherwise healthy, and are younger than age 35 years. The IHS Task Force does not state that migraine with aura is an absolute contraindication to use of combination contraception, and suggests that decisions regarding contraceptive choice be made on a case-by-case basis.

Headaches associated with combination hormonal contraceptives typically will improve as use continues. Reevaluation or discontinuation of combination hormonal contraception is advised for women who develop escalating severity or frequency of headaches, new-onset migraine with aura, or nonmigrainous headaches persisting beyond 3 months of use. For patients with estrogen-withdrawal headaches and menstrual migraines, reducing the hormone-free interval to 3–4 days, or eliminating the hormone-free interval entirely, has been demonstrated to reduce the severity, frequency, and duration of headache. For menstrual migraines, traditional abortive and prophylactic therapies for migraine, including naproxen and mefenamic acid, triptans, and ergot alkaloids, have also been shown to be more effective than placebo. These methods can be first-line therapy for menstrual migraines, particularly in women for whom estrogen use is contraindicated.

In considering the risks of combination hormonal contraception in women with migraine, it is critical to keep the cardiovascular risks of pregnancy (often the result of lack of effective contraception) in mind. The age-adjusted incidence of venous thromboembolic phenomena is 4–50 times greater in pregnant and peripartum women compared with nonpregnant women [74–78]. Pregnancy, delivery, and the postpartum period are also associated with a significantly elevated RR of both ischemic (RR = 8.7) and hemorrhagic (RR = 28.3) stroke, with greatest risk in the postpartum period [79]. Thus, pregnancy likely poses a far greater risk to women's cardiovascular health than does the use of combination hormonal contraception, even in the high-risk group of migraineurs with aura.

References

1. Stewart WF, Wood C, Reed ML, Roy J, Lipton RB, AMPP Advisory Group. Cumulative lifetime migraine incidence in women and men. Cephalalgia. 2008; 28:1170–8.
2. Finer LB, Frohwirth LF, Dauphinee LA, Singh S, Moore AM. Reasons U.S. women have abortions: quantitative and qualitative perspectives. Perspect Sex Reprod Health. 2005;37:110–8.
3. Rosenberg MJ, Waugh MS. Oral contraceptive discontinuation: a prospective evaluation of frequency and reasons. Am J Obstet Gynecol. 1998;179:577–82.
4. Rosenberg MJ, Waugh MS, Long S. Unintended pregnancies and use, misuse and discontinuation of oral contraceptives. J Reprod Med. 1995;40:355–60.
5. Lipton RB, Bigal ME, Diamond M, Freitag F, Reed ML, Stewart WF, AMPP Advisory Group. Migraine prevalence, disease burden, and the need for preventive therapy. Neurology. 2007;68:343–9.
6. MacGregor EA. Migraine and use of combined hormonal contraceptives: a clinical review. J Fam Plann Reprod Health Care. 2007;33:159–69.
7. Headache Classification Subcommittee of the International Headache Society. The International Classification of Headache Disorders, 2nd ed. Cephalalgia. 2004;24 suppl 1:9–160.
8. Charles A. Advances in the basic and clinical science of migraine. Ann Neurol. 2009;65:491–8.
9. Russell MB, Olesen J. A nosographic analysis of the migraine aura in a general population. Brain. 1996; 119(Pt 2):355–61.
10. Merikangas KR, Fenton BT, Cheng SH, Stolar MJ, Risch N. Association between migraine and stroke in a large-scale epidemiological study of the United States. Arch Neurol. 1997;54:362–8.
11. Chang CL, Donaghy M, Poulter N, The World Health Organization Collaborative Study of Cardiovascular Disease and Steroid Hormone Contraception. Migraine and stroke in young women: case–control study. BMJ. 1999;318:13–8.
12. MacClellan LR, Giles W, Cole J, Wozniak M, Stern B, Mitchell BD, et al. Probable migraine with visual aura and risk of ischemic stroke: the stroke prevention in young women study. Stroke. 2007;38:2438–45.
13. Kurth T, Slomke MA, Kase CS, Cook NR, Lee IM, Gaziano JM, et al. Migraine, headache, and the risk of

stroke in women: a prospective study. Neurology. 2005;64:1020–6.
14. Kurth T, Gaziano JM, Cook NR, Logroscino G, Diener HC, Buring JE. Migraine and risk of cardiovascular disease in women. JAMA. 2006;296: 283–91.
15. Etminan M, Takkouche B, Isorna FC, Samii A. Risk of ischaemic stroke in people with migraine: systematic review and meta-analysis of observational studies. BMJ. 2005;330:63–6.
16. Henrich JB, Horwitz RI. A controlled study of ischemic stroke risk in migraine patients. J Clin Epidemiol. 1989;42:773–80.
17. Carolei A, Marini C, De Matteis G, The Italian National Research Council Study Group on Stroke in the Young . History of migraine and risk of cerebral ischaemia in young adults. Lancet. 1996;347:1503–6.
18. Tzourio C, Iglesias S, Hubert JB, Visy JM, Alpérovitch A, Tehindrazanarivelo A, et al. Migraine and risk of ischaemic stroke: a case–control study. BMJ. 1993; 307:289–92.
19. Tzourio C, Tehindrazanarivelo A, Iglésias S, Alpérovitch A, Chedru F, d'Anglejan-Chatillon J, et al. Case–control study of migraine and risk of ischaemic stroke in young women. BMJ. 1995;310: 830–3.
20. Bousser MG, Conard J, Kittner S, de Lignières B, MacGregor EA, Massiou H, The International Headache Society Task Force on Combined Oral Contraceptives & Hormone Replacement Therapy, et al. Recommendations on the risk of ischaemic stroke associated with use of combined oral contraceptives and hormone replacement therapy in women with migraine. Cephalalgia. 2000;20:155–6.
21. Petitti DB, Sidney S, Bernstein A, Wolf S, Quesenberry C, Ziel HK. Stroke in users of low-dose oral contraceptives. N Engl J Med. 1996;335:8–15.
22. Stang PE, Carson AP, Rose KM, Mo J, Ephross SA, Shahar E, et al. Headache, cerebrovascular symptoms, and stroke: the Atherosclerosis Risk in Communities Study. Neurology. 2005;64:1573–7.
23. Lidegaard Ø. Oral contraception and risk of a cerebral thromboembolic attack: results of a case–control study. BMJ. 1993;306:956–63.
24. Lidegaard Ø, Kreiner S. Contraceptives and cerebral thrombosis: a five-year national case control study. Contraception. 2002;65:197–205.
25. Gillum LA, Mamidipudi SK, Johnston SC. Ischemic stroke risk with oral contraceptives: a meta-analysis. JAMA. 2000;284:72–8.
26. Heinemann LA, Lewis MA, Spitzer WO, Thorogood M, Guggenmoos-Holzmann I, Bruppacher R, Transnational Research Group on Oral Contraceptives and the Health of Young Women. Thromboembolic stroke in young women. A European case–control study on oral contraceptives. Contraception. 1998;57:29–37.
27. WHO Collaborative Study of Cardiovascular Disease and Steroid Hormone Contraception. Ischaemic stroke and combined oral contraceptives: results of an international, multicentre, case–control study. Lancet. 1996;348:498–505.
28. Lidegaard O, Lokkegaard E, Jenson A, Skovlund C, Keiding N. Thrombotic stroke and myocardial infarction with hormonal contraception. N Engl J Med. 2012;366:2257–66.
29. World Health Organization. Medical eligibility criteria for contraceptive use. 4th ed. Geneva: World Health Organization; 2009.
30. Donaghy M, Chang CL, Poulter N, on behalf of the European Collaborators of the World Health Organisation Collaborative Study of Cardiovascular Disease and Steroid Hormone Contraception. Duration, frequency, recency, and type of migraine and the risk of ischaemic stroke in women of childbearing age. J Neurol Neurosurg Psychiatry. 2002; 73:747–50.
31. MacGregor EA. Menstrual migraine: a clinical review. J Fam Plann Reprod Health Care. 2007;33: 36–47.
32. World Health Organization Collaborative Study of Cardiovascular Disease and Steroid Hormone Contraception. Cardiovascular disease and use of oral and injectable progestogen-only contraceptives and combined injectable contraceptives. Results of an international, multicenter, case–control study. Contraception. 1998;57:315–24.
33. Schwartz SM, Petitti DB, Siscovick DS, Longstreth Jr WT, Sidney S, Raghunathan TE, et al. Stroke and use of low-dose oral contraceptives in young women: a pooled analysis of two US studies. Stroke. 1998; 29:2277–84.
34. Lidegaard Ø. Oral contraceptives, pregnancy and the risk of cerebral thromboembolism: the influence of diabetes, hypertension, migraine and previous thrombotic disease. Br J Obstet Gynaecol. 1995;102: 153–9.
35. Schürks M, Rist PM, Bigal ME, Buring JE, Lipton RB, Kurth T. Migraine and cardiovascular disease: systematic review and meta-analysis. BMJ. 2009;339:b3914.
36. ACOG Committee on Practice Bulletins-Gynecology. Practice Bulletin ACOG. No. 73: Use of hormonal contraception in women with coexisting medical conditions. Obstet Gynecol. 2006;107:1453–72.
37. Duncan J, Corbett J, Wall M. The incidence of pseudotumor cerebri population studies in Iowa and Louisiana. Arch Neurol. 1988;45(8):875–7.
38. Bousse V, Bruce B, Newman N. Update on the pathophysiology of idiopathic intracranial hypertension. J Neurol Neurosurg Psychiatry. 2012;83:488–94.
39. Robinson JA, Burke AE. Obesity and hormonal contraceptive efficacy. Womens Health. 2013;9(5):453–66.
40. Edelman A, Jensen J. Obesity and hormonal contraception: safety and efficacy. Semin Reprod Med. 2012;30(06):479–85.
41. Granella F, Sances G, Pucci E, Nappi RE, Ghiotto N, Napp G. Migraine with aura and reproductive life events: a case control study. Cephalalgia. 2000; 20:701–7.

42. Loder EW, Buse DC, Golub JR. Headache and combination estrogen-progestin oral contraceptives: integrating evidence, guidelines, and clinical practice. Headache. 2005;45:224–31.
43. Larsson-Cohn U, Lundberg PO. Headache and treatment with oral contraceptives. Acta Neurol Scand. 1970;46:267–78.
44. Loder EW, Buse DC, Golub JR. Headache as a side effect of combination estrogen-progestin oral contraceptives: a systematic review. Am J Obstet Gynecol. 2005;193(3 Pt 1):636–49.
45. Somerville BW, Carey HM. The use of continuous progestogen contraception in the treatment of migraine. Med J Aust. 1970;1:1043–5.
46. Davies P, Fursdon-Davies C, Rees MC. Progestogens for menstrual migraine. J Br Menopause Soc. 2003; 9:134.
47. Croxatto HB, Mäkaräinen L. The pharmacodynamics and efficacy of Implanon. An overview of the data. Contraception. 1998;58:91S–7.
48. Fotherby K. Twelve years of clinical experience with an oral contraceptive containing 30 micrograms ethinyloestradiol and 150 micrograms desogestrel. Contraception. 1995;51:3–12.
49. MacGregor EA, Frith A, Ellis J, Aspinall L, Hackshaw A. Incidence of migraine relative to menstrual cycle phases of rising and falling estrogen. Neurology. 2006;67:2154–8.
50. Sulak PJ, Scow RD, Preece C, Riggs MW, Kuehl TJ. Hormone withdrawal symptoms in oral contraceptive users. Obstet Gynecol. 2000;95:261–6.
51. Silberstein SD. The role of sex hormones in headache. Neurology. 1992;42(3 suppl2):37–42.
52. Silberstein S. Headache and female hormones: what you need to know. Curr Opin Neurol. 2001;14: 323–33.
53. MacGregor EA, Hackshaw A. Prevalence of migraine on each day of the natural menstrual cycle. Neurology. 2004;63:351–3.
54. MacGregor EA, Frith A, Ellis J, Aspinall L, Hackshaw A. Prevention of menstrual attacks of migraine: a double-blind placebo-controlled crossover stud. Neurology. 2006;67:2159–63.
55. MacGregor EA, Hackshaw A. Prevention of migraine in the pill-free interval of combined oral contraceptives: a double-blind, placebo-controlled pilot study using natural oestrogen supplements. J Fam Plann Reprod Health Care. 2002;28:27–31.
56. Edelman A, Gallo MF, Nichols MD, Jensen JT, Schulz KF, Grimes DA. Continuous versus cyclic use of combined oral contraceptives for contraception: systematic Cochrane review of randomized controlled trials. Hum Reprod. 2006;21:573–8.
57. Johannes CB, Linet MS, Stewart WF, Celentano DD, Lipton RB, Szklo M. Relationship of headache to phase of the menstrual cycle among young women: a daily diary study. Neurology. 1995;45: 1076–82.
58. Facchinetti F, Bonellie G, Kangasniemi P, Pascual J, Shuaib A, The Sumatriptan Menstrual Migraine Study Group. The efficacy and safety of subcutaneous sumatriptan in the acute treatment of menstrual migraine. Obstet Gynecol. 1995;86:911–6.
59. Solbach MP, Waymer RS. Treatment of menstruation-associated migraine headache with subcutaneous sumatriptan. Obstet Gynecol. 1993;82:769–72.
60. Sances G, Martignoni E, Fioroni L, Blandini F, Facchinetti F, Nappi G. Naproxen sodium in menstrual migraine prophylaxis: a double-blind placebo controlled study. Headache. 1990;30:705–9.
61. Ashkenazi A, Silberstein S. Menstrual migraine: a review of hormonal causes, prophylaxis and treatment. Expert Opin Pharmacother. 2007;8: 1605–13.
62. Al-Waili NS. Treatment of menstrual migraine with prostaglandin synthesis inhibitor mefenamic acid: double-blind study with placebo. Eur J Med Res. 2000;5:176–82.
63. Mannix LK, Martin VT, Cady RK, Diamond ML, Lener SE, White JD, et al. Combination treatment for menstrual migraine and dysmenorrhea using sumatriptan-naproxen: two randomized controlled trials. Obstet Gynecol. 2009;114:106–13.
64. Massiou H, MacGregor EA. Evolution and treatment of migraine with oral contraceptives. Cephalalgia. 2000;20:170–4.
65. Pringsheim T, Davenport WJ, Dodick D. Acute treatment and prevention of menstrually related migraine headache: evidence-based review. Neurology. 2008; 70:1555–63.
66. de Lignières B, Vincens M, Mauvais-Jarvis P, Mas JL, Touboul PJ, Bousser MG. Prevention of menstrual migraine by percutaneous oestradiol. Br Med J (Clin Res Ed). 1986;293:1540.
67. Dennerstein L, Morse C, Burrows G, Oats J, Brown J, Smith M. Menstrual migraine: a double-blind trial of percutaneous estradiol. Gynecol Endocrinol. 1988;2: 113–20.
68. Menon R, Bushnell CD. Headache and pregnancy. Neurologist. 2008;14:108–19.
69. Contag SA, Mertz HL, Bushnell CD. Migraine during pregnancy: is it more than a headache? Nat Rev Neurol. 2009;5:449–56.
70. Kelman L. Women's issues of migraine in tertiary care. Headache. 2004;44:2–7.
71. Scharff L, Marcus DA, Turk DC. Headache during pregnancy and in the postpartum: a prospective study. Headache. 1997;37:203 10.
72. Aegidius K, Zwart JA, Hagen K, Stovner L. The effect of pregnancy and parity on headache prevalence: the Head-HUNT study. Headache. 2009;49:851–9.
73. Bialer M, Doose DR, Murthy B, Curtin C, Curtin C, Wang SS, Twyman RE, et al. Pharmacokinetic interactions of topiramate. Clin Pharmacokinet. 2004; 43(12):763–80.
74. Marik PE, Plante LA. Venous thromboembolic disease and pregnancy. N Engl J Med. 2008;359:2025–33.

75. Greer IA. Thrombosis in pregnancy: maternal and fetal issues. Lancet. 1999;353:1258–65.
76. Kujovich JL. Hormones and pregnancy: thromboembolic risks for women. Br J Haematol. 2004;126: 443–54.
77. Heit JA, Kobbervig CE, James AH, Petterson TM, Bailey KR, Melton 3rd LJ. Trends in the incidence of venous thromboembolism during pregnancy or postpartum: a 30-year population-based study. Ann Intern Med. 2005;143:697–706.
78. NIH Consensus Development. Prevention of venous thrombosis and pulmonary embolism. JAMA. 1986; 256:744–9.
79. Kittner SJ, Stern BJ, Feeser BR, Hebel R, Nagey DA, Buchholz DW, et al. Pregnancy and the risk of stroke. N Engl J Med. 1996;335:768–74.

Contraception for Women with Epilepsy

8

Anne R. Davis, Alison M. Pack, and Amanda Dennis

Overview of Epilepsy and Epidemiology

Epilepsy is a neurological condition characterized by multiple unprovoked epileptic seizures [1]. Seizures result from a sudden synchronization or surge in electrical activity in the brain. Seizure types include absence, myoclonic, atonic, clonic, tonic, tonic clonic, and focal. The severity of seizures ranges from minimal to disabling. During a seizure an individual can experience a range of brief, involuntary changes in sensation, body movement, or emotion that can occur with or without impaired consciousness. Seizure presentation depends on the specific epilepsy syndrome as well as the location of the epileptogenic network in the brain [2].

The mainstay of treatment is antiepileptic drugs (AEDs), which do not "cure" epilepsy but decrease the likelihood of a seizure occurring. Multiple AEDs are available (Table 8.1). When choosing an AED, physicians consider effectiveness, side effect profile, the long-term implications of treatment, and drug interactions, such as interactions with hormonal therapy. Other comorbid medical conditions are also considered because many persons with epilepsy have headaches or mood disorders and AEDs can be useful for these conditions. Approximately 50 % of persons will respond to the initial AED prescribed. About 33 % of persons will experience drug-resistant or refractory epilepsy [3], which the International League Against Epilepsy (ILAE) defines as the failure to achieve sustained seizure freedom after completing two adequate trials of tolerated, appropriately chosen AEDs [4].

The Institute of Medicine estimates 2.2 million Americans have epilepsy, almost half of which are girls and women [2]. The overall annual incidence of epilepsy in the USA is approximately 48 per 100,000 people [5]. One study in Rochester, Minnesota found that approximately 1 in 26 people will develop epilepsy in their lifetime [6], though this study may not be representative of the US population as it was based on one community. Epilepsy can develop at any age, though some epilepsy syndromes such as juvenile myoclonic epilepsy begin in childhood or adolescence. Epilepsy affects people of all racial, ethnic, and socioeconomic backgrounds [2].

A.R. Davis, M.D., M.P.H. (✉)
Department of Obstetrics and Gynecology, Columbia University Medical Center, New York, NY, USA
e-mail: ard4@columbia.edu

A.M. Pack, M.D., M.P.H.
Department of Neurology, Columbia University Medical Center, New York, NY, USA
e-mail: ap390@columbia.edu

A. Dennis, Dr.P.H., M.B.E.
Ibis Reproductive Health, Cambridge, MA, USA
e-mail: adennis@ibisreproductivehealth.org

R.H. Allen and C.A. Cwiak (eds.), *Contraception for the Medically Challenging Patient*, DOI 10.1007/978-1-4939-1233-9_8, © Springer Science+Business Media New York 2014

Table 8.1 Common antiepileptic drugs (AEDs) and hepatic enzyme inducer effects

Inducers	Non-inducers
• Carbamazepine	• Clobazam
• Felbamate	• Clonazepam
• Lamotrigine[a]	• Ethosuximide
• Oxcarbazepine	• Ezogabine
• Phenobarbital	• Gabapentin
• Phenytoin	• Lacosamide
• Primidone	• Levetiracetam
• Rufinamide	• Pregabalin
	• Tiagabine
	• Topiramate
	• Valproate
	• Vigabatrin
	• Zonisamide

[a]Limited evidence shows decreased levels of progestin, but not ethinyl estradiol during lamotrigine coadministration with an oral contraceptive

Reproductive Physiology, Fertility, and Catamenial Seizures

Women with epilepsy (WWE) face unique concerns related to their reproductive health; increased rates of polycystic ovarian syndrome (PCOS), decreased libido, infertility, and early menopause have all been described [7]. These effects may be secondary to epilepsy itself or related to AED therapy. For example, valproate use is associated with higher rates of PCOS in WWE [8].

Reproductive hormones may influence a woman's seizure presentation. Generally, estrogen has pro-convulsant properties, whereas progesterone, and in particular its metabolite allopregnanolone, are antiepileptic [7]. Some WWE experience catamenial epilepsy, in which the seizure threshold varies with phases of the menstrual cycle. The most commonly accepted definition of catamenial epilepsy is a consistent doubling of seizure frequency during at least one of three menstrual phases: perimenstrual (from cycle day −3 to day +3), periovulatory (day +10 to day +13), or during the luteal phase (day +10 to day +3 of the next cycle). Using this definition, approximately 33 % of women with focal epilepsy experience catamenial seizures [9]. Using other definitions, the prevalence of catamenial patterns among WWE ranges from 10 to 70 % [10].

There is no generally recognized drug treatment specifically for catamenial seizures. One recent double-blind, randomized study compared cyclic natural progesterone therapy (administered as a lozenge) to a placebo for treatment of refractory catamenial and non-catamenial seizures. Overall, results showed no difference in seizure control between progesterone versus placebo groups; however, the subgroup of women with a perimenstrual seizure exacerbation improved more with progesterone than placebo [11]. Whether systemic hormonal contraceptive use benefits catamenial seizures is unknown. Basic education about catamenial seizures is also needed; some WWE and their health care providers are unaware that seizures can be affected by hormonal shifts, and some providers disregard the potential for a catamenial pattern when women report it [12].

Social Effects of Epilepsy for Women, Sexuality, and Reproduction

People with and without epilepsy often display negative, stigmatizing attitudes towards people with the disorder [13]. The stigma attached to epilepsy appears to have a gendered component. Women with epilepsy experience lower health-related quality of life when compared to their male counterparts [14]. They also experience particular negative effects on their romantic, sexual, and reproductive lives, sometimes being considered poor candidates for dating or long-term partnership [15] and being less likely to marry or have children compared to the general population [16, 17]. Relatively high rates of sexual dysfunction, sexual anxiety, and menstrual disorders may play a role [18], along with women's concerns about their ability to safely have children while maintaining their neurological health [19, 20].

Contraception: General Considerations

Determining whether or not to have a child and implementing family-size goals is an essential component of women's health and lives. The average woman in the USA will spend 30 years preventing pregnancy and 5 years seeking pregnancy and then bearing children [21]. For WWE, contraception and pregnancy planning are especially important. Adequate folic acid intake should be established prior to conception and an appropriate medication treatment plan should be chosen to reduce risks to fetal and neonatal health and maintain maternal seizure control during pregnancy and birth. In 1998, the American Academy of Neurology published a Practice Parameter recommending that counseling on contraception be included in care for WWE [22]. This practice parameter acknowledged complexities related to drug interactions but gave little practical advice to guide method choice. No updated practice parameters have since been published.

The use of contraception among WWE is poorly described. National surveys of contraception use in the general population do not assess chronic disorders such as epilepsy. One cross-sectional questionnaire study in an urban, academic medical center ($n = 148$) queried WWE and found that only 53 % of those at risk of unplanned pregnancy used methods with typical failure rates of less than 10 % in the first year of use, most often sterilization or oral contraceptives [23]. The rest relied on condoms, spermicides, natural family planning (timed intercourse), or withdrawal, alone or in combination. Use of long-acting reversible contraception (LARC) was rare. In this same study, 50 % of the 181 pregnancies reported by WWE were unplanned, and poor, Hispanic WWE experienced more unplanned pregnancies than Caucasian WWE of higher socioeconomic status.

WWE experience specific barriers obtaining appropriate contraceptive care. Few health care professionals understand drug interactions between AEDs and contraceptive steroids [24, 25]. Unsurprisingly, WWE report similar confusion [26]. Recent research has explored barriers from women's personal experiences of the health care system. In one qualitative study, WWE reported that neurologists lacked the necessary expertise in contraception and obstetrician/gynecologists (OB/GYNs) lacked adequate knowledge about epilepsy [12]. Furthermore, when WWE raised contraceptive questions with either a neurologist or an OB/GYN, they were often referred to the other specialist. When women obtained contraceptive information from a neurologist, an OB/GYN, or both, the information was often perceived as inadequate, inappropriate, or in conflict with other information they received.

Starting Contraception to Prevent Pregnancy: Focus on Safety and Effectiveness

For all women, a contraceptive method should be as easy to use as possible. Methods that rely on daily or intermittent user actions may pose a particular burden for WWE maintained on complex AED polytherapy. Visits to a clinician for contraception should be minimized since WWE must manage other visits related to epilepsy for years. For these reasons, as well as high effectiveness, LARC methods should be first choice. Women with catamenial epilepsy may benefit from hormonal methods that inhibit ovulation and prevent hormonal withdrawal (see previous section Reproductive Physiology, Fertility, and Catamenial Seizures) [10]. Direct evidence, however, for control of seizures with contraception is lacking. Safety and effectiveness considerations, as well as recommendations by the US Medical Eligibility Criteria for Contraceptive Use (USMEC) from the Centers for Disease Control and Prevention (CDC), guide our discussion. We omit barrier and fertility awareness methods from our discussion since these methods do not raise special clinical issues for WWE. While safe, the relatively high failure rates of these methods make them an especially poor choice given the complex decisions related to pregnancy planning for WWE. Our clinical recommendations are summarized in Fig. 8.1.

Nonhormonal methods are as safe for WWE as their healthy peers. Hormonal methods are familiar, popular, and offer non-contraceptive benefits; however, choosing a hormonal method for WWE can be challenging. Clinicians are especially concerned about the effects of hormones on the disorder itself. Data from the Oxford Family Planning Contraceptive study indicate that use of combined oral contraceptives

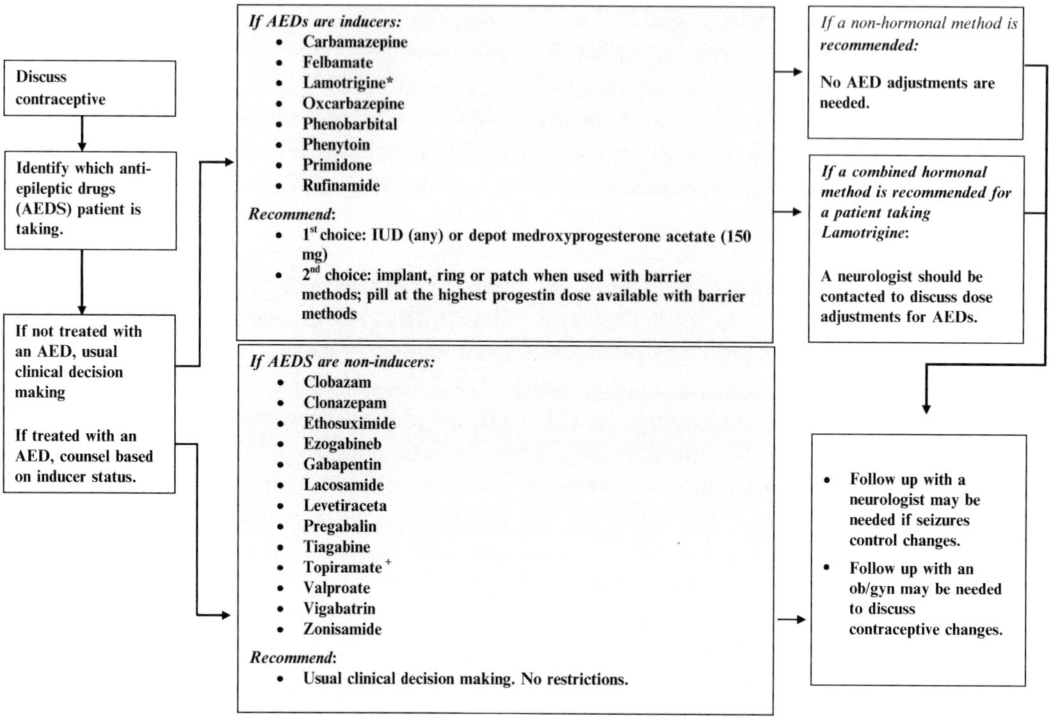

*Lamotrigine lowers C_{max}, AUC, and trough levels of the progestin levonorgestrel. Lamotrigine does not impact levels of ethinyl estradiol [35].
+Topiramate given at a dose of 200 mg a day does not impact levels of norethindrone. Topiramate decreases AUC and C_{max}, but not trough levels, of ethinyl estradiol when given at a dose of 200 mg a day [38].

Fig. 8.1 Clinical algorithm for selecting contraception for women with epilepsy

(COC) does not change the incidence of epilepsy. This cohort study included 17,032 women ages 25–39 years in the UK over an observation period of 20 years. Most women used COCs with "50 micrograms of estrogen." Results were reassuring; neither duration of COC use nor interval since last use was related to a first diagnosis of epilepsy at hospital admission [27]. Clinicians and WWE are appropriately cautious when starting a new medication that may impact seizure control. The Oxford Family Planning Study did not collect information on seizure frequency or intensity during COC use. Indeed, no well-conducted study has yet determined the impact of any contraceptive steroid on seizure frequency, type, or intensity.

It is known, however, that combined hormonal contraceptives (CHC) can impact seizure control and AED side effects via well-understood effects on AED metabolism. This type of interaction is best understood for lamotrigine, a commonly used AED for reproductive-age WWE (Table 8.2) [28]. Lamotrigine is eliminated by conjugation with glucuronic acid, a reaction catalyzed by the uridine 5′-diphosphate (UDP)-glucuronosyltransferases (UGTs) [29]. Among humans, UGT1A4 is the main isoform.

Table 8.2 Clinical considerations for WWE treated with lamotrigine and hormonal contraception

Clinical Concern	Evidence
Antiepileptic drug efficacy	Rapid decreases in lamotrigine levels with associated seizures can occur when estrogen-containing methods are added
Contraceptive efficacy	Decreases levels of progestin, but not EE, with oral contraceptive coadministration
Dosage changes after contraceptive discontinuation	Dosage must be decreased when estrogen-containing methods discontinued
Dosage during pregnancy	Requires close monitoring of levels in pregnancy

EE ethinyl estradiol

Estrogens are also metabolized by glucuronidation. The combination of lamotrigine and CHC increases the metabolism of lamotrigine, likely through induction of the glucuronidation pathway resulting in decreased serum lamotrigine concentrations. In one study, these changes occurred rapidly and resulted in worsening seizure control [30–32]. Lamotrigine levels do not change when taken in combination with progestin-only agents [33]. In practice, if a woman is on a stable dose of lamotrigine and a CHC is added, dose adjustments will likely be necessary to maintain the same lamotrigine concentration. Similarly, when lamotrigine is initiated in a woman taking a CHC, higher doses will be needed to reach therapeutic levels. Women taking CHCs should be counseled about potential symptoms secondary to increased lamotrigine concentrations during the hormone-free interval. Finally, lamotrigine dose reductions need to be considered when a woman stops a CHC.

Contraceptive effectiveness considerations relate to hepatic enzyme induction by some, but not most, commonly used AEDs. Enzyme induction causes enhanced metabolism of contraceptive steroids (see Chap. 20). Many pharmacokinetic (PK) studies examine the degree to which serum levels of ethinyl estradiol (EE) or progestin components of oral contraceptives change during AED administration. Such PK studies are most clinically helpful when no changes occur; then, clinicians can assume AED exposure has no impact on method effectiveness and can follow usual prescribing practices.

When PK data show changes in levels of ethinyl estradiol (EE) or progestin components, clinical decision making becomes more complex because there is no straightforward interpretation of how PK changes impact the risk of pregnancy. We suggest changes in trough levels of contraceptive progestins may be the most useful surrogate marker for pregnancy risk because progestins directly inhibit the luteinizing hormone (LH) surge and subsequent ovulation when maintained above a threshold level. Unfortunately, published PK studies often do not report trough levels. Additionally, data on threshold levels of progestins required for inhibition of ovulation are not readily available to clinicians. A few published AED and contraception interaction studies have included pharmacodynamic measurements of serum follicle-stimulating hormone (FSH), LH, and progesterone as surrogate markers of ovulation but not in a manner to capture unpredictable ovulation. One study demonstrated an increased risk of documented ovulation related to enzyme induction. Davis and colleagues measured ovarian follicular activity with repeated transvaginal ultrasound and serum progesterone in healthy women ($n=10$) who took carbamazepine (CBZ) 600 mg daily or a placebo during use of a low-dose COC containing 20 μg EE and 100 μg levonorgestrel (LNG) [34]. Frank ovulation and increased breakthrough bleeding occurred during CBZ administration compared to placebo administration. Findings from this study indicate that low-dose COCs are not effective when combined with CBZ. These findings may not apply to a higher dose COC or lower doses of CBZ.

For clinical decision making, we categorize AEDs into inducers and non-inducers (see Table 8.1). We define non-inducers as AEDs that cause less than a 10 % change in measured PK parameters of contraceptive progestins. We focus on progestin changes because progestins are more important for contraceptive effectiveness. We assume that if the area under the curve (AUC) and maximum concentration (C_{max}) change less than 10 %, trough levels will be impacted to a similar degree if trough levels are not reported. We assume that a decrease less than 10 % in steroid levels will not meaningfully impact the risk of pregnancy. This is an arbitrary threshold; larger decreases may still provide contraceptive protection, but a conservative approach is warranted to prevent pregnancy for WWE. We define inducers, therefore, as AEDs that cause more than a 10 % decrease in measured PK parameters of the contraceptive progestin.

Lamotrigine and topiramate are unique AEDs in that exposure to either of these drugs has different effects on EE and progestin steroid metabolism. A well-designed crossover study of healthy women ($n=16$) revealed that levonorgestrel C_{max} decreased 12 % and AUC 19 % (0, 24 h) when given with lamotrigine, however, the C_{max} and AUC (0, 24 h) of EE did not change when administered with and without lamotrigine [35]. The exact mechanism to explain this differential effect of lamotrigine on levonorgestrel and not EE is not known. In addition to these PK changes, there was a concerning increase in FSH (4.7-fold) and LH (3.4-fold), and 32 % of participants reported intermenstrual bleeding when lamotrigine was coadministered with the COC (no intermenstrual bleeding occurred without LTG). Endogenous progesterone concentrations remained below the chosen threshold of 5.1 nmol l^{-1}, suggesting that ovulation did not occur; however, progesterone was measured only twice during unspecified times in the pill cycle. In contrast, in a study without formal PK measurement, lamotrigine did not affect individual COC hormone concentrations [36]. Further research with pharmacodynamics and PK outcomes is needed to clarify if, and how, this commonly used drug impacts contraceptive effectiveness.

Like lamotrigine, topiramate has selective effects on COC components. In contrast to lamotrigine, topiramate administration (dose range 100–400 mg) when given in combination with COCs in one observational study ($n=12$) affected ethinyl estradiol but not norethindrone concentrations [37]. Mean AUC values of EE decreased by 18–30 %, and clearance rates of EE increased by 15–33 %. No changes were evident in norethindrone metabolism. This finding is not consistent across studies, however, as healthy volunteers in a randomized trial had only minor changes (<12 %) in AUC or clearance rates of EE [38]. These studies did not measure pharmacodynamic indicators of ovulation risk. It seems unlikely that a selective reduction in EE would decrease contraceptive effectiveness without a decrease in progestin levels.

Intrauterine Devices

Three IUDs are currently available in the USA: the copper IUD, ParaGard (Teva, Israel), and two LNG-releasing IUDs, Mirena (Bayer Healthcare Pharmaceuticals, Wayne, NJ, USA) and Skyla (Bayer Healthcare Pharmaceuticals, Wayne, NJ, USA).

The copper IUD provides an appealing choice because efficacy relies on the local effects of copper ions, which would not be impacted by coadministered AEDs. And while a hormonal method, the predominantly local mechanism of action for either LNG-IUD is probably minimally impacted by enzyme induction. Direct evidence examining the impact of enzyme-inducing drugs on local and systemic LNG levels is lacking; however, one reassuring study in the UK demonstrated a pregnancy rate of 1.1 per 100 women years for 56 women using the 52-mg LNG-IUD and enzyme-inducing AEDs. This pregnancy rate was slightly higher than expected but still very low compared to short-term methods [39]. Overall, we recommend the copper or LNG-IUD as first-line contraception regardless of AED regimen.

Direct evidence of the impact of the LNG-IUD on seizure control is also lacking. One advantage is that progestin-only intrauterine contraception obviates estrogen-mediated decreases in AED levels and associated break-through seizures during use of CHC. In a reassuring study, Ohman and colleagues found comparable lamotrigine levels in 12 women using the LNG-IUD and 20 women not using hormonal contraception [40].

Brain Imaging with an Intrauterine Device

Women with epilepsy may undergo brain magnetic resonance imaging (MRI) intermittently. Clinicians may be concerned that IUD-related artifact could interfere with MRI interpretation as well as possible IUD movement related to magnet exposure. Data on safety and image quality are reassuring. Pelvic MRI image quality is maintained with the copper-containing IUD in place [41–43]; therefore, copper IUD artifact should not degrade brain MRI images. Studies of copper, silver-, and plastic-containing IUDs have not found clinically important IUD movement (deflection, position, or torque) at 0.35, 1.5, and 3.0 T during pelvic MRI (41–44). The 2013 package insert for the copper IUD states that MRI at the level of 1.5 T is acceptable [45].

The package insert for the higher dose LNG-IUD (Mirena) makes no mention of MRI use [46]. However, the 2013 package insert for the lower-dose LNG-IUD (Skyla) states that MRI is safe using a "static magnetic field of 3 T or less, spatial gradient field of 36,000 G/cm (T/m) or less, maximum whole body averaged specific absorption rate (SAR) of 4 W/kg in the First Level Controlled mode for 15 min of continuous scanning"; these are typical MRI conditions for brain imaging [47].

The USMEC rates the copper IUD and the levonorgestrel IUD as category 1 for WWE.

Combined Hormonal Contraception

There are a variety of contraceptive progestins in combined and progestin-only hormonal methods of contraception. Data on interactions are not comprehensive; each AED has not been studied with each progestin. Similarly, interactions with AEDs have been studied for COCs with ethinyl estradiol, but not newer formulations containing 17β estradiol. For purposes of this review, we assume that AEDs classified as inducers and demonstrating lower levels of any progestin or estrogenic steroid will have equal effects on other contraceptive progestins and estrogenic steroids.

Combined oral contraceptives have received the most study with coadministration of AEDs; minimal published data examine patches or rings. Some authors suggest that a non-oral route of administration could circumvent AED/COC interactions by avoiding first-pass metabolism. There is no evidence to support this assertion. Indeed, pregnancies during use of inducing AEDs and contraceptive implants occurred with both older six-rod devices (with phenytoin) as well as the single-rod device currently available (with carbamazepine) [48, 49].

If usual medical eligibility is met, WWE may be offered CHC. Clinicians should carefully ascertain current AED therapy and may prescribe CHC as usual when non-inducing AEDs are coadministered. Commonly used non-inducing AEDs include levetiracetam, gabapentin, valproate, and the newer drug clobazam (see Table 8.1). Clinicians should discuss the teratogenic potential of valproate.

CHCs are not first choice and should be used with caution, and a barrier backup method, in WWE treated with inducing AEDs (see Fig. 8.1). Commonly used inducers include carbamazepine and oxcarbazepine (see Table 8.1). In the case of carbamazepine, a commonly used dose (600 mg daily) resulted in large decreases in AUC, peak and trough levels of EE and levonorgestrel, increased breakthrough bleeding and frank ovulation in ten healthy women using a low-dose COC compared to a placebo (20 mcg EE and 100 mg LNG). Findings from this study support a clinically important risk of method failure previously suggested by case reports of pregnancy from the 1970s of high-dose COC failure [50].

For WWE who strongly prefer CHCs while being treated with inducers, providers should choose CHCs with the highest doses available; guidelines have recommended prescription of formulations containing 50 mcg of EE. This recommendation seems sensible to avoid unscheduled bleeding due to lower EE levels; however, COCs with 50 mcg of EE do not all contain the highest dose of progestin available. Progestins inhibit the LH surge and are the more important COC component for COC efficacy. Practically, access to COC with 50 mcg of EE is limited, since few formulations are currently marketed. If COCs are prescribed with inducers, we recommend choosing a COC with a longer half-life progestin (drospirenone, desogestrel, levonorgestrel) rather than a short-acting progestin (norethindrone) and choosing the highest dose progestin available. Since preovulatory ovarian activity begins during the pill-free interval, a shorter pill-free interval, extended or continuous COC regimen, or continuous patch or ring use is reasonable; however, no evidence supports this strategy. Finally, clinicians should also recall that missed pills are common, further exacerbating any risk of pregnancy related to drug interactions. Clinicians must highlight pregnancy risk and encourage dual method use with a barrier method such as condoms.

The USMEC rates CHC as category 1 with specific recommendations related to drug interactions and AEDs. For inducers, CHC methods are category 3, dual method use is encouraged and preparations with a minimum of 35 mcg of EE are recommended. For WWE using lamotrigine monotherapy, CHC methods are category 3.

Progestin-Only Implant

The progestin-only implant offers a reassuring safety profile for WWE. Clinicians can expect stable LTG levels because the implant is estrogen-free and, in general, progestins increase the seizure threshold. Theoretically, the implant might benefit catamenial seizures since ovulation inhibition and a stable level of etonorgestrel prevents ovulatory and perimenstrual hormone changes believed to trigger hormonally sensitive seizures. No study has yet investigated the role of the implant for this indication.

The progestin implant combines ovulation inhibition and cervical mucus effects for contraception. It is possible that contraceptive effectiveness might be maintained with a coadministered inducer; if etonorgestrel levels fall and ovulation occurs, persistent and continuous cervical mucus effects could provide contraception. Indeed, older implants were effective contraceptives despite ovulation occurring. Unfortunately, no PK or pharmacodynamic evidence exists to support effectiveness of the currently marketed etonogestrel single-rod implant (Nexplanon, Merck, Whitehouse Station, NJ, USA) with inducers. Of concern is a case report of a pregnancy occurring 1.5 years after implant initiation in a WWE treated with 600 mg daily CBZ [49]. Older studies also documented pregnancies with the levonorgestrel implants and coadministration of the inducers phenobarbital and phenytoin [48]. These pregnancies represent true method failures, since user effects do not impact implant effectiveness. The implant is not the first choice for WWE on inducers. As with short-term CHCs, if a WWE chooses the implant and is treated with an inducer, a barrier method should be added.

The USMEC rates the implant category 1. For those on inducers, the implant is rated category 2 owing to concerns about decreased effectiveness.

Injectable Depot Medroxyprogesterone Acetate

Depot medroxyprogesterone acetate (DMPA) is a powerful suppressor of the hypothalamic pituitary axis and completely inhibits ovulation as well as thickens cervical mucus. This method is safe for WWE, and LTG levels should not change as DMPA is estrogen free. High progestin levels and ovulatory suppression offer a theoretical benefit for catamenial epilepsy; however, no evidence supports this use of DMPA. One pilot study conducted nearly 30 years ago explored the use of DMPA for "intractable" (not catamenial) epilepsy ($n=14$) [51]. In this study, participants received both oral and intramuscular medroxyprogesterone acetate in variable doses at variable intervals to achieve amenorrhea, in addition to their AEDs. Seizure frequency decreased, from a mean of 8.3 seizures per month to a mean of 5.1 seizures per month. AED dosing and levels remained stable. These findings have not been duplicated since this report. A more rigorous, controlled study is needed to investigate if intramuscular DMPA affects seizure control.

Epilepsy specialists point out particular concerns for WWE who use DMPA related to bone health. Bone mineral density decreases due to DMPA use in healthy women are reversible and do not increase the risk of fracture [52]. Effects on bone may be compounded when women are taking AEDs known to negatively impact bone. Enzyme-inducing AEDs and valproate are associated with decreased bone mineral density and increased markers of bone turnover [53]. Sustained increased bone turnover results in bone loss. For WWE choosing DMPA and these AEDs, clinicians should approach prolonged use cautiously. No studies have directly examined bone changes in women using DMPA and any AED concurrently. Dual energy X-ray absorptiometry (DXA) scans are recommended for those at significant risk for bone loss. At risk persons include perimenopausal women, persons with prolonged AED use, particularly enzyme inducing AEDs and valproate, and those with other risk factors such as concomitant steroid use [53]. Since BMD loss with DMPA may be recovered, DMPA use alone is not considered a reason monitor BMD.

Progestin levels are high with DMPA compared to other hormonal methods, and hypothalamic and pituitary suppression along with contraceptive effects can persist after the recommended 3-month re-dosing interval. Of all the systemic hormonal methods, DMPA seems most likely to retain effectiveness when combined with enzyme inducers; however, no pharmacodynamic evidence is available regarding use of DMPA with inducers. Some guidelines (including the USMEC) state that DMPA effectiveness is not decreased by use of enzyme inducers; no evidence is cited to support this assertion. Some authors recommend re-dosing DMPA at shorter intervals or when bleeding resumes in order to avoid decreased effectiveness as levels fall; no data are available to address the effectiveness of this strategy.

USMEC rates DMPA category 1 regardless of coadministered AED.

Progestin-Only Pills

Progestin-only pills (POPs) are safe for WWE and they are not expected to alter LTG levels. However, dosing near the same time each day may be challenging for WWE maintained on complex AED polytherapy. Progestin-only pills containing norethindrone are a particularly poor choice for WWE on inducers due to the low dose of norethindrone in this pill and its short half-life. Dosing POPs twice, rather than once, daily is one strategy to improve effectiveness; no evidence supports this approach. Clinicians seeking cycle suppression for catamenial seizures should not choose POPs, since they do not completely suppress ovulation.

USMEC rates POP category 1 with specific recommendations related to drug interactions and AEDs. For inducers, POPs are category 3.

Hysteroscopic and Laparoscopic Sterilization

Usual AED therapy should be continued for the procedure. Intravenous sedation does not increase the risk of seizures, indeed, benzodiazepines are anticonvulsants. The Essure (Bayer Healthcare Pharmaceuticals, Wayne, NJ, USA) coils and Filshie Clips are not likely to impact MRI safety and are not likely to interfere with MR image quality [53]. The Essure product label states that a maximum temperature change of +1.7 C occurred during 15 min of 3 T pelvic MRI, and that MR image quality may be compromised only when the structure being imaged is close to the device; brain images should not be impacted [54]. Providers should anticipate AED dose adjustment if a WWE maintained on LTG discontinues CHC after sterilization.

Women with epilepsy and their partners should receive the full range of contraceptive options in counseling. Providers should keep in mind that some women and men with epilepsy have historically been encouraged to undergo sterilization because they were wrongly viewed as not fit to parent or because of incorrect beliefs that no reversible contraceptive options were effective for women with the disorder [55].

The USMEC does not rate sterilization.

Discontinuing Contraception for Pregnancy

Clinicians who care for WWE should discuss optimal pregnancy planning and potential effects of stopping contraception. AED exposure is associated with a two to threefold increased risk of major congenital malformations compared to the general population with reported rates varying from 3 to 9 % in exposed pregnancies [7]. Higher risks are associated with valproate and polytherapy [7]. The 2009 American Academy of Neurology and American Epilepsy Society Practice Parameter recommend that women with epilepsy take at least 0.4 mg folic acid before and during pregnancy [56]. In addition to reducing risk of major congenital malformations, folic acid supplementation is associated with better cognitive outcomes in children [57].

Seizure control should be considered carefully when choosing a time to stop contraception. Women with epilepsy who remain seizure-free in the 9 months before pregnancy are less likely to seize during pregnancy [58]. Women treated with lamotrigine in combination with CHCs will need dose adjustments (decrease) when the CHC is stopped (see Table 8.2). During pregnancy, AED concentrations, in particular lamotrigine, should be followed closely, as concentrations decrease as pregnancy progresses. A recent analysis found that compared with other monotherapies, pregnant women managed with lamotrigine were less likely to be seizure-free, 58.2 % ($p<0.0001$); had more generalized tonic clonic seizures, 21.1 % ($p<0.0001$); had a greater likelihood of deterioration in seizure control from first to second or third trimesters, 19.9 % ($p<0.01$); and were more likely to require an increase in drug load as the pregnancy progressed, 47.7 % ($p<0.0001$) [59].

Next Steps and Research Priorities

More clinical and social science research could improve contraceptive care for WWE. Specifically, more information is needed to understand the pharmacodynamic effects and associated changes in seizure risk and pregnancy risk during coadministration of AEDs and hormonal contraceptives. The possibility of using hormonal contraception to treat catamenial seizures remains unexplored. A better understanding of the contraceptive experiences, preferences, practices, and health-seeking behaviors of adolescents would improve the reproductive health of many women impacted by epilepsy.

References

1. Fisher R, Acevedo C, Arzimanoglou A, Bogacz A, Cross J, Elger C, et al. An Operational Clinical Definition of Epilepsy [Internet]. International League Against Epilepsy; 2013. http://www.ilae.org/Visitors/Centre/Documents/DefinitionofEpilepsy.pdf.
2. Institute of Medicine (US) Committee on the Public Health Dimensions of the Epilepsies. Epilepsy across the spectrum: Promoting Health and Understanding [Internet]. In: England MJ, Liverman CT, Schultz AM, Strawbridge LM, editors. Washington, DC: National Academies Press; 2012 [cited 2013 Nov 27]. http://www.ncbi.nlm.nih.gov/books/NBK91506/.
3. Kwan P, Brodie MJ. Early identification of refractory epilepsy. N Engl J Med. 2000;342(5):314–9.
4. Kwan P, Arzimanoglou A, Berg AT, Brodie MJ, Allen Hauser W, Mathern G, et al. Definition of drug resistant epilepsy: consensus proposal by the ad hoc task force of the ILAE commission on therapeutic strategies. Epilepsia. 2010;51(6):1069–77.
5. Hirtz D, Thurman DJ, Gwinn-Hardy K, Mohamed M, Chaudhuri AR, Zalutsky R. How common are the "common" neurologic disorders? Neurology. 2007; 68(5):326–37.
6. Hesdorffer DC, Logroscino G, Benn EKT, Katri N, Cascino G, Hauser WA. Estimating risk for developing epilepsy: a population-based study in Rochester, Minnesota. Neurology. 2011;76(1):23–7.
7. Pennell PB. Pregnancy, epilepsy, and women's issues. Continuum (Minneap Minn). 2013;19(3 Epilepsy): 697–714.
8. Morrell MJ, Hayes FJ, Sluss PM, Adams JM, Bhatt M, Ozkara C, et al. Hyperandrogenism, ovulatory dysfunction, and polycystic ovary syndrome with valproate versus lamotrigine. Ann Neurol. 2008;64(2):200–11.
9. Herzog AG, Klein P, Ransil BJ. Three patterns of catamenial epilepsy. Epilepsia. 1997;38(10):1082–8.
10. Verrotti A, D'Egidio C, Agostinelli S, Verrotti C, Pavone P. Diagnosis and management of catamenial seizures: a review. Int J Womens Health. 2012;4:535–41.
11. Herzog AG, Fowler KM, Smithson SD, Kalayjian LA, Heck CN, Sperling MR, et al. Progesterone vs placebo therapy for women with epilepsy: a randomized clinical trial. Neurology. 2012;78(24):1959–66.
12. Dennis A. Identifying and responding to the reproductive decision-making needs of women with epilepsy. Boston, MA: Boston University School of Public Health; 2012.
13. Chung K, Liu Y, Ivey SL, Huang D, Chung C, Guo W, et al. Quality of life in epilepsy (QOLIE): insights about epilepsy and support groups from people with epilepsy (San Francisco Bay Area, USA). Epilepsy Behav. 2012;24(2):256–63.
14. Djibuti M, Shakarishvili R. Influence of clinical, demographic, and socioeconomic variables on quality of life in patients with epilepsy: findings from Georgian study. J Neurol Neurosurg Psychiatry. 2003; 74(5):570–3.
15. Austin JK, Shafer PO, Deering JB. Epilepsy familiarity, knowledge, and perceptions of stigma: report from a survey of adolescents in the general population. Epilepsy Behav. 2002;3(4):368–75.
16. Luef G. Female issues in epilepsy: a critical review. Epilepsy Behav. 2009;15(1):78–82.
17. Elliott JO, Charyton C, Sprangers P, Lu B, Moore JL. The impact of marriage and social support on persons with active epilepsy. Epilepsy Behav. 2011;20(3): 533–8.
18. Harden CL. Sexuality in men and women with epilepsy. CNS Spectr. 2006;11(8 Suppl 9):13–8.
19. Crawford P, Hudson S. Understanding the information needs of women with epilepsy at different lifestages: results of the "Ideal World" survey. Seizure. 2003;12(7):502–7.
20. Pennell PB, Thompson P. Gender-specific psychosocial impact of living with epilepsy. Epilepsy Behav. 2009;15 Suppl 1:S20–5.

21. Gold R, Sonfield A, Richards C, Frost JJ. Next steps for America's family planning program: Leveraging the potential of Medicaid and Title X in an evolving health care system [Internet]. New York, NY: Guttmacher Institute; 2009. p. 44. http://www.guttmacher.org/pubs/NextSteps.pdf.
22. Practice parameter: management issues for women with epilepsy (summary statement). Report of the Quality Standards Subcommittee of the American Academy of Neurology. Neurology. 1998;51(4):944–8.
23. Davis AR, Pack AM, Kritzer J, Yoon A, Camus A. Reproductive history, sexual behavior and use of contraception in women with epilepsy. Contraception. 2008;77(6):405–9.
24. Long L, Montouris G. Knowledge of women's issues and epilepsy (KOWIE-II): a survey of health care professionals. Epilepsy Behav. 2005;6(1):90–3.
25. Morrell MJ, Sarto GE, Shafer PO, Borda EA, Herzog A, Callanan M. Health issues for women with epilepsy: a descriptive survey to assess knowledge and awareness among healthcare providers. J Womens Health Gend Based Med. 2000;9(9):959–65.
26. Pack AM, Davis AR, Kritzer J, Yoon A, Camus A. Antiepileptic drugs: are women aware of interactions with oral contraceptives and potential teratogenicity? Epilepsy Behav. 2009;14(4):640–4.
27. Vessey M, Painter R, Yeates D. Oral contraception and epilepsy: findings in a large cohort study. Contraception. 2002;66(2):77–9.
28. Meador KJ, Penovich P, Baker GA, Pennell PB, Bromfield E, Pack A, et al. Antiepileptic drug use in women of childbearing age. Epilepsy Behav. 2009; 15(3):339–43.
29. Dutton C, Foldvary-Schaefer N. Contraception in women with epilepsy: pharmacokinetic interactions, contraceptive options, and management. Int Rev Neurobiol. 2008;83:113–34.
30. Christensen J, Petrenaite V, Atterman J, SidenIUD P, Ohman I, Tomson T, et al. Oral contraceptives induce lamotrigine metabolism: evidence from a double-blind, placebo-controlled trial. Epilepsia. 2007;48(3): 484–9.
31. Sabers A, Buchholt JM, Uldall P, Hansen EL. Lamotrigine plasma levels reduced by oral contraceptives. Epilepsy Res. 2001;47(1–2):151–4.
32. Sabers A, Ohman I, Christensen J, Tomson T. Oral contraceptives reduce lamotrigine plasma levels. Neurology. 2003;61(4):570–1.
33. Reimers A, Helde G, Brodtkorb E. Ethinyl estradiol, not progestogens, reduces lamotrigine serum concentrations. Epilepsia. 2005;46(9):1414–7.
34. Davis AR, Westhoff CL, Stanczyk FZ. Carbamazepine coadministration with an oral contraceptive: effects on steroid pharmacokinetics, ovulation, and bleeding. Epilepsia. 2011;52(2):243–7.
35. Sidhu J, Job S, Singh S, Philipson R. The pharmacokinetic and pharmacodynamic consequences of the co-administration of lamotrigine and a combined oral contraceptive in healthy female subjects. Br J Clin Pharmacol. 2006;61(2):191–9.
36. Contin M, Albani F, Ambrosetto G, Avoni P, Bisulli F, Riva R, et al. Variation in lamotrigine plasma concentrations with hormonal contraceptive monthly cycles in patients with epilepsy. Epilepsia. 2006;47(9):1573–5.
37. Rosenfeld WE, Doose DR, Walker SA, Nayak RK. Effect of topiramate on the pharmacokinetics of an oral contraceptive containing norethindrone and ethinyl estradiol in patients with epilepsy. Epilepsia. 1997;38(3):317–23.
38. Doose DR, Wang S-S, Padmanabhan M, Schwabe S, Jacobs D, Bialer M. Effect of topiramate or carbamazepine on the pharmacokinetics of an oral contraceptive containing norethindrone and ethinyl estradiol in healthy obese and nonobese female subjects. Epilepsia. 2003;44(4):540–9.
39. Bounds W, Guillebaud J. Observational series on women using the contraceptive Mirena concurrently with anti-epileptic and other enzyme-inducing drugs. J Fam Plann Reprod Health Care. 2002;28(2):78–80.
40. Ohman I, Luef G, Tomson T. Effects of pregnancy and contraception on lamotrigine disposition: new insights through analysis of lamotrigine metabolites. Seizure. 2008;17(2):199–202.
41. Mark AS, Hricak H. Intrauterine contraceptive devices: MR imaging. Radiology. 1987;162(2):311–4.
42. Zieman M, Kanal E. Copper T 380A IUD and magnetic resonance imaging. Contraception. 2007;75(2):93–5.
43. Berger-Kulemann V, Einspieler H, Hachemian N, Prayer D, Trattnig S, Weber M, et al. Magnetic field interactions of copper-containing intrauterine devices in 3.0-Tesla magnetic resonance imaging: in vivo study. Korean J Radiol. 2013;14(3):416–22.
44. Hess T, Stepanow B, Knopp MV. Safety of intrauterine contraceptive devices during MR imaging. Eur Radiol. 1996;6(1):66–8.
45. Federal Drug Administration. Label information: Paragard [Internet]. Washington (DC): Federal Drug Administration; 2013. http://www.accessdata.fda.gov/drugsatfda_docs/label/2013/018680s066lbl.pdf.
46. Federal Drug Administration. Package insert: Mirena [Internet]. Washington (DC): Federal Drug Administration; 2013. http://www.accessdata.fda.gov/drugsatfda_docs/label/2013/021225s032lbl.pdf.
47. Federal Drug Administration. Package insert: Skyla [Internet]. Washington (DC): Federal Drug Administration; 2013. http://www.accessdata.fda.gov/scripts/cder/drugsatfda/index.cfm?fuseaction=Search.Label_ApprovalHistory#labelinfo.
48. Haukkamaa M. Contraception by Norplant subdermal capsules is not reliable in epileptic patients on anticonvulsant treatment. Contraception. 1986;33(6):559–65.
49. Schindlbeck C, Janni W, Friese K. Failure of Implanon contraception in a patient taking carbamazepin for epilepsia. Arch Gynecol Obstet. 2006;273(4):255–6.
50. Kenyon IE. Unplanned pregnancy in an epileptic. Br Med J. 1972;1(5801):686–7.
51. Mattson RH, Cramer JA, Caldwell BV, Siconolfi BC. Treatment of seizures with medroxyprogesterone acetate: preliminary report. Neurology. 1984;34(9): 1255–8.

52. Kaunitz AM, Arias R, McClung M. Bone density recovery after depot medroxyprogesterone acetate injectable contraception use. Contraception. 2008; 77(2):67–76.
53. Pack AM. Treatment of epilepsy to optimize bone health. Curr Treat Options Neurol. 2011;13(4): 346–54.
54. Federal Drug Administration. Label information: Essure [Internet]. Washington (DC): Federal Drug Administration; 2002. http://www.accessdata.fda.gov/cdrh_docs/pdf2/P020014c.pdf.
55. Kevles DJ. In the name of eugenics: genetics and the uses of human heredity. Cambridge, MA: Harvard University Press; 1985. p. 448.
56. Harden CL, Pennell PB, Koppel BS, Hovinga CA, Gidal B, Meador KJ, et al. Practice parameter update: management issues for women with epilepsy–focus on pregnancy (an evidence-based review): vitamin K, folic acid, blood levels, and breastfeeding: report of the Quality Standards Subcommittee and Therapeutics and Technology Assessment Subcommittee of the American Academy of Neurology and American Epilepsy Society. Neurology. 2009;73(2):142–9.
57. Meador KJ, Baker GA, Browning N, Cohen MJ, Bromley RL, Clayton-Smith J, et al. Fetal antiepileptic drug exposure and cognitive outcomes at age 6 years (NEAD study): a prospective observational study. Lancet Neurol. 2013;12(3):244–52.
58. EURAP Study Group. Seizure control and treatment in pregnancy: observations from the EURAP epilepsy pregnancy registry. Neurology. 2006;66(3):354–60.
59. Battino D, Tomson T, Bonizzoni E, Craig J, Lindhout D, Sabers A, et al. Seizure control and treatment changes in pregnancy: observations from the EURAP epilepsy pregnancy registry. Epilepsia. 2013;54(9): 1621–7.

9 Contraception for Women with a History of Solid Organ Transplantation

Colleen M. Krajewski and Anne E. Burke

Introduction

Since the first kidney transplant was performed in 1954, there have been over 575,000 solid organ transplants performed in the USA. Of these, 38 % of transplant patients have been women [1]. In 2012, the most recent year for which complete data are available, a total 10,461 women underwent solid organ transplantation, representing 37 % of all transplants. The majority are kidney and liver transplants (Fig. 9.1). As such, small studies and case series of contraception among women with transplant are largely limited to kidney and liver transplant patients.

The types of solid organ transplantation include kidney, pancreas, liver, intestine, heart, and lung. The annual Scientific Registry of Transplant Recipients (SRTR) details trends in transplant demographics and survival for each organ [2]. For renal transplant, the primary causes of transplantation include diabetes, hypertension, glomerulonephritis, and cystic kidney disease. Graft survival continues to improve, though transplant rates for wait-listed adults have decreased due to a plateau in donation. The proportion of women receiving kidney transplantation is approximately 40 %, and has remained stable over time. Pancreas transplantation, the most common cause of which is overwhelmingly type 1 diabetes, has been declining over the past decade, while outcomes continue to improve. The proportion of female pancreas transplantation patients is stable over time at approximately 40 %, though the rate of transplantation among female transplantation may be increasing. Liver transplantation is preceded by hepatitis C, malignancy, alcoholic liver disease, cholestatic disease, acute hepatic necrosis, and metabolic liver disease. Over the past decade, there have been improvements in survival as well as increases in transplantation, and the proportion of female liver transplant recipients has remained stable at approximately 35 % over time. Likely due to increased medical and surgical treatment for intestinal failure, the numbers of intestine transplant have decreased since 2006, though graft survival continues to improve. The most common etiology of intestine transplant is short gut syndrome. The proportion of women receiving intestine transplant has increased from 53 % in 2001 to 57 % in 2011. Heart transplant rates have increased over the past decade. The most common causes of heart transplant are cardiomyopathy and coronary artery disease, and the number

C.M. Krajewski, M.D., M.P.H. (✉)
Department of Obstetrics and Gynecology, Magee Womens Hospital, University of Pittsburgh School of Medicine, Pittsburgh, PA, USA
e-mail: colleen.krajewski@gmail.com

A.E. Burke, M.D., M.P.H.
Departments of Gynecology and Obstetrics/Population, Family, and Reproductive Health, Johns Hopkins Bayview Medical Center, Bloomberg School of Public Health, Johns Hopkins University School of Medicine, Baltimore, MD, USA
e-mail: aburke@jhmi.edu

R.H. Allen and C.A. Cwiak (eds.), *Contraception for the Medically Challenging Patient*, DOI 10.1007/978-1-4939-1233-9_9, © Springer Science+Business Media New York 2014

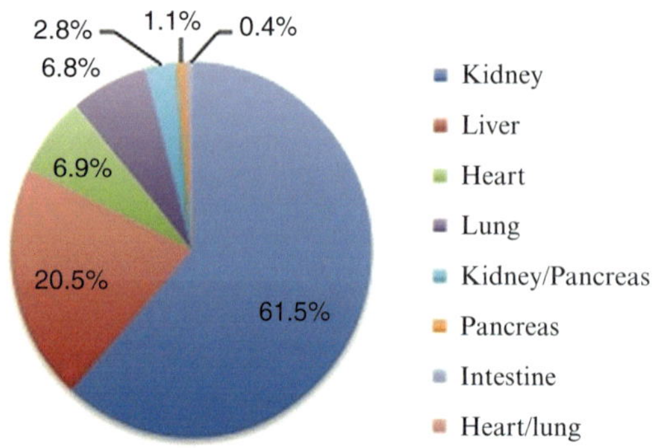

Fig. 9.1 2012 solid organ transplantation types among women

of female heart transplant recipients has increased from 24 to 28 %. Lung transplant has been increasing over time, but not in pace with the rate of additions to the waiting list. The most common causes of lung transplant are chronic obstructive pulmonary disease (COPD), emphysema, pulmonary artery hypertension, cystic fibrosis, and pulmonary fibrosis. The proportion of female lung transplant recipients has decreased from 53.5 % in 2001 to 41.9 % in 2011. Lastly, pediatric transplant rates as well as survival for all solid organ types are generally increasing over time, which is expected to lead to increasing numbers of transplantation patients of reproductive age.

In addition to solid organ transplantation, there are many patients who may be immunosuppressed, either pharmacologically or intrinsically. Patients who undergo bone marrow transplantation are at risk of infection both in the pre-engraftment period and afterwards, due to immunosuppressive medications. In addition, many patients with autoimmune disease, for example, Crohn's disease or rheumatoid arthritis, are on episodic or continuous immunosuppressive medications.[1] While this chapter focuses on solid organ transplantation, much of the concern about post-transplantation contraception has been due to the immunosuppressive state. It therefore seems logical that the underlying science can be extrapolated to similar immunosuppressed conditions.

Decreased fertility often accompanies the end organ failure that precedes transplantation. For many women, the improved fertility following transplantation is a benefit, and ovulation has been described as soon as a month post-transplant [3]. Pregnancy has been described after every type of solid organ transplant [4]. Although pregnancy can be safely achieved, it is important to delay pregnancy following transplantation until stable graft (transplanted organ) function is achieved. Time to stable graft function can vary significantly, with some women achieving stability in as few as 6 months, while others may never reach a state of stable function. In addition, many antirejection agents, such as mycophenolate and azathioprine, are pregnancy Class D, which is defined by the Food and Drug Administration (FDA) as "positive evidence of risk." These can be adjusted in conjunction with a patient's transplant team and obstetric team to minimize fetal exposure, thus necessitating a timed pregnancy. For this reason, a contraceptive visit should be a part of every woman's coordinated pre-transplantation care.

If pregnancy occurs, it comes at higher than average risk to both the mother and her fetus. Several studies have confirmed higher incidence of complications such as cesarean delivery, gestational diabetes, preeclampsia, and preterm delivery. This has been reported in registry data [5], a case–control study [6], and meta-analyses [7, 8].

Internationally, estimates of unplanned pregnancy following solid organ transplantation vary. Iran, China, and Brazil have estimated post-transplant unplanned pregnancy rates to be 49 %, 88 %, and 93 %, respectively [9–11]. There are no comprehensive estimates of the post-transplantation unplanned pregnancy rate in the USA. Medicare data, which excludes elective abortion, reported a pregnancy rate of 33 per 1,000 women with kidney transplant and a live birth rate of 55 % [12]. A voluntary US registry,

[1] It should be noted that the mechanism of immunosuppression for solid organ transplantation is largely the TNF-alpha pathway, which is different than the protease pathway inhibited by HIV. However, the same concepts apply, namely that immunosuppression does not present a contraindication for most contraceptive use, including IUD. For a full discussion of HIV and contraception, please see Chap. 6.

the National Transplantation Pregnancy Registry (NTPR), reported a live birth rate of 50–86 % [5]. The NTPR is unlikely to include a comprehensive estimate of induced abortion, due to stigma and reporting bias. Both estimates likely do not fully include elective abortion, and neither reports on pregnancy intendedness.

The US Medical Eligibility Criteria (USMEC) Guidance

The USMEC has four categories for contraceptive use in specific populations, ranging from category 1 (no restrictions) to category 4 (method generally should not be used). The USMEC divides solid organ transplantation into complicated and uncomplicated (Table 9.1). Every included contraceptive method is USMEC category 2 in a woman with an uncomplicated transplant, meaning the benefits of the method generally outweigh its risks [13]. For a woman with complicated transplantation, defined as graft failure (acute or chronic), rejection, or cardiac allograft vasculopathy, combined hormonal contraception is category 4 due to the risk of cardiovascular events, and initiation of an intrauterine device (IUD) is category 3 due to the theoretical risk of infection with insertion. For a category 3 method, its risks generally outweigh its benefits, but it is safer than pregnancy and can be used if other methods are unavailable or unacceptable to the patient. Importantly, continuation of all methods remains category 2 for a woman with a complicated transplant. This may come up in clinical practice most often in the setting of a patient experiencing rejection or nonspecific infection whose transplant team has requested IUD removal. In these instances, respect for the transplant team should be balanced with education regarding the safety of intrauterine contraception.

In addition, solid organ transplantation is among several conditions identified by the Centers for Disease Control and Prevention (CDC) that expose women to increased risk as a result of unintended pregnancy. In these circumstances, the CDC notes that highly effective contraceptive methods may be the best choice, and women with these conditions should be advised that sole use of barrier or behavior-based methods of contraception may not be the most appropriate choice. Even in a highly motivated patient, methods that require act-specific behavior, such as condoms or fertility awareness, or daily compliance, such as a pill, may still have a risk of unplanned pregnancy that is unacceptably high.

It is important to note that many patients will have underlying health conditions that will persist post-transplantation. For example, lupus, hypertension, or hepatitis can precede solid organ transplant. If such comorbidities are present, USMEC guidelines for these conditions should be followed. On the other hand, conditions such as cystic fibrosis, which can precede lung transplant, have no specific USMEC guidance. In this instance, the innate chloride ion channel defect that leads to nutritional deficiency and subfertility (but not necessarily infertility) can persist post-transplant. Lastly, the transplanted organ's function can vary over time, and should be taken into consideration when considering the choice of contraceptive agent, especially if drug metabolism will be affected. If there is concern for decreased graft function, or drug interaction, consultation with transplant team is recommended prior to starting a systemically absorbed medication.

Table 9.1 USMEC for solid organ transplantation

		Combined pill, patch, ring		Progestin-only pill		Injection		Implant		LNG-IUD		Copper IUD	
Condition	Subcondition	I	C	I	C	I	C	I	C	I	C	I	C
Solid organ transplantation	(a) Complicated	4		2		2		2		3	2	3	2
	(b) Uncomplicated	2+		2		2		2		2		2	

I Initiation, *C* Continuation, *IUD* Intrauterine device

+ Women with Budd-Chiari syndrome should not use combined pill, patch, ring because of the increased risk for thrombosis

Antirejection Therapy and Drug Interactions

Transplant patients are typically on a combination of antirejection medications with dosing that can change over time. The target serum levels of drug concentration are often higher in the immediate post-transplant period than in the maintenance phase, and drug regimens are often adjusted in clinical settings such as rejection or infection. Regimens vary between institutions, and depend on clinical factors such as HLA matching of donor and recipient. Broadly, transplant patients typically receive a combination of a calcineurin inhibitor and antimetabolic agent. Levels of these drugs are typically checked monthly for 2–5 years, and at longer intervals thereafter for a patient in the maintenance phase of therapy. The addition of glucocorticoids varies between centers, with some continuing prednisone indefinitely and others in which taper and withdrawal are routine.

Several small studies of the safety of combined hormonal contraceptives in this population (see section "Combined Hormonal Contraception") have been performed, and none has reported a need to adjust antirejection medications [21–24]. However, none of these studies measured serum levels of contraceptive hormones. There are no published data regarding pharmacokinetic interaction of any antirejection agents and progestins.

Calcineurin inhibitors include cyclosporine and tacrolimus, and are both metabolized through the hepatic CYP450 3A4 pathway. This is also the pathway of estrogen and progestin metabolism. However, no studies have been done to specifically address the pharmacokinetic interaction of calcineurin inhibitors and either estrogen or progestin.

Antimetabolic agents include azathioprine and mycophenolate. Azathioprine is metabolized in the liver by several pathways, including glutathione S-transferase (GST). Mycophenolate is hydrolyzed in the liver, and according to package labeling, it may decrease the serum concentration of ethinyl estradiol—the average area under the curve (AUC) values were unchanged, but there was substantial patient-to-patient variability reported [28].

All new medications, including contraceptives, should be communicated to the transplant care team so that care may be coordinated, and follow-up labs may be scheduled, if indicated.

Specific Methods of Contraception

Overall, the evidence regarding contraceptive use in women with solid organ transplant is limited to small series, case reports, and expert opinion. Studies are largely descriptive in nature, designed to demonstrate tolerability and safety. The relatively rare nature of transplant, combined with the low failure rate of modern contraceptive methods, would make an appropriately powered study of efficacy prohibitive.

Long-Acting Reversible Contraceptives (LARC)

Intrauterine Device (IUD)

The IUD, owing to its high efficacy and minimal or systemic absorption, is an ideal contraceptive device for women with a history of transplantation. Unfortunately, a case report of two failed Copper 7 IUDs in women with a history of solid organ transplantation, combined with lingering fear of infection likely stemming from the Dalkon Shield era, has led to reticence on the part of transplant care providers to recommend its use in their patients. Guidance from the American Society of Transplantation (AST) Consensus Conference on Reproductive Issues and Transplantation, as recently as 2005, recommended against IUD use on the basis of these two cases alone, in a firmly worded statement regarding decreased efficacy and increased infection risk [14].

In reality, in the over 200 patients reported using an IUD with a history of solid organ transplantation, the two cases from 1981 are the only report of failure (Table 9.2). In contrast, in the modern case report literature, there are no failures, infections, or adverse events. While it is difficult to make scientific judgment on the basis of one case report, the positive experience in the

Table 9.2 Summary of LARC use reported in the medical literature to date

Authors	Year	N	IUD type	Location	Findings
Zerner et al.	1981	2	Copper 7	USA	Two pregnancies
Fong and Singh	1999	1	Levonorgestrel	Singapore	Successful treatment of uterine myomas
Xu et al.	2011	178	Not specified	China	No pregnancies
Bahamondes et al.	2011	12	Levonorgestrel	Brazil	No pregnancies; 1 infection in sample of 636 (mixed transplant and non-transplant)
Ramhendar and Byrne	2011	11	Levonorgestrel	Ireland	No pregnancies or pelvic infection

overwhelming majority of reports in this case is reassuring and provides a sound basis to recommend IUDs safely.

There is also no theoretical basis to assume that the IUD would be less effective or pose a higher risk of infection among transplant patients. The main mechanism of action of modern immunosuppressive medications is through the tumor necrosis factor (TNF)-alpha system, whereas the IUD likely works through macrophage function. There are extensive data from women with human immunodeficiency virus (HIV) that IUDs do not increase the risk of pelvic infection in an immunosuppressed population [15, 16]. There is also excellent evidence that the use of IUDs is not associated with increased risk of pelvic inflammatory disease (PID) in the general population [17]. Because of their safety and excellent effectiveness, IUDs can be recommended as first line in women with a history of transplantation.

When initiating an IUD in women with a history of transplantation, there are several issues to consider. One is whether to screen for *N. gonorrhoeae* and *Chlamydia* prior to insertion. There is no data to guide pre-IUD *N. gonorrhoeae* and *Chlamydia* screening in women with a history of transplant. Providers can look to existing guidelines from the CDC, which does not require screening in low-risk women, and allows for screening at the time of insertion in women for whom screening is indicated [18]. Concerns for safety should be balanced with the potential for loss to follow-up when a multi-visit protocol is required for IUD insertion. As urine *N. gonorrhoeae* and *Chlamydia* screening is now considered a standard alternative for testing when a pelvic examination is not being performed, and since transplant patients have labs checked often, it is reasonable to suggest urine *N. gonorrhoeae* and *Chlamydia* testing, if indicated, prior to her contraceptive visit if screening is indicated.

A second issue is whether to provide antibiotic prophylaxis at the time of insertion. A meta-analysis found a low absolute risk of infection with or without antibiotic administration, and no decrease in the risk of PID with antibiotic administration, at the time of IUD insertion (OR 0.89 [95 % confidence interval 0.53–1.51]) [19]. This has not been specifically evaluated in an immunosuppressed population. Nevertheless, we do not recommend the use of antibiotic prophylaxis prior to IUD insertion.

The choice of hormonal vs. copper IUD can be made by the woman; no one type of IUD has been shown to be preferable based on transplant history. Noncontraceptive benefits of the levonorgestrel-containing IUD are relevant in transplant patients as well.

Subdermal Etonogestrel Implant

There are no published reports of the subdermal etonogestrel (ENG) implant used in women with a history of transplantation. Based on the safety profile of other progestins, combined with its very high efficacy, the ENG subdermal implant should be ideal for use in a transplant population. There is no evidence regarding the pharmacokinetic profile of long-acting subdermal implants in women taking transplant medications. Studies of interactions between the etonogestrel implant and other drugs metabolized in the CYP450 pathway are also limited. The authors of a published report of two cases of pregnancy with concomitant use of etonogestrel implant and efavirenz, an antiretroviral drug that is also a CYP450 inducer, suggest that the interaction may lead to a higher likelihood of contraceptive failure in the late second and third years of implant use [20]. Given this limited yet concerning data, it is difficult to make a recommendation regarding the use of the etonogestrel subdermal implant at the current time.

There is no need for a pelvic exam or a sexually transmitted infection (STI) screening prior to implant insertion, though these evaluations may be indicated for other reasons.

Depot Medroxyprogesterone Acetate (DMPA)

This highly effective method of contraception is preferred by many patients, particularly those with chronic diseases, for its ease of use, lack of estrogen, and high rate of amenorrhea. There are no published reports of its use in a transplant population. Notably, there is a "black box" warning from the FDA concerning the bone effects of DMPA with long-term use. This has been widely discredited by family planning experts due to the reversible nature of these bone changes in adult women [21]. However, this may merit additional consideration after transplantation.

Renal osteodystrophy, defined as disturbances in mineral metabolism combined with adynamic bone disease, is an important cause of morbidity and decreased quality of life for patients with chronic kidney disease—the leading cause of transplantation (see Fig. 9.1) [22]. Additionally, transplant patients are often on lifelong glucocorticoid therapy, which is the most common form of secondary osteoporosis. Fracture risk is related to both dose and duration of therapy, and can occur at higher bone mineral density (BMD) levels than women with postmenopausal osteoporosis [23]. Thus, there is a concern that the bone effects of DMPA may not be transient in a transplant population. For this reason, a thorough discussion of the risks and benefits of this method should be undertaken prior to initiation of DMPA, and other methods—LARC in particular—should be considered.

Combined Hormonal Contraception (CHC)

Combined hormonal contraception (CHC), including pill, patch, and ring, has been studied in small series of transplant patients. In a patient on multiple medications, there are two theoretical concerns—one is the effect of CHC on serum levels of transplant medications, and the other is effects of concomitant medications on the efficacy of CHC. This is briefly discussed in a previous section of this chapter. Data are limited, and studies have not been powered to address contraceptive effectiveness in a transplant population.

One study of 26 renal transplant patients showed overall favorable effects of CHC use, with improved hematocrit, no pregnancies, and no reported ovarian cyst formation after 18 months of use [24]. However, several women in this series required adjustment of their antihypertensive medications, and there was one case of deterioration of liver function in a previously stable patient over 10 years post-transplant. A similar study from the same group included ten renal transplant patients using the transdermal patch, and had similar favorable results [25]. A retrospective study of 15 liver transplant patients using combined oral contraceptives (COCs) noted no changes in liver function, glucose metabolism, blood pressure, or BMI. There were no cases of rejection in this small retrospective study [26]. Lastly, the contraceptive vaginal ring has been described in a prospective group of 17 renal and liver transplant patients, in which there were no cases of rejection or need to change immunosuppressive medication, and no cases of contraceptive failure [27]. These small studies provide some reassurance of use of combined hormonal methods in a transplant population, but reinforce the need for caution when using these methods in women with other comorbidities such as hypertension.

Additionally, these methods are adding another medication to a transplant patient's already intensive medication regimen. Many patients in this population are very compliant and the addition of a daily pill is easily incorporated. On the other hand, many patients will desire to avoid an additional daily medication. In a patient with stable graft function, and continued close follow-up with a transplant team, CHC methods are reasonable, and may be preferable due to their favorable side effect profile. However, the estrogen-related risks combined with a 9 % typical-use failure rate may make them less than optimal in patients in whom pregnancy should be planned [28].

When initiating CHC methods, there is no need for pelvic exam or STI testing, although a gynecologic office visit is a prudent time to perform these if indicated. If a patient's graft is functioning well, there is no need for serum chemistries to be performed prior to starting medications. If there is a question of graft function, communication with a patient's transplant team can help to ascertain the need for laboratory screening while taking combined hormonal methods.

Progestin-Only Pill (POP)

The use of POPs has not been described in a transplant population. There is concern for decreased effectiveness due to the need for strict compliance since POPs need to be taken at the same time every day. This may be less of a burden in a highly compliant transplant patient, and so this should be assessed on an individual basis. For patients who prefer pills, yet have estrogen-related contraindications, POPs may be an option.

Emergency Contraception

According to the USMEC, emergency contraception is considered category 1 for all medical conditions. All patients with transplantation, particularly those using daily or behavior-based methods of contraception, should be considered candidates for advanced provision of emergency contraception, and instructed on its use. A single dose of emergency contraception is unlikely to interfere with antirejection medications and, as they do not contain estrogen, should not change a patient's thromboembolic risk.

The Importance of Dual Protection with Barrier Methods

The manufacturers of several antirejection medications recommend that the patient avoid pregnancy, and in the case of mycophenolate mofetil, the manufacturer specifies that women should use sterilization, IUD, or a combination of two less effective forms of contraception (such as COCs with condoms) prior to initiation of therapy [28, 29]. For this reason, barrier methods should be recommended to most patients with transplant as a second method of contraception. While dual protection would ideally be initiated in the preoperative period, this is not always practical due to the unscheduled nature of many transplants. Contraceptive methods should be initiated as soon as possible post-transplant due to the possibly rapid resumption of ovulation. Used alone, barrier methods are not ideal contraceptive methods for women with transplantation given the high typical-user failure rate of 18 % [30].

Fertility Awareness Methods

This method of contraception is often seen as "safe" by transplant care providers due to its lack of drugs with potential interaction. While this method can be practiced with success among dedicated patients, there are several potential concerns. First, transplant patients may not have regular menstrual cycles due to underlying chronic illness or graft dysfunction. Regular cycles are required to practice this method effectively. Second, it is unclear what effect chronic immunosuppression and glucocorticoid therapy have on cervical mucus or basal body temperature monitoring, and thus their ability to reliably predict ovulation. Lastly, a behavior-based method with a high typical user failure rate (24 %) is not optimal for patients who have undergone transplantation or are taking teratogenic medications [27].

Fertility awareness methods are not discussed in detail here. Broadly, these can be grouped into calendar methods and ovulatory methods. Detailed instruction should be provided if this method is chosen.

Research Gaps

As this chapter shows, study of contraceptive use in a transplant population has been limited to IUD and combined hormonal methods, and largely limited to case series. There is also limited data on the incidence of unplanned pregnancy and contraceptive use among transplant patients in the USA. The method of action of the IUD in an immunosuppressed uterus is unknown, but theoretically should be the same as in an immunocompetent uterus. The relatively high number of patients in the IUD studies provides reassurance of their safety, and the next step should be identification of barriers to increased IUD use in a transplant population. There are no studies of the progestin-only pill or injection or the contraceptive subdermal implant in a transplant population.

Conclusion

Women with end organ failure who undergo solid organ transplantation are in need of highly effective contraception. In particular, IUDs are recommended as first line in women with a history of transplantation, due to their superior effectiveness and safety. Unfortunately, negative attitudes persist regarding the use of IUDs among transplant care providers, as evidenced by the 2005 AST consensus statement. Much like women's health providers after the reintroduction of IUDs following the Dalkon Shield recall in the 1990s, transplant care physicians will need to overcome bias in order to improve LARC uptake among women with transplantation.

References

1. 2012 Annual Report of the U.S. Organ Procurement and Transplantation Network and the Scientific Registry of Transplant Recipients: Transplant Data 1994–2003. Department of Health and Human Services, Health Resources and Services Administration, Healthcare Systems Bureau, Division of Transplantation, Rockville, MD; United Network for Organ Sharing, Richmond, VA; University Renal Research and Education Association, Ann Arbor, MI.
2. 2011 Annual Data Report. http://srtr.transplant.hrsa.gov/annual_reports/2011/. Accessed 22 Dec 2013.
3. Farber M. Pregnancy and renal transplantation. Clin Obstet Gynecol. 1978;21:931.
4. Mastrobattista JM, Gomez-Lobo V. Pregnancy after solid organ transplantation. Obstet Gynecol. 2008; 112:919.
5. Coscia LA, Constantinescu S, Moritz MJ, Frank AM, Ramirez CB, Maley WR, et al. Report from the National Transplantation Pregnancy Registry (NTPR): outcomes of pregnancy after transplantation. Clin Transpl. 2010:65–85.
6. Coffin CS, Shaheen AAM, Burak KW, Myers RP. Pregnancy outcomes among liver transplant recipients in the United States: a nationwide case–control analysis. Liver Transpl. 2010;16:56.
7. Deshpande NA, James NT, Kucirka LM, Boyarsky BJ, Garonzik-Wang JM, Montgomery RA, et al. Pregnancy outcomes in kidney transplant recipients: a systematic review and meta-analysis. Am J Transplant. 2011;11:2388.
8. Deshpande NA, James NT, Kucirka LM, Boyarsky BJ, Garonzik-Wang JM, Cameron AM, et al. Pregnancy outcomes of liver transplant recipients: a systematic review and meta-analysis. Liver Transpl. 2012;18(6):621–9.
9. Ghazizadeh S, Lessan-Pezeshki M, Khatami M, Mahdavi M, Razeghi E, Seifi S, et al. Unwanted pregnancy among kidney transplant recipients in Iran. Transplant Proc. 2005;37(7):3085–6.
10. Xu L, Yang Y, Shi JG, Wang H, Qiu F, Peng W, et al. Unwanted pregnancy among Chinese renal transplant recipients. Eur J Contracept Reprod Health Care. 2011;16(4):270–6.
11. Bahamondes MV, Hidalgo MM, Bahamondes L, Monteiro I. Ease of insertion and clinical performance of the levonorgestrel-releasing intrauterine system in nulligravidas. Contraception. 2011;84(5):e11–6.
12. Gill JS, Zalunardo N, Rose C, Tonelli M. The pregnancy rate and live birth rate in kidney transplant recipients. Am J Transplant. 2009;9:1541.
13. Curtis KM, Jamieson DJ, Peterson HB, Marchbanks PA. Adaptation of the World Health Organization's medical eligibility criteria for contraceptive use for use in the United States. Contraception. 2010;82(1):3.
14. McKay DB, Josephson MA, Armenti VT, August P, Coscia LA, Davis CL, et al. Reproduction and transplantation: report on the AST consensus conference on reproductive issues and transplantation. Am J Transplant. 2005;5(7):1592–9.
15. Morrison CS, Sekadde-Kigondu C, Sinei SK, Weiner DH, Kwok C, Kokonya D. Is the intrauterine device appropriate contraception for HIV-1-infected women? BJOG. 2001;108:784.
16. Stringer EM, Kaseba C, Levy J, Sinkala M, Goldenberg RL, Chi BH, et al. A randomized trial of the intrauterine contraceptive device vs hormonal contraception in women who are infected with the human immunodeficiency virus. Am J Obstet Gynecol. 2007;197:144e1.
17. Hubacher D, Lara-Ricalde R, Taylor DJ, Guerra-Infante F, Guzmán-Rodríguez R. Use of copper intrauterine devices and the risk of tubal infertility among nulligravid women. N Engl J Med. 2001; 345:561.
18. U.S. Selected Practice Recommendations for Contraceptive Use, 2013. http://www.cdc.gov/mmwr/preview/mmwrhtml/rr6205a1.htm. Accessed 22 Dec 2013.

19. Grimes DA, Schulz KF. Antibiotic prophylaxis for intrauterine contraceptive device insertion. Cochrane Database Syst Rev. 2001;(2):CD001327. doi:10.1002/14651858.CD001327.
20. Leticee N, Viard J-P, Yamgnane A, Karmochkine M, Benachi A. Contraceptive failure of etonogestrel implant in patients treated with antiretrovirals including efavirenz. Contraception. 2012;85(4):425–7.
21. Kaunitz AM, Grimes DA. Removing the black box warning for depot medroxyprogesterone acetate. Contraception. 2011;84:212.
22. Moe S, Drüeke T, Cunningham J, Goodman W, Martin K, Olgaard K, et al. Definition, evaluation, and classification of renal osteodystrophy: a position statement from kidney disease: improving global outcomes (KDIGO). Kidney Int. 2006;69(11):1945–53.
23. Canalis E, Mazziotti G, Giustina A, Bilezikian JP. Glucocorticoid-induced osteoporosis: pathophysiology and therapy. Osteoporos Int. 2007;18n:1319–28.
24. Pietrzak B, Kaminski P, Wielgos M, Bobrowska K, Durlik M. Combined oral contraception in women after renal transplantation. Neuro Endocrinol Lett. 2006;27:679.
25. Pietrzak B, Bobrowska K, Jabiry-Zieniewicz Z, Kaminski P, Wielgos M, Pazik J. Oral and transdermal hormonal contraception in women after kidney transplantation. Transplant Proc. 2007; 39:2759.
26. Jabiry-Zieniewicz Z, Bobrowska K, Kaminski P, Wielgos M, Zieniewicz K, Krawczyk M. Low-dose hormonal contraception after liver transplantation. Transplant Proc. 2007;39:1530.
27. Paternoster DM, Riboni F, Bertolino M, Garofalo G, Lazzarich E, Surico N, et al. The contraceptive vaginal ring in women with renal and liver transplantation: analysis of preliminary results. Transplant Proc. 2010;42:1162.
28. Azasan Prescribing Information (PI)—azasan-pi.pdf. http://cdn.salix.com/shared/pi/azasan-pi.pdf. Accessed 22 Dec 2013.
29. CellCept. http://www.cellcept.com/cellcept/index-h.htm. Accessed 22 Dec 2013.
30. Trussell J. Contraceptive Efficacy. In: Hatcher RA, Trussell J, Nelson AL, Cates W, Kowal D, Policar M, editors. Contraceptive technology. Revised 20th ed. New York, NY: Ardent Media; 2011.

Contraception in the Setting of Obesity and Bariatric Surgery

10

Katharine Simmons and Alison Edelman

Introduction

Until recently, contraceptive research has generally excluded women over 130 % of ideal body weight. Given that more than half of the population of the USA is now overweight or obese, it has become a public health necessity to address the use and safety of contraception in obese women. The aim of this chapter is to review data on the efficacy, pharmacokinetics, and safety of modern methods of contraception in obese women, and in women undergoing bariatric surgery. We also address the effect of these contraceptive methods on lipid profiles.

Other health conditions associated with obesity, such as diabetes, are reviewed elsewhere in this textbook. Review of condoms, diaphragms, withdrawal and fertility awareness are not addressed in this chapter, as there is no physiological reason that these methods should function differently in obese women. The exceptions to this are that placement of a diaphragm may be more difficult with extreme obesity, and women prone to irregular menstrual cycles or oligomenorrhea will be less successful with fertility awareness. Like all women, obese women wishing to avoid pregnancy should be encouraged to use the best methods for preventing pregnancy, either long-acting reversible or permanent methods.

Epidemiology

The incidence of obesity is increasing rapidly throughout the world, and has become a modern day epidemic. The incidence of obesity among women of reproductive age doubled in the USA between 1980 and 2004, and has tripled in several European nations over the same time frame. Obesity now affects 34 % of reproductive age women in the USA and 12 % in Western Europe, and continues to rise, with nearly 300 million women affected by obesity as of 2008 [1, 2] (Fig. 10.1). Less developed nations are also affected, with obesity rising especially in urban areas [3].

Obesity is defined by the World Health Organization (WHO) as a body mass index (BMI) over 30 kg/m^2; this can be further subdivided (Table 10.1). Some health outcomes vary by degree of obesity, so these classifications are used in this chapter if the information varies by BMI.

Health and Pregnancy in the Obese

Women and men affected by obesity are more likely to experience cardiovascular disease, type 2 diabetes, osteoarthritis, thromboembolic disease, and cancer. Obesity has become the fifth

K. Simmons, M.D. • A. Edelman, M.D., M.P.H. (✉)
Department of Obstetrics and Gynecology, Oregon Health and Science University, Portland, OR, USA
e-mail: simmonka@ohsu.edu; edelmana@ohsu.edu

R.H. Allen and C.A. Cwiak (eds.), *Contraception for the Medically Challenging Patient*, DOI 10.1007/978-1-4939-1233-9_10,

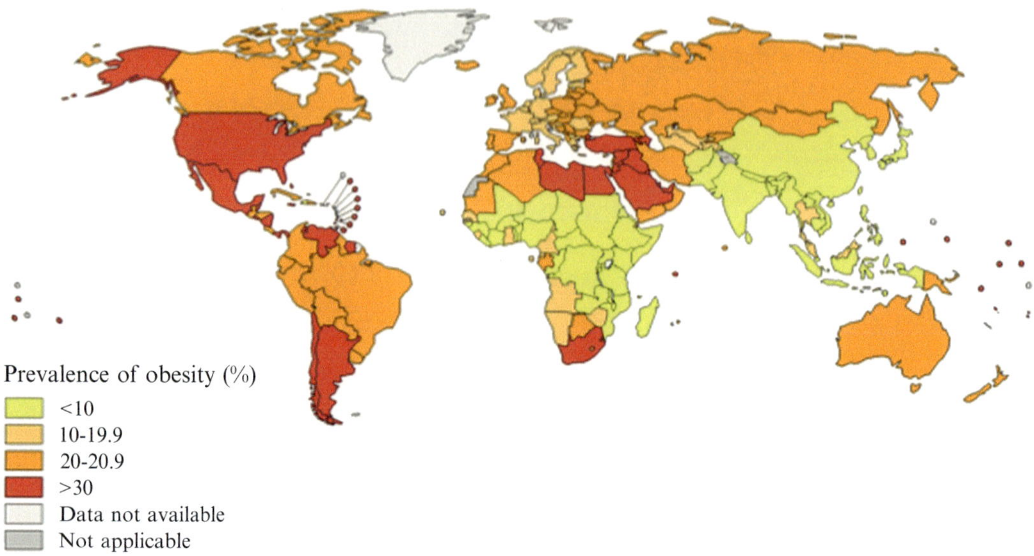

Fig. 10.1 Prevalence of obesity, females ages 20+, age standardized, as of 2008. Reproduced with permission from World Health Organization, Public Health Information and Geographic Information Systems (GIS) 2011. http://gamapserver.who.int/mapLibrary/Files/Maps/Global_Obesity_Females_2008.png

Table 10.1 Weight classification by body mass index (BMI)

Classification of weight	BMI (kg/m^2)
Underweight	<18.5
Normal weight	18.5–24.9
Overweight	25.0–29.9
Class I obesity	30–34.9
Class II obesity	35.0–39.9
Class III obesity	>40.0

leading cause of mortality worldwide [2]. Obesity is associated with a hyperestrogenic state due to the peripheral conversion of androstenedione to estrone and estradiol within adipose tissue. This aromatase reaction is directly related to BMI [4]. Likewise, increased incidence of oligoovulation and anovulation among obese women contribute to this hyperestrogenic state, which increases the risk of abnormal uterine bleeding, endometrial hyperplasia, and endometrial cancer.

In obese women who become pregnant, the large prospective multicenter FASTER trial (First and Second Trimester Evaluation of Risk) demonstrated increased risk of gestational hypertension, diabetes, preeclampsia, anesthesia complications, and an increased rate of cesarean delivery (33.8 % for obese, and 47.4 % for morbidly obese compared to 20.7 % for normal weight) [5]. Fetal complications are also increased, including a higher risk of unexplained stillbirth, fetal growth restriction, neural tube defects, and an increase in childhood obesity [6–8]. Finally, obese women are less likely to return to pre-pregnancy weight following a pregnancy, compounding their weight-associated problems [8].

Bariatric Surgery

Bariatric surgery is the most effective weight loss approach for those with morbid obesity. In addition to weight loss, it has been shown to improve glucose homeostasis, hypertension, hyperlipidemia, sleep apnea, and even to decrease mortality compared to obese controls [9]. Bariatric surgery may be indicated for obese women with class III obesity, and with class II obesity accompanied by serious coexisting health conditions. The incidence of bariatric surgery has increased dramatically over the past two decades, and women account for 83 % of bariatric procedures in reproductive-aged adults [10].

Surgical techniques used today are generally minimally invasive, and mortality from the procedures is less than 1 %. Bariatric procedures can be classified into restrictive or malabsorptive. Malabsorptive procedures such as Roux-en-Y gastric bypass are intended to decrease absorption of calories by shortening the functional length of small intestine. This is the most common procedure performed in the USA and may impair orally administered drugs, like oral contraceptives.

The majority of weight loss and postoperative complications occur within 12–24 months, and the consensus opinion is that women should avoid pregnancy during this time frame due to concern for negative fetal effects from nutritional changes. The American College of Obstetricians and Gynecologists (ACOG) also supports a delay of 12–24 months between bypass surgery and conception [6].

Contraception, Risk of Pregnancy and Obesity

Contraception has always been based on a "one-size-fits all" approach, but as previously mentioned, little is known regarding the interaction between obesity and contraception. Although more data is being accrued, controversy surrounding efficacy still remains. The risk of pregnancy depends on several factors, including baseline fecundity, frequency of intercourse, and use of contraception. Although obese women are more likely to experience ovulatory dysfunction, and may have a slightly lower baseline fecundity than normal weight women [11, 12], sexual behavior, including frequency of intercourse, number of lifetime sexual partners, age at coitarche, and sexual orientation, does not seem to vary by BMI [13, 14].

Obese women access health care, including contraceptive services, less frequently, regardless of insurance status [15]. They have been shown to rely more often on less effective methods such as condoms or withdrawal, or may not use contraception at all due to a decreased perception of fertility risk [13]. Obese women under 30 were four times as likely as normal weight women to report having an unintended pregnancy or abortion [13]. These data emphasize the importance of improving uptake of reliable contraception among obese women.

Contraceptives of Superior Efficacy

Intrauterine Devices

Overview

This section addresses the three intrauterine devices (IUDs) approved by the US Food and Drug Administration (FDA). These IUDs include the levonorgestrel intrauterine device (LNG-IUD) (Mirena, Bayer Healthcare Pharmaceuticals, Wayne, NJ, USA), the copper T380A (copper IUD) (ParaGard, Teva, Israel), and a new smaller LNG-IUD approved in 2013 (Skyla, Bayer Healthcare Pharmaceuticals, Wayne, NJ, USA). This smaller LNG-IUD has just entered the US market, and there is insufficient data on its use in obese populations to review separately in this chapter.

The LNG-IUD was first approved for use in Europe in the early 1990s, and was first marketed in the USA in 2001. The primary mechanisms of action include a sterile inflammatory response that is toxic to sperm, alterations in the viscosity of cervical mucus, and endometrial suppression. Ovulation is not reliably suppressed and therefore this is not one of its primary mechanisms of action. It is approved in the USA for 5 years of use [16]. It is highly effective with a failure rate of 0.2 % over the first year of use.

The copper T380A contains copper wire wrapped around the stem and arms of the polyethylene device. Mechanisms of action include changes in sperm and ova motility, as well as development of a sterile inflammatory response which is hostile to sperm. It is approved for 10 years of use with a failure rate 0.6 % women over the first year of use, and 1.9 % over 10 years, comparable to sterilization [16].

The smaller LNG-IUD (Skyla) contains 13.5 mg of levonorgestrel and has similar mechanisms of action as the original device (Mirena). It is approved for 3 years of use with a cumulative

3-year pregnancy rate of 0.9 %. It was released in the USA in 2013, and there is insufficient data on use in obese populations to review here.

Use and Efficacy in Obese Populations

IUDs provide long lasting, effective contraception regardless of a woman's body weight. As an IUD's mechanism of action is unrelated to systemic hormone levels or ovulation suppression, their efficacy in obese women should be unaffected by body composition. The Contraceptive CHOICE project showed overall failure rates of IUDs (LNG-IUD and Copper T combined data) to be less than one pregnancy per 100 woman years, with no difference in efficacy between women of differing BMIs [17]. This data is based on a sample of nearly 6,000 woman-years of use, approximately 27 % of whom were overweight and 35 % obese.

IUDs require placement by a trained provider. Obesity can make visualization of the cervix and determining uterine position difficult for intrauterine procedures including IUD placements. Optimizing chances for a successful placement can be aided through speculum choice, longer instruments, and retraction of vaginal side walls [18]. Additionally, providers should be aware of their exam table weight restrictions and have access to a bariatric exam table if needed.

Pharmacokinetics

The LNG-IUD contains 52 mg of levonogestrel, which is released into the endometrial cavity initially at a rate of 20 mcg/day and then decreases to a mean of 11 mcg/day after 5 years [19]. BMI is negatively correlated with plasma levels (Table 10.2), but this does not affect the bleeding pattern experienced, nor are plasma levels related to contraceptive efficacy [20]. It is theorized that plasma levels may have some effect on side effects, including acne, headache, and mood changes; however, pharmacologic studies have not examined this relationship to date.

The copper IUD acts locally within the endometrium and its contraceptive effect is not based on systemic pharmacokinetics.

Table 10.2 BMI has a negative correlation with LNG plasma levels in users of the LNG-IUD ($p=0.012$). This does not correlate with contraceptive efficacy[a]

BMI (kg/m^2)	LNG plasma level (pg/mL) (SD)
<20.0	165 (57)
20.0–24.9	152 (59)
25.0–29.9	141 (64)
>30.0	119 (43)

[a]Created with from data from [20]

Safety and Adverse Events

No studies have identified a difference in the safety profile or adverse events experienced by obese as compared to normal BMI IUD users.

Obesity-Related Issues

Weight Gain

Neither the LNG-IUD nor the copper IUD appear to be associated with a risk of weight gain regardless of the baseline weight of the user (normal, overweight, or obese), but women may experience an increase in weight related to aging during long-term IUD use (0.5–1 kg/year) [21, 22].

Hyperlipidemia

The LNG-IUD appears to have no significant effect on lipid metabolism in normal weight women, but small reductions have been reported in total cholesterol (TC) and low density lipoproteins (LDL), with trends towards increased high density lipoproteins (HDL) [23]. Apolipoproteins A and B appear to remain stable with LNG-IUD use [23]. Hyperlipidemia is not a contraindication for LNG-IUD or copper IUD use [24]. Of note, the LNG-IUD is given a category 2 rating (advantages generally outweigh the theoretical or proven risks) by the Centers for Disease Control and Prevention's US Medical Eligibility Criteria for Contraceptive Use (USMEC) for its progestin content for women with known hyperlipidemias.

Menstrual Problems

Obese women commonly experience menstrual irregularities such as abnormal uterine bleeding, oligomenorrhea, secondary amenorrhea, or polycystic ovarian syndrome (PCOS) [25, 26]. The LNG-IUD offers the non-contraceptive benefit of significantly reducing menstrual bleeding, and about half of users will become amenorrheic by 2 years of use. Similar rates of amenorrhea have been reported in obese populations [4].

Endometrial Hyperplasias

All IUDs are associated with a decreased risk of endometrial cancer [27]. For copper IUDs, the causality of this relationship is unclear, but decreased cancer risk may be related to the chronic sterile inflammatory state induced by the copper IUD. Data are more clear for the LNG-IUD, which has been shown to reverse simple (benign) endometrial hyperplasia in over 90 % of cases, and over 65 % of atypical cases (endometrial intraepithelial neoplasia) [4, 28, 29]. It can also be used for endometrial protection in women at risk of developing hyperplasia from oligoovulation or anovulation [29]. The LNG-IUD may be a particularly good choice for contraception in obese women due to this significant non-contraceptive benefit [24].

Bariatric Surgery

Women undergoing bariatric surgery may experience increased fertility postoperatively, and providing effective contraception is crucial to help them avoid pregnancy in the first 2 postoperative years [6, 30, 31]. Intrauterine contraception offers several advantages to women undergoing bariatric surgery. IUDs provide effective, long-lasting contraception during the perioperative and postoperative periods when conception is not advised, with effectiveness that does not vary by weight [17]. The type of bariatric surgery is also unrelated to effectiveness, as oral absorption is not required for contraceptive function. The currently available IUDs do not contain estrogen and therefore can be used in the perioperative period without affecting the risk of venous thrombosis. Some authors have proposed placing IUDs at the time of bariatric surgery to optimize the technical issues with placing IUDs in women with severe obesity [25]. IUDs are well accepted among bariatric surgery populations. In one study of adolescents undergoing bariatric surgery who received preoperative contraceptive counseling, 92 % selected the LNG-IUD for contraception when placement was offered concurrently with the bariatric surgery procedure [25].

Recommendations

Intrauterine devices are considered safe with unrestricted use (category 1) for obese women (Table 10.3) and women undergoing bariatric surgery (Table 10.4), and both IUDs offer non-contraceptive benefits to this population. Hyperlipidemia is not a contraindication for IUD use. IUDs should be considered a first-line contraceptive choice for all women, no matter their weight.

Etonogestrel Contraceptive Implant

Overview

The etonogestrel contraceptive implant (Implanon/Nexplanon, Merck, Whitehouse Station, NJ, USA) is the only form of implantable contraception currently approved in the USA. As is typical of phase II and III clinical trials, studies of the etonogestrel (ENG) implant did not include women over 130 % of ideal body weight [32, 33]. This section reviews the available data on the use of the ENG implant in obese women and women undergoing bariatric surgery.

Use and Efficacy in Obese Populations

To date, no studies have primarily addressed contraceptive efficacy of the ENG implant in overweight and obese women. However, a secondary analysis of the contraceptive CHOICE project examined the ENG implant failure rates in overweight and obese women over 3 years of use [17]. Of 1,168 contraceptive implant users, 28 % were overweight (see Table 10.1) and 35 % were obese. They reported one pregnancy in 1,377 woman years of use, which occurred in an obese woman (BMI 30.7 kg/m^2). This pregnancy occurred 4 days after device insertion and was likely an unrecognized early pregnancy at the time of insertion rather than a true method failure. Cumulative implant failure over 3 years was 0.00 per 100 woman years for normal and overweight

Table 10.3 Recommendations for the use of contraception in obese women

Guidelines for obese women (BMI > 30 kg/m^2)	Cu-IUD/ LNG IUS	ENG implant	DMPA	Combined (OCPs, patch ring)	Oral EC	Condom	Diaphragm/cap
United States Medical Eligibility Criteria (Center for Disease Control) 2010	1	1	1 (2 in adolescents <18)	2	Not rated	1	1[a]
Medical Eligibility Criteria for Contraceptive Use (World Health Organization) 2009	1	1	1 (2 in adolescents <18)	2	Not rated	1	1[a]
UK Medical Eligibility Criteria for Contraceptive Use (Royal College of Obstetricians and Gynaecologists, Faculty of Sexual and Reproductive Health Care) 2009	1	1	1	BMI 30–34 kg/m^2: 2 BMI >35 kg/m^2: 3	Not rated	1	1[a]

Key: 1 = A condition for which there is no restriction for use. 2 = A condition for which the advantages of using the method generally outweigh the theoretical or proven risks. 3 = A condition for which the theoretical or proven risks usually outweigh the advantages of using the method. 4 = A condition that represents an unacceptable health risk if the contraceptive method is use

[a]Severe obesity might make diaphragm placement difficult

Table 10.4 USMEC guidelines for women with a history of bariatric surgery

Guidelines for Obese Women (BMI > 30 kg/m^2)	Cu-IUD/ LNG-IUD	ENG implant	DMPA	Combined (OCPs, patch ring)	Oral EC	Condom	Diaphragm/cap
Restrictive procedures	1	1	1	1	1	1	1
Malabsorptive procedures	1	1	1	1 (patch, ring) 3 (OCPs)	1	1	1

The WHO and UKMEC do not address bariatric surgery
Key: 1 = A condition for which there is no restriction for use. 2 = A condition for which the advantages of using the method generally outweigh the theoretical or proven risks. 3 = A condition for which the theoretical or proven risks usually outweigh the advantages of using the method. 4 = A condition that represents an unacceptable health risk if the contraceptive method is use

women, and 0.23 per 100 woman years in obese women. This study provides evidence that there is not a clinically significant variance in efficacy of the ENG implant by BMI.

Pharmacokinetics

In normal weight women, the implant releases 60–70 mcg of ENG/day in the first 6 weeks of use, and progressively declines to about 30 mcg/day by the third year of use [34, 35]. Serum concentrations of ENG are effective to inhibit ovulation (the primary mechanism of action of the implant) within 24 h of insertion, and reach peak concentration on day 4 after placement (813 pg/mL). Serum concentrations decline over time (1 year: mean 196 pg/mL [range 150–261], 3 years: mean 156 pg/mL [range 111–202]) [34, 36].

Plasma ENG concentration has been shown to have an inverse relationship to body weight in users of the subdermal implant [35]. A small study ($n = 13$) followed a group of obese women over 6 months (median BMI 41, range of 33–52) [37]. Plasma concentrations of ENG were on average 47.6 % lower than in normal weight controls, with projected plasma concentrations calculated for 1, 2, and 3 years of 133 pg/mL, 102 pg/mL, and 98 pg/mL, respectively (Fig. 10.2) [37].

In pharmacodynamics studies of normal weight women, ovulation is inhibited in 97 % of patients when the ENG serum level is greater than 90 pg/mL. With serum levels <90 pg/mL, ovulation was reported in up to 50 % of women [38]. These women may still have some contraceptive benefit from secondary effects of cervical mucus thickening, but contraceptive efficacy may be decreased. With serum levels projected near 90 pg/mL by year 3 in some obese women, there is theoretical concern that contraceptive efficacy may decrease by the third year of use in this population [37]. Increased failure rate in year 3 in obese women has not been demonstrated in any clinical studies. More research is needed to determine if this is a true clinical risk.

Safety and Adverse Events

No studies have identified a difference in the safety profile or adverse events experienced by obese as compared to normal BMI ENG implant users.

Obesity-Related Issues

Weight Gain

Self-perception of weight gain by women appears greater than the actual weight gain documented during implant use. In one trial of normal weight users, 12 % reported weight gain and 2.3 % cited weight gain as reason for discontinuation [39]. The actual amount of mean weight gain has been reported at 1.6 kg over 3 years in normal weight women, with a mean increase in BMI of 0.8 kg/m^2 [36, 40]. Likewise, in the Contraceptive CHOICE Project, weight gain in a study population including overweight and obese women was 2.1 ± 6.7 kg over 12 months. Importantly, after adjusting for race, this amount of weight gain was not significantly higher than that observed with the copper IUD (0.2 ± 5.1 kg) [22]. Weight gain with these long-term contraceptive methods appears more age-associated rather than a contraceptive-related effect [21].

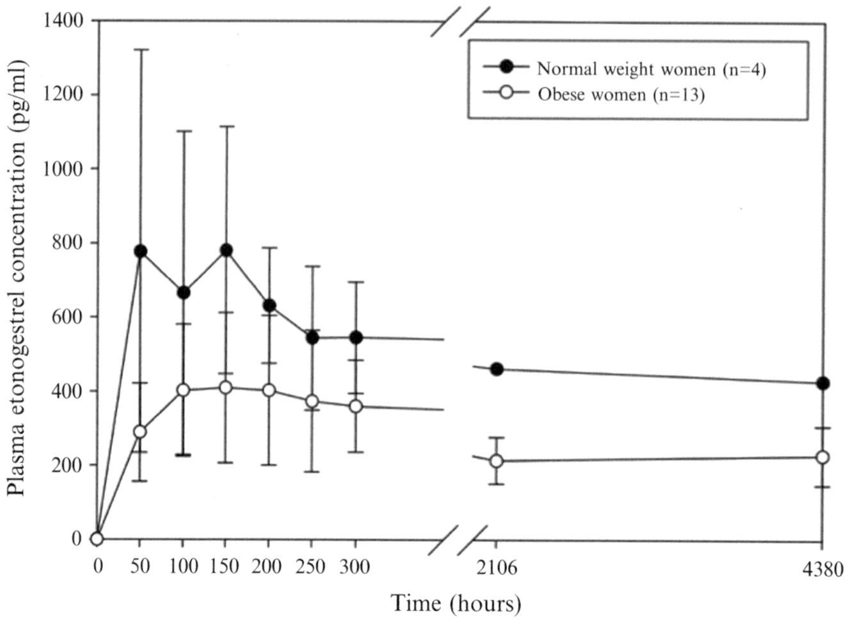

Fig. 10.2 Changes in etonogestrel plasma concentration over 6 months in obese and normal weight users of the ENG implant. Plasma concentrations in obese women at all time points were lower than normal weight controls. Reprinted from Am J Obstet Gynecol, 207/2, Mornar S, Chan L-N, Mistretta S, Neustadt A, Martins S, Gilliam M, Pharmacokinetics of the etonogestrel contraceptive implant in obese women, 110.e1–110.e6, Copyright 2012, with permission from Elsevier

Hyperlipidemia

Several studies have examined the effect of the ENG implant on serum lipid profiles among normal weight women without baseline hyperlipidemia. These studies have demonstrated a mild decrease in TC, LDL, and HDL cholesterol over 2 years of use, with small, clinically insignificant effects on triglyceride (TG) levels [41–43]. A small study of eight obese women (BMI >30) showed no change in TC, HDL, LDL or triglycerides (TG) over 6 months of implant use [44].

Most regulatory agencies rate the ENG implant as category 2 (benefits generally outweigh proven or theoretical risks) for hyperlipidemia based on DMPA studies, not ENG implant studies, where HDL was reduced (Table 10.5). The reduction in HDL reported in ENG implant users is variable and likely not clinically significant, with all subjects remaining in the normal range throughout implant use [42]. Further studies are needed to clarify whether the ENG implant alters lipid profiles in women with baseline hyperlipidemia.

Bariatric Surgery

As the ENG implant does not require oral absorption, malabsorptive bariatric surgery procedures should not affect drug delivery. However, weight loss and other metabolic changes following bariatric surgery can be dramatic, and there is a paucity of data on the pharmacokinetics of the ENG implant in women following bariatric surgery or rapid weight loss. A case report of three patients using the ENG implant before and after bariatric surgery via Roux-en-Y procedure provides most of the available data [45]. In this study, serum ENG concentrations were measured at the time of bariatric surgery (2 months after implant placement), and again at 3 and 6 months postoperatively. At the time of bariatric surgery, serum concentrations of ENG were lower than those reported in normal weight historical controls, which is consistent with prior data that serum levels may be lower in obese women [35]. Serum concentrations of ENG decreased for all three women over time along with weight loss. The lowest serum concentration reported was 125 pg/mL

Table 10.5 Recommendations for the use of contraception in women with hyperlipidemia

Guidelines for known hyperlipidemias	Cu-IUD/ LNG-IUD	ENG implant	DMPA	Combined (OCPs, patch ring)	Oral EC	Condom	Diaphragm/cap
United States Medical Eligibility Criteria (Center for Disease Control) 2010	2	2	2	2/3[a]	Not rated	1	1
Medical Eligibility Criteria for Contraceptive Use (World Health Organization) 2009	1/2	2	2	2/3[a]	Not rated	1	1
UK Medical Eligibility Criteria for Contraceptive Use (Royal College of Obstetricians and Gynaecologists, Faculty of Sexual and Reproductive Health Care) 2009	1/2	2	2	2/3[a]	1	1	1

Key: 1 = A condition for which there is no restriction for use. 2 = A condition for which the advantages of using the method generally outweigh the theoretical or proven risks. 3 A condition for which the theoretical or proven risks usually outweigh the advantages of using the method. 4 = A condition that represents an unacceptable health risk if the contraceptive method is use

[a]Although some types of hyperlipidemias are risk factors for vascular disease, the category should be assessed according to the type, its severity, and the presence of other cardiovascular risk factors

in one woman at 8 months after insertion, at a weight of 130 kg (following 42 kg weight loss). However, one of the other women with very similar preoperative and postoperative weight had serum levels that remained therapeutic and over 200 pg/mL throughout the 6-month study. This suggests that drug elimination rate may play as important a role as volume of distribution in the pharmacokinetics of the ENG implant, such that pharmacokinetics and efficacy cannot be predicted by BMI alone.

Recommendations

All contraceptive eligibility criteria currently recommend the ENG implant as category 1 for obesity (see Table 10.3) and for women undergoing bariatric surgery (see Table 10.4). ACOG especially encourages progestin-only methods such as the implant for obese women due to the increased baseline risk of thromboembolism from obesity and the additional risk of estrogen exposure with combined contraceptive methods [24]. Women experiencing co-morbidities from obesity including hyperlipidemia, vascular disease, or who have multiple cardiovascular risk factors are uniformly given category 2 rating for the ENG-implant despite minimal evidence for any adverse effect in these populations. Further research is needed among women with these conditions.

Permanent Contraception

Overview

Female sterilization is utilized by one in three women worldwide, and over 600,000 tubal sterilization procedures are performed each year in the USA [46]. There are scant data on efficacy and/or complications in obese populations, but these mechanical methods of tubal occlusion should be unaffected by body weight. However, the act of performing these procedures may be more challenging in an obese woman. It is important to consider that LARC methods offer equivalent, if not superior, efficacy to sterilization and should be offered to any woman considering a sterilization procedure [47, 48]. Additionally, vasectomy remains more effective and less invasive than female sterilization procedures, and couples should be counseled on this option, but vasectomy is not addressed here specifically. In this section we review available data on the most common methods of female sterilization in obese women.

Interval Laparoscopic Sterilization

The largest study of sterilization to date, the United States Collaborative Review of Sterilization (CREST), was completed between 1978 and 1987. This study did not include BMI/weight in their analysis of efficacy by method of sterilization, and no studies since have examined rates of sterilization failure by method in obese women [48]. In the absence of data to the contrary and no biologic plausibility, the efficacy is assumed to be the same in women of varying BMI [48, 49].

A secondary analysis of CREST evaluated risk factors for complications in interval sterilization procedures [50]. In this analysis, 13.6 % of 9,475 women undergoing interval sterilization met criteria for obesity. The overall risk of complications (including febrile morbidity, transfusion, reoperation, rehospitalization, conversion to laparotomy) was 1–2 %. Obesity was a risk factor associated with an increased risk of complications (adjusted odds ratio 1.7 [95 % CI, 1.2–2.6]), along with diabetes, general anesthesia, and previous abdominal or pelvic surgery. Application of this data is limited today in that many of these procedures were performed via mini-laparotomy, rather than laparoscopy. Obesity is known to increase surgical risks including wound infection and venous thrombosis during laparotomy. Laparoscopic procedures minimize these risks and many recent studies suggest no increased rate of conversion to laparotomy or other complications in obese versus nonobese women undergoing laparoscopy [51]. With modern laparoscopic techniques, complications of interval sterilization may no longer be increased in obese women.

Hysteroscopic Sterilization

Hysteroscopic sterilization was introduced in the USA in 2002 with the FDA approval of a nickel-titanium coil microinsert (Essure, Bayer Healthcare Pharmaceuticals, Wayne, NJ). This advancement provided women the option of sterilization without undergoing abdominal or laparoscopic surgery. Placement of the microinserts promotes a local tissue reaction leading to scarring and occlusion of the fallopian tubes within 90 days. However, in up to 10 % of patients, physicians are unable to place one or both inserts, and up to 5 % of patients will not develop complete tubal occlusion despite bilateral placement [52]. Anderson et al. examined the relationship between BMI and successful placement of both occlusion devices in 638 women [53]. Though obese patients were more likely to have hysteroscopic sterilization completed in the operating room rather than the office due to patient or surgeon preference, successful placement of the devices and successful tubal occlusion did not vary by BMI or location of procedure. Hysteroscopic sterilization via microinserts is safe and effective in obese populations and offers an alternative to abdominal surgery. In order to optimize visualization of the cervix for completion of hysteroscopy, surgeons should consider correct choice of speculum, retractors and table to maximize success.

Postpartum Tubal Ligation

Postpartum tubal ligation is undertaken either at the time of cesarean section or via mini-laparotomy following vaginal delivery, prior to the onset of uterine involution. The CREST study concluded that postpartum tubal ligation via partial salpingectomy had the lowest rate of failure [48]. Partial salpingectomy in obese women may be difficult at the time of cesarean section due to inability to exteriorize the uterus and tubes. Application of Filshie clips has been suggested in this scenario. Though they do provide effective contraception (failure rate 0.017 over 2 years), Filshie clips placed postpartum are less effective than postpartum partial salpingectomy (failure rate 0.004, $p = 0.04$), and every effort should be made to perform a partial salpingectomy [54, 55].

Performing mini-laparotomy to access tubes may also be challenging depending on the distribution of adipose tissue. These authors have found that visualization of the fundus is improved in obese women with the use of a small Alexis (Applied Medical, Rancho Santa Margarita, California, USA) surgical retractor to compress and retract subcutaneous tissue, sometimes in combination with packing of the bowel with tagged laparotomy sponges. Rates of surgical site infection may be higher in obese women following postpartum mini-laparotomy. For women desiring and planning postpartum permanent contraception who do not receive it, an

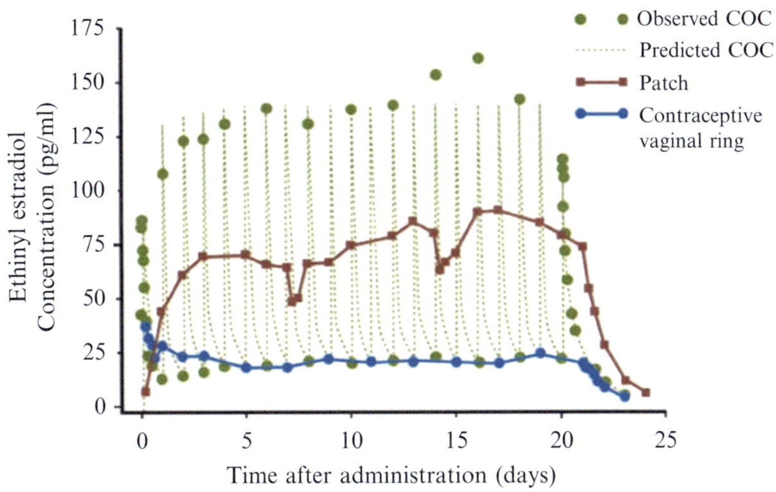

Fig. 10.3 Mean ethinyl estradiol (EE) concentration versus time curves for normal weight subjects using a combined oral contraceptive containing 30 mcg EE/150 mcg LNG ($n = 8$), transdermal contraceptive patch ($n = 6$) and the CVR ($n = 8$). This demonstrates the difference in pharmacokinetics of the three routes of administration. Reprinted from Contraception, 72/3, van den Heuvel MW, van Bragt AJM, Alnabasy AKM, Kaptein MCJ, Comparison of ethintlestradiol pharmacokinetics in three hormonal contraceptive formulations: the vaginal ring, the transdermal patch and an oral contraceptive, 168–174, Copyright 2005, with permission from Elsevier

alternative with similar efficacy includes either an immediate postplacental IUD insertion or implant placement.

Sterilization Considerations in Bariatric Surgery Patients

Significant weight loss after bariatric surgery may improve fertility status, and for some women this may not be a welcome change [9]. Women undergoing bariatric surgery should be counseled on contraceptive options, which include permanent contraception if they have completed childbearing [6, 10, 30, 56]. In some cases, concurrent sterilization with their bariatric surgery may be feasible.

Contraceptives of Intermediate Effectiveness

Combined Hormonal Contraception (Pills, Patch, Ring)

Overview

Combined hormonal contraception refers to methods that contain both estrogen and progestin; this includes combined oral contraceptives (COCs), the contraceptive vaginal ring (CVR) (NuvaRing, Merck, Whitehouse Station, NJ, USA), and the transdermal contraceptive patch (Ortho Evra, Ortho-McNeil Pharmaceutical Inc., Raritan, NJ, USA). The primary mechanism of action of combined hormonal contraceptives is prevention of ovulation by suppression of gonadotropin secretion at the hypothalamic and pituitary levels. The progestin component primarily suppresses luteinizing hormone (LH) release, while the estrogen component suppresses follicle-stimulating hormone (FSH) to prevent formation of a dominant follicle [57]. The inclusion of a cyclic estrogen component, most commonly ethinyl estradiol (EE), offers the additional benefit of menstrual cycle control. Since their introduction in the 1960s, COCs have been the most popular method of contraception in the USA [58]. The development of the CVR and contraceptive patch provided alternate dosing strategies for combined hormonal contraception. Serum levels of EE vary by mode of administration (Fig. 10.3), though the relationship of these levels to BMI and to contraceptive efficacy is still incompletely understood.

Use and Efficacy in Obese Populations

The efficacy of hormonal contraceptives in obese women is dependent both on pharmacokinetic parameters such as drug absorption, distribution, metabolism and excretion, but also on behavioral factors such as compliance, sexual frequency, and a woman's inherent ability to become pregnant (fecundity). Compliance is of particular concern with shorter-acting methods like COCs, CVR, and the contraceptive patch. Additionally, the pharmacokinetic profile of COCs as compared to the CVR and contraceptive patch are different and thus may be affected differently by obesity. Serum levels are important for drug effect, yet minimum serum levels required for contraceptive effectiveness are difficult to determine given the multiple methods of action of most hormonal contraceptives.

COCs

Existing studies conflict regarding whether obesity affects COC efficacy. Many studies suggesting a relationship between higher BMI and COC failure were not designed to differentiate between failure based on pharmacokinetic (PK) factors versus compliance [59]. A recent large, prospective cohort study of over 52,000 women was conducted to study COC failure in two different dosing regimens among normal weight and obese women [60]. Contraceptive failure rates were adjusted for age, parity, and education, and showed a slight but significant increase in failure rates as BMI increased. BMI over 35 was associated with a hazard ratio of 1.5 (1.3–1.8 95 % confidence interval) for contraceptive failure. Although not powered to determine a significant difference in contraceptive failure, the Contraceptive CHOICE project found no efficacy difference by BMI in 1,500 users of combined methods [61]. However, this result was based on a combined group of COCs, CVR, and contraceptive patch users, and results for a COC-only group have not been published. Of note, given their large number of subjects, neither of these studies controlled for compliance using serum levels.

One small study did identify obesity as a risk factor for noncompliance with COCs [62]. It is unclear whether incorrect COC use in this study is generalizable to larger populations, but incorrect pill use may be related to poverty, lower education, or irregular contact with the medical system, which are all also associated with obesity [63, 64]. Noncompliance in studies makes it difficult to discern if obesity actually does have a true impact on contraceptive efficacy.

Dosing strategy of COCs may be related to risk of failure. Several studies suggest that shortening or eliminating the hormone-free interval may be an effective strategy for lowering the risk of contraceptive failure in women regardless of weight [60, 65]. Typical hormone-free intervals (7 days) allow for reactivation of the hypothalamic–pituitary–ovarian (HPO) axis during this time. Pharmacokinetics of COCs in obese women may allow for earlier return of follicular activity following the 7 day hormone-free interval, which has the theoretical result of increasing the risk of contraceptive failure [66].

Overall, it is unclear if obese women have a higher risk of COC failure as compared to normal weight women. If there an influence on efficacy, the absolute risk of failure is low, and COCs still offer superior protection to barrier methods [67].

CVR

There are minimal data on CVR efficacy in obese women. A secondary analysis was performed using the NuvaRing phase III efficacy trials to evaluate contraceptive failure by body weight, though the initial trial was not powered for this analysis [68]. Among 295 women in the highest decile of weight (over 167 lb), there was a 1 % pregnancy rate in a per protocol analysis, and 1.2 % pregnancy rate in an intention to treat analysis. Overall pregnancy rate among 3,259 women (weighing 88–272 lb) in the intention to treat analysis was similar at 0.83 %. No method failures occurred in the 74 heaviest women (189–272 lb). As mentioned earlier, the contraceptive CHOICE project did not report on the risk of contraceptive failure specific to obese CVR users.

Using the limited available data, contraceptive failure rates of the CVR appear to be similar in normal weight and obese women.

Contraceptive Patch

Although not powered to determine a difference in pregnancy rates by body weight, an analysis of the efficacy studies of the contraceptive patch demonstrated that baseline body weight over 90 kg (198 lb) may be related to risk of failure [69]. Women weighing over 90 kg accounted for less than 3 % of the total study population, but 33 % of all on-treatment pregnancies occurred in these women. However, the overall failure rate for the patch across all weight categories was low at 0.8 %. The reported method failures in women over 90 kg suggest that the patch may be less effective in obese women. However, larger studies in obese women are needed, and the patch still provides more effective contraception than barrier methods alone.

Pharmacokinetics

Obesity can affect all aspects of drug metabolism [70]. Obesity adversely affects the PK profile of contraceptive steroid hormones including EE and progestins in COCs, CVR, and the contraceptive patch. However, it remains unclear if the impact on the PK profile is enough to affect drug therapeutics, or in the case of contraceptives, prevention of pregnancy.

COCs

Larger volume of distribution in obese women offers a plausible rationale for lower serum concentrations of lipophilic steroid hormones, which could translate into lower contraceptive efficacy. However, this theory has not been confirmed by PK studies. Rather, the changes in pharmacokinetics appear to be due to a change in drug clearance and drug half-life. Obese women take twice as long to reach steady state as normal BMI women, which might allow for a "window of opportunity" for failure at pill initiation or following a 7-day hormone-free interval [66, 71]. On the other hand, trough levels of contraceptive steroid hormones do not appear to vary by BMI status, which suggests that contraceptive efficacy may be maintained [72].

CVR

Westhoff et al. [73] examined the pharmacokinetics of EE and ENG in normal weight and obese users of the CVR. The obese population had a mean BMI of 34.3 kg/m^2 (SD 3.0) but excluded women over 40 kg/m^2. Over one cycle, EE concentrations were lower in obese women (22 pg/mL vs. 15 pg/mL, $p=0.004$) during all 3 weeks of use. ENG levels were similar between normal weight and obese women (1,256 pg/mL vs. 1,138 pg/mL, respectively, $p=0.39$). Both BMI groups had equivalent suppression of ovarian activity and so contraceptive efficacy does not seem to be compromised. However, obese women did have more days of spotting possibly related to lower EE levels.

Contraceptive Patch

There is minimal published data on pharmacokinetics of the patch in obese women. Initial studies revealed that levels of both EE and norelgestromin decreased as body weight increased, but no further details were published [69].

Safety and Adverse Events

The primary concern with the use of estrogen-containing contraceptives in obese women is an increase in venous thromboembolism (VTE). Obesity doubles the risk of VTE, and the risk is further increased with the use of combined hormonal contraceptives [15]. Many providers incorrectly believe that non-oral combined hormonal contraceptives are "safer" than oral contraceptives because the hormones bypass first-pass hepatic metabolism, and thus do not activate clotting factors. However, the current non-oral formulations contain EE for the estrogen component, and this potent estrogen activates clotting factors whether given orally or not [74, 75]. Therefore, the currently available combined methods are viewed similarly in regard to their safety profiles.

COCs

The absolute risk of VTE remains low even in obese COC users. The incidence of VTE in women using COCs was 60 per 100,000 for class I obesity, and 105 per 100,000 for class II and III obesity, compared to a baseline risk of 12–20 per 100,000 in normal weight women not using hormonal contraception [15]. Additionally, the risk of VTE in pregnant obese women is higher than with OC use (100–200 per 100,000). Relative risks must be considered in prescribing these medications, recognizing that pregnancy may pose greater health risks to an obese patient than use of a combined contraceptive [15, 76–78]. There is no clear evidence for an increased risk of embolic events such as stroke or myocardial infarction in obese users of combined hormonal contraceptives [79].

CVR

Measurements of surrogate markers for the coagulation system (sex hormone binding globulin, protein C, protein S) in vaginal ring users suggest that the ring has similar effect on clot risk as oral dosing of EE [74, 80, 81]. Long-term, prospective studies are needed to confirm whether there are different clinical rates of thromboembolic disease with vaginal or oral dosing, but vaginal dosing cannot be relied upon to lower risk of thromboembolic disease in obese women.

Contraceptive Patch

There is conflicting data on a possible increased risk of thromboembolic disease with the contraceptive patch, though this has not been examined in relation to body weight. Initial case–control studies showed no increased risk of venous thromboembolism or arterial thromboembolic events in patch users compared to users of a norgestimate-containing OC [82]. Likewise, a population based cohort study showed no association with the patch and increased risk of venous or arterial thrombotic events [83]. However, other case–control studies have reported a two-fold higher risk of VTE compared with an oral formulation of the same progestin [84]. Given that obese women are at a baseline elevated risk of VTE, these findings should be interpreted with caution. However, it is important to consider that the relative risk of VTE in pregnancy is higher than has been reported with the contraceptive patch, and so there is not an absolute contraindication to patch use in obese women [15, 78, 85].

Obesity-Related Issues

Weight Gain

Generally, weight gain while using combined hormonal contraception appears to be unrelated to the contraceptive method. However, the bulk of these studies were performed in women of normal weight at baseline. Additionally, the use of any contraception reduces the risk of pregnancy, which has definitely been associated with weight gain.

COCs

Perceived weight gain is the most common reason cited for COC discontinuation, despite lack of evidence for this relationship. Most adults gain weight over time, and given the widespread use of COCs, these medications are often blamed for weight gain. A Cochrane review summarized the weight changes in randomized controlled trials among normal weight women using COCs versus placebo and found no evidence to support a causal relationship between COC use and weight gain [86]. Likewise, in a primate model utilizing normal weight and obese rhesus monkeys, COC use over 8 months resulted in an increase in metabolic activity among all monkeys and no change in food intake or physical activity. Obese monkeys demonstrated an 8.58 % reduction in body weight and a 12.3 % reduction in percent body fat over the study, whereas normal weight monkeys had no change in these parameters [87]. Overall, users should be reassured that there is no definitive evidence for weight gain with COCs.

CVR

Weight gain with the CVR appears to be minimal, comparable to that seen with COCs [88]. Over a 3-month randomized trial, women using the CVR had a 2.5-lb weight gain, and COC users had a 3.1-lb weight gain. Weight gain did not differ by baseline BMI (normal, overweight, obese) or birth control method. Another study demonstrated that fewer women experienced weight gain with the CVR than COCs over 1 year of use (1.7 % vs. 4.5 %)[89]. Available data suggest that weight gain with the CVR is minimal and women with baseline obesity are not at increased risk of weight gain.

Contraceptive Patch

Weight gain with the contraceptive patch is minimal [90]. Mean change in body weight over 13 cycles of patch use was an increase by 0.3 kg. Only 2 % of users reported greater than 10 % body weight increase, and 1.4 % of users reported greater than 10 % body weight decrease [90].

Hyperlipidemia

COCs

Modern low-dose COCs (EE 35 mcg or less) have little effect on lipid metabolism in normal weight women. In a recent randomized controlled trial (RCT) including normal weight and obese women randomized to an OC containing either 30 or 20 mcg of EE, triglycerides and lipid profiles were monitored at baseline and after 3 months of COC use [91]. As expected, baseline LDL was higher and HDL lower for obese compared to normal weight participants. In the obese women, mean LDL decreased by 4.9 mg/dL (±20.6) ($p=0.02$) with COC use, but there was no change in mean TC, HDL or TG over 3 months of use. Such small changes in lipid profiles are unlikely to have clinical significance, and therefore it appears that COCs with 35 mcg or less of EE do not have an effect on lipid profiles in otherwise healthy obese women.

CVR

Exogenous estrogen administration generally improves lipid profiles, whereas progestins, depending on their degree of androgenicity, may counteract this effect [92]. The CVR has lower EE exposure than COCs (see Fig. 10.3) and utilizes a non-androgenic progestin, ENG, both of which could contribute to a different lipid profile than has been observed with COCs. In studies comparing lipid profiles in normal weight users of COCs or the CVR without baseline hyperlipidiema, the CVR does not cause significant change in TC, LDL, HDL, or TG over 12 months of use [89, 92, 93]. Some studies have shown a greater decrease in LDL in users of the CVR compared to COCs users over 6–12 months of use [89], which has unknown clinical significance. Overall, the CVR appears to have a neutral effect on lipid profiles in women without baseline hyperlipidemia. Further research is needed within women with elevated lipid profiles.

Contraceptive Patch

Serum TC and TG were monitored during early safety trials of the patch, and no change in either measurement was noted over 13 treatment cycles [90].

Bariatric Surgery

COCs

Evidence regarding COC efficacy following bariatric surgery is limited, and there is insufficient data to conclude that efficacy is reduced in women following bariatric surgery [10]. However, there is a theoretical risk that oral absorption of COCs may be altered following malabsorptive bariatric surgery procedures, in which ingested pills will bypass a large area of stomach and duodenum.

One study of seven morbidly obese women following jejunoileal bypass surgery demonstrated lower plasma progestin levels in the first 8 h following ingestion of progestin-only pills (3 mg norethisterone and 0.25 mg levonorgestrel) compared to normal weight controls [94]. The difference in serum levels was attributed to decreased absorption following their surgery. However, serum levels in this study did not correlate to ovulatory markers, so it is unclear whether the different drug levels had clinical significance. Additionally, the jejunoileal bypass procedure is no longer performed, and no studies have examined how current procedures involving a smaller volume of bypass affect drug pharmacokinetics.

Other data have been drawn from observational studies. In an observational study with self-reported contraceptive use following bariatric surgery, two of nine women who continued taking the same COC before and after a biliopancreatic diversion procedure became pregnant in the postoperative period [95]. These women also suffered from chronic diarrhea after the procedure, so the exact mechanism for their drug failures is unknown.

Due to the uncertainty of COC pharmacokinetics following bariatric surgery, and due to the importance of avoiding pregnancy in the postoperative period, women should be encouraged to consider non-oral contraceptives including LARCs, which offer significantly improved efficacy. Additionally, obese women planning a major surgery involving immobilization are advised not to use estrogen-containing contraceptives due to increased risk for venous thrombosis [96].

CVR

No studies have specifically addressed CVR use in a population of bariatric surgery patients, and limited data is available in women with a BMI over 40 kg/m^2.

Contraceptive Patch

No studies have examined patch efficacy and pharmacokinetics in women undergoing bariatric surgery.

Recommendations

The USMEC and the WHO MEC give combined methods of contraception a category 2 rating (see Table 10.3) for obesity. The UKMEC stratifies risk by BMI, increasing the rating to category 3 (theoretical or proven risks usually outweigh the benefits of the method) in women over a BMI of 35 kg/m^2 due to the increasing risk of VTE as BMI increases. However, the risk of VTE in obese users of combined contraception is still lower than in pregnancy. While these methods appear overall safe and effective in obese women, they are less effective than LARC methods and should be considered second line options for all women regardless of weight. For women with known hyperlipidemia, the benefits of combined methods generally outweigh risks, unless there are additional cardiovascular risk factors present (see Table 10.5).

Injectable Contraception

Overview

Depot-medroxyprogesterone acetate (DMPA) is a progestin-only contraceptive method with good efficacy, with failure rates reported between 0.7 and 6.0 % for typical use over 3 years [97]. It is administered every 3 months as an intramuscular (IM) injection of 150 mg medroxyprogesterone, but is also available in a subcutaneous injection (104 mg DMPA-SC). It acts primarily by suppression of ovulation [98]. This section reviews evidence on contraceptive efficacy and pharmacokinetics of DMPA in obese and overweight women.

Use and Efficacy in Obese Populations

Ovulation suppression and contraceptive efficacy with DMPA appears unaffected by BMI. DMPA has equal contraceptive efficacy in normal weight and obese women. A large, multicenter trial of 846 DMPA users demonstrated that contraceptive failure with DMPA was not related to body weight among normal or overweight users [99]. In an early PK study comparing thin and obese women (BMI mean 17.9 kg/m^2 vs. 32.3 kg/m^2), there was no difference in return to ovulation following an IM injection of DMPA [100].

More recently, studies have examined contraceptive efficacy in obese women using DMPA-SC. In a phase III 1-year trial with DMPA-SC administered every 3 months, no pregnancies were detected among a population including 36 % overweight or obese women (641 of 1,787), of which 11 % had a BMI over 30 [98]. Likewise, a small study of DMPA-SC use over 6 months among five obese (BMI 30–39.9 kg/m^2) and five extremely obese (BMI >40 kg/m^2) women showed no evidence of ovulation and no method failure [96].

Pharmacokinetics

DMPA IM has a prolonged duration of action over 3 months as it is released from muscle. Serum concentrations vary around a mean of 1,000 pg/mL over 3 months, and then decline [97]. Ovulation resumes when serum levels of DMPA fall under 100 pg/mL. In the subcutaneous formulation, ovulation resumes at serum levels of 200 pg/mL [96].

Serum levels of DMPA following IM injection of 150 mg are equivalent in normal weight and obese women during the first 12 weeks of use [96], and remain equivalent following subsequent doses [101]. Serum levels of DMPA-SC are lower in obese compared to normal weight women, but do not approach the contraceptive threshold for ovulation suppression (200 pg/mL) in women with BMI<40 kg/m^2 [101–103]. However, women with BMI>40 kg/m^2 using the SC formulation have significantly lower serum levels of medroxyprogesterone acetate (MPA) compared to less obese and normal weight women [104]. One woman with a BMI over 40 kg/m^2 had a serum concentration of MPA just under the contraceptive threshold (191 and 183 pg/mL) during the second month of use, though ovulation did not occur. The intramuscular formulation may be preferable in women with BMI over 40 kg/m^2 until the pharmacokinetics and degree of ovulation suppression with DMPA-SC are better understood in the extremely obese population [102]. Intramuscular administration should be assured in obese women by utilizing an adequately long needle.

Safety and Adverse Events

No studies have identified a difference in the safety profile or adverse events experienced by obese as compared to normal BMI DMPA users.

Obesity-Related Issues

Weight Gain

Weight gain is a major concern for women and one of the major reasons for method discontinuation; this is particularly true of DMPA. To help address conflicting reports of weight gain with use of DMPA, a recent Cochrane review evaluated the relationship between progestin-only contraceptive use and body weight change [22]. Only ten studies met their criteria, with little evidence for a DMPA-associated weight change as compared to nonuse of a hormonal contraceptive method. Actual weight gain was low (under 2 kg for many studies), and could not be differentiated from weight gain experienced from aging [105]. Additionally, a woman's baseline BMI does not appear to be predictive of the weight gain women will experience with DMPA use. Overweight and obese users of DMPA do not gain more weight than normal weight women using DMPA [22, 106].

Adolescent users of DMPA may have different patterns of weight gain than those reported in adult women. In normal weight adolescents, an observational study demonstrated that DMPA may cause an increase in total body fat (+10.3 %) and a decrease in lean body mass (−3.4 %) over 6 months of use compared to adolescents not using hormonal contraception [107].

Additionally, a retrospective review found that girls who were obese at the initiation of DMPA gained more weight than normal weight adolescents using DMPA, and gained more weight than all weight categories of adolescents using OCs or non-hormonal contraception [108]. Need for effective contraception and concerns about weight gain must be balanced in adolescent populations, and further research is needed to clarify whether there are long-term consequences for these reported body composition changes.

It is important to acknowledge that weight change on DMPA varies by individual, and population means do not reflect individual variance. This is the main problem with prior studies where population means were reported instead of individual means. The contraceptive CHOICE project noted a range of −7.7 to +21.8 kg over 12 months of DMPA use [109]. Predictors of excessive weight gain on DMPA have been found in adolescent studies, where adolescents who gained more than 5 % of their body weight within the first 6 months of use continued to have excess weight gain [110]. Additionally, African American race has been shown to predict greater weight gain with DMPA and other hormonal contraceptives [110].

Hyperlipidemia

Conflicting data exists on DMPA's effect on serum lipids. A prospective study of normal and obese women examined metabolic markers over 7 months of DMPA use [109]. As expected, obese women (mean BMI 40.7 kg/m^2) at baseline had a lower mean HDL (47 mg/dL) and higher TG (116 mg/dL) than normal weight women (67 mg/dL, 58 mg/dL, respectively). After 7 months of DMPA use, HDL decreased in both normal and obese women, but the difference (−5 mm/dL) was only significant in the obese population. Decreased HDL is associated with increased risk for cardiovascular disease, which may be clinically relevant in obese populations. Women with baseline hyperlipidemias are given a level 2 rating by the WHO, USMEC, and UKMEC for DMPA, based on these reported changes in HDL (see Table 10.5).

However, other studies suggest that these negative effects on lipids may be temporary. A prospective study over 3 years of DMPA use examined lipid profiles in a cohort of women with a mean BMI of 27.2 kg/m^2 (SD 6.9) [111, 112]. Within the first 6 months of use, mean HDL levels decreased from a baseline of 45 to 41 mg/dL, consistent with other studies. However, HDL levels then began rising and returned to baseline after 3 years of use. A subset of women with baseline abnormalities of lipids did not demonstrate an increased risk of worsening their lipid profiles. Further research is needed to clarify the effect of DMPA on serum lipids, but it appears that most observable negative effects (lowering of HDL or raising of LDL) are temporary even with continued use of DMPA.

Bariatric Surgery

There are no data specifically addressing the use of DMPA-IM or SC in women undergoing bariatric surgery. Non-orally administered medications should be unaffected by bariatric surgery. Additionally, as DMPA efficacy appears unaffected by BMI and does not appear to have a significant impact on weight gain, DMPA is a reasonable contraceptive option for women undergoing bariatric surgery.

Recommendations

The US and WHO MEC give DMPA a level 1 rating for obese adult women and women with a history of bariatric surgery, and a level 2 rating for obese adolescents (menarche to age 18) (see Tables 10.3 and 10.4). Progestin-only contraceptives such as DMPA are preferred for obese women as they do not increase thrombotic risks. DMPA can be considered a safe and effective contraceptive option for obese women, with no increased risk of weight gain compared to the baseline population. Benefits of DMPA are considered to outweigh theoretical risks for women with known hyperlipidemias.

Emergency Contraception

Overview

Emergency contraception (EC) is a backup option to decrease the likelihood of pregnancy following unprotected intercourse. Multi-dose regimens of combined OCs (known as the Yuzpe method) have largely been replaced by two oral EC options which are more effective and better tolerated [111, 113]: oral levonorgestrel (LNG) (Plan B OneStep, Teva Pharmaceuticals) and oral ulipristal acetate (UPA) (Ella, HRA Pharma, Paris, France), a selective progesterone receptor modulator. The copper IUD is also effective as emergency contraception.

As EC, LNG is administered as a one-time dose of 1.5 mg within 72 h of unprotected intercourse, and its primary mechanism of action is disruption of ovulation. When administered in normal weight women before the onset of the LH surge in the presence of a 12- to 17-mm ovarian follicle, LNG is able to disrupt or delay ovulation 90 % of the time [111] (Fig. 10.4). However, it is has no effect on ovulation when taken after the onset of the LH surge, and prevents ovulation only in 10 % of cases when taken in the presence of a follicle greater than 18 mm [111]. In an initial WHO trial, when taken within 24, 48, and 72 h of unprotected intercourse, LNG prevented 95 %, 85 %, and 58 % of expected pregnancies, respectively [112, 114]. More recent studies have raised concerns about the calculations used in this trial, and data now suggest that the efficacy of LNG as EC is lower than this, especially in obese women [114].

Ulipristal acetate was approved for use as an EC in Europe in 2009 and the USA in 2010 following two phase III studies demonstrating that UPA was non-inferior to LNG [114]. For women who took EC within 72 h of unprotected intercourse, the pregnancy rate was 1.8 % for UPA, and 2.6 % for LNG. When taken between 72 and 120 h after unprotected intercourse, UPA prevented pregnancy more effectively than LNG ($p=0.037$) [115, 116]. Overall, UPA appears to have 50 % greater efficacy than LNG at pregnancy prevention based on a trial directly com-

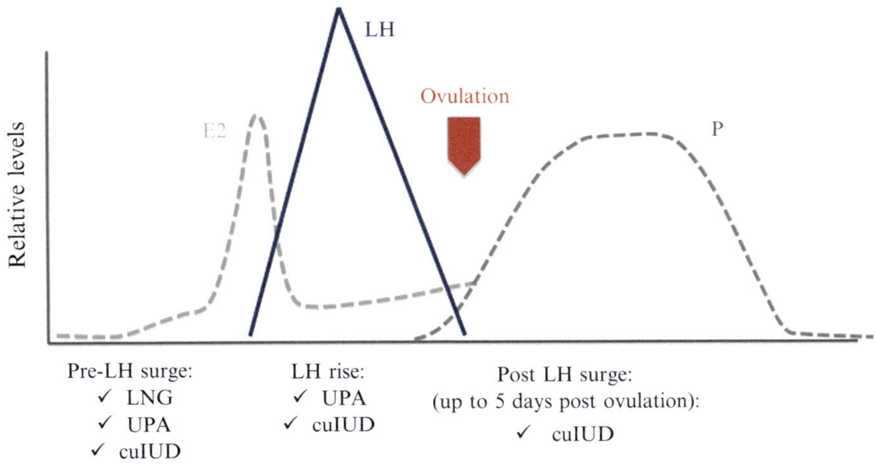

Fig. 10.4 Timing of contraceptive benefit within the menstrual cycle for three methods of emergency contraception in normal weight women. Adapted from [106–108, 110, 112]

paring UPA to LNG [71]. In this section we review data on the efficacy of LNG and UPA in obese women.

Use and Efficacy in Obese Populations

The greatest risk factor for failure of oral EC is body weight, followed by intercourse during the fertile time of the cycle, and repeat acts of unprotected intercourse within the same cycle [71]. Obese women have a three times greater risk of pregnancy following use of oral EC than normal weight women (OR, 3.60; 95 % CI, 1.96–6.53, $p<0.001$). Overweight women (BMI 25–30 kg/m^2) have 1.5 times the risk (OR 1.53, 95 % CI, 0.75–2.95) [114].

Efficacy of LNG appears to be more impaired by body weight than UPA. The limit of contraceptive efficacy for EC LNG is a body weight of 70 kg; LNG efficacy falls to that of placebo when body weight exceeds 70 kg (154 lb), or a BMI of 26 kg/m^2. UPA remains effective at higher body weights, but also loses any benefit as compared to placebo when body weight exceeds 88 kg (194 lb) or a BMI of 35 kg/m^2 [114]. *These data suggest that LNG is an ineffective EC for overweight and obese women, and UPA is less effective in overweight and obese women as compared to normal weight women.* Further data are needed on whether increased dosing of either of these methods would improve efficacy in obese women. LNG and UPA do not have linear pharmacokinetics, so an increase in dose would not necessarily increase serum levels to a contraceptive threshold in obese women.

In women of normal weight, the copper IUD is the most effective method of EC and this should be true for overweight and obese women as well. Copper IUDs do not appear to lose effectiveness with an increase in BMI and have an overall pregnancy rate of <0.1 % when placed postcoitally at any time in the menstrual cycle [115, 116] (see Fig. 10.4).

Pharmacokinetics

Pharmacokinetics of LNG are altered in obese women using LNG-containing OCs, including alterations in clearance, a longer time to achieve steady state, and lower peak serum levels [71]. For use as an EC agent, it is necessary for a single dose of LNG to provide a peak serum level sufficient to inhibit the LH surge. The lower efficacy of LNG in obese women as an EC may be related to these altered pharmacokinetics and an inability to reach adequate serum levels for ovulation inhibition with a single dose of LNG [71]. Pharmacokinetics of UPA or LNG EC in obese women have not been reported.

Safety and Adverse Events

No differences in safety profile or adverse events (other than increased risk of pregnancy) have been reported with LNG or UPA when used as EC.

Bariatric Surgery

Women qualifying for bariatric surgery are likely over a BMI of 35 kg/m^2. The best option for emergency contraception in this population is the copper IUD, as neither oral EC agent has been shown to be superior to placebo in pregnancy prevention in women with a BMI over 35. Additionally, oral absorption of steroid hormones may be altered in women following restrictive bariatric procedures.

Recommendations

The WHO, USMEC, and UKMEC do not have specific recommendations for EC in obese women. The USMEC rates hormonal EC as level 1 for use in women with a history of bariatric surgery, but cautions that efficacy may be lowered in women with a history of malabsorptive procedures. If an obese patient declines copper IUD for EC, using one of the oral EC agents is safe, but may not offer any protection against pregnancy.

Conclusion

Although contraceptive methods have been understudied in obese populations, the use of most methods is generally safer than pregnancy in these women. Additionally, the use of contraception is less likely to cause weight gain over a woman's lifetime as compared to pregnancy. The influence of obesity on contraceptive efficacy is still under investigation for some methods. The only methods with documented inferior efficacy in obese women are hormonal EC (LNG and UPA). Providers should feel reassured in offering obese women a range of contraceptive options, without expectation of increased side effects or weight gain. Due to superior efficacy and satisfaction, the best contraceptive methods for women of any weight are long-acting reversible or permanent methods.

References

1. Ogden C, Carroll M, Kit B, Flegal K. Prevalence of obesity in the United States, 2009–2010. National Center for Health Statistics. 2012;82:1–8.
2. Obesity and overweight [Internet]. World Health Organization [cited 2013 Mar 6]. Available from: http://www.who.int/mediacentre/factsheets/fs311/en/index.html
3. Prentice A. The emerging epidemic of obesity in developing countries. Int J Epidemiol. 2005;35(1):93–9.
4. Vilos GA, Marks J, Tureanu V, Abu-Rafea B, Vilos AG. The levonorgestrel intrauterine system is an effective treatment in selected obese women with abnormal uterine bleeding. J Minim Invasive Gynecol. 2011;18(1):75–80.
5. Weiss JL, Malone FD, Emig D, Ball RH, Nyberg DA, Comstock CH, et al. Obesity, obstetric complications and cesarean delivery rate—a population-based screening study. Am J Obstet Gynecol. 2004;190(4):1091–7.
6. Kominiarek M. Bariatric surgery and pregnancy. ACOG Pract Bull. 2009;105:1–9.
7. Olson G. Obesity and implications for future generations. Am J Obstet Gynecol. 2012;206(3):255–7.
8. Phelan S. Pregnancy: a "teachable moment" for weight control and obesity prevention. Am J Obstet Gynecol. 2010;202(2):135.e1–8.
9. Merhi ZO. Impact of bariatric surgery on female reproduction. Fertil Steril. 2009;92(5):1501–8.
10. Paulen ME, Zapata LB, Cansino C, Curtis KM, Jamieson DJ. Contraceptive use among women with a history of bariatric surgery: a systematic review. Contraception. 2010;82(1):86–94.
11. Gesink Law DC, Maclehose RF, Longnecker MP. Obesity and time to pregnancy. Hum Reprod. 2006;22(2):414–20.
12. van der Steeg JW, Steures P, Eijkemans MJC, Habbema JDF, Hompes PGA, Burggraaff JM, et al. Obesity affects spontaneous pregnancy chances in subfertile, ovulatory women. Hum Reprod. 2007;23(2):324–8.
13. Bajos N, Wellings K, Laborde C, Moreau C, for the CSF Group. Sexuality and obesity, a gender perspective: results from French national random probability survey of sexual behaviours. BMJ. 2010;340:2573–3.
14. Kaneshiro B, Jensen JT, Carlson N, Harvey SM, Nichols M, Edelman A. Body mass index and sexual behavior. Obstet Gynecol. 2008;112(3):586–92.
15. Shaw K, Edelman A. Obesity and oral contraceptives: a clinician's guide. Best Pract Res Clin Endocrinol Metab. 2013;27(1):55–65.
16. Hatcher R, Trussell J, Nelson AL, Cates W. Contraceptive technology. 20th ed. Decatur, GA: Bridging the Gap Foundation; 2011.
17. Xu H, Wade JA, Peipert JF, Zhao Q, Madden T, Secura GM. Contraceptive failure rates of etonogestrel

subdermal implants in overweight and obese women. Obstet Gynecol. 2012;120(1):21–6.
18. Grimes DA, Shields WC. Family planning for obese women: challenges and opportunities. Contraception. 2005;72(1):1–4.
19. Mirena Prescribing Information. United States Food and Drug Administration. 2013. p. 1–29.
20. Seeber B, Ziehr SC, Gschließer A, Moser C, Mattle V, Seger C, et al. Quantitative levonorgestrel plasma level measurements in patients with regular and prolonged use of the levonorgestrel-releasing intrauterine system. Contraception. 2012;86(4):345–9.
21. Ronnerdag M, Odlind V. Health effects of long-term use of the intrauterine levonorgestrel-releasing system. Acta Obst Gynecol Scand. 1999;78: 716–21.
22. Vickery Z, Madden T, Zhao Q, Secura GM, Allsworth JE, Peipert JF. Weight change at 12 months in users of three progestin-only contraceptive methods. Contraception. 2013;88(4):503–8.
23. Ng YW, Liang S, Singh K. Effects of Mirena (levonorgestrel-releasing intrauterine system) and Ortho Gynae T380 intrauterine copper device on lipid metabolism—a randomized comparative study. Contraception. 2009;79(1):24–8.
24. Kaunitz AM. Use of hormonal contraception in women with coexisting medical conditions. ACOG Pract Bull. 2006;73:1–20.
25. Hillman JB, Miller RJ, Inge TH. Menstrual concerns and intrauterine contraception among adolescent bariatric surgery patients. J Women's Health. 2011; 20(4):533–8.
26. Pasquali R, Pelusi C, Genghini S, Cacciari M, Gambineri A. Obesity and reproductive disorders in women. Hum Reprod Update. 2003;9(4):359–72.
27. Curtis KM, Marchbanks PA, Peterson HB. Neoplasia with use of intrauterine devices. Contraception. 2007;75(6):S60–9.
28. Varma R, Soneja H, Bhatia K, Ganesan R, Rollason T, Clark TJ, et al. The effectiveness of a levonorgestrel-releasing intrauterine system (LNG IUS) in the treatment of endometrial hyperplasia—a long-term follow-up study. Eur J Obstet Gynecol Reprod Biol. 2008;139(2):169–75.
29. Gallos ID, Shehmar M, Thangaratinam S, Papapostolou TK, Coomarasamy A, Gupta JK. Oral progestogens vs levonorgestrel-releasingintrauterine system for endometrial hyperplasia:a systematic review and metaanalysis. Am J Obstet Gynecol. 2010;203(6):547.e1–10.
30. Mody SK, Hacker MR, Dodge LE, Thornton K, Schneider B, Haider S. contraceptive counseling for women who undergo bariatric surgery. J Women's Health. 2011;20(12):1785–8.
31. Merhi ZO. Challenging oral contraception after weight loss by bariatric surgery. Gynecol Obstet Invest. 2007;64(2):100–2.
32. Darney PD, Patel A, Rosen K, Shapiro L, Kaunitz AM. Safety and efficacy of a single-rod etonogestrel implant (Implanon): results from 11 international clinical trials. Fertil Steril. 2009;91(5):1646–53.
33. Hohmann HL, Creinin MD. The contraceptive implant. Clin Obstet Gynecol. 2007;50(4):907–17.
34. Le J, Tsourounis C. Implanon: a critical review. Ann Pharmacother. 2001;35:329–36.
35. Huber J. Pharmacokinetics of Implanon. Contraception. 1998;58:85S–90S.
36. Makarainen L, van Beek A, Tuomivaara L, Asplund B, Bennick H. Ovarian function during the use of a single contraceptive implant: Implanon compared with Norplant. Fertil Steril. 1998;69(4):714–21.
37. Mornar S, Chandra A, Mistretta S, Neustadt A, Martinez G, Gilliam M. Pharmacokinetics of the etonogestrel contraceptive implant in obese women. Am J Obstet Gynecol. 2012;207(2):110.e1–6.
38. Diaz S, Pavez M, Moo-Young C, Bardin CW, Croxatto HB. Clinical trial with 3-keto-desogestrel subdermal implants. Contraception. 1991;44(4): 393–408.
39. Davies G, Feng LX, Newton JR. Release characteristics, ovarian activity and menstrual bleeding pattern with a single contraceptive implant releasing 3-ketodesogestrel. Contraception. 1993;47:251–61.
40. Croxatto H, Urbancsek J, Massai MR, Bennick H, van Beek A. A multicentre efficacy and safety study of the singlecontraceptive implant Implanon. Hum Reprod. 1999;14(4):976–81.
41. Biswas A, Viegas OAC, Roy AC. Effect of Implanon® and Norplant® subdermal contraceptive implants on serum lipids—a randomized comparative study. Contraception. 2003;68(3):189–93.
42. Dilbaz B, Ozdegirmenci O, Caliskan E, Dilbaz S, Haberal A. Effect of etonogestrel implant on serum lipids, liver function tests and hemoglobin levels. Contraception. 2010;81(6):510–4.
43. Guazzelli CAF, Barreiros FA, Barbosa R, de Araújo FF, Moron AF. Extended regimens of the vaginal contraceptive ring: cycle control. Contraception. 2009;80(5):430–5.
44. Bender NM, Segall-Gutierrez P, Najera SOL, Stanczyk FZ, Montoro M, Mishell Jr DR. Effects of progestin-only long-acting contraception on metabolic markers in obese women. Contraception. 2013; 88(3):418–25.
45. Ciangura C, Corigliano N, Basdevant A, Mouly S, Declèves X, Touraine P, et al. Etonorgestrel concentrations in morbidly obese women following Roux-en-Y gastric bypass surgery: three case reports. Contraception. 2011;84(6):649–51.
46. Chan LM, Westhoff CL. Tubal sterilization trends in the United States. Fertil Steril. 2010;94(1):1–6.
47. Winner B, Peipert JF, Zhao Q, Buckel C, Madden TE, Allsworth JE, et al. Effectiveness of long-acting reversible contraception. N Engl J Med. 2012; 366(21):1998–2007.
48. Peterson H, Trussell J, Hughes E, Taylor L. The risk of pregnancy after tubal sterilization: findings from the US Collaborative Review of Steriliation (CREST). Am J Obstet Gynecol. 1996;174(4):1161–9.
49. Yan J, Hsu J, Yin C. Comparative study of Filshie clip and Pomeroy method for postpartum sterilization. Int J Gynecol Obstet. 1990;33:263–7.

50. Jamieson DJ, Hillis S, Duerr A, Marchbanks PA, Costello C, Peterson H. Complications of interval laparoscopic tubal sterilization: findings from the United States Collaborative Review of Sterilization. Obstet Gynecol. 2000;96(6):997–1002.
51. Shabanzadeh DM, Sørensen LT. Laparoscopic surgery compared with open surgery decreases surgical site infection in obese patients. Ann Surg. 2012; 256(6):934–45.
52. Connor V. Essure: a review six years later. J Minim Invasive Gynecol. 2009;16(3):282–90.
53. Anderson T, Yunker A, Scheib S, Callahan T. Hysteroscopic sterilization success in outpatient vs office setting is not affected by patient or procedural characteristics. J Minim Invasive Gynecol. 2013;20(6):858–63.
54. Rodriguez MI, Seuc A, Sokal DC. Comparative efficacy of postpartum sterilisation with the titanium clip versus partial salpingectomy: a randomised controlled trial. BJOG. 2012;120(1):108–12.
55. Oligbo N, Revicky V, Udeh R. Pomeroy technique or Filshie clips for postpartum sterilisation? Retrospective study on comparison between Pomeroy procedure and Filshie clips for a tubal occlusion at the time of Caesarean section. Arch Gynecol Obstet. 2009;281(6):1073–5.
56. Krishnan S, Hacker M, Haider S, Thornton K, Trainor L, Lim R, et al. Contraceptive counseling and utilization in women who underwent bariatric surgery. Contraception. 2009;80(2):212.
57. Fritz MA, Speroff L. Clinical gynecologic endocrinology and infertility. 8th ed. Philadelphia: Lippincott Williams & Wilkins; 2010.
58. Mosher WD, Martinez G, Chandra A, Abma J, Wilson SJ. Use of contraception and use of family planning services in the United States: 1982–2002. Center for Disease Control Advance Data. 2004; 350:1–46.
59. Holt V, Cushing-Haugen K, Daling J. Body weight and risk of oral contraceptive failure. Obstet Gynecol. 2002;99(5):820–7.
60. Dinger J, Do Minh T, Buttmann N, Bardenheuer K. Effectiveness of oral contraceptive pills in a large U.S. cohort comparing progestogen and regimen. Obstet Gynecol. 2011;117(1):33–40.
61. McNicholas C, Zhao Q, Secura G, Allsworth JE, Madden T, Peipert JF. Contraceptive failures in overweight and obese combined hormonal contraceptive users. Obstet Gynecol. 2013;121(3):585–92.
62. Westhoff CL, Torgal AH, Mayeda ER, Stanczyk FZ, Lerner J, Benn E, et al. Ovarian suppression in normal-weight and obese women during oral contraceptive use. Obstet Gynecol. 2010;116(2):275–83.
63. McLaren L. Socioeconomic status and obesity. Epidemiol Rev. 2007;29(1):29–48.
64. Westhoff CL, Torgal AT, Mayeda ER, Shimoni N, Stanczyk FZ, Pike MC. Predictors of noncompliance in an oral contraceptive clinical trial. Contraception. 2012;85(5):465–9.
65. Westhoff C, Reape K, Shu H. Impact of body weight on observed pregnancy rates with a low-dose estrogen, 91-day extended regimen oral contraceptive. Contraception. 2009;80(2):196–7.
66. Edelman AB, Carlson NE, Cherala G, Munar MY, Stouffer RL, Cameron JL, et al. Impact of obesity on oral contraceptive pharmacokinetics and hypothalamic. Contraception. 2009;80(2):119–27.
67. Trussell J, Schwarz EB, Guthrie K. Obesity and oral contraceptive pill failure. Contraception. 2009;79(5): 334–8.
68. Westhoff C. Higher body weight does not affect NuvaRing's efficacy (abstract). Obstet Gynecol. 2005;105(4S):56S.
69. Zieman M, Guillebaud J, Weisberg E, Shangold G, Fisher AC, Creasy G. Contraceptive efficacy and cycle control with the Ortho Evra™/Evra™ transdermal system: the analysis of pooled data. Fertil Steril. 2002;77(2):S13–8.
70. Edelman AB, Cherala G, Stanczyk FZ. Metabolism and pharmacokinetics of contraceptive steroids in obese women: a review. Contraception. 2010;82(4): 314–23.
71. Edelman AB, Cherala G, Munar MY, DuBois B, McInnis M, Stanczyk FZ, et al. Prolonged monitoring of ethinyl estradiol and levonorgestrel levels confirms an altered pharmacokinetic profile in obese oral contraceptives users. Contraception. 2013;87(2): 220–6.
72. Westhoff CL, Torgal AH, Mayeda ER, Pike MC, Stanczyk FZ. Pharmacokinetics of a combined oral contraceptive in obese and normal-weight women. Contraception. 2010;81(6):474–80.
73. Westhoff CL, Torgal AH, Mayeda ER, Petrie K, Thomas T, Dragoman M, et al. Pharmacokinetics and ovarian suppression during use of a contraceptive vaginal ring in normal-weight and obese women. Am J Obstet Gynecol. 2012;207(1):39.e1–6.
74. Sitruk-Ware RL, Menard J, Rad M, Burggraaf J, de Kam ML, Tokay BA, et al. Comparison of the impact of vaginal and oral administration of combined hormonal contraceptives on hepatic proteins sensitive to estrogen. Contraception. 2007;75(6):430–7.
75. Goebelmann U, Mashchak CA, Mishell Jr D. Comparison of hepatic impact of oral and vaginal administration of ethinyl estradiol. Am J Obstet Gynecol. 1985;151(7):868–77.
76. Blickstein I. Thrombophilia and women's health: an overview. Obstet Gynecol Clin North Am. 2006; 33(3):347–56.
77. Trussell J, Guthrie KA, Schwarz EB. Much ado about little: obesity, combined hormonal contraceptive use and venous thrombosis. Contraception. 2008;77(3):143–6.
78. Liston F, Davies GAL. Thromboembolism in the obese pregnant woman. Seminars in Perinatology. 2011;35(6):330–4.
79. U.S. Medical Eligibility Criteria for Contraceptive Use, 2010. Center for Disease Control Morbidity

and Mortality Weekly Report. 2010 May 26;59: 1–88.
80. Rad M, Kluft C, Menard J, Burggraaf J, de Kam ML, Meijer P, et al. Comparative effects of a contraceptive vaginal ring delivering a nonandrogenic progestin and continuous ethinyl estradiol and a combined oral contraceptive containing levonorgestrel on hemostasis variables. Am J Obstet Gynecol. 2006; 195(1):72–7.
81. Jensen JT, Burke AE, Barnhart KT, Tillotson C, Messerle-Forbes M, Peters D. Effects of switching from oral to transdermal or transvaginal contraception on markers of thrombosis. Contraception. 2008; 78(6):451–8.
82. Jick S, Kaye JA, Li L, Jick H. Further results on the risk of nonfatal venous thromboembolism in users of the contraceptive transdermal patch compared to users of oral contraceptives containing norgestimate and 35 μg of ethinyl estradiol. Contraception. 2007; 76(1):4–7.
83. Sidney S, Cheetham TC, Connell FA, Ouellet-Hellstrom R, Graham DJ, Davis D, et al. Recent combined hormonal contraceptives (CHCs) and the risk of thromboembolism and other cardiovascular events in new users. Contraception. 2013;87(1):93–100.
84. Dore DD, Norman H, Loughlin J, Seeger JD. Extended case-control study results on thromboembolic outcomes among transdermal contraceptive users. Contraception. 2010;81(5):408–13.
85. Nightingale AL, Lawrenson RA, Simpson EL, Williams TJ, MacRae KD, Farmer RD. The effects of age, body mass index, smoking and general health on the risk of venous thromboembolism in users of combined oral contraceptives. Eur J Contracept Reprod Health Care. 2000;5(4):265–74.
86. Gallo MF, Lopez LM, Schulz KF, Helmerhorst FM. Combination contraceptives: effects on weight (review). Cochrane Database Syst Rev. 2012:1–116.
87. Edelman A, Jensen JT, Bulechowsky M, Cameron J. Combined oral contraceptives and body weight: do oral contraceptives cause weight gain? A primate model. Hum Reprod. 2011;26(2):330–6.
88. O'Connell KJ, Osborne LM, Westhoff C. Measured and reported weight change for women using a vaginal contraceptive ring vs. a low-dose oral contraceptive. Contraception. 2005;72(5):323–7.
89. Mohamed AMM, El-Sherbiny WSM, Mostafa WAI. Combined contraceptive ring versus combined oral contraceptive (30 mcg ethinyl estradiol and 3-mg drospirenone). Int J Gynecol Obstet. 2011; 114(2):145–8.
90. Sibai B, Odlind V, Meador M, Shangold G, Fisher AC, Creasy G. A comparative and pooled analysis of the safety and tolerability of the contraceptive patch (Ortho Evra™/Evra™). Fertil Steril. 2002;77(2): S19–26.
91. Beasley A, Estes C, Guerrero J, Westhoff C. The effect of obesity and low-dose oral contraceptives on carbohydrate and lipid metabolism. Contraception. 2012;85(5):446–52.
92. Tuppurainen M, Klimscheffskij R, Venhola M, Dieben TOM. The combined contraceptive vaginal ring (NuvaRing®) and lipid metabolism: a comparative study. Contraception. 2004;69(5):389–94.
93. Elkind-Hirsch KE, Darensbourg C, Ogden B, Ogden LF, Hindelang P. Contraceptive vaginal ring use for women has less adverse metabolic effects than an oral contraceptive. Contraception. 2007; 76(5):348–56.
94. Victor A, Odlind V, Kral JG. Oral contraceptive absorption and sex hormone binding globulins in obese women: effects of jejunoileal bypass. Gastroenterol Clin North Am. 1987;16(3):483–91.
95. Gerrits E, Ceulemans R, van Hee R, Hendrickz L, Totte E. Contraceptive treatment after biliopancreatic diversion needs consensus. Obes Surg. 2003;13: 378–82.
96. Segall-Gutierrez P, Taylor D, Liu X, Stanzcyk F, Azen S, Mishell Jr DR. Follicular development and ovulation in extremely obese women receiving depo-medroxyprogesterone acetate subcutaneously. Contraception. 2010;81(6):487–95.
97. Mishell Jr D. Pharmacokinetics of depot medroxyprogesterone acetate contraception. J Reprod Med. 1996;51(S5):381–90.
98. Jain J, Jakimiuk AJ, Bode FR, Ross D, Kaunitz AM. Contraceptive efficacy and safety of DMPA-SC. Contraception. 2004;70(4):269–75.
99. Fotherby K, Koetsawang S. Metabolism of injectable formulations of contraceptive steroids in obese and thin women. Contraception. 1982;26(1):51–8.
100. Smit J, Botha J, McFadyen L, Beksinska M. Serum medroxyprogesterone acetate levels in new and repeat users of depot medroxyprogesterone acetate at the end of the dosing interval. Contraception. 2004;69(1):3–7.
101. Lopez LM. Grimes DA, Chen M, Otterness C et al. Hormonal contraceptives for contraception in overweight or obese women. Cochrane Database Syst Rev. 2013; 4. Art No. CD008452. doi: 10.1002/14651858.CD008452.pub3.
102. Curtis KM, Ravi A, Gaffield ML. Progestogen-only contraceptive use in obese women. Contraception. 2009;80(4):346–54.
103. Westhoff C, Jain JK, Milsom I, Ray A. Changes in weight with depot medroxyprogesterone acetate subcutaneous injection 104 mg/0.65 mL. Contraception. 2007;75(4):261–7.
104. Bonny AE, Secic M, Cromer B. A longitudinal comparison of body composition changes in adolescent girls receiving hormonal contraception. J Adolesc Health. 2009;45(4):423–5.
105. Bonny AE, Secic M, Cromer B. Early weight gain related to later weight gain in adolescents on depot medroxyprogesterone acetate. Obstet Gynecol. 2011;117(4):793–7.
106. Gerlach LS, Saldaña SN, Wang Y, Nick TG, Spigarelli MG. Retrospective review of the relationship between weight change and demographic factors following initial depot medroxyprogesterone

acetate injection in adolescents. Clin Therap. 2011; 33(2):182–7.
107. Segall-Gutierrez P, Xiang AH, Watanabe RM, Trigo E, Stanczyk FZ, Liu X, et al. Deterioration in cardiometabolic risk markers in obese women during depot medroxyprogesterone acetate use. Contraception. 2012;85(1):36–41.
108. Berenson A, Rahman M, Wilkenson G. Effect of injectable and oral contraceptives on serum lipids. Obstet Gynecol. 2009;114(4):786–94.
109. Grimes DA, von Hertzen H, Piaggio G, Van Lock P. Randomised controlled trial of levonorgestrel versus the Yuzpe regimen of combined oral contraceptives for emergency contraception. Lancet. 1998; 352:428–33.
110. Croxatto HB, Brache V, Pavez M, Cochon L, Forcelledo ML, Alvarez F, et al. Pituitary–ovarian function following the standard levonorgestrel emergency contraceptive dose or a single 0.75-mg dose given on the days preceding ovulation. Contraception. 2004;70(6):442–50.
111. Glasier AF, Cameron ST, Fine PM, Logan SJ, Casale W, Van Horn J, et al. Ulipristal acetate versus levonorgestrel for emergency contraception: a randomised non-inferiority trial and meta-analysis. Lancet. 2010;375(9714):555–62.
112. Moreau C, Trussell J. Results from pooled Phase III studies of ulipristal acetate for emergency contraception. Contraception. 2012;86(6):673–80.
113. Creinin MD, Schlaff W, Archer DF, Wan L, Frezieres R, Thomas M, et al. Progesterone receptor modulator for emergency contraception. Obstet Gynecol. 2006;108(5):1089–97.
114. Glasier A, Cameron ST, Blithe D, Scherrer B, Mathe H, Levy D, et al. Can we identify women at risk of pregnancy despite using emergency contraception? Data from randomized trials of ulipristal acetate and levonorgestrel. Contraception. 2011; 84(4):363–7.
115. Turok DK, Godfrey EM, Wojdyla D, Dermish A, Torres L, Wu SC. Copper T380 intrauterine device for emergency contraception: highly effective at any time in the menstrual cycle. Hum Reprod. 2013;28(10):2672–6.
116. Cleland K, Zhu H, Goldstuck N, Cheng L, Trussell J. The efficacy of intrauterine devices for emergency contraception: a systematic review of 35 years of experience. Hum Reprod. 2012;27(7):1994–2000.

11 Contraception for Women with Hematologic Abnormalities

Kristina Tocce and S. Lindsey Davis

Iron-Deficiency Anemia

Background/Hematology Review

Iron-deficiency anemia is the most common nutritional disorder worldwide [1]. According to National Health and Nutritional Examination Survey (NHANES) III data from 1988 to 1994, iron-deficiency anemia is present in 2 % of females ages 12–15, 3 % of females ages 16–19, and 5 % of females ages 20–49 in the USA. This is compared to a prevalence of 1 % or less in men of these age groups [2]. Such a finding can be explained largely by causes of iron deficiency specific to women of reproductive age, including menstrual blood losses and increased requirements during pregnancy and childbirth [3]. The average iron loss through menstruation is 0.5–0.68 mg per day over a 28-day cycle, and women lose over 1 g of iron during pregnancy [4]. These and other causes of iron deficiency in the general population can be categorized as increased iron loss (menstruation, gastrointestinal cancer), decreased dietary iron intake (malnutrition, vegan diet), decreased iron absorption (celiac disease, inflammatory bowel disease), and increased iron requirement (pregnancy, lactation) [5]. As occult malignancies can be the source of iron-deficiency anemia, a workup to identify the underlying cause of anemia according to history and risk factors should always be performed [6].

The diagnosis of iron-deficiency anemia is made by evaluating blood markers including hemoglobin/hematocrit, mean corpuscular volume (MCV), serum iron, ferritin, and total iron binding capacity (TIBC). A low hemoglobin or hematocrit is required to confirm anemia, and a low MCV consistent with microcytosis is often seen in iron-deficiency anemia, though it is not universal [7]. Decreased levels of serum iron and ferritin and an elevated TIBC are generally associated with iron-deficiency anemia [8]; however, this evaluation can be complicated by any underlying inflammatory process that may increase ferritin levels as part of acute phase response [9]. In this setting, testing for soluble transferrin receptor levels may be useful, as elevated levels are able to distinguish iron deficiency from anemia of chronic disease [10]. Bone marrow biopsy to evaluate iron stores can be used if these methods are still unable to clarify the diagnosis [11].

Oral supplementation is the mainstay of treatment of iron-deficiency anemia and is effective in the majority of patients at doses of 150–180 mg of elemental iron per day through any of a variety

K. Tocce, M.D., M.P.H. (✉)
Department of Obstetrics and Gynecology, Anschutz Medical Campus, University of Colorado, Aurora, CO, USA
e-mail: kristina.tocce@ucdenver.edu

S.L. Davis, M.D.
Department of Hematology and Medical Oncology, University of Colorado Denver, Aurora, CO, USA
e-mail: Sarah.Davis@ucdenver.edu

R.H. Allen and C.A. Cwiak (eds.), *Contraception for the Medically Challenging Patient*, DOI 10.1007/978-1-4939-1233-9_11, © Springer Science+Business Media New York 2014

of preparations. The commonly used ferrous sulfate preparation contains 65 mg of elemental iron per 325 mg tablet [12]. Effects of iron therapy are appreciated by an increase in hemoglobin levels within 2 weeks, and normalization generally occurs within 2 months [3]. Some recommend continued supplementation for 3 months after resolution of anemia to further replenish iron stores [13]. For those patients intolerant of oral iron supplements, or who have significant ongoing blood loss, chronic kidney disease, or inflammatory bowel disease, IV iron preparations are preferred [14].

Unintended Pregnancy and Maternal/ Fetal Risk

Unintended pregnancy in patients with iron-deficiency anemia carries both maternal and fetal risk. Women may be less able to tolerate blood loss during delivery and may be at higher risk of transfusion. During the first two trimesters of pregnancy, iron-deficiency anemia is associated with a twofold increased risk for preterm delivery and a threefold increased risk for delivering a low birth-weight infant [15]. It has also been documented that even mild iron deficiency in the mother reduces iron stores in the fetus, resulting in a neonatal iron-deficient condition. Iron deficiency in the perinatal period is associated with alternative expression of genes critical for hippocampal development and function [16, 17], and early iron deficiency causes neurocognitive dysfunction both during deficiency and after repletion [18, 19]. Planning pregnancy at a time when iron-deficiency anemia is maximally corrected will decrease these adverse outcomes.

Contraception by Method

Intrauterine Devices

Intrauterine device (IUD) is a safe, highly effective, long-acting, and reversible form of contraception [20–22]. The IUD is currently the most widely used reversible contraceptive method in the world, used by 14.5 % of reproductive-aged women in developing countries and 7.6 % of women in developed countries [23]. In the USA, where the rate of unintended pregnancy is significantly higher than in other developed countries, the rates of IUD use have historically been lower [23, 24]. However, in recent years, the use of the IUD has increased in the USA from 1.3 % in 2002 to 7.7 % in 2009 according to most recent estimates from the National Survey of Family Growth [25]. In the USA, available Food and Drug Administration (FDA) approved IUDs are the levonorgestrel intrauterine systems (LNG-IUD) and the copper T380A IUD.

Hematologic parameters have been studied in users of the LNG-IUD that releases 20 μg of levonorgestrel per day and is approved for 5 years of use (Mirena, Bayer Healthcare Pharmaceuticals, Wayne, NJ, USA) and the copper T380A (ParaGard, Teva, Israel), approved for 10 years. Skyla (Bayer Healthcare Pharmaceuticals, Wayne, NJ, USA) releases 14 μg of levonorgestrel per day and is approved for 3 years of use. Due to its recent FDA approval in 2013, Skyla's effects on hematologic parameters have not yet been investigated.

In four studies [26–29] evaluating hemoglobin changes in normal women, the LNG-IUD was shown to increase hemoglobin concentrations compared to measurements taken prior to insertion. Net gain in hemoglobin concentrations varied depending on length of follow-up, ranging from 0.5 g/dL after 2 years to as much as 1.6 g/dL after 5 years of LNG-IUD use [30]. Use of the LNG-IUD has been shown to reduce the proportion of women with clinical anemia and with depleted iron stores compared to use of the Lippes loop IUD and copper T380A [31]. As a result, the LNG-IUD has been used in the treatment and prevention of iron-deficiency anemia caused by heavy menstrual bleeding.

It is well known that the use of copper IUDs (Cu-IUDs) are associated with an increase in mean blood loss [32]; however, this should not result in clinically significant alterations in hematologic parameters. Two randomized trials have shown slight decreases in hemoglobin concentration among users of Cu-IUDs (specifically copper Multiload 250 and 375 IUDs), ranging from

0.13 g/dL at 1 year to 2.6 g/dL at 5 years [26, 28]. When the first randomized trial examined 7-year follow-up data, hemoglobin levels began to increase and remain slightly above baseline after 2 years of use [27]. Despite the minimal change in hemoglobin measurements, the results of a comparative trial involving the LNG-IUD and the Cu-IUD demonstrated that women using the Cu-IUD discontinued the device due to subjective heavy menstrual bleeding (HMB) ten times more often than women using the LNG-IUD [33].

Mean blood loss (MBL) with copper IUDs has been determined in normal women with the alkaline hematin method; MBL was calculated by spectrophotometric analysis of alkaline hematin extracted from pads and tampons [32]. This observational study demonstrated an increase of MBL of approximately 45 %, but no significant change in the studied hematologic parameters (including ferritin and hemoglobin) during the 3-year observation period. The impact of this MBL on women with iron-deficiency anemia or at risk for this condition has not been studied. Women with gastrointestinal disorders may develop anemia with Cu-IUD use due to decreased mucosal uptake and/or impaired transport of iron from the intestines. In developing countries, the increased MBL may also result in anemia due to poor dietary intake.

Due to the concern about increased blood loss with Cu-IUD use, the WHO and United States Medical Eligibility Criteria for Contraceptive Use (USMEC) classifies Cu-IUD use in women with iron-deficiency anemia as category 2. Category 2 is defined as a condition for which the advantages of using this method generally outweigh the theoretical or proven risks. LNG-IUD use in women with iron-deficiency anemia is category 1 [34], a condition for which there is no restriction for the use of the contraceptive method. In women with HMB, once underlying conditions have been excluded, the USMEC also assigns a category 1 for LNG-IUD use and a category 2 for Cu-IUDs.

HMB is a well-known cause of iron-deficiency anemia [5]. Historically, it has been a common indication for endometrial ablation and hysterectomy. Recently the LNG-IUD has been utilized in the nonsurgical management of HMB. The first landmark study on use of the LNG-IUD for treatment of objectively verified HMB was published in 1990 [35]. This study demonstrated a 90 % reduction in menstrual blood loss 3 months after LNG-IUD insertion, 95 % by 6 months, and 98 % by 12 months. Since then, numerous studies have confirmed these initial findings. Many are randomized controlled trials comparing the LNG-IUD to surgical treatments [36–38]. When compared to endometrial ablation, the LNG-IUD produced similar reductions in menstrual blood loss [36, 38]. Two studies report LNG-IUD use as an alternative to hysterectomy. Both were randomized controlled trials; subjects were assigned either continued conservative (medical) treatments or LNG-IUD for women considering hysterectomy. The proportion of women cancelling their planned hysterectomy in the LNG-IUD arms of the two trials was 82 % [39] and 64 % [40]; this compared with 9 % and 14 % of women respectively assigned to the medical treatment group. A subsequent long-term follow-up study revealed that 46 % of women with menorrhagia treated with a LNG-IUD ultimately underwent hysterectomy within 10 years. Despite this rate of surgical intervention, LNG-IUD treatment was shown to be cost effective [41]. As a result of this work, the LNG-IUD has become a first-line treatment and contraceptive option for women with HMB or iron-deficiency anemia. In 2009 the 20 μg-releasing LNG-IUD was approved by the FDA for the treatment of HMB for women who choose to use intrauterine contraception as their method of contraception [42].

It is unknown if the improved hemoglobin concentrations, anemia prevention and HMB treatment seen with the standard LNG-IUD can be extrapolated to the new lower-dose (14 μg) LNG-IUD. The bleeding pattern with the 14 μg-releasing LNG-IUD may be irregular, and amenorrhea develops in only 6 % of users by 12 months (compared to 20 % of the 20 μg LNG-IUD users) [42, 43]. Studies evaluating potential non-contraceptive health benefits of the lower-dose intrauterine system are needed.

Contraceptive Implants

High effectiveness and ease of maintenance make contraceptive implants an ideal method for many women. Implants are also appropriate for many women who have medical conditions that make combined hormonal contraception contraindicated. The USMEC guidelines consider progestin-only implants to be a safe contraceptive option for women with hypertension, venous thromboembolism (VTE), cardiovascular disease, stroke, migraine headaches (with or without aura), and seizure disorder [34, 44].

Previous research has shown that use of the levonorgestrel subdermal implant (Norplant, Wyeth-Ayerst International Inc, Wayne, PA, USA) generally leads to increased blood levels and iron stores [45]. This implant was voluntarily withdrawn from the US market in 2002 for non-medical reasons; currently, the etonogestrel (ENG) implant (Nexplanon, Merck, Darmstadt, Germany) is the only subdermal contraceptive available in the USA. The ENG implant offers high contraceptive effectiveness for up to 3 years with an excellent safety profile [46]. Although irregular bleeding can occur with the ENG implant, use for up to 2 years had no clinically significant effects on hematologic laboratory parameters [46]. The USMEC allows use of progestin-only implants or pills, or depot medroxyprogesterone acetate (DMPA) without restriction in patients with iron-deficiency anemia [34].

Other Hormonal Methods of Contraception

In 1998, the WHO Task Force for Epidemiological Research on Reproductive Health [47] found that current users of hormonal contraceptive methods (Norplant, DMPA, or combined oral contraceptives [COCs]) generally had higher hemoglobin and ferritin levels than women not using contraception. The differences in mean values for hemoglobin varied between 3 and 6 g/L and for ferritin between 2 and 18 g/L between women using hormonal contraceptive and non-contraceptors. In a longitudinal component of the study, 285 anemic women were followed at 3, 6, and 12 months after initiation of hormonal contraception. Significant mean increases of hemoglobin were observed at 12 months among the users of combined oral contraceptives and DMPA. It was concluded that hemoglobin and ferritin levels are influenced by the use of contraceptives and that the hormonal contraceptives included in this study have a beneficial effect on these parameters.

Since the publication of this task report, DMPA has been shown to decrease iron-deficiency anemia [48] and has been compared to the decrease in mean blood loss seen with LNG-IUD and continuous POP use [49]. In patients with HMB, LNG-IUD use results in a significantly greater MBL decrease (73 %) than either DMPA (49 %) or continuous POPs (33 %) [50]. The difference between the DMPA and POP users was not statistically significant.

Combined oral contraceptives (COCs) containing estrogen and progestin remain the most common method of contraception practiced by women in the USA; 27.5 % of contraceptive users are on COCs [51]. For women with iron-deficiency anemia, the USMEC classifies combined hormonal contraceptive (CHC) use (including pills, patch, and ring) as category 1 [34]. COCs and their effects on hematologic parameters have been studied in healthy women. Markedly increased transferrin levels were seen in COC users; however, serum ferritin, iron, and transferrin saturation levels were not affected [52]. In women with HMB, COCs are often used to treat iron-deficiency anemia [53]. When compared to placebo, COC use consistently and significantly decreases MBL: 64.9 % versus 5.8 % ($p<0.001$) and 64.2 % versus 7.8 % ($p<0.0010$), respectively [54, 55]. However, when compared to oral contraceptives, LNG-IUD use has consistently been shown to result in a larger reduction in MBL [50, 56, 57].

Barrier Methods, Emergency Contraception, and Sterilization

Benefits of hormonal contraception to women with iron-deficiency anemia are clear. However, not all women wish to pursue such methods. Barrier methods (including condoms, spermicides, and diaphragms/cervical caps) and permanent sterilization are certainly viable alternatives. These methods should not impact laboratory parameters or menstrual bleeding patterns and they are assigned to category 1 in the USMEC [34]. Patient counseling should include this information in addition to data regarding the failure rates of each method. There is scant information on emergency contraception (EC) use in patients with iron-deficiency anemia, but anemia is not a contraindication to either oral levonorgestrel or ulipristal acetate. Cu-IUD use for EC is an effective option, but the long-term bleeding pattern with this device may not be optimal for patients with iron-deficiency anemia.

No medical condition absolutely restricts a woman's eligibility for sterilization; however, severe anemia can place a woman at a higher surgical risk. Hysteroscopic bilateral tubal occlusion should be presented as an option that avoids the risks of general anesthesia and abdominal surgery. All women should be counseled appropriately about the permanency of the sterilization and the availability of equally effective, reversible methods of contraception.

Sickle Cell Disease

Background/Hematology Review

Sickle cell disorders are characterized by the presence of abnormal hemoglobin known as hemoglobin S. This hemoglobin is associated with a point mutation in the β-globin gene that results in substitution of a valine for a glutamic acid residue. When hemoglobin S is deoxygenated, it polymerizes with other hemoglobin S molecules, ultimately leading to alteration in the shape of the red blood cell to the classic sickle conformation [58]. These sickled cells in turn cause occlusion and inflammatory response in the microvasculature, resulting in hemolysis and tissue infarction in the acute setting, and vasculopathy and endothelial dysfunction in the chronic setting [59]. The process underlying this chronic vascular injury is complex, but seems to be associated with inflammation from reperfusion injury [60].

The clinical manifestations of these pathophysiologic processes are largely associated with acute tissue infarction and chronic endothelial dysfunction in vascular beds throughout the body. Chief among the tissue infarction events are acute painful crises, which result from microvascular occlusion in areas of bone marrow leading to necrosis and local pain [61]. Polymerization of hemoglobin S in the pulmonary vascular bed can lead to acute chest syndrome, a severe event associated with pulmonary infiltrates, fever, chest pain, and respiratory symptoms that represents the leading cause of death in patients with sickle cell disease [62]. Additional complications of sickle cell diseases associated with acute tissue infarction include avascular necrosis, nephropathy, spontaneous abortion, and splenic infarction [63]. Chronic endothelial dysfunction may be the primary cause of additional manifestations of the sickle cell diseases, including stroke, pulmonary hypertension, priapism, and chronic skin ulceration [59, 64].

The sickle cell disorders are a genetically defined spectrum of diseases that involve one β-globin gene with the hemoglobin S mutation paired with a second abnormal β-globin gene. In the case of homozygous hemoglobin SS disease, both genes code for hemoglobin S [59], while in hemoglobin SC disease, the second gene codes for hemoglobin C [65]. In the sickle-β thalassemias, the second gene has a mutation that results in either decreased production of β-globin (sickle-β^+ thalassemia), or complete absence of β-globin chains (sickle-β^0 thalassemia) [66]. Sickle cell trait is defined by one hemoglobin S gene paired with a normal β-globin gene, and is not considered part of the sickle cell disease spectrum as it is commonly an asymptomatic state [67]. Additional sickle cell disorders are less common. The prevalence of sickle disease in the USA has been estimated at as high as 98,000 persons according to 2008 census data corrected for early mortality related to the disease. Using data from the National Newborn Screening Information System, it is estimated that sickle cell disorders occur in approximately 1:365 African-Americans and 1:16,305 Hispanics in the USA [68].

The distinct molecular characteristics of the sickle cell disorders translate into varied clinical presentations of disease. Patients with hemoglobin SS disease and sickle-β^0 thalassemia have more frequent episodes of pain as compared with patients with hemoglobin SC disease or sickle-β^+ thalassemia [69]. Life expectancy data mirrors this trend, with median age at death of 42 years for males and 48 years for females with hemoglobin SS disease, as compared to median age at death of 60 years for males and 68 years for females with hemoglobin SC disease in one study [70]. The degree of hemoglobin S polymerization within red blood cells has been associated with this variability in clinical outcomes, with higher levels in hemoglobin SS disease and sickle-β^0 thalassemia consistent with a more severe phenotype [71].

Blood transfusion plays a vital role in the management of the complications of sickle cell disease, including symptomatic anemia, acute chest syndrome, acute stroke, multi-organ failure, splenic sequestration, and sepsis [72]. Not only is transfusion thought to improve the delivery of oxygen to the tissues, but it is also thought to benefit patients by decreasing the proportion of red blood cells that contain hemoglobin S [73]. Exchange transfusion through erythrocytopheresis is often utilized as an alternative to simple transfusion in the acute setting when rapid reduction in hemoglobin S is desired (acute neurologic event or severe acute chest syndrome), or if hyperviscosity is a concern [72].

In addition to treating the complications of sickle cell disease, efforts to prevent these disease manifestations are key to management. Chronic therapy with hydroxyurea is one example of such, as this agent has been shown to decrease rates of acute pain events as well as acute chest syndrome in patients with hemoglobin SS disease [74]. Hydroxyurea therapy is thus recommended for patients with hemoglobin SS disease as well as patients with sickle-β^0 thalassemia [72]. Prevention of stroke as a complication of sickle cell disease has been extensively studied in children, with chronic transfusion found to reduce the rate of first and recurrent stroke by up to 90 %. Though it remains unclear if continuing chronic transfusion into adulthood confers continued benefit, this practice is often recommended in the adult population [75].

Unintended Pregnancy and Maternal/Fetal Risk

Observational studies indicate an increased risk of spontaneous abortion and preterm labor in women with hemoglobin SS disease, as well as risk for intrauterine growth restriction and low birth weight in their children [76]. A recent population-based retrospective cohort study of 8.8 million US births determined the maternal mortality rate to be 1.6 per 1,000 deliveries in women with sickle cell disease (SCD), compared to 0.1 per 1,000 in women without SCD. Pregnant women with SCD had a higher risk of developing preeclampsia, eclampsia, venous thromboembolism, cardiomyopathy, intrauterine fetal demise, and intrauterine growth restriction. Cesarean delivery rates were higher in women with SCD. Homozygous SS was the greatest risk factor for antenatal sickle cell crisis, accounting for 89.8 % of all women who developed crisis [77].

Compared to healthy women, women with SCD have higher rates of clinically significant anemia in addition to an increased risk of sickle crises during pregnancy [78]. Prophylactic blood transfusion has not been shown to directly improve maternal or fetal outcomes, but it does decrease the frequency of acute pain events and other complications of sickle cell disease in pregnant women [79]. As such, transfusion is generally recommended only for complications of sickle cell disease as they arise during pregnancy [80]. Due to the high maternal and fetal risks of pregnancy in women with SCD, prevention of unintended pregnancy in this population is of paramount importance.

Contraception by Method

Intrauterine Devices

A recent systematic review of the literature concludes that there is insufficient evidence to comment on the safety of intrauterine contraception in individuals with SCD [81]. Only two small, cross-sectional studies have examined the use of IUDs among women with SCD [82, 83]. These studies were published in 1984 and 1993, respectively. Questionnaires were administered to women with SCD to assess contraceptive use. COCs were the most common method used; IUD use was found in 15 % and 19 %, respectively. IUD type was not specified in either study. Only the 1993 study attempted to determine adverse effects. Dysmenorrhea was reported in 29 %, infection (type of infection was not specified in the study) in 18 %, and increased crises in 4 % of respondents; there were no serious adverse events reported. Since there was no control group in this study, comparative statistics to a non-IUD group or a non-sickle cell group were not possible.

Although the lack of evidence on IUD use among women with SCD represents a major gap in the literature, theoretical concerns about IUD use in this population are few. There is no current evidence to support limiting IUD use among women with SCD [81]. The LNG-IUD is USMEC category 1, indicating that there are no restrictions for this method in women with SCD; the copper IUD is category 2 because of the theoretical concern about increased blood loss with menstruation [34].

Progestin-Only Contraceptives

In the 1970s, progesterone, testosterone, and other related steroids were reported to prevent in vitro sickling of steroid-treated HbSS cells [84–86]. The exact mechanism remains uncertain; however, it has been postulated that progestins may prolong erythrocyte survival by stabilizing the plasma membrane and improving the HgF content in red blood cells. Recent in vitro studies continue to investigate the effects of progesterone on sickle cell osmotic fragility [87], HgF mRNA expression [88], and Ca^{2+} ATPase activity [89].

Significant improvements in hematologic parameters after treatment with progestin-only contraception have been demonstrated in two studies [90, 91]. De Ceulaer et al. found a significant rise in the mean levels of HbF, total hemoglobin, red blood cell count, red blood cell mass, and red blood cell survival in SCD women using DMPA for over 30 weeks. Reticulocyte count, irreversible sickled cell (ISC) counts, and total bilirubin levels were decreased [90]. Nascimento et al. showed a significant increase in the percentage of red blood cells with fetal hemoglobin in subjects using the nomegestrol acetate contraceptive implant [91]. Other authors have published contradictory results, showing no change in hematologic and biochemical markers with DMPA [92], "progestin-only methods" (not differentiating between DMPA, progestin-only pills, or progestin-releasing IUD) [93, 94], and the levonorgestrel implant [95].

In parallel with laboratory markers, studies have evaluated the safety [83, 91, 95, 96] and clinical effects [90–92] of progestin-only contraceptive use in women with sickle cell disease. These studies suggest that progestin-only contraceptives are safe for women with SCD. A recent systemic review found that progestin-only contraception did not increase the risk of sickle cell crisis or other clinical adverse events [81]. However, the internal validity of these studies was fair to low. The randomized trial by De Ceulaer et al. was the single study meeting inclusion criteria for a Cochrane review evaluating steroid hormones for contraception in women with sickle cell disease [97]. The review concluded that DMPA is an appropriate contraceptive option and may also have non-contraceptive health benefits for women with SCD.

The effects of the etonogestrel implant on hematologic parameters and clinical manifestations have not been studied in women with SCD. Only three descriptive studies have reported on implant use in this population: levonogestrel implants were not associated with adverse events or change hematologic/biochemical parameters [95]; nomegestrol acetate implants were found to decrease the incidence and severity of painful crises and increase HbF percentages [91]; nomegestrol acetate implants were shown to have no significant effect on carbohydrate metabolism in sickle cell patients choosing this method [98]. A recent systematic review classified the internal validity of these studies as fair, limited by small sample sizes not powered for detecting a significant difference and lack of comparison groups or paired analysis [81]. These studies did not meet inclusion for the Cochrane review [97].

Although progestin-only methods are classified as USMEC category 1 [34], determining the true hematologic and clinical effects of these methods with well-designed methodology is another important gap in the literature that needs to be filled. Although there is some suggestion that progestin-only contraception may improve hematologic and clinical parameters, there is currently insufficient evidence to recommend progestin-only contraception above other contraceptive options [81]. Once this is better delineated, contraceptive recommendations and quality of life for women with SCD may be significantly improved.

Combined Hormonal Contraception

COCs are a USMEC category 2, indicating that the benefits of using these contraceptive methods (including pills, patch, and ring) usually outweigh the risks for women with SCD [34]. Only four studies have specifically examined COCs in women with SCD. Three were cross-sectional studies [83, 93, 94] and one was a nonrandomized trial [92]. Two of the cross-sectional studies found no differences in hematologic parameters between COC users, progestin-only contraceptive users, and non-hormonal contraceptive users. In the nonrandomized trial with COC, DMPA, and sterilization arms, a reduction in the occurrence of painful crises was noted among COC users over 12 months (decreasing from 100 % at baseline to 45.5 % at 12 months). Although this appeared less pronounced than the improvement seen in the DMPA arm (only 30 % of DMPA users continued to experience some painful crises), no statistical comparisons were reported [92].

The third cross-sectional study attempted to determine whether women with SCD suffer complications from contraceptive use. By self-report on a questionnaire administered to 67 COC users, 6 % identified increased painful crises and 3 % stated they experienced a DVT [83]. Due to self-selection of contraceptive methods, self-reported outcomes with no objective confirmation, no documentation of the length of time using the method in question, and lack of comparative statistics, no definitive conclusions can be made from this study. Increased risk of VTE among users of COCs with SCD remains a primary theoretical concern, particularly in those with pulmonary hypertension, which is a well established complication of sickle cell disease [99]. Use of CHC is category 4 in women with complicated valvular heart disease (pulmonary hypertension, risk for atrial fibrillation, history of subacute bacterial endocarditis) due to the increased risk for arterial thrombosis [34]. This represents yet another major gap in the literature regarding contraception in women with hematologic disorders.

Barriers and Emergency Contraception

Barrier methods (including condoms, spermicides, and diaphragms/cervical caps) and permanent sterilization are also options for patients with SCD. As mentioned above with regard to iron-deficiency anemia, these methods should not impact laboratory parameters or menstrual bleeding patterns and they are assigned to category 1 in the USMEC [34]. Patient counseling should include this information and data regarding the failure rates of each method. There is scant information on emergency contraception (EC) use in patients with iron-deficiency anemia; however, there are no data to discourage the use of either levonorgestrel or ulipristal acetate in women with SCD. Copper IUD use for EC is an effective option, but the long-term bleeding pattern with this device may not be optimal for patients with SCD.

Sterilization

As stated previously, no medical condition absolutely restricts a woman's eligibility for sterilization. However, individuals with SCD who undergo surgery are generally considered to be at greater risk for perioperative complications, such acute chest syndrome, cerebrovascular accidents, and blood transfusion, than otherwise healthy individuals without this hematologic disorder [100]. Hysteroscopic bilateral tubal occlusion should be presented as an option that avoids general anesthesia and abdominal surgery. All women should be counseled appropriately about the permanency of the sterilization and the availability to highly effective, reversible methods of contraception.

Thalassemia

Background/Hematology Review

The thalassemias are a group of diseases associated with decreased or absent production of one or more of the globin chains that comprise the hemoglobin tetramer. The most common hemoglobin in adults, hemoglobin A, consists of two α and two β chains, making α- and β-thalassemias the most clinically relevant entities [101]. Alpha-thalassemia is associated with decreased production of α-globin chains, with severity of disease varying according to the number of functional α genes and amount of α-globin produced [102]. This decrease in α-globin production results in accumulation of remaining globin chains into tetramers. In the fetus, γ chains form tetramers known as hemoglobin Bart's, and in adults β tetramers are known as hemoglobin H. Complete lack of α-globin production produces the most severe form of α-thalassemia and the clinical syndrome of hydrops fetalis [103]. Beta-thalassemia is associated with decreased or absent β-globin production and associated excess of α-globin chains, with severity of clinical presentation directly related to degree of β-globin production [104]. Beta-thalassemia major or β^0-thalassemia is associated with a complete lack of β-globin chains. This disease does not manifest until production of the γ-globulin chains of fetal hemoglobin decreases to allow for replacement by the β-globin chains of adult hemoglobin during the first year of life, but ultimately leads to a severe and chronic anemia [105]. Similar to the clinical presentations of the thalassemias, the specific genetic mutations associated with these disorders are also quite varied [102, 104] (Table 11.1).

The hallmark of the thalassemias is hypochromic and microcytic anemia. In β-thalassemia, this anemia is the result of the precipitation of α-chains in the red blood cells and their precursors, leading to hemolysis and ineffective erythropoiesis. The anemia of α-thalassemia is generally less severe, with hemolysis as the driving cause, and erythropoiesis less affected [106]. In severe forms of the disease, frequent transfusions are required, with a goal hemoglobin level of 9–10 g/dL [105]. Such frequent transfusions lead to serious complications from iron overload, which are responsible for the majority of clinical manifestations associated with the disease. These manifestations are typical of hemochromatosis, with cardiac events related to deposition of iron in the cardiac muscle the primary cause of death in this patient population [107]. In recent years, the development of iron chelation therapy has improved survival rates of patients with thalassemia and iron overload related to transfusion [108].

Table 11.1 Basic thalassemia syndromes [100, 101, 106]

	Genetics[a]	Clinical implications
Alpha-thalassemia		
Carrier	αα/α–	None
Minor/trait	αα/–– or α–/α–	Mild anemia with microcytosis and hypochromia
Hemoglobin H disease	α–/––	Moderate anemia with microcytosis, hemolysis, splenomegaly
Major/hemoglobin Bart's	––/––	Hydrops fetalis
Beta-thalassemia		
Minor/trait	β/β^0 or β/β^+	None to mild anemia with microcytosis
Intermedia	β^+/β^+ or β^+/β^0	Moderate anemia with microcytosis, splenomegaly
Major	β^0/β^0	Severe anemia requiring transfusions from infancy, splenomegaly

[a]β^+, β globin gene with decreased β-chain production; β^0, β globin gene with no β-chain production

Unintended Pregnancy and Maternal/Fetal Risk

In women with thalassemia major, the endocrine organs are sensitive to iron toxicity. This can result in hypogonadotropic hypogonadism and subsequent amenorrhea. Thus, women with thalassemia major tend to have low fertility. However, effective and aggressive iron chelation therapy can preserve reproductive function, and the possibility of spontaneous pregnancy should not be overlooked in women with secondary amenorrhea [109]. Unintended pregnancies can lead to significant morbidity and mortality in this high-risk population. A higher rate of unplanned pregnancy has been found in women with homozygous β-thalassemia when compared to controls [110].

Most research on thalassemia and pregnancy is confined to β-thalassemia major and intermedia; research is scant on reproductive outcomes in women with thalassemia traits. Women with thalassemia major and intermedia are at risk for various complications during pregnancy: cardiac failure, alloimmunization, viral infection, thrombosis, and endocrine and bone disturbances [109]. A multidisciplinary approach with planned preconception assessment, followed by close monitoring of maternal and fetal conditions, helps to ensure optimal obstetrical outcomes.

Contraception by Method

Long-Acting Reversible Contraceptive Methods

Top-tier reversible methods (LNG-IUD, copper IUD, and the ENG implant) are the most effective methods of contraception and do not rely on patient adherence [111]. These methods have few contraindications and are appropriate for use in women with thalassemia. The USMEC classifies LNG-IUD use as category 1 and the copper IUD use as category 2 in women with thalassemia. The category 2 classification is due to concern about the increased risk for menstrual blood loss with copper IUDs [34]. The contraceptive implant and all progestin-only contraceptives are category 1 [34]. However, the entire clinical picture must always be evaluated. For example, osteopenia/osteoporosis is a prominent cause of morbidity in patients with β-thalassemia major [112], making DMPA a less desirable option in patients with osteopathy. Chronic anemia, bone marrow expansion, and iron toxicity lead to unbalanced bone turnover in these women [113, 114].

Combined Hormonal Contraception

Despite scant published research on contraception use in women with thalassemia, no particular type of contraception is contraindicated in these patients [110]. However, an increased risk of thrombosis has been found in women with α-thalassemia syndromes, β-thalassemia major, β-thalassemia intermedia, and hemoglobin E-β-thalassemia. This is due to the presence of circulating defective red blood cells (RBCs); their disrupted membranes expose thrombogenic lipids. The spleen is responsible for removing these disrupted RBCs. Hypersplenism can result and increase blood transfusion requirements, preventing adequate iron control with chelation therapy. Women who have undergone splenectomy therefore experience increased circulating thrombogenic RBCs and platelets [109].

Some authorities suggest that women with thalassemia who take COCs and have had a splenectomy are at increased risk of thrombotic events [115]. This idea is controversial and other authors do not restrict COC use in women with thalassemia [110]. Use of hormone therapy to improve pubertal staging and osteoporosis in women with β-thalassemia major has been studied without comment on increased thrombotic outcomes [116, 117]. Combined hormonal contraceptives (CHC), including pills, patch, and ring, are classified as category 1 in women with thalassemia by the USMEC [34].

Although the USMEC classifies CHC use as category 1, the complete clinical picture must always be considered. Pulmonary hypertension (PH) is an established complication of hemoglobinopathies. Although this has been best studied in sickle cell disease, it is also a concern in patients with β-thalassemia major and intermedia [99]. Use of CHC is category 4 in women with complicated valvular heart disease (pulmonary hypertension, risk for atrial fibrillation, history of subacute bacterial endocarditis) due to the increased risk for arterial thrombosis [34]. Therefore, this can be extrapolated to women who have pulmonary hypertension as a consequence of hemoglobinopathies.

Barrier and Emergency Contraception

Barrier methods (including condoms, spermicides, and diaphragms/cervical caps) and permanent sterilization are also options for patients with thalassemia. These methods should not impact laboratory parameters or menstrual bleeding patterns and they are assigned to category 1 in the USMEC [34]. There is no evidence to discourage the use of either levonorgestrel or ulipristal acetate for emergency contraception in women with thalassemia. The Cu-IUD use for EC is an effective option, but the long-term bleeding pattern with this device may not be optimal for individuals with thalassemia.

Sterilization

As stated previously, no medical condition absolutely restricts a woman's eligibility for sterilization. However, individuals with thalassemia may have an increased risk for surgical complications due to anemia. Hysteroscopic bilateral tubal occlusion should be presented as a permanent option, and all women should be counseled appropriately about the availability of highly effective, reversible methods of contraception. Male partner sterilization can also be considered.

Von Willebrand Disease

Background/Hematology Review

Von Willebrand factor (VWF) is a multimeric plasma protein that complexes with factor VIII to facilitate platelet adhesion and aggregation. Von Willebrand disease (VWD) is an inherited disorder associated with decreased quantity or function of this protein, often resulting in hemorrhagic complications [118]. VWD is further divided into three subtypes according to the nature of the abnormality affecting VWF. Type 1 VWD is associated with a decreased concentration of VWF in the blood, type 2 disease encompasses a variety of functional deficits that interfere with the normal function of VWF, and type 3 disease is associated with a near-complete deficiency of VWF [119]. The clinical presentation of VWD varies according to the subtype, with type 3 disease being the most severe. This subtype is often associated with severe bleeding of both the mucous membranes and soft tissues and joints due to abnormal platelet function as well as decreased factor VIII activity in the setting of significant VWF deficiency [120]. In addition to these inherited types of VWD, there is also an acquired form. Acquired VWD is most commonly associated with monoclonal gammopathies, lymphoproliferative disorders, and myeloproliferative disorders, but can also be related to autoimmune disease. The pathologic mechanisms underlying acquired VWD are varied, but the clinical presentation is similar to that of the inherited forms [121].

Management of VWD is based on replacement of normal functioning VWF for treatment or prevention of bleeding. Transient increases in autologous VWF and factor VIII can be induced with desmopressin (DDAVP), which is able to increase both factors by 3–5 times baseline levels within 1 h [122]. This therapy is of greatest benefit in type 1 VWD, as functional deficits associated with type 2 disease and severely decreased levels associated with type 3 disease are less likely to respond to such therapy. For these subtypes, fresh-frozen plasma and cryoprecipitate are options, though are somewhat limited by the risk for fluid overload associated with the high-volume replacement required to achieve clinically significant levels. Concentrated factor supplements that contain both factor VIII and VWF are more widely used [123].

More than 70 % of women with VWD suffer from HMB [124]. Endometriosis may result from heavy menstrual blood loss, as it leads to retrograde menstruation thought to cause endometriosis [124]. Because of their bleeding tendency, women with VWD are more symptomatic compared to women without VWD and present early with gynecologic problems [125]. Adolescent HMB has long been recognized to be associated with inherited bleeding disorders; studies of this population show the prevalence of inherited bleeding disorders (IBD) to be 10–57 % [126, 127]. VWD is the most common IBD [128] and was first described in a 13-year-old girl who died of uncontrolled menstrual bleeding [129]. The American College of Obstetricians and Gynecologists (ACOG) recommends screening for VWD in adolescents presenting with severe HMB; it also specifies that VWD and other inherited and acquired disorders of coagulation and hemostasis should be considered in the differential diagnosis of all patients being evaluated for HMB, regardless of age [130].

There is a high rate of surgical interventions for HMB in this population, including hysterectomy. A hysterectomy rate of 23–26 % has been reported among women with VWD [131, 132]. Hysterectomy is often performed at a relatively young age; an international survey reports hysterectomy as early as 14 years of age [131].

Unintended Pregnancy and Maternal/Fetal Risk

For patients with VWD, morbidity and mortality centers on the occurrence of hemorrhage. During pregnancy, levels of both factor VIII and VWF increase, and patients with VWD may reach normal levels in the third trimester. These levels will rapidly fall after delivery, and patients are at increased risk for bleeding within the first 24 h. Factor VIII and VWF levels less than 50 are associated with increased risk of bleeding, and patients with such levels should be supplemented with desmopressin (DDAVP) or factor concentrates as appropriate. This supplementation should continue for 3–5 days after delivery [133].

Women should be counseled prior to conception as to the inheritance patterns of VWD; since VWD can be transmitted as an autosomal dominant or recessive trait, the fetus can have up to a 50 % risk of being affected [130]. In order to prevent unintended pregnancies and the subsequent complications that can arise with delivery, pregnancy loss or abortion, contraception should be discussed with all VWD patients of reproductive age as a part of routine health care.

Contraception by Method

Intrauterine Devices

Due to the heavier and/or longer menstruation that may result with the copper IUD in healthy women, this device is not a common method of contraception utilized in women with VWD [128]. As discussed previously for iron-deficiency anemia, the 20 μg-releasing LNG-IUD has been shown to suppress endometrial growth and induce a state of atrophic endometrium [134]. This translates into a reduction in average menstrual blood loss of 74 % by 3 months and 97 % after 12 months of use [135]. Extrapolation of this data from its use in healthy women has made the LNG-IUD a promising contraceptive option for women with VWD and has led to a number of small studies that evaluated the use of LNG-IUD in women with IBDs. These studies have utilized the 20 μg-releasing LNG-IUD. It is unknown if these results apply to the recently FDA-approved 14 μg-releasing LNG-IUD.

The first study to look at the LNG-IUD for the treatment of HMB specifically in women with IBDs was published in 2004 [136]. In this prospective pilot study, 16 women with IBDs who had subjective and objective HMB that was not responsive to medical management (defined as COC, desmospressin, or tranexamic acid) were followed for 9 months after LNG-IUD insertion. Thirteen of the women had VWD and all received prophylactic hemostatic treatment with desmopressin at the time of LNG-IUD insertion. The LNG-IUD was found to be effective at reducing pictorial blood-loss assessment chart (PBAC) scores and increasing hemoglobin and ferritin in all subjects. All women reported that their bleeding improved and 56 % became amenorrheic. Reported side effects were minimal.

Three additional publications have shown favorable results of LNG-IUD use in women with various inherited bleeding disorders. In a survey of seven women with hemostatic disorders who received a LNG-IUD for menstrual management, the number of bleeding days was reduced in three of the four women with VWD. These women had all attempted treatment with COCs; one patient was also on warfarin [137]. In a retrospective case series that described the long-term efficacy (mean follow-up was 33 months) of the LNG-IUD in 26 English women, the median PBAC scores were decreased, hemoglobin levels were increased, and quality of life measures were improved after LNG-IUD insertion. Thirteen of the 26 women included in this review had VWD [138]. Finally, a retrospective chart review of 28 women with hemostatic disorders (5 with VWD) showed improvement in menorrhagia in 68 % after LNG-IUD insertion [139]. Of note, seven women experienced return of symptoms at a median of 3 years post insertion. This deterioration was reversed when the LNG-IUD was removed and a new device placed. This strategy may be useful and should be considered for individuals whose symptoms return after initial clinical improvement [124].

Recently, a small retrospective review was published in the hematology literature that attempted to determine the expulsion rate of LNG-IUD in women with IBDs; 13 of the 20 patients had VWD [140]. The authors hypothesized that the expulsion and malposition rate would be higher among women with IBDs compared to the reported 1-year rates of 5–10 % in healthy women [135, 141]. Of the 20 patients, 3 IUDs were expelled and 2 were removed due to malposition, for a total of 25 % (95 % CI 11.2–46.9 %). An additional five were removed due to pain ($n=1$) and failure to satisfactorily reduce menstrual bleeding ($n=4$), making the overall discontinuation in this population 50.0 % (95 % CI 29.9–70.1 %) within 2 years. In the 50 % who maintained the IUD, increases in hemoglobin were consistent with the results found in prior studies of LNG-IUD use in healthy women and in women with bleeding disorders [35, 136]. These results may not be generalizable: the sample size is small and factors such as the experience of the inserter were not taken into account. However, even if only 50 % on women with VWD maintain and experience hematologic improvement with the LNG-IUD, its use should be considered a top-tier method of contraception for women with VWD, since surgical treatment of HMB carries additional risks in this population.

A potential concern at the time of IUD insertion is the risk of bleeding in patients with VWD. In the study described above, the majority of patients did not receive prophylaxis medications (e.g., desmopressin) at the time of insertion [140]. This differs from the previous studies [136–138] and prior recommendations, where adequate hemostatic coverage was recommended, especially in women with severe forms of VWD [124]. Clinical efficacy of prophylaxis medication for IUD insertion has not been adequately studied and management must be made on a case-by-case basis.

In addition to HMB, there is also the risk of significant bleeding with ovulation in women with VWD. Hemoperitoneum and broad ligament hematomas from ovarian cyst rupture may result in severe cases [124]. More commonly, ovulation can be associated with significant mid-cycle pain. Although the USMEC recommendations are the same for women with IBDs and those without [34], the risks and benefits of various contraceptive options may differ in women with VWD and individualized assessment is required.

Since the contraceptive effect of the LNG-IUD is mainly due to its local effect, ovulatory cycles with follicular rupture usually occur in women using this method [42]. Studies to date have not addressed the incidence, management, and clinical outcomes of ovarian cysts in women with VWD who are utilizing the LNG-IUD for contraception and treatment of HMB. Inhibiting ovulation and decreasing menstrual bleeding may require a multifactorial approach in women with VWD. This may include the simultaneous use of multiple contraceptive methods and/or combinations of contraceptives with prophylactic hemostatic medications.

Progestin-Only Methods

Even less thoroughly investigated than the LNG-IUD are the other progestin-only methods (including contraceptive implants, progestin-only pills, and DMPA). The etonogestrel implant provides effective contraception but carries a theoretical risk of irregular light vaginal bleeding in addition to localized bleeding at the time of insertion and removal in women with VWD [128]. In clinical studies of the contraceptive implant in healthy women, irregular bleeding was the single most common reason (10.8 %) for implant discontinuation [142]. The risks should be weighed with the benefit of potential amenorrhea, which was achieved in on average in 22.2 % of healthy women during each 90-day reference period [142]. Injected depot medroxyprogesterone acetate (DMPA) can also result in amenorrhea (in almost 60 % of healthy women by 12 months) and an unpredictable bleeding pattern [128]. Neither the implant nor DMPA has been studied in patients with inherited bleeding disorders.

Progestin-only pills (POPs) are also associated with irregular bleeding and have not been evaluated in women with inherited bleeding disorders. The POP available in the USA is low dose, 0.35 mg of norethindrone daily. High doses of oral norethindrone may be a useful treatment of acute HMB in women with VWD [124] based on a single trial that compared a 21-day course of 5 mg of norethindrone three times daily to the 20 μg LNG-IUD [143]. A significant reduction in menstrual blood loss was seen in both groups (a mean reduction of 103 mL (94 %) was seen in the LNG-IUD group and 95 mL (87 %) in the norethindrone group). In addition to being less effective, the oral progestin was less acceptable to patients. After three cycles, only 22 % of subjects wished to continue norethindrone, compared to 76 % of subjects wishing to continue LNG-IUD use. High-dose progestin therapy can cause side effects including fatigue, mood changes, weight gain, bloating, and irregular bleeding [124].

For women choosing to use a progestin only-method, if persistent, bothersome irregular bleeding occurs, the appropriate clinical workup must be performed. If there is no identifiable pathology, the clinician's first choice to alleviate the irregular bleeding is typically a 21-day course of COCs or estrogen followed by a 7-day break. Although another often-utilized strategy is non-steroidal anti-inflammatory drug (NSAID) administration, NSAID use is contraindicated in women with VWD due to its anti-aggregatory effect on platelet function [144].

Combined Hormonal Contraception

CHCs (available as a pill, ring, or patch) are effective in preventing ovulation and improving HMB and dysmenorrhea. They induce atrophy of the endometrium, resulting in a reduction in menstrual blood loss in women with and without menorrhagia [145, 146]. Higher-dose COCs (50-μg ethinyl estradiol [EE]) have been shown to significantly reduce menstrual blood loss in women with objective menorrhagia [147]. Low-dose monophasic COCs (≤30 μg EE) and their reduction in menstrual blood loss have been assessed in only one randomized controlled trial [148]. A significant reduction in blood loss was observed in the COC group, similar to the results in the other treatment groups (low-dose danazol and mefenamic acid groups).

In 2012, a novel quadriphasic combination oral contraceptive pill containing estradiol valerate (E2V) and dienogest (DNG) (Natazia, Bayer Healthcare Pharmaceuticals, Wayne, NJ, USA) was the first COC to receive FDA approval for the treatment of HMB in women without organic pathology who choose an oral contraceptive as their method of contraception [149]. In contrast with traditional combination oral contraceptives, the progestin component of E2V/DNG stabilizes the endometrium [150]. Pooled analysis of two multinational, randomized, double-blind, placebo-controlled trials showed that after 6 months of E2V/DNG use, the median menstrual blood loss was decreased by 88 % compared to 24 % in placebo users. Statistically significant improvements in hematologic parameters (hemoglobin, hematocrit, and ferritin) were also seen [151].

The efficacy of COCs in reducing the menstrual blood loss in women with VWD has not been rigorously evaluated since women with VWD and other bleeding disorders are usually excluded from these studies. However, due to the reduced MBL seen in healthy individuals, various COC preparations are often used in an attempt improve the bleeding and hematologic profiles of patients with VWD. In a survey of 44 women with types 2 and 3 VWD unresponsive to DDAVP, COCs were reported to be effective in 88 % of women [131]. A questionnaire administered to 99 type 1 patients revealed less positive results: hormonal interventions for menorrhagia were ≤50 % effective, with "standard" dose COCs effective in only 24 % of cases [152]. Types and dosages of COCs were not specified in this patient survey.

Traditionally, COCs are taken once daily for 21 days followed by a hormone free week during which uterine bleeding occurs. Recently, continuous administration of COCs has been utilized successfully in the treatment of endometriosis, dysmenorrhea, and other menstrual-related symptoms [153, 154]. Continuous administration permits avoidance of menstruation and authors have advocated the use of this strategy in VWD-related HMB, particularly in adolescents that do not respond to cyclic COC therapy [124]. As with any woman considering COC use, potential side effects should be discussed. Thrombosis may be less of a concern with VWD patients since they have a low inherited thrombotic risk [124].

Management of HMB in adolescents commonly requires more than one treatment modality [155]. Combination therapy can provide effective contraception while treating HMB and preventing hemorrhagic sequelae from ovulation. First-line treatment options include CHCs, LNG-IUD, and specific hemostatic therapies, including tranexamic acid (which competitively inhibits multiple plasminogen binding sites, decreasing plasmin formation and fibrinolysis), desmopressin, and clotting factor replacement. The selection of management options depends on clinical presentation, patient preferences, and toleration of side effects. A multidisciplinary team that includes a hematologist and gynecologist will ensure that optimal medical treatment strategies are utilized and premature surgical intervention is avoided for women with VWD.

Barriers and Emergency Contraception

Barrier methods should not impact laboratory parameters or menstrual bleeding patterns and they are assigned to category 1 in the USMEC [34]. Patient counseling should include this information and data regarding the failure rates of each method. There is scant information on emergency contraception (EC) use in this population. Oral methods (levonorgestrel or ulipristal acetate) are preferable to the copper IUD. In women with VWD, the risk of HMB with the copper IUD should be discussed and tranexamic acid used concomitantly to prevent this complication [128].

Sterilization

As stated in prior sections, no medical condition absolutely restricts a woman's eligibility for sterilization. However, certain conditions place a woman at high surgical risk and in these cases, careful consideration should be given to the risks and benefits of other acceptable alternatives [34]. Women with VWD should be made aware of the increased bleeding risks with surgery and alternative methods should be discussed, including reversible contraception and male sterilization. Hysteroscopic bilateral tubal occlusion can also be presented as an option that avoids abdominal surgery, although this modality has not been studied or reported on women with VWD.

In a report of nine laparoscopic sterilization procedures among women with inherited bleeding disorders, there was one conversion to mini-laparotomy and salpingectomy to control bleeding from a fallopian tube. A wound hematoma developed in another patient [156]. A team approach between hematology, anesthesiology, and gynecology is essential prior to any surgical procedure in VWD patients. Factor levels may need to be monitored in the perioperative periods and adequate hemostatic coverage should be provided.

Treatment with COCs for 1–2 months prior to surgery may decrease the risk of transfusion in patients with VWD. In a case series report, three women with type 1 VWD who required transfusions with prior surgeries, exhibited normal or near normal coagulation test results while taking COCs. They then underwent laminectomy, cholecystectomy, and hysterectomy, respectively, and did not require fresh frozen plasma, cryoprecipitate, or other blood components [157].

Hematologic Malignancies

Background/Hematology Review

Hematologic malignancies are cancers of the hematopoietic system, which can be classified according to the lineage of cells affected. The myeloid neoplasms affect erythroid cells, granulocytic cells (neutrophils, eosinophils, basophils), megakaryocytes, monocytes, and mast cells, as well as their precursors. Within this group, acute processes refer to those aggressive neoplasms with at least 20 % blasts in the peripheral blood or bone marrow. Acute myeloid leukemia is the most common. The less aggressive category of myeloproliferative neoplasms includes chronic myeloid leukemia [158]. In contrast to the myeloid disorders, the lymphoid neoplasms affect B- and T-lymphocytes and their precursors. In this group, diseases are first categorized as Hodgkin or non-Hodgkin lymphomas, and then further distinguished according to B-cell versus T-cell lineage [159]. The hematologic malignancies are more precisely characterized according to molecular subtype [160].

Hematologic malignancies are generally a rare occurrence in women of childbearing age. This is largely due to the low prevalence of these diseases in this patient population. The most recent Surveillance, Epidemiology, and End Results (SEER) data estimates a 0.13 % probability of a woman developing leukemia from birth to age 39, and a similarly low probability of 0.15 % between ages 40 and 59. The probability of developing non-Hodgkin lymphoma is similar at 0.09 % in women up to age 39, though it increases a bit in the 40- to 59-year age group with a probability of 0.31 % [161]. Hodgkin lymphoma is an exception to this rule, with an incidence of up to 4.7 % in women of child-bearing age [162].

The treatments for hematologic malignancies vary according to specific disease type, though the majorities involve combinations of chemotherapy agents. In addition, hematopoietic stem cell transplant may be required in the setting of aggressive or refractory disease, and radiation therapy is indicated in some lymphomas. Both the underlying malignancy and the treatment for it can affect fertility in male and female patients. In the female population, chemotherapy has been found to cause ovarian fibrosis and follicle destruction, and can result in amenorrhea [163]. In a retrospective study of women with Hodgkin lymphoma, 14 % were amenorrheic prior to initiation of therapy, with resumption of menstrual cycles after initiation of therapy, and an additional 18 % became amenorrheic while on chemotherapy. Notably, the median age in the latter group was higher than that of the overall patient population evaluated (30 years versus 23 years) [164].

Unintended Pregnancy and Maternal/ Fetal Risk

Most of the reproductive literature on Hodgkin lymphoma (HL) focuses on fertility preservation prior to and during treatment. Currently, ABVD (doxorubicin, bleomycin, vinblastine, dacarbazine) and escalated BEACOPP (bleomycin, etoposide, doxorubicin, cyclophosphamide, vincristine, procarbazine, prednisone) are the most frequently used regimens for treating Hodgkin lymphoma [165, 166]. Of the two regimens, ABVD is not associated with a greater risk of premature menopause. In a case–control study of 36 survivors attempting pregnancy, there was no evidence of impairment in fertility compared to controls [167]. In contrast, over 50 % of women receiving escalated BEACOPP were found to have permanent amenorrhea [168].

For all patients with hematologic malignancies, regardless of type and treatment regimen, safe and effective contraception should be provided to avoid unintended pregnancies (see Chap. 14). Maternal and fetal outcomes with chemotherapy during pregnancy are not well studied and pregnant women face difficult decisions regarding continuation of pregnancy and treatment options. One small study followed 90 women diagnosed with lymphoma during pregnancy; 33 % deferred treatment until after delivery and 9 % terminated the pregnancy [169]. Of the 56 women with lymphoma who received chemotherapy in the second and third trimesters; minimal maternal complications and fetal effects were seen [169].

Contraception by Method

Combined Hormonal Contraception

Since hematologic malignancy is a rare occurrence in women of childbearing age, there is little research on contraception in this population.

However, several studies have been published that examine the role of COCs and gonadotropin-releasing hormone analogs (GnRH-a) in preserving fertility in women with hematologic cancer. It has been hypothesized that the rate of follicular destruction is accelerated by chemotherapy and the subsequent decreases in estradiol and inhibin production results in increased FSH production [169]. By inducing pituitary desensitization, the administration of COCs or GnRH-a may prevent the increased levels of FSH and therefore protect follicles. Standard recommendations for administering GnRH-a or COCs during treatment of hematologic cancer have not been established based on these preliminary studies.

An important consideration when considering COC use in patients with hematologic malignancies is hypercoagulability. Malignancy is a recognized secondary hypercoagulable state [170] and the Society of Family Planning recommends that women of childbearing age who are being treated for cancer avoid all CHC if possible because they may further increase the risk of VTE already elevated due to the cancer [171]. Whether using COCs solely to prevent pregnancy or as a means to prevent premature ovarian failure as a result of chemotherapy, the risk–benefit ratio should be considered on a case-by-case basis since these cancers are not listed in the USMEC.

Progestin-Only Methods

Progestin-only contraception (including oral, injectable, and implantable) has not been associated with thrombotic events in healthy individuals [172–174]. A recent meta-analysis of eight observational studies also concluded that there is no increased risk of venous thromboembolism in healthy users of progestin-only contraception compared to nonusers of contraception [175]. Unfortunately, there are insufficient data to evaluate the risk of VTE with progestin-only methods in patients at high risk for VTE [171]. Treatment plans should be made on a case-by-case basis. Women with osteopathy following chemotherapy should avoid DMPA [171]. The benefit of single-dose oral LNG for EC most likely outweighs the risks for these patients; there is no evidence to restrict ulipristal acetate use.

Intrauterine Devices

Copper IUD and LNG-IUD can be utilized in this population for contraception and EC; however, the safety and effectiveness of these devices by women who are immunosuppressed by chemotherapy have not been adequately studied. Case reports have documented IUD failures in immunosuppressed patients [176, 177], but this remains a theoretical concern. These case reports were published in 1976 and 1981 and did not utilize the IUDs that are currently available. Please see Chap. 9 for further discussion.

Sterilization

The same theoretical concern exists for effectiveness of hysteroscopic sterilization. During this procedure, a 4-cm microinsert (Essure, Bayer Healthcare Pharmaceuticals, Wayne, NJ, USA) is placed into each fallopian tube. Once deployed, the stainless steel inner coil and the expanding nickel–titanium outer coil anchor the implant. Wound in and around the inner coil are polyethylene terephthalate (PET) fibers. These PET fibers stimulate benign tissue growth that surrounds and infiltrates the device over time. This results in the fallopian tube occlusion and permanent sterilization. Patients are evaluated for bilateral tubal occlusion at 3 months by hysterosalpingogram (HSG) [178]. Insufficient tissue reaction or prolonged times to occlusion are theoretical concerns in immunosuppressed patients.

The potential benefits of hysteroscopic sterilization most likely outweigh the risks in this patient population. Laparoscopic bilateral tubal ligation is another option for sterilization, but elective surgeries are typically avoided during treatment of a malignancy. Prior to performing either form of sterilization, consultation with the patient's oncologist is appropriate. Highly effective reversible methods of contraception and male sterilization should also be considered and discussed.

Barrier Methods and Emergency Contraception

Barrier methods (including condoms, spermicides, and diaphragms/cervical caps) are options for women with hematologic malignancy.

There is no evidence to discourage the use of either levonorgestrel or ulipristal acetate for emergency contraception in women with hematologic malignancy. The Cu-IUD use for EC is an option, but the effectiveness has not been investigated in this patient population.

Conclusion

For women with iron-deficiency anemia, sickle cell anemia, thalassemia, and Von Willebrand disease, contraception can also be utilized to improve heavy menstrual bleeding and hematologic laboratory values. Each patient's complete clinical picture must be assessed, since certain complications of hematologic disorders may make particular contraceptive methods suboptimal. LNG-IUDs are typically safe for even the most complicated patients and have clearly been shown to decrease menstrual bleeding and improve hematologic laboratory values in healthy patients. Current research is leading to similar conclusions in women with hematologic abnormalities. Barrier methods and sterilization do not have the benefit of improving bleeding profiles and hematologic parameters. Although barrier methods are less effective at preventing pregnancy, they are certainly safe in this patient population. The risks of bleeding and anesthesia are minimized with hysteroscopic sterilization; but menstrual bleeding patterns will not be favorably altered. The risks and benefits of any sterilization surgery must be carefully considered in women with hematologic abnormalities.

References

1. WHO/CDC. Worldwide prevalence of anemia, 1993-2005. Geneva: World Health Organization; 2008.
2. Looker AC, Dallman PR, Carroll MD, Gunter EW, Johnson CL. Prevalence of iron deficiency in the United States. JAMA. 1997;277(12):973–6.
3. Ross EM. Evaluation and treatment of iron deficiency in adults. Nutr Clin Care. 2002;5(5):220–4.
4. Coad J, Conlon C. Iron deficiency in women: assessment, causes and consequences. Curr Opin Clin Nutr Metab Care. 2011;14(6):625–34.
5. Alleyne M, Horne MK, Miller JL. Individualized treatment for iron-deficiency anemia in adults. Am J Med. 2008;121(11):943–8.
6. Killip S, Bennett JM, Chambers MD. Iron-deficiency anemia. Am Fam Physician. 2007;75(5):671–8.
7. Bermejo F, Garcia-Lopez S. A guide to diagnosis of iron deficiency and iron-deficiency anemia in digestive diseases. World J Gastroenterol. 2009;15(37): 4638–43.
8. Short MW, Domagalski JE. Iron-deficiency anemia: evaluation and management. Am Fam Physician. 2013;87(2):98–104.
9. Weiss G, Goodnough LT. Anemia of chronic disease. N Engl J Med. 2005;352(10):1011–23.
10. Skikne BS, Punnonen K, Caldron PH, Bennett MT, Rehu M, Gasior GH, et al. Improved differential diagnosis of anemia of chronic disease and iron-deficiency anemia: a prospective multicenter evaluation of soluble transferrin receptor and the sTfR/log ferritin index. Am J Hematol. 2011;86(11):923–7.
11. Hughes DA, Stuart-Smith SE, Bain BJ. How should stainable iron in bone marrow films be assessed? J Clin Pathol. 2004;57(10):1038–40.
12. Johnson-Wimbley TD, Graham DY. Diagnosis and management of iron-deficiency anemia in the 21st century. Therap Adv Gastroenterol. 2011;4(3):177–84.
13. Goddard AF, James MW, McIntyre AS, Scott BB, British Society of Gastroenterology. Guidelines for the management of iron deficiency anaemia. Gut. 2011;60(10):1309–16.
14. Auerbach M, Ballard H. Clinical use of intravenous iron: administration, efficacy, and safety. Hematology Am Soc Hematol Educ Program. 2010; 2010:338–47.
15. Scholl TO, Hediger ML, Fischer RL, Shearer JW. Anemia vs iron deficiency: increased risk of preterm delivery in a prospective study. Am J Clin Nutr. 1992;55(5):985–8.
16. Carlson ES, Stead JD, Neal CR, Petryk A, Georgieff MK. Perinatal iron deficiency results in altered developmental expression of genes mediating energy metabolism and neuronal morphogenesis in hippocampus. Hippocampus. 2007;17(8):679–91.
17. Radlowski EC, Johnson RW. Perinatal iron deficiency and neurocognitive development. Front Hum Neurosci. 2013;7:585.
18. Beard JL, Connor JR. Iron status and neural functioning. Annu Rev Nutr. 2003;23:41–58.
19. Jorgenson LA, Sun M, O'Connor M, Georgieff MK. Fetal iron deficiency disrupts the maturation of synaptic function and efficacy in area CA1 of the developing rat hippocampus. Hippocampus. 2005; 15(8):1094–102.
20. Winner B, Peipert JF, Zhao Q, Buckel C, Madden T, Allsworth JE, et al. Effectiveness of long-acting reversible contraception. N Engl J Med. 2012; 366(21):1998–2007.
21. Thonneau PF, Almont T. Contraceptive efficacy of intrauterine devices. Am J Obstet Gynecol. 2008; 198(3):248–53.

22. American College of Obstetricians and Gynecologists. ACOG Practice Bulletin No. 121: long-acting reversible contraception: Implants and intrauterine devices. Obstet Gynecol. 2011;118(1): 184–96.
23. d'Arcangues C. Worldwide use of intrauterine devices for contraception. Contraception. 2007;75(6 Suppl):S2–7.
24. Finer LB, Zolna MR. Unintended pregnancy in the United States: incidence and disparities, 2006. Contraception. 2011;84(5):478–85.
25. Finer LB, Jerman J, Kavanaugh ML. Changes in use of long-acting contraceptive methods in the United States, 2007-2009. Fertil Steril. 2012;98(4):893–7.
26. Andersson K, Odlind V, Rybo G. Levonorgestrel-releasing and copper-releasing (Nova T) IUDs during five years of use: a randomized comparative trial. Contraception. 1994;49(1):56–72.
27. Sivin I, Stern J, Coutinho E, Mattos CE, el Mahgoub S, Diaz S, et al. Prolonged intrauterine contraception: a seven-year randomized study of the levonorgestrel 20 mcg/day (LNg 20) and the Copper T380 Ag IUDS. Contraception. 1991;44(5):473–80.
28. Sivin I, Stern J, Diaz J, Diaz MM, Faundes A, el Mahgoub S, et al. Two years of intrauterine contraception with levonorgestrel and with copper: a randomized comparison of the TCu 380Ag and levonorgestrel 20 mcg/day devices. Contraception. 1987;35(3):245–55.
29. Ronnerdag M, Odlind V. Health effects of long-term use of the intrauterine levonorgestrel-releasing system. A follow-up study over 12 years of continuous use. Acta Obstet Gynecol Scand. 1999;78(8): 716–21.
30. Hubacher D, Grimes DA. Noncontraceptive health benefits of intrauterine devices: a systematic review. Obstet Gynecol Surv. 2002;57(2):120–8.
31. Faundes A, Alvarez F, Brache V, Tejada AS. The role of the levonorgestrel intrauterine device in the prevention and treatment of iron-deficiency anemia during fertility regulation. Int J Gynaecol Obstet. 1988;26(3):429–33.
32. Larsson G, Milsom I, Jonasson K, Lindstedt G, Rybo G. The long-term effects of copper surface area on menstrual blood loss and iron status in women fitted with an IUD. Contraception. 1993; 48(5):471–80.
33. Luukkainen T, Allonen H, Haukkamaa M, Holma P, Pyörälä T, Terho J, et al. Effective contraception with the levonorgestrel-releasing intrauterine device: 12-month report of a European multicenter study. Contraception. 1987;36(2):169–79.
34. Centers for Disease Control and Prevention. U S. medical eligibility criteria for contraceptive use, 2010. MMWR Recomm Rep. 2010;59(RR-4):1–86.
35. Andersson JK, Rybo G. Levonorgestrel-releasing intrauterine device in the treatment of menorrhagia. Br J Obstet Gynaecol. 1990;97(8):690–4.
36. Chrisman C, Ribeiro P, Dalton VK. The levonorgestrel-releasing intrauterine system: an updated review of the contraceptive and noncontraceptive uses. Clin Obstet Gynecol. 2007;50(4):886–97.
37. Marjoribanks J, Lethaby A, Farquhar C. Surgery versus medical therapy for heavy menstrual bleeding. Cochrane Database Syst Rev. 2006;2, CD003855.
38. Kaunitz AM, Meredith S, Inki P, Kubba A, Sanchez-Ramos L. Levonorgestrel-releasing intrauterine system and endometrial ablation in heavy menstrual bleeding: a systematic review and meta-analysis. Obstet Gynecol. 2009;113(5):1104–16.
39. Barrington JW, Bowen-Simpkins P. The levonorgestrel intrauterine system in the management of menorrhagia. Br J Obstet Gynaecol. 1997;104(5):614–6.
40. Lahteenmaki P, Haukkamaa M, Puolakka J, Riikonen U, Sainio S, Suvisaari J, et al. Open randomised study of use of levonorgestrel releasing intrauterine system as alternative to hysterectomy. BMJ. 1998; 316(7138):1122–6.
41. Heliovaara-Peippo S, Hurskainen R, Teperi J, Aalto AM, Grénman S, Halmesmäki K, et al. Quality of life and costs of levonorgestrel-releasing intrauterine system or hysterectomy in the treatment of menorrhagia: a 10-year randomized controlled trial. Am J Obstet Gynecol. 2013;209(6):535.e1–14.
42. Information, M.F.P. February 17, 2014. Available from: http://labeling.bayerhealthcare.com/html/products/pi/Mirena_PI.pdf.
43. Information, S.F.P. Available from: http://labeling.bayerhealthcare.com/html/products/pi/Skyla_PI.pdf.
44. Bonnema RA, McNamara MC, Spencer AL. Contraception choices in women with underlying medical conditions. Am Fam Physician. 2010;82(6): 621–8.
45. Meckstroth KR, Darney PD. Implantable contraception. Obstet Gynecol Clin North Am. 2000;27(4): 781–815.
46. Funk S, Miller MM, Mishell Jr DR, Archer DF, Poindexter A, Schmidt J, et al. Safety and efficacy of Implanon, a single-rod implantable contraceptive containing etonogestrel. Contraception. 2005;71(5): 319–26.
47. Effects of contraceptives on hemoglobin and ferritin. Task Force for Epidemiological Research on Reproductive Health, United Nations Development Programme/United Nations Population Fund/World Health Organization/World Bank Special Programme of Research, Development and Research Training in Human Reproduction, World Health Organization, Geneva, Switzerland. Contraception. 1998;58(5):262–73.
48. Cullins VE. Noncontraceptive benefits and therapeutic uses of depot medroxyprogesterone acetate. J Reprod Med. 1996;41(5 Suppl):428–33.
49. Matteson KA, Rahn DD, Wheeler II TL, Casiano E, Siddiqui NY, Harvie HS, et al. Nonsurgical management of heavy menstrual bleeding: a systematic review. Obstet Gynecol. 2013;121(3):632–43.
50. Kucuk T, Ertan K. Continuous oral or intramuscular medroxyprogesterone acetate versus the levonorg-

estrel releasing intrauterine system in the treatment of perimenopausal menorrhagia: a randomized, prospective, controlled clinical trial in female smokers. Clin Exp Obstet Gynecol. 2008;35(1):57–60.
51. Urata YN, Lyra EC, Katayama ML, Basso RA, Assis PE, Cardoso AP, et al. Calcitriol supplementation effects on Ki67 expression and transcriptional profile of breast cancer specimens from post-menopausal patients. Clin Nutr. 2014;33(1):136–42.
52. Casabellata G, Di Santolo M, Banfi G, Stel G, Gonano F, Cauci S. Evaluation of iron deficiency in young women in relation to oral contraceptive use. Contraception. 2007;76(3):200–7.
53. Maguire K, Westhoff C. The state of hormonal contraception today: established and emerging noncontraceptive health benefits. Am J Obstet Gynecol. 2011;205(4 Suppl):S4–8.
54. Fraser IS, Römer T, Parke S, Zeun S, Mellinger U, Machlitt A, et al. Effective treatment of heavy and/or prolonged menstrual bleeding with an oral contraceptive containing estradiol valerate and dienogest: a randomized, double-blind Phase III trial. Hum Reprod. 2011;26(10):2698–708.
55. Jensen JT, Parke S, Mellinger U, Machlitt A, Fraser IS. Effective treatment of heavy menstrual bleeding with estradiol valerate and dienogest: a randomized controlled trial. Obstet Gynecol. 2011;117(4): 777–87.
56. Endrikat J, Shapiro H, Lukkari-Lax E, Kunz M, Schmidt W, Fortier M. A Canadian, multicentre study comparing the efficacy of a levonorgestrel-releasing intrauterine system to an oral contraceptive in women with idiopathic menorrhagia. J Obstet Gynaecol Can. 2009;31(4):340–7.
57. Shaaban MM, Zakherah MS, El-Nashar SA, Sayed GH. Levonorgestrel-releasing intrauterine system compared to low dose combined oral contraceptive pills for idiopathic menorrhagia: a randomized clinical trial. Contraception. 2011;83(1):48–54.
58. Bunn HF. Pathogenesis and treatment of sickle cell disease. N Engl J Med. 1997;337(11):762–9.
59. Rees DC, Williams TN, Gladwin MT. Sickle-cell disease. Lancet. 2010;376(9757):2018–31.
60. Hebbel RP, Vercellotti G, Nath KA. A systems biology consideration of the vasculopathy of sickle cell anemia: the need for multi-modality chemo-prophylaxsis. Cardiovasc Hematol Disord Drug Targets. 2009;9(4):271–92.
61. Charache S, Page DL. Infarction of bone marrow in the sickle cell disorders. Ann Intern Med. 1967; 67(6):1195–200.
62. Vichinsky EP, Neumayr LD, Earles AN, Williams R, Lennette ET, Dean D, et al. Causes and outcomes of the acute chest syndrome in sickle cell disease. National Acute Chest Syndrome Study Group. N Engl J Med. 2000;342(25):1855–65.
63. Steinberg MH. Management of sickle cell disease. N Engl J Med. 1999;340(13):1021–30.
64. Stuart MJ, Nagel RL. Sickle-cell disease. Lancet. 2004;364(9442):1343–60.
65. Ballas SK, Lewis CN, Noone AM, Krasnow SH, Kamarulzaman E, Burka ER. Clinical, hematological, and biochemical features of Hb SC disease. Am J Hematol. 1982;13(1):37–51.
66. Gonzalez-Redondo JM, Kutlar A, Kutlar F, McKie VC, McKie KM, Baysal E, et al. Molecular characterization of Hb S(C) beta-thalassemia in American blacks. Am J Hematol. 1991;38(1):9–14.
67. Castro O, Rana SR, Bang KM, Scott RB. Age and prevalence of sickle-cell trait in a large ambulatory population. Genet Epidemiol. 1987;4(4):307–11.
68. Hassell KL. Population estimates of sickle cell disease in the US. Am J Prev Med. 2010;38(4 Suppl): S512–21.
69. Platt OS, Thorington BD, Brambilla DJ, Milner PF, Rosse WF, Vichinsky E, et al. Pain in sickle cell disease. Rates and risk factors. N Engl J Med. 1991; 325(1):11–6.
70. Platt OS, Brambilla DJ, Rosse WF, Milner PF, Castro O, Steinberg MH, et al. Mortality in sickle cell disease. Life expectancy and risk factors for early death. N Engl J Med. 1994;330(23):1639–44.
71. Brittenham GM, Schechter AN, Noguchi CT. Hemoglobin S polymerization: primary determinant of the hemolytic and clinical severity of the sickling syndromes. Blood. 1985;65(1):183–9.
72. Lottenberg R, Hassell KL. An evidence-based approach to the treatment of adults with sickle cell disease. Hematology Am Soc Hematol Educ Program, 2005:58–65.
73. Wayne AS, Kevy SV, Nathan DG. Transfusion management of sickle cell disease. Blood. 1993;81(5): 1109–23.
74. Charache S, Terrin ML, Moore RD, Dover GJ, Barton FB, Eckert SV, et al. Effect of hydroxyurea on the frequency of painful crises in sickle cell anemia. Investigators of the Multicenter Study of Hydroxyurea in Sickle Cell Anemia. N Engl J Med. 1995;332(20):1317–22.
75. Josephson CD, Su LL, Hillyer KL, Hillyer CD. Transfusion in the patient with sickle cell disease: a critical review of the literature and transfusion guidelines. Transfus Med Rev. 2007;21(2): 118–33.
76. Hassell, K. Pregnancy and sickle cell disease. Hematol Oncol Clin North Am, 2005. 19(5): p. 903-16, vii-viii.
77. Alayed N, Kezouh A, Oddy L, Abenhaim HA. Sickle cell disease and pregnancy outcomes: population-based study on 8.8 million births. J Perinat Med. 2013:1–6.
78. Sun PM, Wilburn W, Raynor BD, Jamieson D. Sickle cell disease in pregnancy: twenty years of experience at Grady Memorial Hospital, Atlanta. Georgia Am J Obstet Gynecol. 2001;184(6):1127–30.
79. Koshy M, Burd L, Wallace D, Moawad A, Baron J. Prophylactic red-cell transfusions in pregnant patients with sickle cell disease. A randomized cooperative study. N Engl J Med. 1988;319(22): 1447–52.

80. Koshy M, Chisum D, Burd L, Orlina A, How H. Management of sickle cell anemia and pregnancy. J Clin Apher. 1991;6(4):230–3.
81. Haddad LB, Curtis KM, Legardy-Williams JK, Cwiak C, Jamieson DJ. Contraception for individuals with sickle cell disease: a systematic review of the literature. Contraception. 2012;85(6):527–37.
82. Samuels-Reid JH, Scott RB, Brown WE. Contraceptive practices and reproductive patterns in sickle cell disease. J Natl Med Assoc. 1984;76(9): 879–83.
83. Howard RJ, Lillis C, Tuck SM. Contraceptives, counselling, and pregnancy in women with sickle cell disease. BMJ. 1993;306(6894):1735–7.
84. Isaacs WA, Effiong CE, Ayeni O. Steroid treatment in the prevention of painful episodes in sickle-cell disease. Lancet. 1972;1(7750):570–1.
85. Isaacs WA, Hayhoe FG. Steroid hormones in sickle-cell disease. Nature. 1967;215(5106):1139–42.
86. Adadevoh BK, Isaacs WA. The effect of megestrol acetate on sickling. Am J Med Sci. 1973;265(5): 367–70.
87. Yoong WC, Tuck SM, Michael AE. Binding of ovarian steroids to erythrocytes in patients with sickle cell disease; effects on cell sickling and osmotic fragility. J Steroid Biochem Mol Biol. 2003;84(1):71–8.
88. da Silva Santos Duarte A, Sales TS, Mengel JO, Costa FF, Saad ST. Progesterone upregulates GATA-1 on erythroid progenitors cells in liquid culture. Blood Cells Mol Dis. 2002;29(2):213–24.
89. Olawoye TO. Erythrocyte membrane Ca2+ ATPase: reactivities of human A, AS, and S erythrocytes with steroid hormones. Biochem Med Metab Biol. 1989; 42(3):179–84.
90. De Ceulaer K, Gruber C, Hayes R, Serjeant GR. Medroxyprogesterone acetate and homozygous sickle-cell disease. Lancet. 1982;2(8292):229–31.
91. Nascimento Mde L, Ladipo OA, Coutinho EM. Nomegestrol acetate contraceptive implant use by women with sickle cell disease. Clin Pharmacol Ther. 1998;64(4):433–8.
92. de Abood M, de Castillo Z, Guerrero F, Espino M, Austin KL. Effect of Depo-Provera or Microgynon on the painful crises of sickle cell anemia patients. Contraception. 1997;56(5):313–6.
93. Yoong WC, Tuck SM, Pasi KJ, Owens D, Perry DJ. Markers of platelet activation, thrombin generation and fibrinolysis in women with sickle cell disease: effects of differing forms of hormonal contraception. Eur J Haematol. 2003;70(5):310–4.
94. Yoong WC, Tuck SM, Yardumian A. Red cell deformability in oral contraceptive pill users with sickle cell anaemia. Br J Haematol. 1999;104(4): 868–70.
95. Ladipo OA, Falusi AG, Feldblum PJ, Osotimehin BO, Otolorin EO, Ojengbede OA. Norplant use by women with sickle cell disease. Int J Gynaecol Obstet. 1993;41(1):85–7.
96. O'Brien SH, Klima J, Reed S, Chisolm D, Schwarz EB, Kelleher KJ. Hormonal contraception use and pregnancy in adolescents with sickle cell disease: analysis of Michigan Medicaid claims. Contraception. 2011;83(2):134–7.
97. Manchikanti A, Grimes DA, Lopez LM, Schulz KF. Steroid hormones for contraception in women with sickle cell disease. Cochrane Database Syst Rev. 2007;2, CD006261.
98. Barbosa IC, Ladipo OA, Nascimento ML, Athayde C, Hirsch C, Lopes R, et al. Carbohydrate metabolism in sickle cell patients using a subdermal implant containing nomegestrol acetate (Uniplant). Contraception. 2001;63(5):263–5.
99. Machado RF, Farber HW. Pulmonary hypertension associated with chronic hemolytic anemia and other blood disorders. Clin Chest Med. 2013;34(4): 739–52.
100. Koshy M, Weiner SJ, Miller ST, Sleeper LA, Vichinsky E, Brown AK, et al. Surgery and anesthesia in sickle cell disease Cooperative Study of Sickle Cell Diseases. Blood. 1995;86(10):3676–84.
101. Nathan DG, Gunn RB. Thalassemia: the consequences of unbalanced hemoglobin synthesis. Am J Med. 1966;41(5):815–30.
102. Higgs DR, Vickers MA, Wilkie AO, Pretorius IM, Jarman AP, Weatherall DJ. A review of the molecular genetics of the human alpha-globin gene cluster. Blood. 1989;73(5):1081–104.
103. Lehmann H. Different types of alpha-thalassaemia and significance of haemoglobin Bart's in neonates. Lancet. 1970;1(7663):78–80.
104. Thein SL. Genetic insights into the clinical diversity of beta thalassaemia. Br J Haematol. 2004;124(3): 264–74.
105. Olivieri NF. The beta-thalassemias. N Engl J Med. 1999;341(2):99–109.
106. Weatherall DJ. Pathophysiology of thalassaemia. Baillieres Clin Haematol. 1998;11(1):127–46.
107. Rund D, Rachmilewitz E. Beta-thalassemia. N Engl J Med. 2005;353(11):1135–46.
108. Borgna-Pignatti C, Rugolotto S, De Stefano P, Zhao H, Cappellini MD, Del Vecchio GC, et al. Survival and complications in patients with thalassemia major treated with transfusion and deferoxamine. Haematologica. 2004;89(10):1187–93.
109. Leung TY, Lao TT. Thalassaemia in pregnancy. Best Pract Res Clin Obstet Gynaecol. 2012;26(1):37–51.
110. Psihogios V, Rodda C, Reid E, Clark M, Clarke C, Bowden D. Reproductive health in individuals with homozygous beta-thalassemia: knowledge, attitudes, and behavior. Fertil Steril. 2002;77(1):119–27.
111. American College of Obstetricians and Gynecologists Committee on Gynecologic Practice; Long-Acting Reversible Contraception Working Group. Long-Acting Reversible Contraception Working, ACOG Committee Opinion no. 450: Increasing use of contraceptive implants and intrauterine devices to reduce unintended pregnancy. Obstet Gynecol. 2009;114(6):1434–8.
112. Baldini M, Forti S, Orsatti A, Marcon A, Ulivieri FM, Airaghi L, et al. Thalassemic osteopathy: a new

marker of bone deposition. Blood Cells Mol Dis. 2014;52(2–3):91–4.
113. Skordis N, Toumba M. Bone disease in thalassaemia major: recent advances in pathogenesis and clinical aspects. Pediatr Endocrinol Rev. 2011;8 Suppl 2: 300–6.
114. Perisano C, Marzetti E, Spinelli MS, Callà CA, Graci C, Maccauro G. Physiopathology of bone modifications in beta-thalassemia. Anemia. 2012; 2012:320737.
115. Jensen CE, Tuck SM, Wonke B. Fertility in beta thalassaemia major: a report of 16 pregnancies, preconceptual evaluation and a review of the literature. Br J Obstet Gynaecol. 1995;102(8):625–9.
116. El-Beshlawy A, Youssry I, El-Saidi S, El Accaoui R, Mansi Y, Makhlouf A, et al. Pulmonary hypertension in beta-thalassemia major and the role of L-carnitine therapy. Pediatr Hematol Oncol. 2008; 25(8):734–43.
117. Chatterjee R, Katz M, Bajoria R. Use of hormone replacement therapy for correction of high turnover bone disease in hypogonadal beta-Thalassemia major patients presenting with osteoporosis: comparison with idiopathic premature ovarian failure. Hemoglobin. 2011;35(5–6):653–8.
118. Rodeghiero F, Castaman G, Dini E. Epidemiological investigation of the prevalence of von Willebrand's disease. Blood. 1987;69(2):454–9.
119. Sadler JE, Budde U, Eikenboom JC, Favaloro EJ, Hill FG, Holmberg L, et al. Update on the pathophysiology and classification of von Willebrand disease: a report of the Subcommittee on von Willebrand Factor. J Thromb Haemost. 2006;4(10):2103–14.
120. Lak M, Peyvandi F, Mannucci PM. Clinical manifestations and complications of childbirth and replacement therapy in 385 Iranian patients with type 3 von Willebrand disease. Br J Haematol. 2000;111(4): 1236–9.
121. Mohri H. Acquired von Willebrand syndrome: features and management. Am J Hematol. 2006;81(8): 616–23.
122. Mannucci PM, Ruggeri ZM, Pareti FI, Capitanio A. 1-Deamino-8-d-arginine vasopressin: a new pharmacological approach to the management of haemophilia and von Willebrands' diseases. Lancet. 1977; 1(8017):869–72.
123. Mannucci PM. Treatment of von Willebrand's disease. N Engl J Med. 2004;351(7):683–94.
124. Kadir RA, Chi C. Women and von Willebrand disease: controversies in diagnosis and management. Semin Thromb Hemost. 2006;32(6):605–15.
125. James AH. More than menorrhagia: a review of the obstetric and gynaecological manifestations of bleeding disorders. Haemophilia. 2005;11(4): 295–307.
126. Bevan JA, Maloney KW, Hillery CA, Gill JC, Montgomery RR, Scott JP. Bleeding disorders: a common cause of menorrhagia in adolescents. J Pediatr. 2001;138(6):856–61.
127. Jayasinghe Y, Moore P, Donath S, Campbell J, Monagle P, Grover S. Bleeding disorders in teenagers presenting with menorrhagia. Aust N Z J Obstet Gynaecol. 2005;45(5):439–43.
128. Burton C, Chi C, Kadir R. Gynaecological problems and choices for contraception in women with inherited bleeding disorders. J Fam Plann Reprod Health Care. 2008;34(2):93–8.
129. Nilsson IM. Von Willebrand's disease—fifty years old. Acta Med Scand. 1977;201(6):497–508.
130. Committee on Adolescent Health. C and P Committee on Gynecologic, Committee opinion no. 580 von Willebrand disease in women. Obstet Gynecol. 2013;122(6):1368–73.
131. Foster PA. The reproductive health of women with von Willebrand Disease unresponsive to DDAVP: results of an international survey. On behalf of the Subcommittee on von Willebrand Factor of the Scientific and Standardization Committee of the ISTH. Thromb Haemost. 1995;74(2):784–90.
132. Kirtava A, Drews C, Lally C, Dilley A, Evatt B. Medical, reproductive and psychosocial experiences of women diagnosed with von Willebrand's disease receiving care in haemophilia treatment centres: a case-control study. Haemophilia. 2003;9(3):292–7.
133. Pacheco LD, Costantine MM, Saade GR, Mucowski S, Hankins GD, Sciscione AC. von Willebrand disease and pregnancy: a practical approach for the diagnosis and treatment. Am J Obstet Gynecol. 2010;203(3):194–200.
134. Silverberg SG, Haukkamaa M, Arko H, Nilsson CG, Luukkainen T. Endometrial morphology during long-term use of levonorgestrel-releasing intrauterine devices. Int J Gynecol Pathol. 1986;5(3):235–41.
135. Stewart A, Cummins C, Gold L, Jordan R, Phillips W. The effectiveness of the levonorgestrel-releasing intrauterine system in menorrhagia: a systematic review. BJOG. 2001;108(1):74–86.
136. Kingman CE, Kadir RA, Lee CA, Economides DL. The use of levonorgestrel-releasing intrauterine system for treatment of menorrhagia in women with inherited bleeding disorders. BJOG. 2004;111(12): 1425–8.
137. Lukes AS, Reardon B, Arepally G. Use of the levonorgestrel-releasing intrauterine system in women with hemostatic disorders. Fertil Steril. 2008;90(3):673–7.
138. Chi C, Huq FY, Kadir RA. Levonorgestrel-releasing intrauterine system for the management of heavy menstrual bleeding in women with inherited bleeding disorders: long-term follow-up. Contraception. 2011;83(3):242–7.
139. Schaedel ZE, Dolan G, Powell MC. The use of the levonorgestrel-releasing intrauterine system in the management of menorrhagia in women with hemostatic disorders. Am J Obstet Gynecol. 2005;193(4): 1361–3.
140. Rimmer E, Jamieson MA, James P. Malposition and expulsion of the levonorgestrel intrauterine system

among women with inherited bleeding disorders. Haemophilia. 2013;19(6):933–8.
141. Kriplani A, Singh BM, Lal S, Agarwal N. Efficacy, acceptability and side effects of the levonorgestrel intrauterine system for menorrhagia. Int J Gynaecol Obstet. 2007;97(3):190–4.
142. Information NFP. Available from http://www.nexplanon.com/en/consumer/main/prescribing-information/.
143. Irvine GA, Campbell-Brown MB, Lumsden MA, Heikkilä A, Walker JJ, Cameron IT. Randomised comparative trial of the levonorgestrel intrauterine system and norethisterone for treatment of idiopathic menorrhagia. Br J Obstet Gynaecol. 1998;105(6):592–8.
144. Mansour D, Bahamondes L, Critchley H, Darney P, Fraser IS. The management of unacceptable bleeding patterns in etonogestrel-releasing contraceptive implant users. Contraception. 2011;83(3):202–10.
145. Callard GV, Litofsky FS, DeMerre LJ. Menstruation in women with normal or artificially controlled cycles. Fertil Steril. 1966;17(5):684–8.
146. Ramcharan S, Pellegrin FA, Ray RM, Hsu JP, The Walnut Creek Contraceptive Drug Study. A prospective study of the side effects of oral contraceptives. Volume III, an interim report: a comparison of disease occurrence leading to hospitalization or death in users and nonusers of oral contraceptives. J Reprod Med. 1980;25(6 Suppl):345–72.
147. Nilsson L, Rybo G. Treatment of menorrhagia. Am J Obstet Gynecol. 1971;110(5):713–20.
148. Fraser IS, McCarron G. Randomized trial of 2 hormonal and 2 prostaglandin-inhibiting agents in women with a complaint of menorrhagia. Aust N Z J Obstet Gynaecol. 1991;31(1):66–70.
149. Information, N.F.P. February 17, 2014. Available from http://labeling.bayerhealthcare.com/html/products/pi/natazia_pi.pdf.
150. Rafie S, Borgelt L, Koepf ER, Temple-Cooper ME, Lehman KJ. Novel oral contraceptive for heavy menstrual bleeding: estradiol valerate and dienogest. Int J Women's Health. 2013;5:313–21.
151. Fraser IS, Parke S, Mellinger U, Machlitt A, Serrani M, Jensen J. Effective treatment of heavy and/or prolonged menstrual bleeding without organic cause: pooled analysis of two multinational, randomised, double-blind, placebo-controlled trials of oestradiol valerate and dienogest. Eur J Contracept Reprod Health Care. 2011;16(4):258–69.
152. Kouides PA, Phatak PD, Burkart P, Braggins C, Cox C, Bernstein Z, et al. Gynaecological and obstetrical morbidity in women with type I von Willebrand disease: results of a patient survey. Haemophilia. 2000;6(6):643–8.
153. Cressman BE, Waldrop E, Holleman S, Kuehl TJ. Extending the duration of active oral contraceptive pills to manage hormone withdrawal symptoms. Obstet Gynecol. 1997;89(2):179–83.
154. Vercellini P, De Giorgi O, Mosconi P, Stellato G, Vicentini S, Crosignani PG. Cyproterone acetate versus a continuous monophasic oral contraceptive in the treatment of recurrent pelvic pain after conservative surgery for symptomatic endometriosis. Fertil Steril. 2002;77(1):52–61.
155. Chi C, Pollard D, Tuddenham EG, Kadir RA. Menorrhagia in adolescents with inherited bleeding disorders. J Pediatr Adolesc Gynecol. 2010;23(4):215–22.
156. Kadir RA, Economides DL, Sabin CA, Pollard D, Lee CA. Assessment of menstrual blood loss and gynaecological problems in patients with inherited bleeding disorders. Haemophilia. 1999;5(1):40–8.
157. Alperin JB. Estrogens and surgery in women with von Willebrand's disease. Am J Med. 1982;73(3):367–71.
158. Vardiman JW, Thiele J, Arber DA, Brunning RD, Borowitz MJ, Porwit A, et al. The 2008 revision of the World Health Organization (WHO) classification of myeloid neoplasms and acute leukemia: rationale and important changes. Blood. 2009;114(5):937–51.
159. Morton LM, Turner JJ, Cerhan JR, Linet MS, Treseler PA, Clarke CA, et al. Proposed classification of lymphoid neoplasms for epidemiologic research from the Pathology Working Group of the International Lymphoma Epidemiology Consortium (InterLymph). Blood. 2007;110(2):695–708.
160. Swerdlow SH, Campo E, Harris NL, Jaffe ES, Pileri SA, Stein H, et al., editors. World Health Organization classification of tumors of haematopoietic and lymphoid tissues. Lyon, France: IARC Press; 2008.
161. Siegel R, Naishadham D, Jemal A. Cancer statistics, 2013. CA Cancer J Clin. 2013;63(1):11–30.
162. Howlader N, Krapcho M, Neyman N, Aminou R, Waldron W, Altekruse SF, Kosary CL, Ruhl J, Tatalovich Z, Cho H, Mariotto A, Eisner MP, Lewis DR, Chen HS, Feuer EJ, Cronin KA, Edwards BK, editors. SEER cancer statistics review, 1975–2008. Bethesda, MD: National Cancer Institute; 2010.
163. Schilsky RL, Lewis BJ, Sherins RJ, Young RC. Gonadal dysfunction in patients receiving chemotherapy for cancer. Ann Intern Med. 1980;93(1):109–14.
164. Whitehead E, Shalet SM, Blackledge G, Todd I, Crowther D, Beardwell CG, et al. The effect of combination chemotherapy on ovarian function in women treated for Hodgkin's disease. Cancer. 1983;52(6):988–93.
165. Biasoli I, Falorio S, Luminari S, Spector N, Federico M, et al. Fertility in female survivors of Hodgkin's lymphoma. Rev Bras Hematol Hemoter. 2012;34(1):48–53.
166. Borchmann P, Engert A. The past: what we have learned in the last decade. Hematology Am Soc Hematol Educ Program. 2010;2010:101–7.
167. Hodgson DC, Pintilie M, Gitterman L, Dewitt B, Buckley CA, Ahmed S, et al. Fertility among female Hodgkin lymphoma survivors attempting pregnancy

following ABVD chemotherapy. Hematol Oncol. 2007;25(1):11–5.
168. Behringer K, Breuer K, Reineke T, May M, Nogova L, Klimm B, et al. Secondary amenorrhea after Hodgkin's lymphoma is influenced by age at treatment, stage of disease, chemotherapy regimen, and the use of oral contraceptives during therapy: a report from the German Hodgkin's Lymphoma Study Group. J Clin Oncol. 2005;23(30):7555–64.
169. Evens AM, Advani R, Press OW, Lossos IS, Vose JM, Hernandez-Ilizaliturri FJ, et al. Lymphoma occurring during pregnancy: antenatal therapy, complications, and maternal survival in a multicenter analysis. J Clin Oncol. 2013;31(32):4132–9.
170. Schafer AI. The hypercoagulable states. Ann Intern Med. 1985;102(6):814–28.
171. Patel A, Schwarz EB. Society of Family Planning. Cancer and contraception. Release date May 2012. SFP Guideline #20121. Contraception. 2012;86(3):191–8.
172. Cardiovascular disease and use of oral and injectable progestogen-only contraceptives and combined injectable contraceptives. Results of an international, multicenter, case-control study. World Health Organization Collaborative Study of Cardiovascular Disease and Steroid Hormone Contraception. Contraception. 1998;57(5):315–24.
173. Vasilakis C, Jick H, del Mar Melero-Montes M. Risk of idiopathic venous thromboembolism in users of progestagens alone. Lancet. 1999;354(9190):1610–1.
174. Lidegaard O, Løkkegaard E, Svendsen AL, Agger C. Hormonal contraception and risk of venous thromboembolism: national follow-up study. BMJ. 2009;339:b2890.
175. Mantha S, Karp R, Raghavan V, Terrin N, Bauer KA, Zwicker JI. Assessing the risk of venous thromboembolic events in women taking progestin-only contraception: a meta-analysis. BMJ. 2012;345:e4944.
176. Zerner J, Doil KL, Drewry J, Leeber DA. Intrauterine contraceptive device failures in renal transplant patients. J Reprod Med. 1981;26(2):99–102.
177. Zerner J, Miller BA, Festino MJ. Failure of an intrauterine device concurrent with administration of corticosteroids. Fertil Steril. 1976;27(12):1467–8.
178. Hodges KR, Swaim LS. Hysteroscopic sterilization in the office setting. Obstet Gynecol Clin North Am. 2013;40(4):671–85.

Contraceptive Options for Women with Thrombophilia and Thromboembolic Disease

12

Jennifer Salcedo, Aparna Sridhar, and Tina Rizack

Introduction

Hemostasis involves a complex process of blood clot formation at the site of vessel injury. It is a delicate balance between bleeding and clotting. Both clot formation and clot lysis are linked to initially stop bleeding, and later to facilitate tissue remodeling. Excessive clot formation or reduced clot lysis can lead to excessive thrombosis. Platelets are generally the first line of defense and are activated at the site of vascular injury to form a platelet plug and trigger the clotting cascade. Tissue factor is generated at the site of the wound and interacts with factor VII to generate factor X (the extrinsic pathway), which initiates clotting. The intrinsic pathway (factors VIII, IX, XI) then amplifies this process. Antithrombin, tissue factor pathway inhibitor, and the protein C pathway are involved in the termination phase of coagulation. They are critical in mediating the extent of clot formation. The final process in hemostasis is to organize and remove the clot and restore vessel patency. This is another complex process involving plasminogen binding to fibrin and tissue plasminogen activator (tPA) leading to active proteolytic plasmin, which then cleaves fibrin, fibrinogen, and many other plasma proteins and clotting factors. If any factors are missing or dysfunctional, nonphysiologic thrombosis can occur.

Thromboembolism, of which venous thromboembolism (VTE) is the most prevalent, is related to risk factors that may be genetic or acquired, permanent or transient. The risk of thromboembolism varies throughout a woman's life, with increased risk associated with estrogen exposure. Both pregnancy and the puerperium are hypercoagulable states that prepare the body for the bleeding challenges of delivery. The incidence of thromboembolism during the postpartum period is up to five times higher than during pregnancy and approximately 22- to 84-fold higher than in nonpregnant women [1, 2]. While the risk of VTE is highest immediately following delivery and declines sharply thereafter, it remains 5 to 7 times higher from 4 to 6 weeks postpartum compared to nonpregnant, nonpostpartum women, generally reaching baseline levels by 6 weeks in average-risk women [1, 2]. Increased risk of VTE associated with pregnancy is a result of both obstruction of the venous flow

J. Salcedo, M.D., M.P.H., M.P.P., F.A.C.O.G. (✉)
Department of Obstetrics and Gynecology,
John A. Burns School of Medicine,
University of Hawaii at Manoa, Honolulu, HI, USA
e-mail: jlsalced@hawaii.edu

A. Sridhar, M.D., M.P.H., F.A.C.O.G.
Department of Obstetrics and Gynecology,
University of California Los Angeles,
Los Angeles, CA, USA
e-mail: asridhar@mednet.ucla.edu

T. Rizack, M.D., M.P.H.
Program in Women's Oncology, Women and Infants Hospital, Alpert Medical School of Brown University,
Providence, RI, USA
e-mail: trizack@wihri.org

R.H. Allen and C.A. Cwiak (eds.), *Contraception for the Medically Challenging Patient*,
DOI 10.1007/978-1-4939-1233-9_12, © Springer Science+Business Media New York 2014

from an enlarged uterus and the hypercoagulable state associated with pregnancy. Many coagulation factors increase during normal pregnancy. Additionally, fibrinolysis decreases. Estrogen-containing contraception also increases the risk of VTE. This is seen in both high-dose (50 mcg or more) and low-dose (less than 50 mcg) estrogen-containing combined hormonal contraceptive (CHC) preparations [3, 4]. Hormone therapy and hormone receptor modulators, such as tamoxifen and raloxifene, also increase the risk of VTE.

A woman's history of VTE, or risk factors for VTE, significantly impacts the choice of contraception. However, the elevated risk of VTE in pregnancy, even in the first trimester, makes effective contraception and appropriate preconception management imperative. This chapter reviews the risks for thromboembolism both outside of and during pregnancy, and the appropriate selection and use of contraception in women with a history of VTE or thrombophilia. In addition, assessment of women for clotting disorders is reviewed.

Scope of the Problem

VTE is estimated to have an overall annual incidence of 117 per 100,000 persons [5]. It is associated with major complications such as acute death from pulmonary embolism (PE), which occurs in 1–25 % of patients with VTE, and post-thrombotic syndrome, which can be disabling [6]. The incidence of VTE increases with age: at 25 years the risk is 51/100,000, at 50 it is 123/100,000, at 60 it is 207/100,000, at 70 it is 351/100,000, and at 80 it is 703/100,000 [7]. VTE is a significant issue for women due to an increased risk from pregnancy and the puerperium, as well as from the use of CHC and hormone therapy (HT).

VTE remains among the top causes of maternal death in the developed world. Pregnancy increases the risk of VTE fivefold. During the puerperium, the risk is increased by as much as 60-fold [8]. The overall incidence of VTE during pregnancy is 1–2 per 1,000 births, with an average morality rate of 0.41 % [9]. Significant risk factors for VTE in pregnancy include maternal age greater than 25 years, black race, smoking, thrombophilia, cardiovascular disease, obesity, cesarean delivery, postpartum hemorrhage, and blood transfusion. Risk factors for maternal death from VTE include black race, hypertension, cesarean delivery, and transfusion [10]. Infertility treatments, particularly when ovarian hyperstimulation syndrome and conception occur together, also expose women to a significant risk of VTE [9].

The use of CHCs approximately doubles the risk of VTE in average-risk women. Additionally, VTE risk may be higher in some formulations of CHCs than others, based on the type of progestin and route of administration [9]. Importantly, a synergistic effect exists between thrombophilias and various reproductive risks.

Patient Assessment

An identifiable risk factor, either inherited or acquired, can be established in about 80 % of patients with VTE after thorough assessment, including a detailed family history. Many patients have more than one risk factor. It is important to document the age of onset, location of any prior thromboses, and results of objective diagnostic studies for the diagnosis of VTE. Precipitating conditions such as prior surgeries, trauma, pregnancy, heart failure, travel, and immobility should be ascertained. Medications, especially the use of combined hormonal contraceptives, tamoxifen and raloxifene, or hormone therapy, should be clearly established. Additionally, a careful obstetric history should be obtained, with particular attention to recurrent fetal loss, which may suggest the possibility of an inherited thrombophilia or antiphospholipid antibody syndrome (APS). A family history that identifies one or more first-degree relatives with VTE is strongly suggestive of an inherited thrombotic disorder. History of prior or current malignancies, and adherence to routine age-appropriate cancer screening, such as pap smears, mammograms, and colonoscopy, should be reviewed.

The initial laboratory testing for a patient with VTE should include a complete blood count, coagulation studies, serum chemistries to evaluate liver and renal function, and urinalysis. Current data

Table 12.1 Thrombophilia testing[a]

Thrombophilia	Test	Test reliable during pregnancy?	Test reliable during acute thrombosis?	Test reliable in setting of anticoagulation?
Factor V Leiden mutation	Activated protein C resistance assay[b]	Yes	Yes	No[c]
Prothrombin G20210A mutation	DNA analysis	Yes	Yes	Yes
Protein C deficiency	Protein C activity (<60 %)	Yes	No	No
Protein S deficiency	Functional assay (<55 %)	No[d]	No	No
Antithrombin deficiency	Antithrombin activity (<60 %)	Yes	No	No

[a]Adapted from [25]
[b]Follow with confirmatory DNA analysis if abnormal
[c]DNA analysis is reliable in the setting of anticoagulation
[d]If necessary to test during pregnancy, recommended cutoff values for free protein S antigen levels in the second and third trimesters are <30 % and <24 %, respectively

does not support an extensive search for occult malignancy, but signs and symptoms that suggest an underlying malignancy should be pursued.

Approximately 24–37 % of all patients with a DVT have an identifiable inherited thrombophilia, and the majority of these patients have a history of familial thrombosis [11–13]. Currently, there is no consensus regarding which patients with a VTE to test for inherited thrombophilias and consultation with a hematologist is reasonable. To date there have been no randomized controlled trials assessing the benefit of testing for thrombophilia on the risk of recurrent VTE [14]. In general, testing is suggested if identifying an inherited thrombophilia would influence the duration of anticoagulant therapy or other patient management, such as selection of contraception or preconception care. For patients with an initial idiopathic (unprovoked) DVT, testing is generally favored, particularly for those with a strong family history. This should include the five major inherited defects: protein C and protein S, factor V Leiden, prothrombin 20210A gene mutation, and antithrombin III. If screening is positive, family members should then be offered screening. Deficiencies of protein C, protein S, and antithrombin are more likely in patients with initial thrombosis prior to age 50, a family history of VTE, recurrent thrombosis, thrombosis in association with CHCs or pregnancy, and thrombosis in unusual vascular beds (e.g., portal, hepatic, mesenteric, or cerebral vein thrombosis), and in patients with warfarin-induced skin necrosis [15–17]. Factor V Leiden, the prothrombin 20210A gene mutation, and APS should be tested for in idiopathic VTE in patients less than 50, and all women with hormone therapy-associated events. Testing for APS should include these antiphospholipid antibodies (aPL): IgG and IgM anticardiolipin antibodies (aCL) by enzyme-linked immunosorbent assay (ELISA), IgG and IgM anti-β_2-glycoprotein I (anti-β_2GPI) antibodies by ELISA (although testing for anti-β_2GPI antibodies may be reserved for patients suspected of APS in whom the IgG and IgM aCL and lupus anticoagulant testing are negative) [18], and lupus anticoagulant testing (dilute Russell viper venom time and activated partial thromboplastin time). Transient elevations in aPL are common and repeat testing of elevated markers after 12 weeks is recommended for confirmation of a positive test [19].

Screening for the factor V Leiden mutation is performed through a second-generation activated protein C resistance assay, with subsequent DNA analysis for diagnosis if the assay is abnormal. The resistance assay may be performed during pregnancy, but is unreliable in the setting of anticoagulation. In contrast, testing for the prothrombin gene mutation is conducted via DNA analysis, which is unaffected by pregnancy, acute thrombosis, and anticoagulation. Antithrombin deficiency is diagnosed by a measurement of antithrombin activity less than 50 % of normal [20]. Such testing is reliable during pregnancy, but not in the settings of acute thrombosis and anticoagulation (Table 12.1). Testing for protein C deficiency is performed by measuring protein C activity (either through clotting or chromogenic assays), which is reliable during pregnancy, but not in the settings of acute thrombosis or anticoagulation [21]. Protein S deficiency is diagnosed using activity assays and measurement of free protein S antigen levels, with levels less than 55 % of normal generally used as a cutoff. Testing is unreliable in the settings of acute thrombosis and anticoagulation. Additionally, testing in pregnant women is less reliable, leading to recommendations for stricter cutoffs for free protein S antigen levels in the second and third trimesters of less than 30 % and less than 24 %, respectively [22–24].

Baseline Risks of Clotting Disorders and Risks of Clotting Disorders in Pregnancy

Second only to a personal history of VTE, the presence of a thrombophilia significantly elevates a woman's risk of VTE both during pregnancy and outside of the pregnant state. Thrombophilias are present in 20–50 % of women who experience VTE during pregnancy and the postpartum period [25–28]. This section briefly explores the prevalence, diagnosis, risks, and treatment of thrombophilias both during and outside of pregnancy.

Antiphospholipid Antibody Syndrome

Antiphospholipid antibody syndrome (APS) is an autoimmune disorder characterized by the presence of characteristic clinical features, such as VTE and certain obstetric complications, and specified levels of persistent circulating antiphospholipid antibodies [29]. There are no clear data on the prevalence of APS. The diagnosis of APS requires the presence of one clinical criterion and one laboratory criterion. Clinical criteria include one or more clinical episodes of arterial, venous, or small-vessel thrombosis in any tissue or organ; one or more unexplained deaths of a morphologically normal fetus after the 10th week of gestation; one or more births of a morphologically normal fetus before the 34th week of gestation due to preeclampsia or placental insufficiency; or three or more unexplained consecutive pregnancy losses before the 10th week of gestation for which maternal anatomic and hormonal abnormalities and parental chromosomal causes have been excluded [30]. Small-vessel thromboses generally include thromboses of the glomerular, skin, retinal, bowel, hepatic, and pulmonary vessels [31]. Laboratory criteria include the presence of lupus anticoagulant, anticardiolipin antibodies (IgG or IgM), or anti-β2-glycoprotein I antibodies (IgG or IgM) detected on two or more occasions at least 12 weeks apart [32]. Venous thrombotic events are the most commonly present clinical criteria, comprising 65–70 % of total events, while cerebrovascular accidents involving the middle cerebral artery are the most common manifestation of arterial thrombosis [33, 34]. The presence of antiphospholipid antibodies is associated with obstetric complications including fetal loss, placental abruption, severe preeclampsia, and intrauterine growth restriction (IUGR). The management of affected patients during pregnancy requires treatment with either unfractionated heparin or low-molecular-weight heparin (LMWH) through a minimum of 6 weeks postpartum. The addition of low-dose aspirin may be helpful to reduce pregnancy loss among women with APS [35, 36].

Factor V Leiden and Other Factor V Mutations

The factor V Leiden (FVL) mutation has a prevalence of approximately 5 % among European populations and 3 % among African Americans [37]. Its prevalence is nearly zero among Asian and black African populations. The mutation inhibits the proteolysis of factor V by activated protein C. Women may be either heterozygous or homozygous for the mutation. The annual risk of VTE in carriers is approximately 0.45–0.58 %, compared to a 0.16 % annual incidence in the general population [38–40]. This risk varies significantly by age, with a rate of approximately 0.25 % per year in patients 15–30 years old that increases to approximately 1.1 % for patients over 60 [38, 39].

Due to the high prevalence of the mutation relative to other inherited thrombophilias, women who are heterozygous for the mutation account for approximately 40 % of VTE cases during pregnancy. However, the risk of VTE during pregnancy for heterozygotes without a personal or a close family history of VTE is approximately 0.5–1.2 %. This risk increases to 1.5 % in the setting of a first-degree relative with a history of VTE, and may reach 10 % among heterozygotes with a personal history of VTE [41–43]. In contrast, homozygotes for the mutation without a personal or a first-degree relative history of VTE have a 1–2 % risk of VTE in pregnancy, which increases to 17 % for women with such a history [41, 44].

Prothrombin Gene Mutation

The G20210A prothrombin gene mutation is present in approximately 3 % of people of European ancestry and accounts for 17 % of VTE cases in pregnancy [44]. It is a point mutation that results in increased levels of prothrombin [37]. Women heterozygous for the mutation without a personal or a close family history of VTE have a less than 1 % risk of VTE in pregnancy, while women with such a history have at least a 10 % risk [42, 44]. Homozygosity for the mutation confers a 2–3 % risk of VTE in pregnancy when no personal or first-degree relative history of VTE is present, while the presence of such a history substantially increases the risk to more than 20 % [21, 44, 45]. Additionally, the rare combination of factor V Leiden and prothrombin gene mutations results in 4 % to 5 % risk of VTE in pregnancy, even when no personal or family history of VTE is present [41].

Antithrombin Deficiency

Antithrombin deficiency is rare, occurring in approximately 1 in 2,500 people [20, 46]. It can be caused by any of more than 250 mutations that either decrease gene transcription, leading to a reduction in both antigen and activity, or alter function, leading to decreased activity in the setting of normal antigen levels [20, 37]. Additionally, antithrombin deficiency can be acquired in the settings of liver impairment, sepsis, disseminated intravascular coagulation (DIC), and severe nephrotic syndrome [21]. Outside of pregnancy, the risk of VTE is increased more than 25-fold over the general population to approximately 1.1 % per year, while VTE risk in pregnancy is approximately 3–7 % without a personal or a strong family history of VTE, and may be as high as 40 % with such a history [17, 20, 41, 47, 48].

Protein C Deficiency

Protein C deficiency occurs in approximately 0.2 % of women and is generally defined as protein C activity of less than 50–60 % of normal [20, 37, 49]. It may result from any of more than 160 mutations that lead to reductions in either antigen and activity or activity only, resulting in a highly variable phenotype [37]. In nonpregnant women, the relative risk of VTE is 6.5–12.5, with as many as 50 % of women experiencing thrombosis by age 50 [20, 37, 49, 50]. VTE risk in pregnancy is similar to that of FVL heterozygotes [47, 51]. Rare homozygosity for mutations leading to protein C deficiency results in neonatal purpura fulminans, which requires lifelong anticoagulation [52].

Protein S Deficiency

Protein S deficiency is rare, occurring in approximately 0.03–0.13 % of women. It can result from either a silenced gene or a mutation, leading to decreased free protein S antigen levels and activity [37]. The associated risk of VTE is similar to that of both factor V Leiden heterozygosity and protein C deficiency [17]. Homozygosity for protein S deficiency results in neonatal purpura fulminans, similar to homozygous protein C deficiency [52].

MTHFR and Hyperhomocysteinemia

Homozygosity for the methylenetetrahydrofolate reductase (MTHFR) gene mutations C677T and

A1298C occurs in 10–16 % and 4–6 % of Caucasians of Northern European descent, respectively. These mutations result in single-amino acid substitutions that impair folate binding and decrease the activity of the MTHFR enzyme, which leads to elevated levels of homocysteine. In turn, hyperhomocysteinemia has been associated with moderately increased risk of VTE in some geographic regions. However, a recent meta-analysis found that the increased risk of VTE associated with hyperhomocysteinemia in prospective studies was only half that previously seen in retrospective studies. Additionally, the C677T genotype was not associated with increased risk for VTE in North America, presumably due to effect modification due to the higher dietary intake of folate and riboflavin in North America, compared to Europe and other continents [53]. Significantly, approximately 40 % of white women are heterozygous for MTHFR polymorphism, which is generally associated with normal levels of homocysteine [21]. Consequently, given current evidence, the classifications of MTHFR mutations and hyperhomocysteinemia as thrombophilias for the purpose of contraceptive and pregnancy management should be avoided, and all patients should be recommended to achieve adequate vitamin intake as part of their health maintenance.

Other Thrombophilias

A large number of additional potentially thrombophilic polymorphisms are being uncovered, at an ever-increasing pace. Protein Z is a vitamin K-dependent plasma protein that serves as a cofactor for the inhibition of factor Xa by protein Z-dependent protease inhibitor (ZPI). Concomitant protein Z deficiency has been shown to dramatically increase the severity of the prothrombotic phenotype of factor V Leiden in some animal studies [54]. Additionally, in some human studies, deficiency of protein Z has been linked with thrombosis, stroke, and fetal loss. However, more studies are needed to strengthen the existing evidence [55–57].

Thrombophilia and Pregnancy Outcomes

Inherited Thrombophilias

Unlike APS, no causal link has yet been established between inherited thrombophilias and adverse pregnancy outcomes other than VTE, and available evidence currently prohibits definitive conclusions regarding such an association. Specifically, prospective studies have found no increased risk of first-trimester pregnancy loss in carriers of the FVL or prothrombin G20210A gene mutations [58, 59]. However, retrospective studies have demonstrated a modest increase in fetal loss after 10 weeks, and particularly after 22 weeks, in women with FVL [60–63]. Interestingly, FVL has been associated in retrospective studies with a protective effect against pregnancy loss before 10 weeks, and a higher rate of implantation after in vitro fertilization [21, 64, 65]. Similarly, studies have reached inconsistent conclusions regarding the association of the prothrombin gene mutation and pregnancy loss, with stronger, but still modest increases in pregnancy loss seen with increasing gestational ages in several meta-analyses [21, 60, 66]. Multiple studies have failed to note an increased risk of IUGR with FVL, the prothrombin G20210A mutation, or MTHFR mutations [59, 67–72]. Nonetheless, FVL studies have been underpowered to definitively exclude an association with early-onset severe preeclampsia or severe IUGR [21]. Antithrombin deficiency has been associated with increased rates of fetal loss, particularly after 28 weeks' gestation, as well as IUGR, abruption, and preterm delivery. However, given its low prevalence, information regarding the strength of the association between antithrombin deficiency and adverse pregnancy outcomes is limited [21, 64, 73]. Possible links have been noted between protein C deficiency and abruption and preeclampsia, as well as between protein S deficiency and late fetal loss and preeclampsia [60, 64, 74]. However, very small sample sizes in these studies limit the ability to draw firm conclusions [21].

Treatment of Thrombophilia and History of VTE in Pregnancy and the Postpartum Period

There are no large trials addressing the optimal use and dose of anticoagulants in pregnancy. Consequently, recommendations for their use are based primarily on case series and expert opinion, and significant leeway is left for clinician discretion based on risk-modifying factors such as family history, immobility, obesity, and the presence of obstetric complications [25]. According to the American College of Obstetricians and Gynecologists (ACOG), therapeutic anticoagulation during pregnancy and the postpartum period is currently recommended for women with acute VTE during the current pregnancy, those at high risk for thrombosis due to the presence of a mechanical heart valve or a history of two or more episodes of VTE, and those on long-term anticoagulation (with or without a thrombophilia) [42]. The use of prophylactic or therapeutic anticoagulation is recommended for women with two or more episodes of VTE who are not otherwise on long-term anticoagulation, whether or not a thrombophilia is present. Prophylactic or intermediate-dose anticoagulation is recommended for women with a high-risk thrombophilia and a single episode of VTE (personally or in a first-degree relative), who are not on long-term anticoagulation, and for those with a low-risk thrombophilia with a history of a single VTE, who are not on long-term anticoagulation. For the purpose of these recommendations, high-risk thrombophilias include antithrombin deficiency, double heterozygosity for prothrombin G20210A mutation and FVL, FVL homozygosity, or prothrombin G20210A mutation homozygosity. Low-risk thrombophilias include FVL heterozygosity, prothrombin G20210A heterozygosity, and protein C or protein S deficiency (Table 12.2).

Table 12.2 Classification of thrombophilias[a]

High-risk thrombophilias	Low-Risk Thrombophilias
Antithrombin deficiency	FVL heterozygosity
Double heterozygosity (FFL and prothrombin mutation)	Prothrombin mutation heterozygosity
FVL homozygosity	Protein C deficiency
Prothrombin mutation homozygosity	Protein S deficiency

[a]Adapted from [25]

Prophylactic anticoagulation is recommended for women with a history of a single episode of VTE associated with a transient risk factor that was pregnancy or estrogen related without the presence of a thrombophilia, and those with a history of a single previous idiopathic VTE who are not receiving long-term anticoagulation therapy. Prophylactic anticoagulation or surveillance is recommended for women with a high-risk thrombophilia without a history of VTE. In contrast, surveillance only is recommended for women with a history of single episode of VTE that was associated with a risk factor that is no longer present, such as surgery (excluding pregnancy- or estrogen-related risk factors) in whom no thrombophilia is present, as well as women with low-risk thrombophilias without a history of VTE. Importantly, given that the highest risk for VTE surrounding pregnancy is in the postpartum period, the level of anticoagulation selected for at least 6 weeks after delivery should be greater than or equal to antepartum treatment [25].

Neither unfractionated heparin nor low-molecular-weight heparin (LMWH) cross the placenta, and both are considered safe in pregnancy. However, LMWH is generally preferred due to its association with fewer bleeding episodes, more predictable therapeutic response, lower risk of heparin-induced thrombocytopenia, longer half-life, and less risk of bone mineral density loss [75–79]. Higher doses and more frequent administration are usually required in pregnancy for both unfractionated and LMWH due to the increase in maternal blood volume and glomerular filtration rate, which result in shorter half-lives and lower peak plasma concentrations of the medications [80–87]. Warfarin is generally avoided in pregnancy due to its link with embryopathy when exposure occurs at 6–12 weeks of gestation. Nevertheless, it is still considered for women with mechanical heart valves, due to their high risk of thrombosis even when on heparin or LMWH [88, 89]. Warfarin, LMWH, and unfractionated heparin are all compatible with breastfeeding, as they do not accumulate in breast milk and do not cause anticoagulation in the infant [90–92].

Treatment of Thrombophilia and History of VTE Outside of Pregnancy

Studies performed before the routine use of anticoagulants demonstrated a 20 % risk of fatal pulmonary embolism (PE) in patients with untreated deep venous thrombosis (DVT), highlighting the importance of anticoagulation for women in this clinical situation [93]. For women with a first VTE associated with a reversible or a time-limited risk factor (such as trauma, surgery, immobility, or estrogen use), the American College of Chest Physicians generally recommends 3 months of anticoagulation treatment. Those with an idiopathic first VTE are recommended to receive at least 3 months of anticoagulation, with annual (or more frequent) evaluation of the risks and benefits of continuing anticoagulation therapy. In contrast, women who experience a first VTE in the setting of ongoing cancer, APS, or an inherited thrombophilia, and those experiencing recurrent VTEs, are generally recommended to receive 12 months to lifetime anticoagulation [94, 95]. It is important to consider that for idiopathic and primary VTE, regardless of the duration of initial anticoagulation treatment, recurrence is highest in the 6–9 months following discontinuation of therapy. Additionally, the benefits of anticoagulation in these patients beyond 1 year begin to be diluted by the cumulative major bleeding risk of 2–3 % per year [94]. However, if anticoagulation is discontinued, aggressive prophylaxis should be considered during any high-risk situation, such as surgery or prolonged immobility.

The recommended duration of treatment for women with PE is the same as for DVT. However, patients with PE have a higher rate of mortality from recurrent VTE over the subsequent 6 months (1.4 % vs. 0.4 %), which may influence decisions regarding duration of therapy [94]. Due to the complexity of decision making for individual patients about the risks and benefits of continuing anticoagulation, other factors, such as a woman's modifiable risk factors for VTE, risk for pregnancy, and use of hormonal therapy for contraception or gynecologic treatment, should be considered when determining duration of anticoagulation treatment [96].

History of DVT/PE Without Diagnosed Thrombophilia

In addition to inherited and acquired thrombophilias, there are many other factors known to increase the risk of VTE. Such risk factors may be structural or situational, modifiable or permanent. For example, Paget-Schroetter syndrome, an inherited anatomic abnormality that causes musculoskeletal venous compression at the thoracic inlet, is associated with spontaneous upper extremity VTE. Similarly, May-Thurner syndrome, a common anatomic variant, is a hemodynamically significant compression of the left common iliac vein between the overlying right common iliac artery and the underlying vertebral body, which is associated with unprovoked left iliofemoral DVT and chronic venous insufficiency [97]. May-Thurner syndrome is most often seen in women between the ages of 20 and 50 [98, 99]. Diagnosis can be difficult because the thrombus may present high in the pelvis. Patients often have reduced left common iliac diameters or severe degrees of iliac vein compression [100, 101]. Episodes of DVT may be recurrent and poorly responsive to anticoagulation [102]. Treatment may require catheter-directed thrombolysis, venous angioplasty, or intravascular stenting, especially in those with limb-threatening thrombosis [98, 99, 103]. Congenital venous malformations of the inferior vena cava (IVC) may also lead to DVTs that can be bilateral and recurrent [104–106].

Malignancy causes a hypercoagulable state by producing substances with procoagulant activity, such as tissue factor and procoagulant, which leads to VTE in approximately 5 % of patients. Surgery further increases thrombotic risk [107–109]. Additionally, all forms of major trauma result in increased risk of thrombosis. Among patients with major trauma who underwent venographic studies, 58 % had a DVT of the lower extremities, of which 18 % were proximal. The incidence of DVT is particularly elevated following major head injuries and fractures of the pelvis, tibia, and femur [110–113]. Minor trauma occurring in the preceding 3 weeks also increases the risk of DVT by 3- to 5-fold among average risk patients, and up to 50-fold in FVL carriers [114].

Obesity predisposes patients to venous stasis, increased prothrombotic factors, and impaired fibrinolytic activity, and may be associated with decreased mobility. Obesity has been shown to be a significant risk factor for VTE in a number of studies, and this risk is potentiated by smoking, combined hormonal contraceptives, and increased age [115–123]. Obese patients with a body mass index greater than 40 have an increased risk of a first VTE with a hazard ratio of 2.7. Data from the National Discharge Survey showed a relative risk (RR) for DVT of 2.5 (95 % CI 2.49–2.51) and for PE, a RR of 2.21 (95 % CI 2.20–2.23) for such women, which was more pronounced for those under the age of 40 [124, 125].

Smoking increases the RR of thrombosis from 1.3 to 3.3. This risk increases with number of pack-years smoked [115, 123, 126–128]. Women who smoke and use CHCs have an 8.8-fold higher risk of thrombosis compared to nonsmokers using CHCs [129, 130]. Other risk factors for VTE include immobilization, heart failure, renal disease, cardiac disease, inflammatory bowel disease, and seasonal variation (highest risk in winter and lowest in summer) [131, 132].

Use of Contraception in Women with Thrombophilias or History of VTE

Scant information is available on the use of different contraceptive modalities in women with a history of thromboembolism or thrombophilia. One study found that, of women with isolated APS under hematologic specialty care who were not pregnant or attempting to conceive, 17 % were using no method of contraception, while 38 % were using condoms, and 19 % were using natural family planning methods. Additionally, of women in the same study with both lupus and APS who were not pregnant or attempting to conceive, 18 % were using no method of contraception, while 47 % were using condoms, and 13 % were using natural family planning methods. Of women with isolated APS in this study, 40 % reported that they were given no information regarding contraception following their diagnosis, while 47 % reported being instructed to avoid combined oral contraceptives due to the elevated risk of thrombosis. Of women with both systemic lupus erythematosus (SLE) and antiphospholipid antibody positivity, 35 % reported receiving no information regarding contraception, while 53 % reported receiving instructions to avoid combined oral contraceptives (COCs). Additionally, two women with APS had continued to use COCs, unaware of the potential thrombotic hazards. Importantly, while these women were often advised to avoid COCs, few were provided with information on effective alternatives, and most were relying on contraceptive methods with very high failure rates in typical use. Further, nearly 20 % of women with these disorders who were not pursuing pregnancy were using no contraceptive method. This study demonstrates a large unmet need for effective contraception in women with histories of VTE, and other women at high risk, which places these women at even higher risk for VTE associated with unintended pregnancy [133].

Risks of Contraception

Combined Hormonal Contraception (CHC)

The Centers for Disease Control and Prevention, through the US Medical Eligibility Criteria for Contraceptive Use (USMEC), classifies the use of CHC (estrogen-containing pill, patch, and ring) as category 4 in most circumstances involving prior VTE and thrombophilia, meaning that such conditions represent unacceptable health risks if the contraceptive methods are used [134] (Table 12.3). Specifically, use of CHC in women with known thrombogenic mutations or a history

Table 12.3 The US medical eligibility for contraceptive use, 2010[a]

Condition	COC/P/R	POP	DMPA	Implants	LNG-IUD	Cu-IUD	ECPs	Condom	Spermicide	Diaphragm/cap
History of DVT/PE, not on anticoagulant therapy at higher risk for recurrent DVT/PE[b]	4	2	2	2	2	1	2[c]	1	1	1
History of DVT/PE, not on anticoagulant therapy, without risk factors for recurrent DVT	3	2	2	2	2	1	2[c]	1	1	1
Acute DVT/PE	4	2	2	2	2	2	–	1	1	1
DVT/PE, established on anticoagulant therapy for at least 3 months, at higher risk for recurrent DVT/PE[d]	4	2	2	2	2	2	–	1	1	1
DVT/PE, established on anticoagulant therapy for at least 3 months, at lower risk for recurrent DVT/PE	3	2	2	2	2	2	–	1	1	1
Family history of DVT/PE in first-degree relative	2	1	1	1	1	1	–	1	1	1
Major surgery with prolonged immobilization	4	2	2	2	2	1	–	1	1	1
Major surgery without prolonged immobilization	2	1	1	1	1	1	–	1	1	1
Minor surgery without immobilization	1	1	1	1	1	1	–	1	1	1
Known thrombogenic mutations[e]	4	2	2	2	2	1	–	1	1	1
Varicose veins	1	1	1	1	1	1	–	1	1	1
Superficial thrombophlebitis	2	1	1	1	1	1	–	1	1	1

COC combined oral contraception, *P* combined patch, *R* combined ring, *DMPA* depot medroxyprogesterone acetate, *LNG-IUD* levonorgestrel intrauterine device, *Cu-IUD* copper intrauterine device, *ECPs* emergency contraceptive pills, *DVT* deep vein thrombosis, *PE* pulmonary embolus

[a]Adapted from [134]

[b]Higher risk for recurrent DVT/PE, as determined by positivity for at least one of the following risk factors: history of estrogen-associated DVT/PE, pregnancy-associated DVT/PE, idiopathic DVT/PE, known thrombophilia (including antiphospholipid syndrome), active cancer (metastatic, on therapy, or within 6 months of clinical remission) excluding non-melanoma skin cancer, and history of recurrent DVT/PE

[c]ECP use is category 2 for history of severe cardiovascular complications, including thromboembolic conditions

[d]Higher risk for recurrent DVT/PE, as determined by positivity for at least one of the following risk factors: known thrombophilia (including antiphospholipid syndrome), active cancer (metastatic, on therapy, or within 6 months of clinical remission) excluding non-melanoma skin cancer, and history of recurrent DVT/PE

[e]Including Factor V Leiden; prothrombin mutation; protein C, protein S, and antithrombin deficiencies

of VTE who are not currently on anticoagulation therapy, and who are considered at high risk for recurrent VTE, is classified as category 4 [134]. For the purposes of the USMEC, the presence of any of the following risk factors constitutes high-risk status for VTE recurrence: history of estrogen-associated or pregnancy-associated VTE, history of idiopathic VTE, known thrombophilia (including APS), active cancer or cancer within 6 months of remission (excluding non-melanoma skin cancer), and history of recurrent VTE. In contrast, women with a history of DVT or PE without any of the high-risk factors previously discussed are considered category 3 for the use of CHC, meaning that the theoretical or the proven risks generally outweigh the advantages of using the methods. Use of CHC by women with an acute DVT or PE, or by those with a history of DVT or PE who have been on anticoagulant therapy for at least 3 months, is also category 4 for women at high risk for VTE recurrence. In contrast, women with a history of VTE who are currently anticoagulated and who have absence of the high-risk factors for recurrence are given a category 3 classification for use of CHC. Women without a personal history of thrombophilia or VTE, but with a family history of VTE in a first-degree relative, are considered category 2, in which the advantages of using CHC generally outweigh the theoretical or the proven risks of the methods. Similarly, current superficial thrombophlebitis is considered category 2 for use of these methods, while the presence of varicose veins is considered category 1, a clinical situation in which there is no restriction for use of the contraceptive methods [134]. While the attributable risk of VTE associated with the use of CHC is similar in women with and without thrombophilia, the substantially higher absolute risk of VTE in those with thrombophilia led to the USMEC recommendations to avoid CHC use in that population [135]. Additionally, history of VTE in a first-degree relative (particularly if it was idiopathic or occurred at a young age) is concerning for an undiagnosed thrombophilia even in an asymptomatic patient, given the high prevalence of both the index and other thrombophilias in affected families.

However, it is important for clinicians to understand that available studies compare the risk of VTE in women using CHC with similar non-users, excluding pregnant women and those in the postpartum period. Consequently, such studies neglect that replacing CHC with less reliable contraceptive methods in young women with thrombophilia exposes them to higher risks of unintended pregnancy, and consequently to an increase in pregnancy-related VTE. Taking into account the relative effectiveness of COCs and barrier methods, one study estimated that for women with thrombophilia, a similar overall risk of VTE exists with the use of COCs as with the use of condoms (due to higher pregnancy rates in condom users), which is substantially higher than the risk with use of long-acting reversible contraception (LARC) [135, 136]. Additionally, despite its strength as a quick-reference tool, the USMEC is unable to adequately assess individual risk for VTE based on the type of thrombophilia present, or its association with other non-modifiable and modifiable risk factors, such as the coexistence of multiple thrombophilias, obesity, age, and outcomes during prior periods of hormonal exposure, such as pregnancy and estrogen-containing contraceptive use [7, 135, 137–139].

VTE Risk in Anticoagulated Women Using Hormonal Contraception

No published studies have evaluated the risk of recurrent VTE in women using CHCs while on anticoagulant therapy [140]. Published data is limited to one case report of a transverse sinus thrombosis occurring in a woman with a known thrombophilia on chronic warfarin therapy who was using a levonorgestrel IUD [141]. Diversity of expert opinion also exists on this issue. While some hematology specialists consider the use of CHCs in anticoagulated women with a history of VTE to be contraindicated (consistent with the associated USMEC category 3 and 4 classifications), others consider the use of CHCs appropriate in some circumstances (particularly when LARC and DMPA are declined or contraindicated) secondary to the idea that therapeutic anticoagulation may overcome the elevated VTE risk associated with estrogen use. We suggest that the decision to initiate CHC in such cases be made on an individualized basis in consultation with a hematologist.

Management of Perioperative Contraception

To date there is limited evidence to recommend the discontinuation of CHC prior to or after elective surgery. However, surgery is a known risk factor for thrombosis and compounds the risk of thrombosis with CHC. In patients undergoing low-risk surgery the decision to continue CHC may be appropriate. The decision to discontinue CHC must be balanced against the risk of pregnancy, but should be considered in patients with other strong risk factors such as prior VTE, high-risk procedures (such as major abdominal-pelvic surgeries, major orthopedic surgeries, colorectal surgery, major trauma, spinal cord, or cancer surgery), or anticipated prolonged postoperative immobility. In these patients, CHC should be discontinued 4–6 weeks before surgery and restarted after the elevated risk of VTE has resolved [142, 143]. In such circumstances, bridging with non-estrogen contraceptive methods should be strongly considered.

Combined Oral Contraceptives (COCs)

The USMEC recommendations for combined oral contraceptive (COC) use in women with thrombophilia or history of VTE are primarily based on case-control studies that have reported increased relative risks of lower extremity VTE during COC use in women with hereditary thrombophilic defects. For example, one study found an annual risk of VTE of 5.7 per 10,000 among FVL heterozygote nonusers of contraception, compared with 28.5 per 10,000 among FVL heterozygous women using CHC, making the VTE risk for CHC users with the mutation similar to the risk of mutation carriers in pregnancy without a history of thrombosis [144]. Similarly, another investigation found that the odds ratio for VTE in COC users heterozygous for FVL was 41.0 (95 % CI 13.5–125), compared to an odds ratio of 58.6 (95 % CI 12.8–267) in COC users with the prothrombin gene mutation, and 86.5 (95 % CI 10.0–747) for double carriers, all relative to nonusers without a thrombophilic mutation [145]. Using logistic regression, Spannagl et al. found an adjusted odds ratio for VTE of 10.2 (95 % CI 3.8–27.6) for FVL carrier COC users, compared with non-FVL carrier nonusers, but with a confidence interval that overlapped substantially with the elevated risk for VTE of 6.7 (95 % CI 3.3–13.7) for obese women in the study without a thrombophilia [146]. There is very little evidence regarding the increased risk for VTE when COCs are used by women with APS. One small study found that in women with a primary or a secondary APS diagnosis there were seven thrombotic events in a total of 32 COC users (22 %), which is more than double the background risk of thrombosis in nonpregnant women with APS without additional risk factors. However, these results may not be generalizable to all women with APS, as they represented women with active disease and recent hospitalization [133].

The absolute risk of lower extremity VTE in women with thrombophilia who use COCs appears to be notably different between different thrombophilia types. It is estimated that for all thrombophilias considered together, the annual risk of VTE in COC users is 4.62 %, compared to 1.54 % for never-users of COCs. However, the annual risk of VTE while using COCs ranged from 2.42 % for protein S-deficient women to 5.14 % for antithrombin-deficient women to 7.06 % for protein C-deficient women. These rates compare with a VTE incidence during the postpartum period of approximately 14.3 % in such patients [48].

Significantly less information is available regarding the association between COC use in women with and without thrombophilias and upper extremity DVTs. Upper extremity DVTs are quite rare generally, representing approximately 4 % of all DVTs. Further, primary upper extremity DVTs, meaning those that occur outside of malignancy and indwelling catheter use, represent only 30 % of upper extremity cases [147, 148]. The limited available studies have been inconsistent in their findings of a statistically significant association between COC use and upper extremity DVTs in women without thrombophilias, while one study noted an odds ratio of 13.6 for such DVTs in FVL and prothrombin gene mutation carriers using these methods, compared to an odds ratio of 4.2 in mutation carriers not using COCs. However, the confidence intervals overlapped significantly [149, 150].

Limited information is also available regarding the association of COC use with cerebral sinus thrombosis, a rare event that occurs in approximately four per million reproductive-aged women annually, and has a wide range of clinical presentations, which may include headache, focal deficits, seizures, and impaired consciousness [151, 152]. Women with thrombophilias are thought to have a 3- to 4-fold increased risk of cerebral sinus thrombosis at baseline, compared to women without thrombophilia, while women with thrombophilias taking COCs are likely to have 30- to 149-fold increased risk compared to nonusers without thrombophilia [151, 152]. Additionally, while thrombophilias alone have not been found to be significantly associated with ischemic stroke, COC use has been associated with elevated risk of ischemic stroke compared to nonuse, and COC use by women with thrombophilias further elevates this risk. Specifically, several case-control studies have found odds ratios for ischemic stroke of approximately 2 for COC users, compared to nonusers, with odds ratios of 11–23 for thrombophilia carriers using COCs, relative to non-carrier, nonusers [153–155].

Given an absolute risk of VTE of 0.5 per 10,000 per year for women younger than 45, it is estimated that COCs would need to be withheld from approximately 50 women with antithrombin, protein C, or protein S deficiency; 200–400 women with FVL or prothrombin gene mutations; and 2,500 women with a family history of VTE without a diagnosed thrombophilia, respectively, to prevent one VTE event. This compares to the need to withhold COCs from approximately 5,000 women in the general population to prevent such an event [156, 157]. Additionally, it is important to consider that cumulative event rates for VTE by the age of 50 are similar in women with thrombophilia who have used COCs versus those who have never used COCs, with event-free survival curves demonstrating that VTE events simply occur earlier in COC users [158].

While COCs containing 50 mcg or more of ethinyl estradiol (EE) have been associated with a higher risk of VTE than their lower dose EE-containing counterparts, the association of different progestins with VTE risk is less clear, particularly among women with thrombophilia [6]. Several studies have noted an increased risk of VTE associated with the use of third-generation progestin-containing COCs (levonorgestrel derivatives) such as desogestrel, gestodene, and norgestimate, relative to the second-generation progestin-containing COCs (gonanes derived from testosterone), such as levonorgestrel. Additionally, a similarly elevated risk has been seen with the use of the fourth-generation progestin (non-ethylated estrane) drospirenone, relative to levonorgestrel [139, 159–163]. For example, a meta-analysis of cohort and case-control studies assessing the risk of VTE among women using COCs before 1996 found an adjusted odds ratio for VTE for third-generation progestin-containing COCs of 1.7 (95 % CI 1.4–2.0), compared to second-generation progestin-containing COCs [164]. Such studies indicating an increased VTE risk among users of later generation progestin-containing COCs, as well as several highly publicized cases of VTE, led the US Food and Drug Administration (FDA) to issue a *Drug Safety Communication* stating that the use of drospirenone-containing COCs may be associated with a higher risk of VTE than other COCs. This warning was associated with additions to product labeling, despite the FDA's conclusion that it was unable to confirm causality [165].

An association between drospirenone-containing COCs and elevated VTE risk is biologically plausible, given that aldosterone has been found to upregulate the protein C receptor in human vascular endothelium, which may indicate that the antimineralocorticoid effects of drospirenone could be associated with relative hypercoagulability [166]. However, studies linking drospirenone and other later generation progestins with elevated VTE risk have been strongly criticized for methodological concerns, including failure to account for the known increased VTE risk during the first several months of COC use (or upon re-starting COCs after a hiatus), lack of statistical significance of study results, information and detection biases, errors in accounting for duration of COC use, and failure to account for confounding factors such as age and obesity [167]. Additionally, several large studies have failed to find an association between newer generation progestin-containing COCs and elevated VTE risk relative to older COCs. For instance, a cohort study of almost 60,000 European women found no evidence of an increased risk of VTE among users of drospirenone or other new progestin-containing COCs relative to users of levonorgestrel-containing COCs when accounting for the "starter effect" and controlling for confounding by factors such as duration of use, obesity, and family history of VTE [168]. Similarly, a study of almost 67,000 women undertaken using a US claims database found no evidence of an increased risk of VTE among users of drospirenone-containing COCs relative to users of COCs containing other progestin types [169].

Importantly, if an elevated VTE risk is present for later generation progestin-containing COCs relative to earlier generation progestins, the absolute risk increase is likely on the order of 1.22–7.22 cases per 10,000 woman-years for average-risk women, and is uncertain in women with thrombophilias or history of VTE [170]. This potential risk elevation should be weighed against the evidence of a lower typical-use failure rate of drospirenone-containing COCs compared to their earlier generation COC counterparts, which is presumed secondary to their substantially longer half-life, which may be more forgiving to missed or mistimed pills [171].

Contraceptive Patch

Highly publicized reports in 2004 of several fatal VTE events in patch users led to the addition of a specific FDA warning in the product prescribing information regarding an increase in estrogen exposure of patch users compared to users of COCs [172–174]. Specifically, the mean area under the curve for estrogen exposure in a cycle of patch use is approximately 1.6 times higher than with COC use, and 3.4 times higher than with contraceptive ring use. In contrast, the highest peak estrogen concentration is seen instead in COC users [175]. Interestingly, placing the patch on the abdomen has been found to result in 20 % less absorption of EE compared with the arm, buttock, or torso, which were all equivalent [176]. In a study directly evaluating the effects of different routes of CHC exposure on the intermediate outcome of clotting parameters, it was demonstrated that when COC users were switched to the patch or the ring, sex-hormone-binding globulin (SHBG) increased significantly from baseline in patch users, but not in ring users. Additionally, protein S decreased significantly from baseline in patch users, but increased significantly in ring users, while the activated protein C resistance ratio (APC-r ratio) did not change significantly from baseline in either group. Therefore, COC users who switched to the ring exhibited beneficial changes in biomarkers of thrombosis, while those who switched from COCs to the patch displayed a shift favoring clot formation [172].

Nevertheless, there is conflicting evidence on the risk of VTE in patch users compared to COC users. For instance, a US insurance claims database-based nested case-control analysis found a VTE incidence ratio of 2.4 (95 % CI 1.1–5.5) for patch compared to norgestimate-containing COC users after adjusting for high-risk factors [177]. This study was then extended to include 24 months of additional health care claims data and found that the patch was associated with a twofold higher risk of VTE (OR 2.0, 95 % CI 1.2–3.3) [178]. Similarly, a historical national registry-based cohort study from Denmark compared the risk of VTE in women using the patch with those using levonorgestrel-containing COCs and found an adjusted relative risk of 2.3 (95 % CI 1.0–5.2) [179]. Compared with users of norgestimate-containing COCs, the adjusted ratio was 2.2 (95 % CI 1.0–5.0) for patch users [179]. In contrast, another study using a similar claims-based case control design found the VTE risk with the patch to be equivalent to that of norgestimate-containing COCs with an odds ratio of 0.9 (0.5–1.6) in the initial study, and 1.0 (0.7–1.5) in the expanded study. Similarly, this study found no VTE risk difference between patch users and users of levonorgestrel-containing COCs for women 39 years old and younger [180]. According to the authors of the latter studies, their results likely differ from those of studies finding a difference in VTE risk between patch and COC users due to their studies' inclusion of only new users of both contraceptive methods, which reduced the potential for a survivor cohort effect (e.g., healthy user bias). Along the same lines, these authors stated that failure to include only new users in the initial studies was likely to have resulted in a lower reported risk of VTE among the norgestimate-containing COC users, compared to users of the newly available patch. This suggestion is supported by the fact that the incidence of VTE among the norgestimate-containing COC users in the initial studies (18.3 per 100,000 woman-years) was substantially lower than that in the latter studies (41.8 per 100,000 woman-years), while the VTE incidence among patch users was similar (40.8 per 100,000 woman-years versus 52.8 per 100,000 woman-years) [181, 182]. No published studies have compared VTE risk among patch users and COC users for women with thrombophilia or history of VTE.

While not directly comparable to hormonal contraceptives, studies of transdermal hormone therapy (HT) in the USA and Europe have generally pointed toward decreased risk of VTE relative to oral preparations (CO 556) [183, 184]. Such findings are supported by a 2010 meta-analysis that found pooled risk ratios for VTE of 1.9 (95 % CI 1.3–2.3) and 1.0 (95 % CI 0.9–1.1) among oral and transdermal estrogen users, respectively, compared to nonusers of HT. However, the estrogen component of transdermal HT formulations is estradiol, which has different effects than ethinyl estradiol, the potent synthetic estrogen used in most contraceptives, and lower doses of estrogen are used in HT. In addition, studies comparing VTE risk among users of transdermal and oral HT have been limited to case-control studies, and no randomized controlled studies comparing the two have been published to date.

Given an estimated VTE incidence of 6 per 10,000 exposure years in women using levonorgestrel-containing COCs and 14 per 10,000 exposure years in women using the contraceptive patch, approximately 1,250 women using the patch would need to switch to COCs to prevent one VTE in a year [179]. In addition, the potential for an elevated VTE risk with contraceptive patch use should be weighed against the fact that patient adherence to prescribing instructions with the weekly contraceptive patch has been found to be significantly better than with daily COCs. For example, one study found that the percentage of cycles with perfect use was significantly higher with the patch (88.7 %) than with pill (79.2 %) [185]. Consequently, it is estimated that due to improved adherence, use of the contraceptive patch instead of COCs would result in three fewer unintended pregnancies per 100 users over a 2-year period [186].

Contraceptive Vaginal Ring

Ethinyl estradiol exposure among users of the contraceptive vaginal ring is significantly less than among COC users, with peak estrogen concentration values of less than half those with COCs [187]. However, studies evaluating the effect of the vaginal ring on coagulation parameters relative to COCs are conflicting [172, 188, 189]. A large prospective multinational cohort study found a similar risk of venous and arterial thromboembolism among users of the vaginal ring and COCs [171]. However, no randomized trials have compared VTE risk between COC and ring users or between patch users and ring users, and no studies have evaluated changes in clotting parameters or VTE risk among women with thrombophilias or history of VTE.

Progestin-Only Contraception

In contrast to CHC, the USMEC classifies the use of progestin-only contraceptives as category 2 for most women with a history of VTE, including those at both low and high risk of recurrence as well as those with acute VTE or known thrombophilia. According to the USMEC, the advantages of using these methods generally outweigh the theoretical or the proven risks [134]. In support of this classification, the USMEC states that although there is no direct evidence of the use of progestin-only contraceptives in women with acute DVT or PE, including those on anticoagulation therapy, and findings on the risk of VTE for otherwise healthy women on these methods is inconsistent, any increased risk over the baseline is likely to be substantially less than with combined hormonal methods. Use of progestin-only methods in women without a personal history of venous thromboembolism, but with a history of DVT or PE in a first-degree relative, is category 1, meaning that there are no restrictions on the use of these methods. However, for women with SLE and either unknown or positive antiphospholipid antibodies, use of progestin-only contraceptives is category 3, indicating that the theoretical or the proven risks generally outweigh the advantages of such methods. This category 3 classification for women with antiphospholipid antibody positivity is based on the fact that antiphospholipid antibody positivity generally confers an increased risk of both venous and arterial thrombosis [134]. However, available evidence does not seem to support an elevated risk of thrombosis in high-risk women with the use of progestin-only methods [190, 191].

In the general population, multiple studies have failed to demonstrate a statistically significant increase in VTE in users of progestin-only contraception compared with nonusers [192–194]. Additionally, a meta-analysis that included eight observational studies found an adjusted relative risk of VTE for users versus nonusers of 1.03 (95 % CI 0.76–1.39) [190]. Importantly, in women who experienced a first VTE while using COCs, future use of progestin-only contraception was not found to elevate the risk of recurrent VTE compared to nonuse [195].

Progestin-Only Pills (POPs)

The amount of progestin in progestin-only pills (POPs) is considerably less than that commonly found in COCs. For instance, norethindrone, the only POP marketed in the USA, contains only 0.35 mg daily, approximately one-third of the dose commonly found in norethindrone-containing COCs [196]. The progestin dose in POPs is also less than that found in intramuscular injections of depot medroxyprogesterone acetate (DMPA), in which peak plasma concentrations reach 2,500–7,000 pg/mL and remain higher than 430 pg/mL for the 3 months following injection [197].

In the general population, use of POPs, including those consisting of third-generation progestins, has not been associated with increased risk of VTE versus nonuse [198]. Additionally, desogestrel and levonorgestrel progestin-only contraceptive pills available in Europe, unlike their estrogen-containing counterparts discussed previously, were found to have comparable and favorable effects on clotting parameters, including increased protein S and increased t-PA [191]. Further, in a retrospective cohort study of women at high risk for VTE due to personal history of VTE, an inherited or an acquired thrombophilia, or, less often, history of a severe or a fatal VTE in a first-degree relative, use of the POP chlormadinone acetate was found not to elevate the risk of VTE relative to nonuse [199].

Depot Medroxyprogesterone Acetate (DMPA)

While summary measures evaluating the relative risk of VTE in users of progestin-only contraceptives as a class, including DMPA, have failed to demonstrate an elevated risk compared to nonusers, subgroup analysis of DMPA in a recent meta-analysis demonstrated a mildly increased VTE risk among users, compared to nonusers (OR 2.67, 95 % CI 1.29–5.53) [190]. However, only two articles were available to evaluate this risk, depicting a total of 31 VTE events [200, 201]. Additionally, no information is available on VTE risk of DMPA use relative to that of other progestin-only methods in high-risk women, such as those with a history of VTE or thrombophilia.

Long-Acting Reversible Contraceptive (LARC) Methods

Intrauterine devices and contraceptive implants, also called long-acting reversible contraceptives (LARCs), are the most effective reversible contraceptives. These contraceptive methods do not require ongoing effort on the part of the user for effective use, which makes these types of contraceptives ideal for women with chronic medical conditions.

Etonogestrel Implant

Etonogestrel, a metabolite of desogestrel, is the active ingredient in the only contraceptive implant currently available in the USA. The USMEC suggests that the benefits of using implantable contraception outweigh the risks in women with a history of venous thromboembolism (category 2). The guidelines further recommend that women with a history of VTE associated with estrogen, pregnancy, known thrombophilias (including APS), recurrent VTE, and active cancer benefit from the usage of implants for contraception with minimal risks (category 2). Additionally, the USMEC recommends no restriction to the use of implants (category 1) for women with a family history of VTE. Contraceptive implants can also be used for women undergoing minor surgical procedures or major surgeries without prolonged immobilization without any restrictions (category 1) [134]. The USMEC highlights the safety of progestinonly contraceptives among women with acute DVT and PE and those on anticoagulation therapy [194, 202, 203]. Two studies evaluated the effect of etonogestrel on the hemostatic system and coagulation cascade [204, 205]. Both studies suggested that etonogestrel in isolation does not demonstrate a prothrombotic pattern.

There is no data on the risk of hematoma formation at the insertion site of contraceptive implants among women who are on anticoagulation. Studies evaluating the administration of intramuscular DMPA injections and influenza vaccination in anticoagulated patients have shown that injections usually are safe [206, 207]. There is theoretical risk of hematoma formation with intramuscular injections, however. Nevertheless, minor dental procedures for such patients are usually done without discontinuation of anticoagulation treatment, as discontinuation of such drugs can unnecessarily increase medical risk [208]. Given the demonstrated safety of these invasive procedures, insertion of contraceptive implants should not be withheld from anticoagulated patients without clinical or laboratory evidence of significantly supratherapeutic anticoagulation.

Levonorgestrel Intrauterine Device (LNG-IUD)

The USMEC classifies the use of LNG-IUD for the purposes of contraception as category 2 in most of the circumstances involving current or prior VTE and thrombophilia, meaning that the benefits of using the intrauterine device for contraception overweigh the risks. This includes women with a history of VTE who are not on anticoagulation therapy, with and without risk factors for recurrence. According to the USMEC, history of estrogen-related venous thromboembolic events, known thrombophilias (including APS), pregnancy-associated VTEs, and active cancer (excluding breast cancer) do not pose significant risk for LNG-IUD use for contraception purposes. The USMEC bases its recommendations on studies which suggest that the risk of VTE with the use of progestin-only contraceptives are inconsistent and any small increased risk is substantially less than that of combined hormonal contraceptives [194, 202, 203].

The higher dose LNG-IUD (Mirena, Bayer Healthcare Pharmaceuticals, Wayne, NJ, USA) has been investigated as a treatment for heavy menstrual bleeding among women with inherited bleeding disorders and hemostatic disorders, and among women on oral anticoagulation therapy [141, 209, 210]. It is clear from these studies and a related systematic review that LNG-IUD use does not pose any major bleeding risks in women on chronic anticoagulation therapy [140]. In addition, the LNG-IUD may be the preferred treatment for heavy menstrual bleeding for many women on long-term anticoagulation therapy. The USMEC further suggests no restrictions on the use of LNG-IUD among women undergoing minor surgical procedures and major surgeries without prolonged immobilization, and those with superficial thrombosis (category 1) [134]. There is no contraindication for LNG-IUD use among women with a family history of VTE [211].

Copper Intrauterine Device

The USMEC recommends no restrictions on the use of the copper IUD for women with a history of VTE who are not on anticoagulant therapy (category 1). This includes women with estrogen-associated VTE, pregnancy-related VTE, known thrombophilia (including APS), and active cancer [134]. A Finnish study noted no cases of PE among copper IUD users under the age of 40 years over 1,383,000 women-years of use [212]. The USMEC classifies the use of copper IUD for the purposes of contraception as category 2 in women with acute VTE, and those who are on anticoagulant therapy for at least 3 months [134]. This means that the benefits of using the copper IUD are thought to overweigh the risks of the method. However, literature regarding the use of the copper IUD in women on anticoagulant therapy is scant. It is known that some women using the copper IUD may experience heavier menstrual bleeding, increased duration of bleeding, or an increase in dysmenorrhea, leading to discontinuation of the method [213]. Average blood loss per menstrual cycle may increase by 55 % [214]. Since women with bleeding disorders and those on anticoagulant therapy are likely to experience a higher prevalence of gynecological problems such as dysmenorrhea, intermenstrual bleeding, and heavy menstrual bleeding, the use of the copper IUD by women in these circumstances is often suboptimal when equally effective LARC options, such as the LNG-IUD and etonogestrel implant, that decrease menstrual blood loss are available [215]. However, additional studies are needed to establish evidence-based guidelines for the use of copper IUD among women with underlying bleeding disorders (see Chap. 11 for more information). The USMEC places no additional restrictions on the use of copper IUDs for emergency contraception in women with a history of VTE or thrombophilia, and this highly effective method of emergency contraception should be provided to such patients when needed.

Barrier Methods

The USMEC places no restrictions on the use of barrier methods in women with a history of VTE, superficial thromboses, or thrombophilia [211]. Due to the theoretical concern that anticoagulated women may be at higher risk for STI acquisition given the increased potential for bleeding and abrasions with intercourse, dual method use with barrier methods should be encouraged, as for all women at risk for sexually transmitted infections. However, given the higher typical-use failure rates (up to 18 %) of barrier methods, compared to short-term hormonal and LARC methods, their use as primary contraceptives should be discouraged in women with a history of VTE or thrombophilia who have elevated risk of morbidities associated with unplanned pregnancy [216].

Emergency Contraceptive Pills (ECPs)

The 2010 USMEC provides recommendations only for the use of levonorgestrel ECPs and combined oral contraceptives used as ECPs (although combined oral contraceptives are no longer used as first-line ECPs). The benefits of ECP use outweigh the potential risks of unintended pregnancy for all patients. Specifically, ECPs are classified as category 2 for women with thromboembolic conditions [134, 211]. A review by the UK's Committee on Safety of Medicines of all the adverse events that occurred during the first 13 years and four million uses of COCs for emergency contraception noted 61 pregnancies, three cases of VTE (including one death), and three cases of cerebrovascular accidents. However, in none of the three VTE cases was the relationship between the administration of ECPs and the VTE event straightforward [217]. Other studies have affirmed the safety of progestins among women with VTE on anticoagulation [202]. Thus, a short exposure to COCs or levonorgestrel ECPs for the purpose of emergency contraception is generally not contraindicated in women with a history of VTE or thrombophilia. Further, no cases of VTE have been associated with ulipristal acetate (UPA) administration or any other progesterone receptor modulator [218]. In addition, UPA has been noted to defer or prevent ovulation more effectively than levonorgestrel, particularly during the late follicular phase [219]. UPA should thus be strongly considered for women with a history of VTE or thrombophilia when ECPs are indicated.

Sterilization

Female Sterilization Methods

The two most common methods of female sterilization in the USA are postpartum tubal sterilization using a mini-laparotomy approach and laparoscopic interval sterilization. A third and relatively newer method of sterilization, a nickel-titanium coil microinsert (Essure, Bayer Healthcare Pharmaceuticals, Wayne, NJ, USA) that involves a transcervical approach and may be performed in office settings, is gaining popularity as well. In 1996, the CDC conducted a large prospective multicenter observational study of over 10,000 women undergoing transabdominal sterilization who were followed for 14 years. The study suggested that postpartum sterilization had the lowest cumulative pregnancy rates at 5 and 10 years compared to interval sterilization methods such as bipolar cauterization of fallopian tubes or use of silastic band tubal rings [220]. The long-term effectiveness of transcervical sterilization still needs to be fully assessed. Studies of women who have undergone successful bilateral coil placement and who demonstrate complete bilateral occlusion have demonstrated cumulative failure rates of only 0.25 % over 5 years [221]. However, a recent decision analysis found that of all women who initiate this sterilization method, only 85–86 % are effectively sterilized at 3 months [222]. Given that current sterilization methods are associated with failure rates comparable to those of LARC methods, but are associated with increased risk of procedural complications (dependent on the specific technique and anesthesia used) that are elevated in women with a history of VTE or thrombophilia, the risks, benefits, and alternatives to sterilization should be carefully considered.

Challenges for Surgical Sterilization in Women with Clotting Disorders

Surgical sterilization can last anywhere from 30 min to 1 h. Most surgical sterilizations are performed under general anesthesia. Transcervical sterilization procedures can be performed in the office setting with preoperative nonsteroidal anti-inflammatory drug (NSAID) administration and paracervical block for pain control. Although regional anesthesia is associated with a significant decrease in VTE compared to general anesthesia, women on anticoagulation are not good candidates for regional anesthesia due to the risk of hematoma formation [223]. In women who are currently on oral anticoagulation for thromboprophylaxis, oral anticoagulants should be stopped 5 days before the planned laparoscopic surgical procedure [224]. Additionally, non-urgent surgical procedures such as surgical sterilization should be delayed if a thrombotic event occurred in the last 3 months [224]. Risk assessment for thromboembolism adapted from Bonnar and colleagues suggests that women with a personal or a family history of VTE or thrombophilia are at moderate risk for thromboembolism [225]. Consequently, ACOG recommends low-dose unfractionated heparin (5,000 units every 12 h), 40 mg enoxaparin daily, graduated compression stockings, or intermittent pneumatic compression devices as successful perioperative prevention strategies in such women. Unfractionated heparin (5,000 units) every 12 h or low-molecular-weight heparin 40 mg every day can be continued until the patient is discharged [226, 227]. For women on oral anticoagulation therapy, appropriate bridging anticoagulation with the administration of a short-acting anticoagulant such as low-molecular-weight heparin should be started pre- and postoperatively and continued until the patient is again therapeutic on the oral agent.

Male Sterilization Methods

Vasectomy has proven to be one of the most highly effective and reliable contraceptive methods, with a first-year failure rate of 0.15 % [216]. For women with limited contraceptive options due to a history of VTE or thrombophilia who are in stable monogamous relationships and have completed childbearing, vasectomy of the male partner should be strongly considered. Unlike female sterilization, vasectomy is almost always performed under local anesthesia using a no-scalpel approach. This is a safe, reliable technique with minimal side effects. However, the couple should be counseled that vasectomy is not immediately effective and women must use an effective adjunct contraceptive method until azoospermia is confirmed via post-vasectomy semen analysis.

Use of Contraceptive Methods for Management of Gynecological Conditions

Many women use contraceptive methods for their non-contraceptive benefits (see Chaps. 11 and 13). Improvements in menstrual cycle regularity, heavy menstrual bleeding, dysmenorrhea, premenstrual syndrome, acne, fibroids, and pelvic pain due to endometriosis are some of the potential non-contraceptive benefits of hormonal contraceptive methods. The USMEC clarifies that its recommendations refer to the use of contraceptive methods for contraceptive purposes only, and do not consider the use of such methods for the treatment of medical conditions, for which the risk-to-benefit ratio may differ significantly. Women of reproductive age who are on oral anticoagulation may experience prolonged and heavy menstrual bleeding. Specifically, a study conducted in the UK found that the mean duration of menstrual bleeding increased from 5 days before starting anticoagulation therapy to 7 days after the commencement of treatment. Additionally, the number of women experiencing passage of blood clots, intermenstrual bleeding, postcoital bleeding, and intraperitoneal hemorrhage related to hemorrhagic ovarian cysts is increased [228]. These challenges highlight the importance of using available hormonal contraceptive options to treat underlying menstrual bleeding abnormalities in anticoagulated women, in addition to their use in preventing unwanted and mistimed pregnancies.

Medication Interactions

Drug Interactions

Warfarin is metabolized by the cytochrome p450 system in the liver, primarily by cytochrome P4502C9. It is not known to be an inducer or an inhibitor of any enzymes in the cytochrome p450 system and would not be anticipated to change the efficacy of hormonal contraception (also see Chap. 20). Further, there is little evidence for clinically significant effects of hormonal contraception on warfarin metabolism [229, 230]. For example, one pharmacokinetic crossover study in ten women found no significant induction or inhibition of CYP2C9 by a triphasic COC after two cycles in healthy women [230]. Similarly, in anticoagulated women with prosthetic heart valves who received DMPA prior to hospital discharge for hemorrhagic ovarian cysts, INR values were found to remain in the therapeutic range, with the exception of rare, sporadic, INR increases that resolved with warfarin dose changes and were not accompanied by bleeding complications [206].

An isolated case report of a woman with antithrombin deficiency and history of VTE on warfarin reported an INR increase from 2.1 to 8.1 3 days following receipt of a two-dose levonorgestrel ECP regimen. Authors of this report suggest a possible mechanism of displacement of warfarin by levonorgestrel from the F1S-binding site of human alpha 1 acid glycoprotein, the main transport protein for drugs in plasma. This is a different mechanism than enzyme induction or inhibition which has not been demonstrated over the long term with concurrent use of the medications [231]. Similar to warfarin, there are no known pharmacokinetic drug interactions of heparin or LMWH with hormonal contraceptives, and no published cases or studies in the literature [140]. Given case reports of INR changes possibly precipitated by new or changed hormonal contraceptive use, some providers may choose to monitor coagulation parameters more closely in such clinical situations.

Bone Density Concerns with Concurrent Use of DMPA and Anticoagulants

Long-term use of DMPA, heparins, and warfarin has individually been associated with decreased bone mineral density (BMD) (also see Chap. 16). Consequently, a reasonable concern exists regarding the possibility of a clinically significant loss of BMD, with the potential for increased fracture risk, when DMPA is used for long-term contraception in the setting of prolonged anticoagulation. However, no studies have evaluated the effects of concurrent use of DMPA and anticoagulation on women's BMD or fracture risk, assessed the evolution of such potential effects over time, or evaluated the extent of BMD recovery after discontinuation of one or both medications. Consequently, in the absence of information about combined medication effects on BMD, anticipated effects of the individual medications must be evaluated, with attention to their respective durations of use, and an individualized risk assessment for BMD changes and fracture risk made in the setting of the patient's overall clinical context.

Clinical trials evaluating BMD loss in users of unfractionated and low-molecular-weight heparin have generally been burdened by low numbers and have been focused primarily on pregnant women. Consequently, a wide range of fracture rates have been reported and diverse methodologies have been employed in evaluating for such fractures. Available evidence suggests that the risk of osteoporosis is lower with LMWH than with heparin, but subclinical decreases in BMD have also been reported with long-term use of LMWH. Additionally, it is uncertain if all LMWHs decrease BMD loss equally [79, 232–234]. The lesser BMD loss noted with LMWH, compared to unfractionated heparin, may be due to the fact that unfractionated heparin causes bone loss both by decreasing formation and increasing resorption, while LMWHs tend to impact only bone formation.

Warfarin's impairment of vitamin K metabolism is associated with under-carboxylation of the non-collagenous bone-matrix protein osteocalcin, which is required in its fully carboxylated state for normal bone formation. Accordingly, long-term use of warfarin has been associated with reduced BMD and has been shown to increase fracture risks of the ribs and vertebra, but not of the hip. It is suggested that the difference in fracture risks among sites is due to the compensatory increase in hip strength associated with the adaption of cortical bone structure to the higher mechanical stimuli of the hip joint, relative to the ribs and vertebrae [235–237]. However, such studies have generally been limited to children, men, and the elderly.

Given the effects of DMPA and anticoagulants on BMD discussed above, several general guidelines for the use of DMPA as a contraceptive are recommended. First, the benefits of DMPA use as a short-term bridge to a more effective method, such as LARC or sterilization, in women receiving long-term anticoagulation are likely to outweigh combined medication effects on BMD in most circumstances. Similarly, women receiving anticoagulation for brief durations, such as acute treatment for VTE, or periods of prophylactic-dose anticoagulation, are likely to benefit from long-term use of DMPA as a contraceptive, if more effective methods, such as LARC, are undesired. For women in whom long-term anticoagulation is planned, particularly with unfractionated heparin or warfarin, and concurrent long-term DMPA use is considered, significant caution should be used when other risk factors for osteoporosis or fracture are present, and alternative contraception should be strongly considered. In women without additional risk factors for decreased BMD or fracture, or women with such risk factors who opt to continue long-term DMPA use with long-term anticoagulation, consideration should be given to BMD evaluation after 2 years, with transition to an alternative contraceptive method advised if significant abnormalities are noted. In all women in whom DMPA and anticoagulation are used concurrently, particular attention should be paid to adequate intake of calcium and vitamin D, as well as adequate participation in weight-bearing exercises, smoking cessation, and nutrition consultation or supplementation as appropriate.

Research Gaps

Despite what we know about VTE, significant research gaps exist in both the diagnosis and treatment of women with VTE and thrombophilias. There is limited data on determining who should be tested for thrombophilias and how testing impacts management. Additionally, thrombophilia data to date is largely based on Caucasian populations and data on non-Caucasian populations is lacking. Uncertainty exists on the risk of VTE with later generation progestin-containing

CHCs and the transdermal route of hormone administration. Further, little information is available on the VTE risks of CHC use specific to each thrombophilia, and there is no published data on VTE risk when CHCs are used by women with a history of VTE or thrombophilia who are on anticoagulation therapy. The optimal duration and intensity of anticoagulation for both treatment and prophylaxis of pregnancy-related VTE with low-molecular-weight heparin (LMWH) are unknown, as is the best way to dose LMWH. In addition, information is limited on adverse pregnancy outcomes related to thrombophilia and the extent to which prophylactic or therapeutic anticoagulation mitigates such risks.

Conclusion

Thromboembolic diseases, including VTE, are one of the leading causes of maternal mortality in the USA. However, for women at high risk of VTE due to thrombophilia or other risk factors, there is a large unmet need for appropriate contraceptive care. While combined hormonal contraception elevates VTE risk above that of nonusers, the highest risk periods for VTE are often during pregnancy and postpartum. Consequently, health care providers caring for women with VTE, or at high risk for VTE, should make every effort to address their contraceptive needs in an individualized and evidence-based fashion. This chapter reviewed current evidence on the safety of contraceptive use among women at high risk for thromboembolic disease and provides a framework for managing common contraceptive issues as they arise. Despite current research gaps, it is clear that most women under care for a current or a past VTE can safely use several effective contraceptive methods, including LARC. Given the low typical-use failure rates of LARC methods, presenting such methods as first line contraceptive agents should be routine in this population, as it should be for all women. Diligent attention to the contraceptive and preconception planning needs of women in this high-risk population will promote significant strides toward reducing unintended and mistimed pregnancy and its associated morbidity and mortality.

References

1. Heit JA, Kobbervig CE, James AH, Petterson TM, Bailey KR, Melton III LJ. Trends in the incidence of venous thromboembolism during pregnancy or postpartum: a 30-year population-based study. Ann Intern Med. 2005;143(10):697–706. PubMed PMID: 16287790. Epub 2005/11/17. eng.
2. Jackson E, Curtis KM, Gaffield ME. Risk of venous thromboembolism during the postpartum period: a systematic review. Obstet Gynecol. 2011;117(3):691–703. PubMed PMID: 21343773. Epub 2011/02/24. eng.
3. Kujovich JL. Hormones and pregnancy: thromboembolic risks for women. Br J Haematol. 2004;126(4):443–54. PubMed PMID: 15287937. Epub 2004/08/04. eng.
4. Gomes MP, Deitcher SR. Risk of venous thromboembolic disease associated with hormonal contraceptives and hormone replacement therapy: a clinical review. Arch Intern Med. 2004;164(18):1965–76. PubMed PMID: 15477430. Epub 2004/10/13. eng.
5. Silverstein MD, Heit JA, Mohr DN, Petterson TM, O'Fallon WM, Melton III LJ. Trends in the incidence of deep vein thrombosis and pulmonary embolism: a 25-year population-based study. Arch Intern Med. 1998;158(6):585–93. PubMed PMID: 9521222. Epub 1998/04/01. eng.
6. Rosendaal FR, Van Hylckama VA, Tanis BC, Helmerhorst FM. Estrogens, progestogens and thrombosis. J Thromb Haemost. 2003;1(7):1371–80. PubMed PMID: 12871270. Epub 2003/07/23. eng.
7. Naess IA, Christiansen SC, Romundstad P, Cannegieter SC, Rosendaal FR, Hammerstrom J. Incidence and mortality of venous thrombosis: a population-based study. J Thromb Haemost. 2007;5(4):692–9. PubMed PMID: 17367492. Epub 2007/03/21. eng.
8. Pomp ER, Lenselink AM, Rosendaal FR, Doggen CJ. Pregnancy, the postpartum period and prothrombotic defects: risk of venous thrombosis in the MEGA study. J Thromb Haemost. 2008;6(4):632–7. PubMed PMID: 18248600. Epub 2008/02/06. eng.
9. ESHRE Capri Working Group. Venous thromboembolism in women: a specific reproductive health risk. Human Reprod Update. 2013;19(5):471–82. PubMed PMID: 23825156. Epub 2013/07/05. eng.
10. Abbasi N, Balayla J, Laporta DP, Kezouh A, Abenhaim HA. Trends, risk factors and mortality among women with venous thromboembolism during labour and delivery: a population-based study of 8 million births. Arch Gynecol Obstet. 2013;289:275–84. PubMed PMID: 23864199. Epub 2013/07/19. Eng.
11. Makris M, Rosendaal FR, Preston FE. Familial thrombophilia: genetic risk factors and management. J Intern Med Suppl. 1997;740:9–15. PubMed PMID: 9350176. Epub 1997/01/01. eng.
12. Mateo J, Oliver A, Borrell M, Sala N, Fontcuberta J. Laboratory evaluation and clinical characteristics of 2,132 consecutive unselected patients with venous thromboembolism—results of the Spanish

Multicentric Study on Thrombophilia (EMET-Study). Thromb Haemost. 1997;77(3):444–51. PubMed PMID: 9065991. Epub 1997/03/01. eng.
13. Ridker PM, Goldhaber SZ, Danielson E, Rosenberg Y, Eby CS, Deitcher SR, et al. Long-term, low-intensity warfarin therapy for the prevention of recurrent venous thromboembolism. N Engl J Med. 2003;348(15):1425–34. PubMed PMID: 12601075. Epub 2003/02/26. eng.
14. Cohn D, Vansenne F, de Borgie C, Middeldorp S. Thrombophilia testing for prevention of recurrent venous thromboembolism. Cochrane Database Syst Rev. 2009;1, CD007069. PubMed PMID: 19160316. Epub 2009/01/23. eng.
15. Heijboer H, Brandjes DP, Buller HR, Sturk A, ten Cate JW. Deficiencies of coagulation-inhibiting and fibrinolytic proteins in outpatients with deep-vein thrombosis. N Engl J Med. 1990;323(22):1512–6. PubMed PMID: 2146503. Epub 1990/11/29. eng.
16. McColl MD, Ramsay JE, Tait RC, Walker ID, McCall F, Conkie JA, et al. Risk factors for pregnancy associated venous thromboembolism. Thromb Haemost. 1997;78(4):1183–8. PubMed PMID: 9364982. Epub 1997/11/19. eng.
17. Friederich PW, Sanson BJ, Simioni P, Zanardi S, Huisman MV, Kindt I, et al. Frequency of pregnancy-related venous thromboembolism in anticoagulant factor-deficient women: implications for prophylaxis. Ann Intern Med. 1996;125(12):955–60. PubMed PMID: 8967705. Epub 1996/12/15. eng.
18. Giannakopoulos B, Passam F, Ioannou Y, Krilis SA. How we diagnose the antiphospholipid syndrome. Blood. 2009;113(5):985–94. PubMed PMID: 18755986. Epub 2008/08/30. eng.
19. Vila P, Hernandez MC, Lopez-Fernandez MF, Batlle J. Prevalence, follow-up and clinical significance of the anticardiolipin antibodies in normal subjects. Thromb Haemost. 1994;72(2):209–13. PubMed PMID: 7831653. Epub 1994/08/01. eng.
20. Carraro P. Guidelines for the laboratory investigation of inherited thrombophilias. Recommendations for the first level clinical laboratories. European Communities Confederation of Clinical chemistry and Laboratory Medicine, Working Group on Guidelines for Investigation of Disease. Clin Chem Lab Med. 2003;41:382–91.
21. Creasy RK, Resnik R, Iams JD. Creasy and Resnik's maternal-fetal medicine: principles and practice, xvii. 6th ed. Philadelphia: Saunders/Elsevier; 2009. 1282 pp.
22. Paidas MJ, Ku DH, Lee MJ, Manish S, Thurston A, Lockwood CJ, et al. Protein Z, protein S levels are lower in patients with thrombophilia and subsequent pregnancy complications. J Thromb Haemost. 2005;3:497–501.
23. Goodwin AJ, Rosendaal FR, Kottke-Marchant K, Bovill EG. A review of the technical, diagnostic, and epidemiologic considerations for protein S assays. Arch Path Lab Med. 2002;126:1349–66.
24. Fardella P, Parra M, Conte G, Flores C, Munoz H, Soto L, et al. Free protein S (PS) in normal pregnancy: a comparison between two analytical methods. Rev Med Chil. 2005;133:633–8. Spanish.
25. ACOG Practice Bulletin No. 138. Inherited thrombophilias in pregnancy. Obstet Gynecol. 2013; 122(3):706–17. PubMed PMID: 23963422. Epub 2013/08/22. eng.
26. James AH, Tapson VF, Goldhaber SZ. Thrombosis during pregnancy and the postpartum period. Am J Obstet Gynecol. 2005;193:216–9.
27. James AH, Jamison MG, Brancazio LR, Myers ER. Venous thromboembolism during pregnancy and the postpartum period: incidence, risk factors, and mortality. Am J Obstet Gynecol. 2006;194: 1311–5.
28. James AH. Venous thromboembolism in pregnancy. Arterioscler Thromb Vasc Biol. 2009;29:326–31.
29. Wilson WA, Gharavi AE, Koike T, Lockshin MD, Branch DW, Piette JC, et al. International consensus statement on preliminary classification criteria for definite antiphospholipid syndrome: report of an international workshop. Arthritis Rheum. 1999;42(7):1309–11. PubMed PMID: 10403256. Epub 1999/07/14. eng.
30. Practice Bulletin No. 132. Antiphospholipid syndrome. Obstet Gynecol. 2012;120(6):1514–21. PubMed PMID: 23168789. Epub 2012/11/22. eng.
31. Asherson RA, Cervera R. Microvascular and microangiopathic antiphospholipid-associated syndromes ("MAPS"): semantic or antisemantic? Autoimmun Rev. 2008;7(3):164–7. PubMed PMID: 18190872. Epub 2008/01/15. eng.
32. Miyakis S, Lockshin MD, Atsumi T, Branch DW, Brey RL, Cervera R, et al. International consensus statement on an update of the classification criteria for definite antiphospholipid syndrome (APS). J Thromb Haemost. 2006;4(2):295–306. PubMed PMID: 16420554. Epub 2006/01/20. eng.
33. Khamashta MA, Cuadrado MJ, Mujic F, Taub NA, Hunt BJ, Hughes GR. The management of thrombosis in the antiphospholipid-antibody syndrome. N Engl J Med. 1995;332(15):993–7. PubMed PMID: 7885428. Epub 1995/04/13. eng.
34. Silver RM, Draper ML, Scott JR, Lyon JL, Reading J, Branch DW. Clinical consequences of antiphospholipid antibodies: an historic cohort study. Obstet Gynecol. 1994;83(3):372–7. PubMed PMID: 8127528. Epub 1994/03/01. eng.
35. Bates SM, Greer IA, Middeldorp S, Veenstra DL, Prabulos AM, Vandvik PO. VTE, thrombophilia, antithrombotic therapy, and pregnancy: Antithrombotic Therapy and Prevention of Thrombosis, 9th ed. American College of Chest Physicians Evidence-Based Clinical Practice Guidelines. Chest. 2012;141(2 Suppl):e691S–736S. PubMed PMID: 22315276. Pubmed Central PMCID: PMC3278054. Epub 2012/02/15. eng.
36. Empson M, Lassere M, Craig JC, Scott JR. Recurrent pregnancy loss with antiphospholipid antibody: a systematic review of therapeutic trials. Obstet Gynecol. 2002;99(1):135–44. PubMed PMID: 11777524. Epub 2002/01/05. eng.

37. Franco RF, Reitsma PH. Genetic risk factors of venous thrombosis. Hum Genet. 2001;109:369–84.
38. Middeldorp S, Henkens CM, Koopman MM, Van Pampus EC, Hamulyak K, Van der Meer J, et al. The incidence of venous thromboembolism in family members of patients with factor V Leiden mutation and venous thrombosis. Ann Intern Med. 1998;128:15–20.
39. Middeldorp S, Meinardi JR, Koopman MM, Van Pampus EC, Hamulyak K, Van der Meer J, et al. A prospective study of asymptomatic carriers of the factor V Leiden mutation to determine incidence of venous thromboembolism. Ann Intern Med. 2001; 135:322–7.
40. Nordstrom M, Lindblad B, Bergqvist D, Kjellstrom T. A prospective study of the incidence of deep-vein thrombosis within a defined urban population. J Intern Med. 1992;232:155–60.
41. Zotz RG, Gerhardt A, Scharf RE. Inherited thrombophilia and gestational venous thromboembolism. Best Pract Res Clin Haematol. 2003;16:243–59.
42. Bates SM, Greer IA, Middeldorp S, Veenstra DL, Prabulos AM, Vandvik PO. VTE, thrombophilia, antithrombotic therapy, and pregnancy: antithrombotic therapy and prevention of thrombosis, 9th ed. American College of Chest Physicians evidence-based clinical practice guidelines. Chest. 2012;41: 691s–736s.
43. Pabinger I, Grafenhofer H, Kaider A, Kyrle PA, Quehenberger P, Manhalter C, et al. Risk of pregnancy-associated recurrent venous thromboembolism in women with a history of venous thrombosis. J Thromb Haemost. 2005;3:949–54.
44. Gerhardt A, Scharf RE, Beckmann MW, Struve S, Bender HG, Pillny M, et al. Prothrombin and factor V mutations in women with a history of thrombosis during pregnancy and the puerperium. N Engl J Med. 2000;342:374–80.
45. Field SL, Brighton TA, McNeil HP, et al. Recent insights into antiphospholipid antibody-mediated thrombosis. Baillieres Best Pract Res Clin Haematol. 1999;12:407–22.
46. Hellgren M, Tengborn L, Abildgaard U. Pregnancy in women with congenital antithrombin III deficiency: experience of treatment with heparin and antithrombin. Gynecol Obstet Invest. 1982;14: 127–41.
47. De Stefano V, Leone G, Mastrangelo S, Tripodi A, Rodeghiero F, Castaman G, et al. Thrombosis during pregnancy and surgery in patients with congenital deficiency of antithrombin III, protein C, protein S. Thromb Haemost. 1994;71:799–800.
48. Van Boven HH, Vandenbroucke JP, Briet E, Rosendaal FR. Gene-gene and gene-environment interactions determine risk of thrombosis in families with inherited antithrombin deficiency. Blood. 1999;94:2590–4.
49. Vossen CY, Preston FE, Conard J, Fontcuberta J, Makris M, van der Meer FJ, et al. Hereditary thrombophilia and fetal loss: a prospective follow-up study. J Thromb Haemost. 2004;2:592–6.
50. Anderson Jr FA, Spencer FA. Risk factors for venous thromboembolism. Circulation. 2003;107(23 Suppl 1):I9–16. PubMed PMID: 12814980. Epub 2003/06/20. eng.
51. Conard J, Horellou MH, Van Dreden P, Lecompte T, Samama M. Thrombosis and pregnancy in congenital deficiencies in AT III, protein C or protein S: study of 78 women. Thromb Haemost. 1990;63: 319–20.
52. Marlar RA, Neumann A. Neonatal purpura fulminans due to homozygous protein C or protein S deficiencies. Semin Thromb Hemost. 1990;16:299–309.
53. Den Heijer M, Lewington S, Clarke R. Homocysteine, MTHFR and risk of venous thrombosis: a meta-analysis of published epidemiological studies. J Thromb Haemost. 2005;3:292–9.
54. Broze Jr GJ. Protein Z-dependent regulation of coagulation. Thromb Haemost. 2001;86(1):8–13. PubMed PMID: 11487045. Epub 2001/08/07. eng.
55. Corral J, Gonzalez-Conejero R, Hernandez-Espinosa D, Vicente V. Protein Z/Z-dependent protease inhibitor (PZ/ZPI) anticoagulant system and thrombosis. Br J Haematol. 2007;137(2):99–108. PubMed PMID: 17391489. Epub 2007/03/30. eng.
56. Vasse M, Guegan-Massardier E, Borg JY, Woimant F, Soria C. Frequency of protein Z deficiency in patients with ischaemic stroke. Lancet. 2001;357(9260):933–4. PubMed PMID: 11289354. Epub 2001/04/06. eng.
57. Gris JC, Quere I, Dechaud H, Mercier E, Pincon C, Hoffet M, et al. High frequency of protein Z deficiency in patients with unexplained early fetal loss. Blood. 2002;99(7):2606–8. PubMed PMID: 11895801. Epub 2002/03/16. eng.
58. Dizon-Townson D, Miller C, Sibai B, Spong CY, Thom E, Wendel G, et al. The relationship of the factor V Leiden mutation and pregnancy outcomes for mother and fetus. National Institute of Child Health and Human Development Maternal-Fetal Medicine Units Network. Obstet Gynecol. 2005;106:517–24.
59. Silver RM, Zhao Y, Spong CY, Sibai B, Wendel G, Wenstrom K, et al. Prothrombin gene G20210A mutation and obstetric complications. Eunice Kennedy Shriver National Institute of Child Health and Human Development Maternal-Fetal Medicine Units (NICHD MFMU) Network. Obstet Gynecol. 2010;115:14–20.
60. Rey E, Kahn SR, David M, Shrier I. Thrombophilic disorders and fetal loss: a meta-analysis. Lancet. 2003;361:901–8.
61. Gris JC, Quere I, Monpeyroux F, Mercier E, Ripart-Neveu S, Tailland ML, et al. Case-control study of the frequency of thrombophilic disorders in couples with late foetal loss and no thrombotic antecedent: The Nimes Obstetricians and Haematologists Study 5 (NOHA5). Thromb Haemost. 1999;81:891–9.
62. Dudding TE, Attia J. The association between adverse pregnancy outcomes and maternal factor V Leiden genotype: a meta-analysis. Thromb Haemost. 2004;91:700–11.

63. Lissalde-Lavigne G, Fabbro-Peray P, Quere I, Mercier E, Ripart-Neveu S, Balducchi JP, et al. Factor V Leiden and prothrombin G20210A polymorphisms as risk factors for miscarriage during a first intended pregnancy: the matched case-control "NOHA First" study. J Thromb Haemost. 2005;3:2178–84.
64. Roque H, Paidas MJ, Funai EF, Kuczynski E, Lockwood CJ. Maternal thromophilias are not associated with early pregnancy loss. Thromb Haemost. 2004;91:290–5.
65. Gopel W, Ludwig M, Junge AK, Kohlmann T, Diedrich K, Möller J. Selection pressure for the factor V-Leiden mutation and embryo implantation. Lancet. 2001;358:1238–9.
66. Kovalevsky G, Gracia CR, Berlin JA, Sammel MD, Barnhart KT. Evaluation of the association between hereditary thrombophilias and recurrent pregnancy loss: a meta-analysis. Arch Intern Med. 2004;164: 558–63.
67. Kupferminc MJ, Eldor A, Steinman N, Many A, Bar-Am A, Jaffa A, et al. Increased frequency of genetic thrombophilia in women with complications of pregnancy. N Engl J Med. 1999;340:9–13.
68. D'Elia AV, Driul L, Giacomello R, Colaone R, Fabbro D, Di Leonardo C, et al. Frequency of factor V, prothrombin and methylenetetrahydrofolate reductase gene variants in preeclampsia. Gynecol Obstet Invest. 2002;53:84–7.
69. Howley HE, Walker M, Rodger MA. A systematic review of the association between factor V Leiden or prothrombin gene variant and intrauterine growth restriction. Am J Obstet Gynecol. 2005;192:694–708.
70. Franchi F, Cetin I, Todros T, Antonazzo P, Nobile de Santis MS, Cardaropoli MS, et al. Intrauterine growth restriction and genetic predisposition to thrombophilia. Haematologica. 2004;89:444–9.
71. Verspyck E, Borg JY, Le Cam-Duchez V, Goffinet F, Degre S, Fournet P, et al. Thrombophilia and fetal growth restriction. Eur J Obstet Gynecol Reprod Biol. 2004;113:36–40.
72. Infante-Rivard C, Rivard GE, Yotov WV, Genin E, Guiguet M, Weinberg C, et al. Absence of association of thrombophilia polymorphisms with intrauterine growth restriction. N Engl J Med. 2002;347:19–25.
73. Preston FE, Rosendaal FR, Walker ID, Briët E, Berntorp E, Conard J, et al. Increased fetal loss in women with heritable thrombophilia. Lancet. 1996; 48:913–6.
74. Alfirevic Z, Roberts D, Martlew V. How strong is the association between maternal thrombophilia and adverse pregnancy outcome? A systematic review. Eur J Obstet Gynecol Reprod Biol. 2002;101:6–14.
75. Flessa HC, Kapstrom AB, Glueck HI, Will JJ. Placental transport of heparin. Am J Obstet Gynecol. 1965;93:570–3.
76. Harenberg J, Schneider D, Heilmann L, Wolf H. Lack of anti-factor Xa activity in umbilical cord vein samples after subcutaneous administration of heparin or low molecular mass heparin in pregnant women. Haemostasis. 1993;23:314–20.
77. Greer IA, Nelson-Piercy C. Low-molecular-weight heparins for thromboprophylaxis and treatment of venous thromboembolism in pregnancy: a systematic review of safety and efficacy. Blood. 2005;106: 401–7.
78. Sanson BJ, Lensing AW, Prins MH, Ginsberg JS, Barkagan ZS, Lavenne-Pardonge E. Safety of low-molecular weight heparin in pregnancy: a systematic review. Thromb Haemost. 1999;81:668–72.
79. Pettila V, Leinonen P, Markkola A, Hiilesmaa V, Kaaja R. Postpartum bone mineral density in women treated for thromboprophylaxis with unfractionated heparin or LMW heparin. Thromb Haemost. 2002;87:182–6.
80. James AH, Abel DE, Brancazio LR. Anticoagulants in pregnancy. Obstet Gynecol Surv. 2006;61:59–69.
81. Brancazio LR, Roperti KA, Stierer R, Laifer SA. Pharmacokinetics and pharmacodynamics of subcutaneous heparin during the early third trimester of pregnancy. Am J Obstet Gynecol. 1995;173: 1240–5.
82. Casele HL, Laifer SA, Woelkers DA, Venkataramanan R. Changes in the pharmacokinetics of the low-molecular-weight heparin enoxaparin sodium during pregnancy. Am J Obstet Gynecol. 1999;181:1113–7.
83. Barbour LA, Oja JL, Schultz LK. A prospective trial that demonstrates dalteparin requirements increase in pregnancy to maintain therapeutic levels of anticoagulation. Am J Obstet Gynecol. 2004;191:1024–9.
84. Lykke JA, Gronlykke T, Langhoff-Roos J. Treatment of deep venous thrombosis in pregnant women. Acta Obstet Gynecol Scand. 2008;87:1248–51.
85. Norris LA, Bonnar J, Smith MP, Steer PJ, Savidge G. Low molecular weight heparin (tinzaparin) therapy for moderate risk thromboprophylaxis during pregnancy. A pharmacokinetic study. Thromb Haemost. 2004;92:791–6.
86. Lebaudy C, Hulot JS, Amoura Z, Costedoat-Chalumeau N, Serreau R, Ankri A, et al. Changes in enoxaparin pharmacokinetics during pregnancy and implications for anti-thrombotic therapeutic strategy. Clin Pharmacol Ther. 2008;84:370–7.
87. Fox NS, Laughon SK, Bender SD, Saltzman DH, Rebarber A. Anti-factor Xa plasma levels in pregnant women receiving low molecular weight heparin thromboprophylaxis. Obstet Gynecol. 2008;112: 884–9.
88. Iturbe-Alessio I, Fonseca MC, Mutchinik O, Santos MA, Zajarias A, Salazar E. Risks of anticoagulant therapy in pregnant women with artificial heart valves. N Engl J Med. 1986;315:1390–3.
89. Elkayam U, Bitar F. Valvular heart disease and pregnancy part I: native valves. J Am Coll Cardiol. 2005;46:223–30.
90. Clark SL, Porter TF, West FG. Coumarin derivatives and breast-feeding. Obstet Gynecol. 2000;95: 938–40.
91. Orme ML, Lewis PJ, de Swiet M, Serlin MJ, Sibeon R, Baty JD, et al. May mothers given warfarin breast-feed their infants? Br Med J. 1977;1:1564–5.

92. Richter C, Sitzmann J, Lang P, Weitzel H, Huch A, Huch R. Excretion of low molecular weight heparin in human milk. Br J Clin Pharmacol. 2001;52: 708–10.
93. Barritt DW, Jordan SC. Anticoagulant drugs in the treatment of pulmonary embolism. A controlled trial. Lancet. 1960;1:1309–12.
94. Myers TM. Long-term anticoagulation prophylaxis following acute thromboembolism. Dis Mon. 2005;51:158–65.
95. Kearon C, Akl EA, Comerota AJ, Prandoni P, Bounameaux H, Goldhaber SZ, et al. Antithrombotic therapy for VTE disease: antithrombotic therapy and prevention of thrombosis, 9th ed. American College of Chest Physicians evidence-based clinical practice guidelines. Chest. 2012;141:e419s–94s.
96. Le Moigne E, Delluc A, Tromeur C, Nowak E, Mottier D, Lacut K, et al. Risk of recurrent venous thromboembolism among young women after a first event while exposed to combined oral contraception versus not exposed to: a cohort study. Thromb Res. 2013;132:51–5.
97. Kibbe MR, Ujiki M, Goodwin AL, Eskandari M, Yao J, Matsumura J. Iliac vein compression in an asymptomatic patient population. J Vasc Surg. 2004;39(5):937–43. PubMed PMID: 15111841. Epub 2004/04/28. eng.
98. O'Sullivan GJ, Semba CP, Bittner CA, Kee ST, Razavi MK, Sze DY, et al. Endovascular management of iliac vein compression (May-Thurner) syndrome. J Vasc Interv Radiol. 2000;11(7):823–36. PubMed PMID: 10928517. Epub 2000/08/06. eng.
99. Patel NH, Stookey KR, Ketcham DB, Cragg AH. Endovascular management of acute extensive iliofemoral deep venous thrombosis caused by May-Thurner syndrome. J Vasc Interv Radiol. 2000;11(10):1297–302. PubMed PMID: 11099239. Epub 2000/12/01. eng.
100. Carr S, Chan K, Rosenberg J, Kuo WT, Kothary N, Hovsepian DM, et al. Correlation of the diameter of the left common iliac vein with the risk of lower-extremity deep venous thrombosis. J Vasc Interv Radiol. 2012;23(11):1467–72. PubMed PMID: 23101919. Epub 2012/10/30. eng.
101. Narayan A, Eng J, Carmi L, McGrane S, Ahmed M, Sharrett AR, et al. Iliac vein compression as risk factor for left- versus right-sided deep venous thrombosis: case-control study. Radiology. 2012;265(3):949–57. PubMed PMID: 23175547. Pubmed Central PMCID: 3504322. Epub 2012/11/24. eng.
102. Sharaf M. Recurrent left-leg venous thrombosis in a woman despite a therapeutic international normalized ratio. CMAJ. 2005;173(9):1032. PubMed PMID: 16247096. Pubmed Central PMCID: 1266323. Epub 2005/10/26. eng.
103. Lamont JP, Pearl GJ, Patetsios P, Warner MT, Gable DR, Garrett W, et al. Prospective evaluation of endoluminal venous stents in the treatment of the May-Thurner syndrome. Ann Vasc Surg. 2002;16(1):61–4. PubMed PMID: 11904806. Epub 2002/03/21. eng.
104. Chee YL, Culligan DJ, Watson HG. Inferior vena cava malformation as a risk factor for deep venous thrombosis in the young. Br J Haematol. 2001; 114(4):878–80. PubMed PMID: 11564079. Epub 2001/09/21. eng.
105. Ruggeri M, Tosetto A, Castaman G, Rodeghiero F. Congenital absence of the inferior vena cava: a rare risk factor for idiopathic deep-vein thrombosis. Lancet. 2001;357(9254):441. PubMed PMID: 11273066. Epub 2001/03/29. eng.
106. Lambert M, Marboeuf P, Midulla M, Trillot N, Beregi JP, Mounier-Vehier C, et al. Inferior vena cava agenesis and deep vein thrombosis: 10 patients and review of the literature. Vasc Med. 2010;15(6):451–9. PubMed PMID: 21183652. Epub 2010/12/25. eng.
107. White RH, Zhou H, Romano PS. Incidence of symptomatic venous thromboembolism after different elective or urgent surgical procedures. Thromb Haemost. 2003;90(3):446–55. PubMed PMID: 12958614. Epub 2003/09/06. eng.
108. Lee AY, Gent M, Julian JA, Bauer KA, Eriksson BI, Lassen MR, et al. Bilateral vs ipsilateral venography as the primary efficacy outcome measure in thromboprophylaxis clinical trials: a systematic review. J Thromb Haemost. 2004;2(10):1752–9. PubMed PMID: 15456486. Epub 2004/10/01. eng.
109. Maxwell GL, Synan I, Dodge R, Carroll B, Clarke-Pearson DL. Pneumatic compression versus low molecular weight heparin in gynecologic oncology surgery: a randomized trial. Obstet Gynecol. 2001;98(6):989–95. PubMed PMID: 11755543. Epub 2002/01/05. eng.
110. Geerts WH, Code KI, Jay RM, Chen E, Szalai JP. A prospective study of venous thromboembolism after major trauma. N Engl J Med. 1994;331(24):1601–6. PubMed PMID: 7969340. Epub 1994/12/15. eng.
111. Montgomery KD, Geerts WH, Potter HG, Helfet DL. Thromboembolic complications in patients with pelvic trauma. Clin Orthop Relat Res. 1996;329:68–87. PubMed PMID: 8769438. Epub 1996/08/01. eng.
112. Geerts WH, Jay RM, Code KI, Chen E, Szalai JP, Saibil EA, et al. A comparison of low-dose heparin with low-molecular-weight heparin as prophylaxis against venous thromboembolism after major trauma. N Engl J Med. 1996;335(10):701–7. PubMed PMID: 8703169. Epub 1996/09/05. eng.
113. McLaughlin DF, Wade CE, Champion HR, Salinas J, Holcomb JB. Thromboembolic complications following trauma. Transfusion. 2009;49 Suppl 5:256S–63S. PubMed PMID: 19954488. Epub 2009/12/04. eng.
114. van Stralen KJ, Rosendaal FR, Doggen CJ. Minor injuries as a risk factor for venous thrombosis. Arch Intern Med. 2008;168(1):21–6. PubMed PMID: 18195191. Epub 2008/01/16. eng.
115. Holst AG, Jensen G, Prescott E. Risk factors for venous thromboembolism: results from the Copenhagen City Heart Study. Circulation. 2010;121(17):1896–903. PubMed PMID: 20404252. Epub 2010/04/21. eng.

116. Goldhaber SZ, Savage DD, Garrison RJ, Castelli WP, Kannel WB, McNamara PM, et al. Risk factors for pulmonary embolism. The Framingham Study. Am J Med. 1983;74(6):1023–8. PubMed PMID: 6859053. Epub 1983/06/01. eng.
117. Hansson PO, Eriksson H, Welin L, Svardsudd K, Wilhelmsen L. Smoking and abdominal obesity: risk factors for venous thromboembolism among middle-aged men: "the study of men born in 1913". Arch Intern Med. 1999;159(16):1886–90. PubMed PMID: 10493318. Epub 1999/09/24. eng.
118. Kucher N, Tapson VF, Goldhaber SZ. Risk factors associated with symptomatic pulmonary embolism in a large cohort of deep vein thrombosis patients. Thromb Haemost. 2005;93(3):494–8. PubMed PMID: 15735800. Epub 2005/03/01. eng.
119. Samama MM. An epidemiologic study of risk factors for deep vein thrombosis in medical outpatients: the Sirius study. Arch Intern Med. 2000;160(22): 3415–20. PubMed PMID: 11112234. Epub 2000/12/09. eng.
120. Pomp ER, le Cessie S, Rosendaal FR, Doggen CJ. Risk of venous thrombosis: obesity and its joint effect with oral contraceptive use and prothrombotic mutations. Br J Haematol. 2007;139(2):289–96. PubMed PMID: 17897305. Epub 2007/09/28. eng.
121. Delluc A, Mottier D, Le Gal G, Oger E, Lacut K. Underweight is associated with a reduced risk of venous thromboembolism. Results from the EDITH case-control study. J Thromb Haemost. 2009;7(4):728–9. PubMed PMID: 19192117. Epub 2009/02/05. eng.
122. Severinsen MT, Kristensen SR, Johnsen SP, Dethlefsen C, Tjonneland A, Overvad K. Anthropometry, body fat, and venous thromboembolism: a Danish follow-up study. Circulation. 2009;120(19):1850–7. PubMed PMID: 19858417. Epub 2009/10/28. eng.
123. Wattanakit K, Lutsey PL, Bell EJ, Gornik H, Cushman M, Heckbert SR, et al. Association between cardiovascular disease risk factors and occurrence of venous thromboembolism. A time-dependent analysis. Thromb Haemost. 2012;108(3):508–15. PubMed PMID: 22782466. Pubmed Central PMCID: 3482827. Epub 2012/07/12. eng.
124. Tsai AW, Cushman M, Rosamond WD, Heckbert SR, Polak JF, Folsom AR. Cardiovascular risk factors and venous thromboembolism incidence: the longitudinal investigation of thromboembolism etiology. Arch Intern Med. 2002;162(10):1182–9. PubMed PMID: 12020191. Epub 2002/05/22. eng.
125. Stein PD, Beemath A, Olson RE. Obesity as a risk factor in venous thromboembolism. Am J Med. 2005;118(9):978–80. PubMed PMID: 16164883. Epub 2005/09/17. eng.
126. Severinsen MT, Overvad K, Johnsen SP, Dethlefsen C, Madsen PH, Tjonneland A, et al. Genetic susceptibility, smoking, obesity and risk of venous thromboembolism. Br J Haematol. 2010;149(2):273–9. PubMed PMID: 20148880. Epub 2010/02/13. eng.
127. Goldhaber SZ, Grodstein F, Stampfer MJ, Manson JE, Colditz GA, Speizer FE, et al. A prospective study of risk factors for pulmonary embolism in women. JAMA. 1997;277(8):642–5. PubMed PMID: 9039882. Epub 1997/02/26. eng.
128. Blondon M, Wiggins KL, McKnight B, Psaty BM, Rice KM, Heckbert SR, et al. The association of smoking with venous thrombosis in women. A population-based, case-control study. Thromb Haemost. 2013;109(5):891–6.
129. Farmer RD, Lawrenson RA, Todd JC, Williams TJ, MacRae KD, Tyrer F, et al. A comparison of the risks of venous thromboembolic disease in association with different combined oral contraceptives. Br J Clin Pharmacol. 2000;49(6):580–90. PubMed PMID: 10848722. Pubmed Central PMCID: 2015039. Epub 2000/06/10. eng.
130. Pomp ER, Rosendaal FR, Doggen CJ. Smoking increases the risk of venous thrombosis and acts synergistically with oral contraceptive use. Am J Hematol. 2008;83(2):97–102. PubMed PMID: 17726684. Epub 2007/08/30. eng.
131. Boulay F, Berthier F, Schoukroun G, Raybaut C, Gendreike Y, Blaive B. Seasonal variations in hospital admission for deep vein thrombosis and pulmonary embolism: analysis of discharge data. BMJ. 2001;323(7313):601–2. PubMed PMID: 11557707. Pubmed Central PMCID: 55575. Epub 2001/09/15. eng.
132. Lindqvist PG, Epstein E, Olsson H. Does an active sun exposure habit lower the risk of venous thrombotic events? A D-lightful hypothesis. J Thromb Haemost. 2009;7(4):605–10. PubMed PMID: 19335448. Epub 2009/04/02. eng.
133. Lakasing L, Khamashta M. Contraceptive practices in women with systemic lupus erythematosus and/or antiphospholipid syndrome: What advice should we be giving? J Fam Plann Reprod Health Care. 2001;27:7 12.
134. Curtis KM, Tepper NK, Marchbanks PA. U.S. medical eligibility criteria for contraceptive use, 2010. J Women's Health. 2011;20(6):825–8. PubMed PMID: 21671772. Epub 2011/06/16. eng.
135. Middeldorp S. Thrombosis in women: what are the knowledge gaps in 2013? J Thromb Haemost. 2013;11:180–91.
136. Van Vlijmen EF, Veeger NJ, Middeldorp S, Hamulyak K, Prins MH, Buller HR, et al. Thrombotic risk during oral contraceptive use and pregnancy in women with factor-V-Leiden or prothrombin mutation; a rational approach to contraception. Blood. 2011;8:2055–61.
137. Nordstrom M, Lindblad B, Bergqvist D, Kjellstrom T. A prospective study of the incidence of deep-vein thrombosis within a defined urban population. J Intern Med. 1992;2:155–60.
138. Anderson FA, Wheeler HB, Goldberg AB, Hosmer DW, Patwardhan NA, Jovanovic B, et al. A population-based perspective of the hospital incidence and case-fatality rates of deep vein thrombosis

and pulmonary embolism. The Worcester DVT Study. Arch Intern Med. 1991;5:933–8.
139. Van Hylckama VA, Helmerhorst FM, Vandenbroucke JP, Doggen CJ, Rosendaal FR. The venous thrombotic risk of oral contraceptives, effects of oestrogen dose and progestogen type: results of the MEGA case-control study. BMJ. 2009;339:b2921.
140. Culwell KR, Curtis KM. Use of contraceptive methods by women with current venous thrombosis on anticoagulant therapy: a systematic review. Contraception. 2009;80:337–45. PubMed PMID: 19751856.
141. Schaedel ZE, Dolan G, Powell MC. The use of the levonorgestrel-releasing intrauterine system in the management of menorrhagia in women with hemostatic disorders. Am J Obstet Gynecol. 2005;193:1361–3. PubMed PMID: 16202726. Epub 2005/10/06. eng.
142. Ueng J, Douketis JD. Prevention and treatment of hormone-associated venous thromboembolism: a patient management approach. Hematol Oncol Clin North Am. 2010;24(4):683–94. vii-viii. PubMed PMID: 20659653. Epub 2010/07/28. eng.
143. Geerts WH, Pineo GF, Heit JA, Bergqvist D, Lassen MR, Colwell CW, et al. Prevention of venous thromboembolism: the seventh ACCP conference on antithrombotic and thrombolytic therapy. Chest. 2004;126(3 Suppl):338S–400S. PubMed PMID: 15383478. Epub 2004/09/24. eng.
144. Vandenbroucke JP, Koster T, Briet E, Reitsma PH, Bertina RM, Rosendaal FR. Increased risk of venous thrombosis in oral-contraceptive users who are carriers of factor V Leiden mutation. Lancet. 1994;344: 1453–7.
145. Legnani C, Palareti G, Guazzaloca G, Cosmi B, Lunghi B, Bernardi F, et al. Venous thromboembolism in young women: role of thrombophilic mutations and oral contraceptive use. Eur Heart J. 2002;23:984–90.
146. Spannagl M, Heinemann LA, Schramm W. Are factor V Leiden carriers who use oral contraceptives at extreme risk of venous thromboembolism? Eur J Contracept Reprod Health Care. 2000;5:105–12.
147. Bolgiano EB, Foxwell MM, Browne BJ, Barish RA. Deep venous thrombosis of the upper extremity. J Emerg Med. 1990;8:85–91.
148. Mustafa S, Stein PD, Patel KC, Otten TR, Holmes R, Silbergleit A. Upper extremity deep venous thrombosis. Chest. 2003;123:1953–6.
149. Vaya A, Mira Y, Mateo J, Falco C, Villa P, Estelles A, et al. Prothrombin G20210A and oral contraceptive use increase upper-extremity deep venous thrombosis risk. Thromb Haemost. 2003;89:452–8.
150. Martinelli I, Battaglioli T, Bucciarelli P, Passamonti SM, Mannucci PM. Risk factors and recurrence rate of primary deep vein thrombosis of the upper extremities. Circulation. 2004;110:566–70.
151. Martinelli I, Sacchi E, Landi F, Taioli E, Duca F, Mannucci PM. High risk of cerebral-vein thrombosis in carriers of a prothrombin-gene mutation and in users of oral contraceptives. N Engl J Med. 1998;338: 1793–7.
152. de Bruijn SF, Stam J, Koopman MM, Vandenbroucke JP. Case-control study of risk of cerebral sinus thrombosis in oral contraceptive users and in carriers of hereditary prothrombotic conditions. The Cerebral Venous Sinus Thrombosis Study Group. BMJ. 1998;316:589–92.
153. Martinelli I, Battaglioli T, Burgo I, Di Domenico S, Mannucci PM. Oral contraceptive use, thrombophilia and their interaction in young women with ischemic stroke. Haematologica. 2006;91:844–7.
154. Pezzini A, Grassi M, Iacoviello L, Del Zotto E, Archetti S, Giossi A, et al. Inherited thrombophilia and stratification of ischaemic stroke risk among users of oral contraceptives. J Neurol Neurosurg Psychiatry. 2007;78:271–6.
155. Slooter AJ, Rosendaal FR, Tanis BC, Kemmeren JM, Van der Graaf Y. Prothrombotic conditions, oral contraceptives, and the risk of ischemic stroke. J Thromb Haemost. 2005;3:1213–7.
156. Cohn DM, Roshani S, Middeldorp S. Thrombophilia and venous thromboembolism: implications for testing. Semin Thromb Hemost. 2007;6:573–81.
157. Middeldorp S. Evidence-based approach to thrombophilia testing. J Thromb Thrombolysis. 2011;3:275.
158. Van Vlijmen EF, Brouwer JL, Veeger NJ, Eskes TK, De Graeff PA, Van der Meer J. Oral contraceptives and the absolute risk of venous thromboembolism in women with single or multiple thrombophilic defects. Arch Intern Med. 2007;167:282–9.
159. Effect of different progestogens in low oestrogen oral contraceptives on venous thromboembolic disease. World Health Organization Collaborative Study of Cardiovascular Disease and Steroid Hormone Contraception. Lancet. 1995;346:1582–88.
160. Jick H, Jick SS, Gurewich V, Myers MW, Vasilakis C. Risk of idiopathic cardiovascular death and nonfatal venous thromboembolism in women using oral contraceptives with differing progestogen components. Lancet. 1995;346:1589–93.
161. Bloemenkamp KW, Rosendaal FR, Helmerhorst FM, Buller HR, Vandenbroucke JP. Enhancement by factor V Leiden mutation of risk of deep-vein thrombosis associated with oral contraceptives containing a third-generation progestogen. Lancet. 1995;346: 1593–6.
162. Lidegaard O, Lokkegaard E, Svendsen AL, Agger C. Hormonal contraception and risk of venous thromboembolism: national follow-up study. BMJ. 2009;339:b2890.
163. Davtyan C. Four generations of progestins in oral contraceptives. Proceedings of UCLA healthcare 2012;16.
164. Kemmeren JM, Algra A, Grobbee DE. Third generation oral contraceptives and risk of venous thrombosis: meta-analysis. BMJ. 2001;323:1–9.
165. Food and Drug Administration. FDA drug safety communication: updated information about the risks

of blood clots in women taking birth control pills containing drospirenone. Rockville, MD: U.S. Food and Drug Administration; 2012.
166. Ducros E, Berthaut A, Mirshahi SS, Faussat AM, Soria J, Agarwal MK, et al. Aldosterone modifies hemostasis via upregulation of the protein-C receptor in human vascular endothelium. Biochem Biophys Res Commun. 2008;373:192–6.
167. Shapiro S, Dinger J. Risk of venous thromboembolism among users of oral contraceptives: a review of two recently published studies. J Fam Plan Reprod Health Care. 2010;36:33–8.
168. Dinger JC, Heinemann LJ, Kuhl-Habich D. The safety of a drospirenone-containing oral contraceptive: final results from the European Active Surveillance Study on Oral Contraceptives (EURAS-OC) based on 142,475 women-years of observation. Contraception. 2007;75:344–54.
169. Seeger JD, Loughlin J, Eng PM, Clifford CR, Cutone J, Walker AM. Risk of thromboembolism in women taking ethinylestradiol/drospirenone and other oral contraceptives. Obstet Gynecol. 2007;110:587–93.
170. ACOG Committee Opinion Number 540. Risk of venous thromboembolism among users of drospirenone-containing oral contraceptive pills. Obstet Gynecol. 2012;120(5):1239–42. PubMed PMID: 23090561. Epub 2012/10/24. eng.
171. Dinger J, Minh TD, Buttmann N, Bardenheuer K. Effectiveness of oral contraceptive pills in a large U.S. cohort comparing progestogen and regimen. Obstet Gynecol. 2011;117:33–40.
172. Jensen JT, Burke AE, Barnhart KT, Tillotson C, Messerle-Forbes M, Peters D. Effects of switching from oral to transdermal or transvaginal contraception on markers of thrombosis. Contraception. 2008;78:451–8.
173. Srivastava A, Weiss M. First patch death; Coroner confirms it. New York Post. 2004 April 28, 2004:13.
174. Edelman S, Krancs M. 'Patch' shock grows: kin ID new 'victims'. New York Post. 2004 May 16, 2004:1.
175. Van den Heuvel MW, Van Bragt AJ, Alnabawy AK, Kaptein MC. Comparison of ethinylestradiol pharmacokinetics in three hormonal contraceptive formulations: the vaginal ring, the transdermal patch and an oral contraceptive. Contraception. 2005;72:168–74.
176. Abrams LS, Skee DM, Natarajan J, Wong FA, Anderson GD. Pharmacokinetics of a contraceptive patch (Evra/Ortho Evra) containing norelgestromin and ethinyloestradiol at four application sites. Br J Clin Pharmacol. 2002;53:141–6.
177. Cole JA, Norman H, Doherty M, Walker AM. Venous thromboembolism, myocardial infarction, and stroke among transdermal contraceptive system users. Obstet Gynecol. 2007;109:339–46.
178. Dore DD, Norman H, Loughlin J, Seeger JD. Extended case-control study results on thromboembolic outcomes among transdermal contraceptive users. Contraception. 2010;81:408–13.
179. Lidegaard O, Nielsen LH, Skovlund CW, Lokkegaard E. Venous thrombosis in users of non-oral hormonal contraception: follow-up study, Denmark 2001-10. BMJ. 2012;344:e2990.
180. Jick SS, Hagberg KW, Hernandez RK, Kaye JA. Postmarketing study of ORTHO EVRA and levonorgestrel oral contraceptives containing hormonal contraceptives with 30 mcg of ethinyl estradiol in relation to nonfatal venous thromboembolism. Contraception. 2010;81:16–21.
181. Jick SS, Kaye JA, Russmann S, Jick H. Risk of nonfatal venous thromboembolism in women using a contraceptive transdermal patch and oral contraceptives containing norgestimate and 35 mcg of ethinyl estradiol. Contraception. 2006;73:223–8.
182. Jick S, Kaye JA, Li L, Jick H. Further results on the risk of nonfatal venous thromboembolism in users of the contraceptive transdermal patch compared to users of oral contraceptives containing norgestimate and 35 mcg of ethinyl estradiol. Contraception. 2007;76:4–7.
183. Laliberte F, Dea K, Duh MS, Kahler KH, Rolli M, Lefebvre P. Does the route of administration for estrogen hormone therapy impact the risk of venous thromboembolism? Estradiol transdermal system versus estrogen-only hormone therapy. Menopause. 2011;18:1052–9.
184. Canonico M, Oger E, Plu-Bureau G, Conard J, Meyer G, Levesque H, et al. Hormone therapy and venous thromboembolism among postmenopausal women: impact of the route of estrogen administration and progestogens: the ESTHER study. Circulation. 2007;115:840–5.
185. Archer DF, Cullins V, Creasy GW, Fisher AC. The impact of improved compliance with a weekly contraceptive transdermal system (Ortho Evra) on contraceptive efficacy. Contraception. 2004;69:189–95.
186. Sonnenberg FA, Burkman RT, Speroff L, Westhoff C, Hagerty CG. Cost-effectiveness and contraceptive effectiveness of the transdermal contraceptive patch. Am J Obstet Gynecol. 2005;192:1–9.
187. Timmer CJ, Mulders TM. Pharmacokinetics of etonogestrel and ethinyl estradiol released from a combined contraceptive vaginal ring. Clin Pharmacokinet. 2000;39:233–42.
188. Fleischer K, Van Vliet HA, Rosendaal FR, Rosing J, Tchaikovski S, Helmerhorst FM. Effects of the contraceptive patch, the vaginal ring and an oral contraceptive on APC resistance and SHBG: a cross over study. Thromb Res. 2009;123:429–35.
189. Magnusdottir EM, Bjarnadottir RI, Onundarson PT, Gudmundsdottir BR, Geirsson RT, Magnusdottir SD, et al. The contraceptive vaginal ring (NuvaRing) and hemostasis: a comparison study. Contraception. 2004;69:461–7.
190. Mantha S, Karp R, Raghavan V, Terrin N, Bauer KA, Zwicker JI. Assessing the risk of venous thromboembolic events in women taking progestin-only contraception: a meta-analysis. BMJ. 2012;345:e4944.
191. Winkler UH, Howie H, Buhler K, Korver T, Geurts TB, Coelingh Bennink HJ. A randomized controlled double-blind study of the effects on hemostasis of

two progestogen-only pills containing 75 mcg desogestrel or 30 mcg levonorgestrel. Contraception. 1998;57:385–92.

192. World Health Organization. Cardiovascular disease and use of oral and injectable progestogen-only contraceptives and combined injectable contraceptives. Results of an international, multicenter, case-control study. Contraception. 1998;57:315–24.
193. Heinemann LA, Assmann A, DoMinh T, Garbe E. Oral progestogen-only contraceptives and cardiovascular risks: results from the Transnational Study on Oral Contraceptives and the Health of Young Women. Eur J Contracep Reprod Health Care. 1999;4:67–73.
194. Vasilakis C, Jick H, Mar Melero-Montes M. Risk of idiopathic venous thromboembolism in users of progestogens alone. Lancet. 1999;354:1610–1. PubMed PMID: 10560680. Epub 1999/11/24. eng.
195. Vaillant-Roussel H, Ouchchane L, Dauphin C, Philippe P, Ruivard M. Risk factors for recurrence of venous thromboembolism associated with the use of oral contraceptives. Contraception. 2011;84:e23–30.
196. Stanczyk FZ, Mroszczak EJ, Ling T, Runkel R, Henzl M, Miyakawa I, et al. Plasma levels and pharmacokinetics of norethindrone and ethinylestradiol administered in solution and as tablets to women. Contraception. 1983;28:241–51.
197. Nanda K, Amaral E, Hays M, Viscola MA, Mehta N, Bahamondes L. Pharmacokinetic interactions between depot medroxyprogesterone acetate and combination antiretroviral therapy. Fertil Steril. 2008;90:965–71.
198. Lidegaard O, Nielsen LH, Skovlund CW, Skjeldestad FE, Lokkegaard E. Risk of venous thromboembolism from use of oral contraceptives containing different progestogens and oestrogen doses: Danish cohort study, 2001-9. BMJ. 2011;343:d6423.
199. Conard J, Plu-Bureau G, Bahi N, Horellou MH, Pelissier C, Thalabard JC. Progestogen-only contraception in women at high risk of venous thromboembolism. Contraception. 2004;70:437–41.
200. Van Hylckama VA, Helmerhorst FM, Rosendaal FR. The risk of deep venous thrombosis associated with injectable depot-medroxyprogesterone acetate contraceptives or a levonorgestrel intrauterine device. Arterioscler Thromb Vasc Biol. 2010;30: 2297–300.
201. Barsoum MK, Heit JA, Ashrani AA, Leibson CL, Petterson TM, Bailey KR. Is progestin an independent risk factor for incident venous thromboembolism? A population-based case-control study. Thromb Res. 2010;126:373–8.
202. Cardiovascular disease and use of oral and injectable progestogen-only contraceptives and combined injectable contraceptives. Results of an international, multicenter, case-control study. World Health Organization Collaborative Study of Cardiovascular Disease and Steroid Hormone Contraception. Contraception. 1998;57(5):315–24. PubMed PMID: 9673838. Epub 1998/07/23. eng.
203. Heinemann LA, Assmann A, DoMinh T, Garbe E. Oral progestogen-only contraceptives and cardiovascular risk: results from the Transnational Study on Oral Contraceptives and the Health of Young Women. Eur J Contracept Reprod Health Care. 1999;4(2):67–73. PubMed PMID: 10427481. Epub 1999/07/31. eng.
204. Egberg N, van Beek A, Gunnervik C, Hulkko S, Hirvonen E, Larsson-Cohn U, et al. Effects on the hemostatic system and liver function in relation to Implanon® and Norplant®: a prospective randomized clinical trial. Contraception. 1998;58(2):93–8.
205. Vieira CS, Ferriani RA, Garcia AA, Pintao MC, Azevedo GD, Gomes MK, et al. Use of the etonogestrel-releasing implant is associated with hypoactivation of the coagulation cascade. Hum Reprod (Oxford, England). 2007;22(8):2196–201. PubMed PMID: 17569674.
206. Sonmezer M, Atabekoglu C, Cengiz B, Dokmeci F, Cengiz SD. Depot-medroxyprogesterone acetate in anticoagulated patients with previous hemorrhagic corpus luteum. Eur J Contracept Reprod Health Care. 2005;10(1):9–14. PubMed PMID: 16036292. Epub 2005/07/23. eng.
207. Raj G, Kumar R, McKinney WP. Safety of intramuscular influenza immunization among patients receiving long-term warfarin anticoagulation therapy. Arch Intern Med. 1995;155(14):1529–31. PubMed PMID: 7605155. Epub 1995/07/24. eng.
208. Jeske AH, Suchko GD. Lack of a scientific basis for routine discontinuation of oral anticoagulation therapy before dental treatment. J Am Dent Assoc. 2003;134(11):1492–7. PubMed PMID: 14664269. Epub 2003/12/11. eng.
209. Kingman CE, Kadir RA, Lee CA, Economides DL. The use of levonorgestrel-releasing intrauterine system for treatment of menorrhagia in women with inherited bleeding disorders. BJOG. 2004;111(12): 1425–8. PubMed PMID: 15663130. Epub 2005/01/25. eng.
210. Pisoni CN, Cuadrado MJ, Khamashta MA, Hunt BJ. Treatment of menorrhagia associated with oral anticoagulation: efficacy and safety of the levonorgestrel releasing intrauterine device (Mirena coil). Lupus. 2006;15(12):877–80. PubMed PMID: 17211994. Epub 2007/01/11. eng.
211. Medical eligibility criteria for contraceptive use: a WHO Family Planning Cornerstone. Geneva: World Health Organization; 2010.
212. Hirvonen E, Idanpaan-Heikkila J. Cardiovascular death among women under 40 years of age using low-estrogen oral contraceptives and intrauterine devices in Finland from 1975 to 1984. Am J Obstet Gynecol. 1990;163(1 Pt 2):281–4. PubMed PMID: 2372033. Epub 1990/07/01. eng.
213. Rivera R, Chen-Mok M, McMullen S, Milsom I, Andersson K, Jonasson K, Lindstedt G, et al. Analysis of client characteristics that may affect early discontinuation of the TCu-380A IUD. Contraception. 1999;60(3):155–60.

214. Milsom I, Andersson K, Jonasson K, Lindstedt G, Rybo G. The influence of the Gyne-T 380S IUD on menstrual blood loss and iron status. Contraception. 1995;52(3):175–9.
215. Kadir RA, Davies J. Hemostatic disorders in women. J Thromb Haemost. 2013;11 Suppl 1:170–9. doi:10.1111/jth.12267.
216. Hatcher R. Contraceptive technology. 20th ed. Atlanta, GA: Bridging the Gap Communications; 2011.
217. Glasier A. Emergency postcoital contraception. N Engl J Med. 1997;337(15):1058–64.
218. Gemzell-Danielsson K, Rabe T, Cheng L. Emergency contraception. Gynecol Endocrinol. 2013;29 Suppl 1:1–14. PubMed PMID: 23437846. Epub 2013/03/06. eng.
219. Brache V, Cochon L, Deniaud M, Croxatto HB. Ulipristal acetate prevents ovulation more effectively than levonorgestrel: analysis of pooled data from three randomized trials of emergency contraception regimens. Contraception. 2013;88(5): 611–8. PubMed PMID: 23809278. Epub 2013/07/03. eng.
220. Peterson HB, Xia Z, Hughes JM, Wilcox LS, Tylor LR, Trussell J. The risk of pregnancy after tubal sterilization: findings from the U.S. Collaborative Review of Sterilization. Am J Obstet Gynecol. 1996;174(4):1161–8. discussion 1168–70.
221. Rios-Castillo JE, Velasco E, Arjona-Berral JE, Monserrat Jordan JA, Povedano-Canizares B, Castelo-Branco C. Efficacy of Essure hysteroscopic sterilization–5 years follow up of 1200 women. Gynecol Endocrinol. 2013;29(6):580–2. PubMed PMID: 23557170. Epub 2013/04/06. eng.
222. Gariepy AM, Creinin MD, Schwarz EB, Smith KJ. Reliability of laparoscopic compared with hysteroscopic sterilization at 1 year: a decision analysis. Obstet Gynecol. 2011;118(2 Pt 1):273–9. PubMed PMID: 21775842. Pubmed Central PMCID: PMC3272841. Epub 2011/07/22. eng.
223. Roderick P, Ferris G, Wilson K, Halls H, Jackson D, Collins R, Baigent C, et al. Towards evidence-based guidelines for the prevention of venous thromboembolism: systematic reviews of mechanical methods, oral anticoagulation, dextran and regional anaesthesia as thromboprophylaxis. Health Technol Assess. 2005;9(49):iii–iv. ix-x, 1–78.
224. Lentz GM. Comprehensive gynecology. Philadelphia: Mosby Elsevier; 2012. Available from: http://uclibs.org/PID/226901.
225. Bonnar J. Can more be done in obstetric and gynecologic practice to reduce morbidity and mortality associated with venous thromboembolism? Am J Obstet Gynecol. 1999;180(4):784–91.
226. ACOG Practice Bulletin No. 84. Prevention of deep vein thrombosis and pulmonary embolism. Obstet Gynecol. 2007;110(2 Pt 1):429–40.
227. Geerts WH, Pineo GF, Heit JA, Bergqvist D, Lassen MR, Colwell CW, Ray JG, et al. Prevention of venous thromboembolism: the seventh ACCP conference on antithrombotic and thrombolytic therapy. 20040922 DCOM-20041026(0012–3692 (Print)). eng.
228. Huq FY, Tvarkova K, Arafa A, Kadir RA. Menstrual problems and contraception in women of reproductive age receiving oral anticoagulation. Contraception. 2011;84(2):128–32. PubMed PMID: 21757053. Epub 2011/07/16. eng.
229. De Teresa E, Vera A, Ortigosa J, Pulpon LA, Arus AP, De Artaza M. Interaction between anticoagulants and contraceptives: an unsuspected finding. BMJ. 1979;2:1260–1.
230. Shelepova T, Nafziger AN, Victory J, Kashuba AD, Rowland E, Zhang Y, et al. Effect of a triphasic oral contraceptive on drug-metabolizing enzyme activity as measured by the validated Cooperstown 5+1 cocktail. J Clin Pharmacol. 2005;45:1413–21.
231. Ellison J, Thomson AJ, Greer IA, Walker ID. Drug points: apparent interaction between warfarin and levonorgestrel used for emergency contraception. BMJ. 2000;321:1382.
232. Shaughnessy SG, Hirsh J, Bhandari M, Muir JM, Young E, Weitz JI. A histomorphometric evaluation of heparin-induced bone loss after discontinuation of heparin treatment in rates. Blood. 1999;93:1231–6.
233. Casele HL, Haney EI, James A, Rosene-Montella K, Carson M. Bone density changes in women who receive thromboprophylaxis in pregnancy. Am J Obstet Gynecol. 2006;195:1109–13.
234. Rajgopal R, Bear M, Butcher MK, Shaughnessy SG. The effects of heparin and low molecular weight heparins on bone. Thromb Res. 2008;122:293–8.
235. Philip WJ, Martin JC, Richardson JM, Reid DM, Webster J, Douglas AS. Decreased axial and peripheral bone density in patients taking long-term warfarin. QJM. 1995;88:635–40.
236. Barnes C, Newall F, Ignjatovic V, Wong P, Cameron F, Jones G, et al. Reduced bone density in children on long-term warfarin. Pediatr Res. 2005;57:578–81.
237. Sugiyama T, Takaki T, Sakanaka K, Sadamaru H, Mori K, Kato Y, et al. Warfarin-induced impairment of cortical bone material quality and compensatory adaptation of cortical bone structure to mechanical stimuli. J Endocrinol. 2007;194:213–22.

Using Contraceptives for Gynecologic Conditions

13

David R. Kattan and Ronald T. Burkman

Introduction

This chapter covers several common gynecologic conditions that can be encountered among women in the reproductive age group and the role contraceptives may play in the treatment of these disorders. Although there are purported non-contraceptive benefits associated with the use of contraceptive medications in the presence of some of these disorders, the data supporting such effects vary. Further, some types of contraception may not be appropriate in certain circumstances.

Classification of Abnormal Uterine Bleeding

In 2011, the International Federation of Gynecology and Obstetrics (FIGO) introduced a nomenclature system to more precisely characterize uterine bleeding [1]. Known as the PALM-COEIN classification, it has been adopted by the American College of Obstetricians and Gynecologists (ACOG). Abnormal bleeding etiologies are divided into structural (PALM) and nonstructural causes (COEIN). PALM includes *P*olyps, *A*denomyosis, *L*eiomyomata, and *M*alignancy/hyperplasia. *C*oagulopathy, *O*vulatory dysfunction, *E*ndometrial, *I*atrogenic, and *N*ot yet classified make up COEIN.

The US Medical Eligibility Criteria for Contraceptive Use (USMEC) from the Centers for Disease Control and Prevention (CDC) recommend that unexplained vaginal bleeding that is suspicious for a serious condition or pregnancy be evaluated before prescribing contraception [2]. The concern is that the contraceptive method could also cause irregular bleeding which may mask the underlying pathology or diagnosis. The USMEC rates the appropriateness of contraceptive methods for several benign gynecologic conditions (Table 13.1).

Abnormal Uterine Bleeding-Adenomyosis (AUB-A)

Adenomyosis is characterized by the ectopic location of endometrial tissue within the myometrium. While a definitive diagnosis of this condition can only be made histologically, a clinical history of heavy menses, dysmenorrhea, and an examination noting an enlarged, globular uterus, combined with radiographic findings suggestive of adenomyosis, is often sufficient [3]. Therapies that target the heavy menses seen with adenomyosis are likely to be beneficial.

D.R. Kattan, M.D., M.P.H. • R.T. Burkman, M.D. (✉)
Department of Obstetrics and Gynecology, Baystate Medical Center, Tufts University School of Medicine, Springfield, MA, USA
e-mail: david.kattanmd@bhs.org; rtb@bhs.org

R.H. Allen and C.A. Cwiak (eds.), *Contraception for the Medically Challenging Patient*,
DOI 10.1007/978-1-4939-1233-9_13,

Table 13.1 Benign gynecologic conditions and eligibility criteria for contraception[a]

Condition	CHC	POP	Injection	Implant	LNG-IUD	CU-IUD	
Heavy or prolonged vaginal bleeding (includes regular and irregular patterns)	1	2	2	2	1/2[b]	2	
Endometriosis	1	1	1	1	1	2	
Benign ovarian tumors (including cysts)	1	1	1	1	1	1	
Severe dysmenorrhea	1	1	1	1	1	2	
Uterine fibroids	1	1	1	1	2	2	
Distorted uterine cavity (any congenital or acquired uterine abnormality distorting the uterine cavity in a manner that is incompatible with IUD insertion)	N/A	N/A	N/A	N/A	4	4	
Past PID with subsequent pregnancy	1	1	1	1	1	1	
Past PID without subsequent pregnancy	1	1	1	1	2	2	
Current PID	1	1	1	1	4/2[b]	4/2[b]	
Current purulent cervicitis, chlamydia, or gonorrhea	1	1	1	1	4/2[b]	4/2[b]	
Other STIs (excluding hepatitis and HIV)	1	1	1	1	2	2	
Vaginitis (including *Trichomonas vaginalis* and bacterial vaginosis)	1	1	1	1	2	2	
Increased risk for STIs	1	1	1	1	2–3/2[b]	2–3/2[b]	If very high risk for chlamydia or gonorrhea exposure, initiation is category 3, otherwise 2

1 = no restrictions on use	3 = risks outweigh benefits
2 = benefits outweigh risks	4 = contraindicated

CHC combined hormonal contraception, *PO* progestin-only pills, *LNG-IUD* levonorgestrel intrauterine device, *Cu-IUD* copper intrauterine device

[a]Adapted from [101]

[b]Initiation vs. continuation

Recently, there have been several studies demonstrating the levonorgestrel intrauterine device, LNG-IUD (Mirena, Bayer Healthcare Pharmaceuticals, Wayne, NJ, USA), as an effective therapy for AUB-A. A new smaller LNG-IUD was approved in 2013 (Skyla, Bayer Healthcare Pharmaceuticals, Wayne, NJ, USA), and there are insufficient data on its use for gynecologic conditions to review in this chapter. A prospective, non-randomized trial reported in 2012 examined the effects of the LNG-IUD and the copper T380A IUD (ParaGard, Teva, Israel) for 74 women with and without clinical evidence of adenomyosis [4]. Twenty-three women with a diagnosis of adenomyosis by transvaginal ultrasound criteria all received the LNG-IUD, 25 without adenomyosis but who desired an IUD for contraception also received the LNG-IUD, and 26 without adenomyosis who desired an IUD for contraception received the copper IUD. Subjects were followed for 12 months. Outcomes of interest were days of menstrual bleeding, dysmenorrhea (visual-analog [VAS] pain scores 0–10), and hemoglobin levels. Women in the LNG-IUD with adenomyosis group saw significant decreases in the number of bleeding days, dysmenorrhea pain scores, and a significant increase in hemoglobin level when compared to baseline (6.64–3.68 days, 5.69–3.17, and 10.9–11.7 g/dL, respectively, all $p<0.001$). Those in the LNG-IUD without adenomyosis group saw similar results, although their baseline bleeding days and pain score levels were lower than the group with adenomyosis. Women without adenomyosis who received the copper T380A IUD saw statistically significant increases in their number of bleeding days and pain scores, as well as a statistically significant decrease in their hemoglobin levels (4.66–5.57 days, 3.94–5.11, and 12.5–12.1 g/dL, respectively, all $p<0.001$). Such a decrease in hemoglobin level is not likely to be clinically significant. In a 2009 study performed in China, 94 women diagnosed with adenomyosis based on symptoms of dysmenorrhea and transvaginal ultrasound findings received an LNG-IUD and were followed for 3 years [5]. The primary outcome was menstrual pain as measured on a VAS from 0 to 100. Pain scores decreased significantly during the study from a mean of 77.9 at baseline to 11.8 at 36 months. The uterine volume of participants was also seen to decrease significantly over time, suggesting suppression of adenomyosis present in the myometrium. Over 70 % of women were satisfied with their treatment. Another study enrolled 29 women to receive the LNG-IUD who reported heavy, painful menses and had MRI findings of adenomyosis and followed subjects over time for changes in bleeding pattern and menstrual pain scores [6]. Heavy menses resolved in all 29 women, with 2 reporting regular menses with normal flow, 10 reporting unpredictable spotting, 9 reporting oligomenorrhea, and 8 reporting amenorrhea 6 months after insertion. VAS pain scores decreased from a mean of 8 out of 10 at baseline to 1.75, 6 months after insertion. A systematic review concluded that the LNG-IUD was equally effective as surgical therapy in improving the quality of life for women with AUB, including AUB-A [7]. Taken together, these investigations all support the use of the LNG-IUD as an effective treatment for AUB-A.

There are scant data regarding the use of combined oral contraceptives (COCs) specifically for AUB-A, but as the evidence clearly suggests that COCs reduce menstrual bleeding and dysmenorrhea (discussed in section "Dysmenorrhea"), they are a reasonable therapeutic option for patients with AUB-A. A study of 118 women with uterine fibroids and heavy menses, 40 of which were using a COC, found that 32 % of subjects had histological evidence of adenomyosis on hysteroscopic biopsy [8]. Immunohistochemical evaluation of all subjects' biopsies determined that COC use was associated with inhibition of vascular endothelial growth factor, aromatase, and Cox-2, all of which are thought to increase menstrual flow. The findings provide biochemical evidence that COCs are useful medications for women with AUB-A.

Data regarding depot medroxyprogesterone acetate (DMPA) use for AUB-A are few. However, taking into account that DMPA reduces menstrual flow over time, it is a reasonable treatment option for women with AUB-A. The etonogestrel subdermal implant also has not been well studied for AUB-A, but its similar effect on reduced menstrual flow gives credence to its use for the treatment of AUB-A as long as patients accept the irregular bleeding profile.

Abnormal Uterine Bleeding-Leiomyomata (AUB-L)

Leiomyomata, or uterine fibroids, are also often implicated as the reason for menstrual disorders in women. Heavy menses are the most common symptom reported by women with uterine fibroids [9]. Mass effect on the uterine venous system is thought to lead to venous dilation within the myometrium and endometrium [10]. When menses occur, these enlarged vessels do not respond normally to the usual hemostatic mechanisms of the uterus, and abnormally heavy bleeding results. Uterine fibroids are classified by their location in the uterus. *Subserosal* fibroids are found immediately beneath the peritoneal surface of the uterus and distort its surface. *Intramural* fibroids are located entirely within the myometrium of the uterus. *Submucosal* fibroids are found immediately beneath the endometrium and distort the intrauterine cavity. Regardless of the location within the uterus, fibroids can cause heavy menstrual bleeding; however, submucosal fibroids are most frequently associated with bleeding [11].

Most recently, attention has been paid to the value of using the LNG-IUD for management of AUB-L. A systematic review of IUD use for women with uterine fibroids was performed in 2010 [12]. Eleven studies met the inclusion criteria of the review, with all 11 showing significant decreases in menstrual blood flow among LNG-IUD users. Serum levels of hemoglobin, hematocrit, and ferritin rose for LNG-IUD users in studies that examined these outcomes. Since this review was published, other studies have demonstrated similar results. A randomized trial that enrolled 58 women with AUB-L compared treatment with the LNG-IUD and COCs [13]. Menstrual blood flow was significantly lower in the LNG-IUD group, with a 90 % reduction compared to 13 % in the COC group. Additionally, hemoglobin levels increased by 2 g/dL in the LNG-IUD group compared to 0.1 g/dL in the COC group. Another prospective study of 102 women with leiomyomas and AUB-L administered the LNG-IUD to all subjects [14]. The primary outcome, menstrual bleeding, decreased significantly over the year of the study, with 89 % of participants being satisfied with the LNG-IUD. These findings have been comparable in other investigations [15, 16]. A 2013 systematic review concluded that the LNG-IUD reduces menstrual blood flow in women with uterine fibroids, but also noted that there are few published randomized controlled trials focusing on this problem [17].

Though not as effective as the LNG-IUD, COCs are often used for management of AUB-L. A 2002 Italian non-randomized trial compared COCs to placebo in 121 women with asymptomatic fibroids [18]. The COC group had a significant reduction of menstrual flow by more than 2 days and an increase of 2.5 % in hematocrit, while the placebo group did not see any significant change from baseline for either measure. As COCs are widely used for heavy menses, they are a reasonable therapy for AUB-L.

The evidence behind using DMPA for uterine fibroids is positive, but scant. One prospective study observed 20 women with uterine fibroids and AUB-L who received DMPA over the course of 6 months [19]. At the end of the investigation, 30 % of subjects reported amenorrhea, 70 % reported an improvement in bleeding pattern, and 15 % had improved hemoglobin levels. The possible therapeutic effect of the etonogestrel implant on AUB-L has not been studied.

Abnormal Uterine Bleeding: Coagulopathies (AUB-C)

Defects in the coagulation pathway can lead to abnormal uterine bleeding. According to ACOG, up to 20 % of women with heavy menstrual bleeding may have an underlying coagulopathy [20]. A patient's history which includes findings such as heavy menses since menarche, frequent nosebleeds, easy bruising, and difficulty stopping bleeding from cuts in their skin should raise the possibility of a coagulation disorder, and laboratory testing to determine that the diagnosis is commonly indicated.

One common coagulopathy is von Willebrand disease (vWD), which affects up to 13 % of women with heavy menstrual bleeding. Inherited in an autosomally dominant or recessive fashion, many variants of the disease exist and involve a quantitative or a qualitative deficiency in von Willebrand factor (vWF). When vWF is absent or deficient, platelet adhesion does not occur normally and other coagulation factors may degrade [21]. If von Willebrand disease is suspected, consultation with a hematologist is prudent.

Since a consequence of untreated coagulopathy in women is heavy menses, treatments that target AUB-C aim to reduce or eliminate menstrual blood loss. The LNG-IUD has been studied in the context of coagulopathies. In a prospective pilot study of 16 women with known coagulation disorders and AUB-C, all the subjects were provided with an LNG-IUD and were followed for 9 months to determine the effect on menstrual blood loss [22]. All 16 reported significant improvements in menstrual blood flow as measured by a Pictorial Bleeding Assessment Chart (PBAC) score, where higher scores indicated greater amounts of bleeding. At the start of the study, the median PBAC score was 213; this decreased to a median PBAC score of 47 after 9 months of LNG-IUD use ($p<0.0001$). Fifty-six percent of the study population reported amenorrhea at the study's conclusion.

COCs are also effective treatment options. In a prospective study of 25 women with vWD and menorrhagia, 22 of the 25 subjects had a significant decrease in menstrual bleeding when administered COCs [23]. As COCs also inhibit the formation of hemorrhagic corpus luteum cysts, they are widely used option for women suffering from AUB-C. DMPA and the etonogestrel implant have not been studied for use in women with AUB-C, but resulting decreased menstrual blood loss and ovulation suppression with their use make them reasonable options. See Chap. 11 for further discussion of contraception for women with bleeding disorders.

Dysmenorrhea

Painful menstrual periods, or dysmenorrhea, are categorized by its underlying cause. *Primary* dysmenorrhea, which is the focus of this section of the chapter, is caused by excessive prostaglandin production within the uterus. Conversely, *secondary* dysmenorrhea results from a source other than excessive prostaglandin production, such as uterine leiomyomata, endometriosis, and adenomyosis. The use of contraceptives to treat these conditions is discussed in other parts of this chapter.

During the beginning of the luteal phase of the menstrual cycle, the increase in progesterone levels leads to production of prostaglandins in the endometrium. If pregnancy does not occur, progesterone levels decrease at the end of the menstrual cycle and the endometrium begins to separate from the uterus. As the endometrium is shed, prostaglandins are released which in turn enhance uterine contractions. As blood flow to the uterus decreases from enhanced uterine contractions, tissue ischemia and a sensation of pain result. Moreover, prostaglandins that enter the systemic circulation during this process may cause symptoms such as headache, nausea, vomiting, and diarrhea.

Dysmenorrhea is a common phenomenon. A survey of teenage women in Brazil found that 73 % reported symptoms of painful menses [24]. In this study, two-thirds of respondents said that dysmenorrhea negatively affected their activities of daily life. In another survey, which asked undergraduate college and medical students in Hong Kong about their menses, 80 % of participants noted painful periods [25]. Seventy-five percent of participants reported disruption of their ability to study and 60 % said that dysmenorrhea negatively affected their physical activity. In another survey of young Italian women, 84 % answered that they had experienced dysmenorrhea, with 32 % of the women stating that their menstrual pain symptoms had caused them to miss time at school [26]. On a societal scale, dysmenorrhea is associated with significant lost working hours and economic activity [27].

Contraceptives that reduce or eliminate menses have been found to be effective in alleviating the symptoms of dysmenorrhea. The LNG-IUD is a promising therapy for treatment of primary dysmenorrhea. Although published data for treatment of primary dysmenorrhea are scant, the LNG-IUD is associated with a 90 % reduction in menstrual flow and induces amenorrhea after 24 months of use in 60 % of users [28, 29]. Like other modalities that decrease menstrual flow, the LNG-IUD likely reduces painful menstrual symptoms for a majority of women who use it because of this mechanism of action.

In particular, studies have consistently demonstrated that COCs reduce menstrual pain in a majority of women who use them. However, there is a paucity of information regarding the mechanism by which COCs reduce dysmenorrhea. One group of investigators measured uterine tonicity before and after COC use in women reporting dysmenorrhea and established that uterine contractile force and painful menstrual symptoms were decreased when COCs were used [30]. A longitudinal study that followed a cohort of Swedish women found that COC users had significantly less dysmenorrhea than non-COC users [31]. A prospective study of women seeking family planning care in the USA showed that COC users were eight times more likely to have a significant reduction in their dysmenorrhea symptoms than non-COC users [32]. More recently, double-blind, randomized controlled trials have demonstrated a benefit of COC use for dysmenorrhea. In one such trial, 76 adolescent women who reported moderate or severe dysmenorrhea were randomized to receive a placebo or a COC for 3 months [33]. During the third month of the study period, the subjects were asked to rate their menstrual pain scores using the Moos Menstrual Distress Questionnaire, a 0–10 scale. Those that received COCs reported a mean pain rating of 3.7 versus 5.4 in the placebo group ($p=0.004$). COC users also reported fewer days of pain and severe pain than placebo users, although the difference did not reach significance. Another randomized, controlled trial investigated two different COC formulations, one containing desogestrel and the other levonorgestrel [34]. Although the primary outcome of the study was tolerability of each pill, subjects in both arms of the study experienced comparable decreases in the occurrence of dysmenorrhea from baseline: 57–40 % in the desogestrel group and 55–38 % in the levonorgestrel group. As shown in this study, no investigations have demonstrated a difference in successful treatment of dysmenorrhea symptoms among various COC formulations.

Investigators have also evaluated the continuous use of COCs in treatment of dysmenorrhea. A 2012 randomized, double-blind, controlled trial examined differences in dysmenorrhea symptoms in 38 women diagnosed with primary dysmenorrhea who were assigned to continuous regimen of COCs versus a traditional cyclic regimen [35]. While the continuous regimen was superior to a cyclic regimen after 1 and 3 months, there was no significant difference between groups in dysmenorrhea pain scores at 6 months. Both groups experienced a significant decrease of menstrual pain scores when compared with baseline scores.

There are limited studies that have evaluated the effectiveness of the contraceptive patch and ring for treating primary dysmenorrhea. A randomized, controlled trial comparing the contraceptive ring to a COC formulation demonstrated comparable decreases in dysmenorrhea symptoms in both groups [31]. It would be therefore expected that their effects on dysmenorrhea would be similar to COCs.

Depot medroxyprogesterone acetate (DMPA) has also been extensively used for treatment of dysmenorrhea. Most studies examining DMPA as a treatment for dysmenorrhea do so in the context of endometriosis and will be discussed elsewhere in this chapter. However, as more than half of women experience amenorrhea after three doses of DMPA, it appears that DMPA decreases dysmenorrhea symptoms in general by reducing or eliminating menstrual flow [36].

The etonogestrel subdermal implant offers beneficial effects against primary dysmenorrhea symptoms as well. One study of 330 American women who used the implant for at least 1 year found a decrease in dysmenorrhea prevalence from 59 % at baseline to 21 % after treatment [37]. In another study of 635 subjects, 35 % reported dysmenorrhea at baseline, with 82 % of women reporting improvement of symptoms at the end of device use [38]. Since decreased menstrual flow and amenorrhea are common among etonogestrel implant users, this is likely the reason for improvement in painful menstrual symptoms.

The USMEC rates all contraceptive methods, except the copper IUD, as category 1 or no restrictions on use for severe dysmenorrhea (see Table 13.1). The copper IUD is rated category 2 or benefits likely outweigh risks due to the fact that dysmenorrhea may worsen.

Endometriosis

Endometriosis is a common chronic condition that affects 6–10 % of women in the reproductive age group in the USA. However, among infertile women, the prevalence is 20–50 % and in women with chronic pelvic pain the prevalence is 71–87 % [39]. Among women with endometriosis desiring contraception, there are no contraindications to the use of any method. However, hormonal approaches including combination hormonal methods or progestin-only methods such as DMPA and the LNG-IUD may be preferable. In addition, a number of studies have examined the use of various hormonal approaches to possibly prevent the occurrence of endometriosis, as initial treatment or as an adjunct to surgical treatment.

The use of the LNG-IUD also has been shown to effectively relieve endometriosis-related pain. In a study of 34 women with laparoscopically confirmed endometriosis who subsequently used an LNG-IUD, among subjects followed for 3 years, most experienced a reduction in pain [40]. However, 40 % of subjects withdrew from the study due to persistent pain, bleeding, or weight gain. In another study of 84 women comparing users of the LNG-IUD versus use of a GnRH analog, both groups showed a significant reduction in pain [41]. There are no proven theories on how this device reduces pain, although it is likely that the levonorgestrel released by the device has a direct effect on endometriotic implants.

Most of the studies involving combination hormonal methods related to endometriosis have been carried out with combined oral contraceptives. Since they prevent ovulation and reduce menstrual flow, it has been suggested that this may reduce or eliminate the risk of retrograde menstruation with implantation of endometrial cells on the pelvic peritoneum. However, there is insufficient data to indicate that they have a major effect on the incidence of the disorder [42]. For example, data involving over 17,000 women in the Oxford Family Planning Association cohort study who were followed for up to 23 years demonstrated a relative risk of endometriosis among users of combined oral contraceptives compared to nonusers of 0.4 (95 % confidence interval [CI], 0.2–0.7) [43]. There was no association with occurrence of the disorder and duration of use. More importantly, the relative risk was 1.8 (95 % CI, 1.0–3.1) among former oral contraceptive users, suggesting that the findings may only reflect masking of symptoms during oral contraceptive use as opposed to a true protective effect.

In women with pelvic pain and known or suspected endometriosis who desire future fertility, there is some evidence that the use of DMPA, combined oral contraceptives, as well as the LNG-IUD reduces pain. However, there are not a large number of studies evaluating this issue and many have small sample sizes. In a randomized trial of 300 women with laparoscopically diagnosed endometriosis, the use of DMPA or leuprolide acetate, a GnRH analog, had equivalent effects in substantially reducing endometriosis-related pain symptoms [44]. Similarly, another trial involving 274 women with surgically diagnosed endometriosis comparing these two drugs also showed similar efficacy in the reduction of pain [45]. Of note, the bone loss with DMPA use was less than that with leuprolide acetate use in both studies.

Combined oral contraceptives, given either cyclically or in a continuous fashion, have also been shown to reduce endometriosis-associated pain. For example, in a randomized placebo-controlled trial of 100 subjects, users of COCs as well as those on placebo showed some decrease in dysmenorrhea after four cycles [46]. However, the pain reduction in the oral contraceptive group was significantly greater. It also appears that the use of a continuous oral contraceptive, either initially or when cyclical use fails, may be beneficial. For example in a study of 50 women who had inadequate pain relief on cyclic COCs, the use of a continuous method resulted in over 75 % of subjects being at least satisfied with their pain control after 2 years [42].

The use of COCs or the LNG-IUD has been shown to suppress the recurrence of symptoms in women who have undergone surgical treatment of endometriosis. Relative to oral contraceptives, symptoms are reasonably controlled during use and both the cyclical and continuous approaches work equally well [47, 48]. Based on limited data, it also appears that the LNG-IUD reduces dysmenorrhea following endometriosis surgery [49].

Similar to dysmenorrhea, the USMEC rates all contraceptive methods, except the copper IUD, as category 1 or no restrictions on use for endometriosis (see Table 13.1). The copper IUD is rated category 2 or benefits likely outweigh risks due to the fact that dysmenorrhea may worsen.

Uterine Leiomyomata

Uterine leiomyomata, also known as myomas or fibroids, are benign smooth muscle tumors that are extremely common, with the incidence reported as high as 70 % in African-American women and 40 % in Caucasian women by age 50 [50]. Although most are asymptomatic, they can produce pelvic pain or pressure and infertility depending on their size and location as well as abnormal uterine bleeding. Further, there is some evidence that their growth is at least partially hormone dependant, with both estrogen and progesterone promoting development [51]. Relative to contraceptive use, the major issues are whether given methods affect the occurrence of myomas or their growth and alter symptoms such as pain or abnormal bleeding, or whether myomas in some way affect contraceptive effectiveness.

As is noted in the discussion of the management of abnormal uterine bleeding associated with fibroids, oral contraceptives and DMPA have been used as treatment options. Further, given the frequency of myomas, substantial numbers of women requesting contraception likely have myomas and have been treated with a variety of approaches including hormonal methods. To date, epidemiologic studies are inconsistent regarding whether the use of hormonal contraceptive methods affects the occurrence or the growth of these tumors. For example, in a nested case-control study within the Oxford Family Planning cohort study, the authors determined that the use of oral contraceptives reduced the risk of myomas and that the extent of risk reduction was related to duration of use [52]. That is, each 5 years of use resulted in a 17 % reduction in risk of the tumor. They also determined that the intrauterine device (all types though most were likely inert such as the Lippes loop) use did not affect the occurrence of myomas. Conversely, the Nurses Health Study II cohort of 95,601 premenopausal nurses found little change in the occurrence of myomas among combined oral contraceptive users [53]. Duration of use did not affect the occurrence of myomas. However, use at an early age (13–16 years) compared to never use of oral contraceptives was associated with a modest increased risk of myomas (relative risk 1.26, 95 % CI 1.05, 1.51). Of note, a prospective cohort of 2,279 cases of myomas in the US Black women noted a 40 % reduction in the risk of myomas for women using DMPA [54]. For the most part, no consistent patterns of detection or reduction in myoma size were noted for users of other forms of hormonal contraception. None of the studies reviewed here were able to assess whether the growth of existing myomas was affected in any way. Although the contraceptive patch and vaginal ring have not been studied, it is likely their effects on myomas would be similar to oral contraceptives.

There is some evidence that use of the LNG-IUD appears to decrease both bleeding and reduce uterine volume in women using the method for abnormal bleeding due to myomas, but does not reduce uterine volume in women using the device for contraception [55]. In this cohort study, 87 women with myomas were divided into three groups: women with idiopathic menorrhagia, women with menorrhagia due to the myomas, and women without myomas using the device only for contraception. After 36 months, 44.5 % of the women with menorrhagia due to myomas were amenorrheic ($p<0.027$). Women in both of the groups with menorrhagia had statistically significant reductions in uterine volume; the women using the device only for contraception did not. Of interest, the reduction was not due to a decrease in myoma size but rather appeared to affect only myometrium.

There is no evidence that the use of combined hormonal contraceptives, the implant, or DMPA in women with myomas leads to any adverse change in contraceptive efficacy. However, efficacy may be affected if intrauterine devices are used in women who have greatly distorted uterine cavities, which can occur in association with myomas. In such situations, the rate of expulsion may be as high as 20 %, which, if unrecognized, may result in pregnancy. However, much of this data are in non-comparative studies or in studies without statistical significance [2]. The USMEC assigns IUD use in the presence of uterine fibroids as category 2, or the benefits outweigh the risks, due to the possible increased risk of expulsion (see Table 13.1). If contraception is not needed and the LNG-IUD is being used to treat abnormal bleeding, it would be appropriate to try the device in women with large myomatous uteri particularly if other nonsurgical therapies have failed. The insertion of the IUD in a woman with an enlarged fibroid uterus may be more difficult as the path to the fundus could be tortuous. If any difficulty is encountered, ultrasound guidance can be considered.

Benign Functional Ovarian Cysts

Benign functional ovarian cysts are a common problem in reproductive-aged women. It is estimated that about 250,000 women are discharged from the US hospitals annually with a diagnosis related to a benign ovarian cyst [56, 57]. Since combination hormonal contraceptives inhibit the ovulation process which can lead to benign cyst formation, it has been postulated that their use may interfere with ovarian cyst formation and may even lead to resolution of existing cysts. However, with the introduction of modern hormonal contraceptives with reduced dosages of the estrogen and progestin components, the question has been raised whether these changes affect cyst formation or resolution. It should be noted that studies to date have involved combined oral contraceptives. Thus, it is unknown whether results would be different among users of either the contraceptive patch or the vaginal ring.

The prevention of benign ovarian cysts, given their frequency, would be an obvious benefit for users of combined oral contraceptives. Although results from earlier studies with higher dose COCs indicated a protective effect against development of functional ovarian cysts [57, 58], some studies with lower dose COCs have not shown similar results. A cohort study with only 32 subjects with the diagnosis of ovarian cysts suggested that the use of higher dose (>35 μg of ethinyl estradiol [EE]) COCs compared to nonuse had a greater protective effect than preparations with lower doses [59]. However, the results were not statistically significant. A case-control study examining the risk of developing functional ovarian cysts with use of either a monophasic or a triphasic COC (EE dose not reported) compared with nonuse suggested a slight protective effect with the monophasic preparation and an increased risk with the triphasic preparation [60]. However, these results also were not statistically significant. A randomized trial involving 42 subjects followed over 6 months showed that users of a "higher" progestin dose monophasic oral contraceptive (35 μg ethinyl estradiol, 1.0 mg norethindrone) had a greater protective effect against formation of functional ovarian cysts compared to women with a "lower" progestin dose monophasic pill (35 μg ethinyl estradiol, 0.5 mg norethindrone), users of a multiphasic preparation with the same amount of estrogen, or nonusers of hormonal contraception [61]. The results in this last study also did not reach statistical significance. In conclusion, based on scant data, current oral contraceptives may have limited, if any, effect on reducing the risk of functional ovarian cysts. Also, since many of these studies involve diagnosis of cysts by serial ultrasounds, often these cysts are small (3 cm or less), vary in size depending upon when the ultrasound is completed, are not associated with symptoms, and therefore are of little clinical significance [62, 63].

There is some evidence, based on very limited data, that the use of progestin-only pills as well as the implant may be associated with some increased risk for functional ovarian cysts, though their clinical significance is questionable. In a study of 21 women on a progestin-only oral contraceptive compared to 21 women not using hormonal contraception, about one-half of the oral contraceptive users developed an ovarian cyst detected by ultrasound within two cycles of use [64]. Only one of the non-hormonal contraceptive users developed a cyst. In a cohort study that involved 116 users of the etonogestrel implant, about 25 % of users developed an ultrasound-detected functional cyst during the first year of use [65]. These cysts appeared to be small (only one in this group exceeded 40 mm), asymptomatic, and transient. The USMEC does not restrict the use of any contraceptives in the presence of benign ovarian cysts (see Table 13.1).

Since oral contraceptives suppress gonadotrophins, there has been interest in determining whether their use would help resolve existing functional ovarian cysts. A recent Cochrane literature review examined eight clinical trials involving 686 women [63]. None of the trials showed a beneficial effect of COCs in the treatment of existing functional cysts compared to no treatment. Further, most cysts resolved within a few menstrual cycles even without treatment. As an example, one trial randomized 80 women with functional cysts to a high-dose monophasic COC, a low-dose COC, a multiphasic COC, or a placebo [66]. The rates of cyst resolution were similar in all four groups.

Premenstrual Syndrome and Premenstrual Dysphoric Disorder

It is estimated that about 40 % of women will experience luteal phase symptoms which may be physical (breast tenderness, bloating), cognitive (confusion, poor concentration), or mood related (irritability, mood swings, anxiety) [67, 68]. For most, the symptoms will be mild and characterized as premenstrual syndrome (PMS) while for about 3–5 % of women the symptoms will be severe enough to interfere with some aspects of daily living. This last group will usually be classified as having the premenstrual dysphoric disorder (PMDD). PMDD as classified by the American Psychiatric Association DSM V system requires a prospective documentation of both behavioral and physical symptoms with five or more symptoms present in the week before menses followed by resolution within a few days after menses. Although the etiology of both PMS and PMDD is unknown, it has been suggested that fluctuating reproductive hormone levels may play a role since suppressing ovarian activity can relieve symptoms.

Combination oral contraceptives have been studied as treatment for both PMS and PMDD. Although frequently used to treat PMS, randomized clinical trials have shown only modest differences between COCs and placebo. Further, the number of participants in such studies has been small and study duration short, often only 3 months. For example, one study initially recruited 82 symptomatic subjects but only 23 in the triphasic COC group and 36 in the placebo group completed the 3-month trial [69]. Both groups showed similar improvement in the most of the symptoms monitored, with the exception that the COC group had improved breast tenderness and bloating to a greater extent ($p<0.03$) compared to placebo. COCs containing the progestin drospirenone have recently been evaluated since this progestin is similar in structure to spironolactone which has been used to treat PMS [70]. However, as demonstrated in a randomized controlled trial of 82 subjects comparing a drospirenone-containing oral contraceptive to placebo over three cycles, only minor differences in outcome were shown between the two groups [71]. Further, based on a 26-cycle trial comparing a desogestrel-containing COC to one containing drospirenone for efficacy, side effects, and other factors, there were no differences between them relative to improvement of PMS symptoms [72]. Thus, it is unclear whether the use of COCs, even those containing drospirenone, conveys any benefit over placebo in the management of most women with PMS. Also, current COC users report the same frequency of PMS-like symptoms as women not using such agents, especially during the hormone-free interval. One option is to reduce the hormone-free interval from the traditional 7 to 4 days or use COCs continuously. A systematic review concluded that women experienced decreased menstrual pain, headaches, and bloating in continuous COC use compared to cyclical [73].

In contrast, combined oral contraceptives for PMDD show more promise. COCs containing 3 mg of drospirenone and 20 μg of ethinyl estradiol appear to improve some of the symptoms of women with PMDD. As reviewed in the Cochrane database, five trials involving 1,290 subjects have demonstrated more symptom improvement in COC users comprising these two hormones compared to placebo [74]. For example, a multicenter, double-blind, randomized trial was conducted with 450 subjects with PMDD who received either a COC containing drospirenone or a placebo [70]. A 50 % decline in symptom scores occurred in 48 and 36 % of the COC and placebo groups, respectively ($p=0.015$). Despite data showing improvement with this particular preparation, the Cochrane database authors also note that it is unknown whether other oral contraceptives exhibit similar effects and whether the improvement persists for more than three cycles of treatment. COCs are likely better at improving the physical symptoms of PMS and PMDD compared to the emotional symptoms [74]. If emotional symptoms are predominant, then selective serotonin reuptake inhibitors (SSRIs) are the initial treatment of choice for severe PMS and PMDD.

Sexually Transmitted Infections and Pelvic Inflammatory Disease

Sexually transmitted infections (STIs) exert a major public health burden in the USA (Table 13.2). In 2011, the CDC estimated that 2.86 million *Chlamydia trachomatis* infections occurred in the USA, with more than a million of those cases being unknown or unreported [75]. As of 2009, the CDC also estimated that about 1.1 million people in the USA have human immunodeficiency virus (HIV) infection, with more than 200,000 not knowing that they are infected. In that year, HIV infection was the eighth highest cause of death in American women aged 25–44 years. Other than mortality, consequences like infertility and pelvic inflammatory disease (PID) present strong motivation to prevent STIs.

Table 13.2 Most common STIs in the USA (Annual New Infections in 2012) [76, 77]

Chlamydia	1,422,976
Gonorrhea	334,826
Genital herpes	228,000[a]
Vaginal trichomoniasis	219,000[a]
HIV	47,500[b]
Syphilis	16,667

[a]Estimate
[b]2010 estimate

Condoms have the strongest evidence supporting their use in the prevention of STI transmission [78]. As a barrier method, condoms limit skin and mucous membrane contact between sexual partners and eliminate exposure to semen and vaginal secretions when used correctly. As such, condoms should be recommended for use by all women who are not certain of their partner's or their own infection status.

Condoms are available for use by both men and women. An advantage to both male and female condoms as methods of contraception and STI prevention is that no prescription is required prior to their use. Both male and female condoms can be used immediately before sexual activity, so it requires little planning for initiation. Male condoms are placed over the penis, while female condoms are inserted into the vagina and held in place by polyurethane rings that are at each end of the condom. In the USA, there are numerous male condom types and sizes, and they are widely available. Conversely, there is one type of female condom approved for use in the USA. There have been no randomized trials comparing the effectiveness of male and female condoms in terms of pregnancy or STI prevention. However, available evidence suggests that male condoms may be more effective in pregnancy prevention. Estimates of pregnancy rates with perfect and typical use of male condoms are 2 % and 18 %, respectively, while estimates of pregnancy rates with perfect and typical use of female condoms are 5 % and 21 %, respectively [79, 80].

Hormonal contraception and IUDs do not prevent the transmission of STIs. In fact, COCs have been associated with increased risk of chlamydial infection in some studies, even when controlling for number of sexual partners (relative risk 1.8) [81, 82]. Possible explanations for these findings include evidence from animal models that estrogen and progesterone use may enhance the growth of chlamydia infection [83]. It is important to note, however, that COC use has also been associated with reduction in PID risk by 50–80 % in other studies [84]. Suspected reasons for protection against PID include increased cervical mucus thickness with COC use, leading to decreased ability for pathogens to ascend into the cervix and uterus from the vagina. COC use does not seem to increase the risk of HIV infection or trichomonas infection [85, 86]. Conversely, COC use in women with high-risk human papillomavirus (HPV) types is associated with greater progression to invasive cervical cancer when compared to non-COC use. A 2002 study conducted by the World Health Organization (WHO) pooled data from eight case-control studies to compare the odds of invasive cervical cancer or carcinoma in situ among COC users and never users [87]. COC use of 5–9 years was associated with a 2.82 times greater odds (95 % CI 1.46–5.42) of progression to invasive cancer or carcinoma in situ. Using COCs for greater than 10 years was associated with a 4.03 times greater odds (95 % CI 2.09–8.02) of progression to invasive cancer or carcinoma in situ. Since the publication of this study, the relationship between COC use and cervical cancer has been examined by several other investigations. One such study enrolled 1,135 Thai women aged 20–37, tested them for HPV infection at baseline, and followed them for 18 months at 6-month intervals [88]. While subjects who used COCs cleared HPV infection less often than non-COC users in the study (relative risk 0.67, 95 % CI 0.49–0.93), there was no significant difference in new HPV acquisition between groups. Increased persistence of HPV infection in COC users has also been demonstrated in other studies [89]. However, other studies have not found a link between COC use and high-grade cervical dysplasia [90–92]. A reanalysis of pooled data regarding 16,573 women with cervical cancer and 35,509 women without cervical cancer determined that the risk of cervical cancer declined after stopping COC use and returned to the risk seen by never users after 10 years [93]. Taking this evidence into account, the USMEC regard COC use in women with cervical dysplasia as having greater advantages than potential risk (category 2), recognizing the overall contraceptive and non-contraceptive benefits of COC use [2].

The exact relationship between DMPA and STIs is unclear. Some investigations have established DMPA use as a risk factor for increased chlamydia infection, reporting a relative risk of 1.6 (95 % CI, 1.1–2.4) when compared with non-users [82]. Other studies have not found such an association [94]. DMPA does not increase the risk of trichomonas infection [86]. DMPA has been the focus of several African studies examining its link with HIV infection. In a prospective observational study of 1,341 couples consisting of an HIV-infected man and a non-infected woman, the risk of HIV acquisition was two times greater in women who used DMPA versus non-hormonal contraception [95]. A South African study of 5,567 women examined their risk of HIV acquisition as it related to hormonal contraception use [85]. Although not statistically significant, there was a trend suggesting greater risk of HIV infection among DMPA users. Reanalysis of a cohort study that had originally not found an increased risk of HIV infection with DMPA use demonstrated an increased risk when the data was subjected to a different statistical method of analysis [96]. In contrast, there have also been studies that did not show an elevated risk of HIV infection with DMPA use [97, 98]. Two studies that examined the possible effects of removing DMPA from family planning services in Africa warn that such an action would cause greater numbers of death from maternal mortality [99, 100]. The USMEC issued an update in 2012 to address this issue, stating that the use of DMPA was safe in women at increased risk for HIV acquisition but that they should be strongly advised to use condoms for HIV prevention (see Chap. 6 on HIV/AIDs for more details) [101].

Historically, IUD use was linked to greater risk of PID. In 1992, however, the WHO published the results of 22,908 IUD insertions and found that the risk of PID after IUD insertion was higher than non-IUD users for only the first 20 days after insertion [102]. A 2000 systematic review determined that, in fact, current positive STI status, and not IUD use, placed women at higher risk of developing PID [103]. A more recent study performed in West Africa produced similar conclusions, demonstrating that IUD use does not lead to a higher risk of PID [104]. A large retrospective cohort study of 57,218 IUD insertions in California demonstrated a PID risk of only 0.54 % within 90 days after insertion [105]. The same study determined that screening for cervical infections at any time was equivalent to non-screening in terms of PID risk. The 2013 US Selected Practice Recommendations (USSPR) for IUD insertion do not require additional cervical infection screening beyond what is already recommended by the CDC, namely that women under 25, those with new sexual partners, or those who have multiple sexual partners should be screened annually [106]. If the woman has not been screened as per CDC guidelines, then tests can be sent on the same day as IUD insertion. Like COCs, the LNG-IUD may be protective against the development of PID as its primary contraceptive method of action is cervical mucus thickening. As IUDs are not associated with greater PID risk, their use should be encouraged in women who seek reliable, highly effective contraceptive methods regardless of the STI risk. Of course, if the patient has an active cervical infection or PID, then IUD insertion should be deferred until after treatment (see Table 13.1). The USSPR also notes that women at high risk for gonorrhea or chlamydia infection (e.g., those with a currently infected partner) generally should have testing and treatment prior to IUD insertion.

In the event that a patient is diagnosed with PID and has an IUD in place, the USSPR supports treatment of PID without removal of the IUD for at least 48–72 h. After reassessment of the patient at this point, consideration of IUD removal can be made if there is no improvement in the patient's status. Antibiotics should be continued even if the IUD is removed to ensure adequate treatment of PID. In cases where a patient with PID requests IUD removal, antibiotics should be initiated prior to removal to prevent possible bacteremia resulting from the removal procedure. The patient should be counseled about alternative contraceptive methods and options for emergency contraception should be provided when appropriate [106]. Similarly, gonorrhea, chlamydia, and trichomonas can be treated with the IUD in place.

Conclusion

More than just agents used to prevent pregnancy, contraception use is beneficial in many gynecological conditions like abnormal uterine bleeding, endometriosis, and dysmenorrhea. However, evidence suggests that contraceptives may not be effective in other contexts, like benign ovarian cyst prevention or STI prevention (with the exception of condoms). Published data should guide non-contraceptive uses of these medications to ensure that women receive maximal benefit and face minimal harm.

References

1. Munro MG, Critchley HO, Broder MS, Fraser IS, Disorders FWGoM. FIGO classification system (PALM-COEIN) for causes of abnormal uterine bleeding in nongravid women of reproductive age. Int J Gynaecol Obstet. 2011;113(1):3–13.
2. U. S. Medical Eligibility Criteria for Contraceptive Use, 2010. MMWR Recomm Rep. 2010; 59(RR-4):1 86.
3. Committee on Practice B-G. Practice bulletin no. 128: diagnosis of abnormal uterine bleeding in reproductive-aged women. Obstet Gynecol. 2012; 120(1):197–206.
4. Kelekci S, Kelekci KH, Yilmaz B. Effects of levonorgestrel-releasing intrauterine system and T380A intrauterine copper device on dysmenorrhea and days of bleeding in women with and without adenomyosis. Contraception. 2012;86(5):458 63.
5. Sheng J, Zhang WY, Zhang JP, Lu D. The LNG-IUS study on adenomyosis: a 3-year follow-up study on the efficacy and side effects of the use of levonorgestrel intrauterine system for the treatment of dysmenorrhea associated with adenomyosis. Contraception. 2009;79(3):189–93.
6. Bragheto AM, Caserta N, Bahamondes L, Petta CA. Effectiveness of the levonorgestrel-releasing intrauterine system in the treatment of adenomyosis diagnosed and monitored by magnetic resonance imaging. Contraception. 2007;76(3):195–9.

7. Marjoribanks J, Lethaby A, Farquhar C. Surgery versus medical therapy for heavy menstrual bleeding. Cochrane Database Syst Rev. 2006;2, CD003855.
8. Maia Jr H, Casoy J, Pimentel K, Correia T, Athayde C, Cruz T, et al. Effect of oral contraceptives on vascular endothelial growth factor, Cox-2 and aromatase expression in the endometrium of uteri affected by myomas and associated pathologies. Contraception. 2008;78(6):479–85.
9. Olufowobi O, Sharif K, Papaionnou S, Neelakantan D, Mohammed H, Afnan M. Are the anticipated benefits of myomectomy achieved in women of reproductive age? A 5-year review of the results at a UK tertiary hospital. J Obstet Gynaecol. 2004;24(4): 434–40.
10. Stewart EA, Nowak RA. Leiomyoma-related bleeding: a classic hypothesis updated for the molecular era. Hum Reprod Update. 1996;2(4):295–306.
11. Wegienka G, Baird DD, Hertz-Picciotto I, Harlow SD, Steege JF, Hill MC, et al. Self-reported heavy bleeding associated with uterine leiomyomata. Obstet Gynecol. 2003;101(3):431–7.
12. Zapata LB, Whiteman MK, Tepper NK, Jamieson DJ, Marchbanks PA, Curtis KM. Intrauterine device use among women with uterine fibroids: a systematic review. Contraception. 2010;82(1):41–55.
13. Sayed GH, Zakherah MS, El-Nashar SA, Shaaban MM. A randomized clinical trial of a levonorgestrel-releasing intrauterine system and a low-dose combined oral contraceptive for fibroid-related menorrhagia. Int J Gynaecol Obstet. 2011;112(2):126–30.
14. Socolov D, Blidaru I, Tamba B, Miron N, Boiculese L, Socolov R. Levonorgestrel releasing-intrauterine system for the treatment of menorrhagia and/or frequent irregular uterine bleeding associated with uterine leiomyoma. Eur J Contracept Reprod Health Care. 2011;16(6):480–7.
15. Xie ZW, Zhang YN, Wan S, Xu WZ, Chen J. Levonorgestrel-releasing intrauterine device is an efficacious contraceptive for women with leiomyoma. J Int Med Res. 2012;40(5):1966–72.
16. Kriplani A, Awasthi D, Kulshrestha V, Agarwal N. Efficacy of the levonorgestrel-releasing intrauterine system in uterine leiomyoma. Int J Gynaecol Obstet. 2012;116(1):35–8.
17. Sangkomkamhang US, Lumbiganon P, Laopaiboon M, Mol BW. Progestogens or progestogen-releasing intrauterine systems for uterine fibroids. Cochrane Database Syst Rev. 2013;2, CD008994.
18. Orsini G, Laricchia L, Fanelli M. Low-dose combination oral contraceptives use in women with uterine leiomyomas. Minerva Ginecol. 2002;54(3):253–61.
19. Venkatachalam S, Bagratee JS, Moodley J. Medical management of uterine fibroids with medroxyprogesterone acetate (Depo Provera): a pilot study. J Obstet Gynaecol. 2004;24(7):798–800.
20. American College of O, Gynecologists. ACOG committee opinion no. 557: management of acute abnormal uterine bleeding in nonpregnant reproductive-aged women. Obstet Gynecol. 2013;121(4):891–6.
21. American College of O, Gynecologists Committee on Adolescent Health C, American College of O, Gynecologists Committee Gynecologic P. ACOG Committee Opinion No. 451: Von Willebrand disease in women. Obstet Gynecol. 2009;114(6):1439–43.
22. Kingman CE, Kadir RA, Lee CA, Economides DL. The use of levonorgestrel-releasing intrauterine system for treatment of menorrhagia in women with inherited bleeding disorders. BJOG. 2004;111(12): 1425–8.
23. Foster PA. The reproductive health of women with von Willebrand Disease unresponsive to DDAVP: results of an international survey. On behalf of the Subcommittee on von Willebrand Factor of the Scientific and Standardization Committee of the ISTH. Thromb Haemost. 1995;74(2):784–90.
24. Pitangui AC, Gomes MR, Lima AS, Schwingel PA, Albuquerque AP, de Araujo RC. Menstruation disturbances: prevalence, characteristics, and effects on the activities of daily living among adolescent girls from Brazil. J Pediatr Adoles Gynecol. 2013;26(3): 148–52.
25. Chia CF, Lai JH, Cheung PK, Kwong LT, Lau FP, Leung KH, et al. Dysmenorrhoea among Hong Kong university students: prevalence, impact, and management. Hong Kong Med J. 2013;19(3):222–8.
26. Grandi G, Ferrari S, Xholli A, Cannoletta M, Palma F, Romani C, et al. Prevalence of menstrual pain in young women: what is dysmenorrhea? J Pain Res. 2012;5:169–74.
27. Dawood MY. Ibuprofen and dysmenorrhea. Am J Med. 1984;77(1A):87–94.
28. Ronnerdag M, Odlind V. Health effects of long-term use of the intrauterine levonorgestrel-releasing system. A follow-up study over 12 years of continuous use. Acta Obstet Gynecol Scand. 1999;78(8):716–21.
29. Varma R, Sinha D, Gupta JK. Non-contraceptive uses of levonorgestrel-releasing hormone system (LNG-IUS)—a systematic enquiry and overview. Eur J Obstet Gynecol Reprod Biol. 2006;125(1): 9–28.
30. Lalos O, Joelsson I. Effect of salbutamol on the non-pregnant human uterus in vivo. A hysterometric study in dysmenorrheic women. Acta Obstet Gynecol Scand. 1981;60(4):349–52.
31. Milsom I, Lete I, Bjertnaes A, Rokstad K, Lindh I, Gruber CJ, et al. Effects on cycle control and body-weight of the combined contraceptive ring, NuvaRing, versus an oral contraceptive containing 30 microg ethinyl estradiol and 3 mg drospirenone. Hum Reprod. 2006;21(9):2304–11.
32. Robinson JC, Plichta S, Weisman CS, Nathanson CA, Ensminger M. Dysmenorrhea and use of oral contraceptives in adolescent women attending a family planning clinic. Am J Obstet Gynecol. 1992;166(2):578–83.
33. Davis AR, Westhoff C, O'Connell K, Gallagher N. Oral contraceptives for dysmenorrhea in adolescent girls: a randomized trial. Obstet Gynecol. 2005;106(1):97–104.

34. Winkler UH, Ferguson H, Mulders JA. Cycle control, quality of life and acne with two low-dose oral contraceptives containing 20 microg ethinylestradiol. Contraception. 2004;69(6):469–76.
35. Dmitrovic R, Kunselman AR, Legro RS. Continuous compared with cyclic oral contraceptives for the treatment of primary dysmenorrhea: a randomized controlled trial. Obstet Gynecol. 2012;119(6):1143–50.
36. French L. Dysmenorrhea. Am Fam Physician. 2005;71(2):285–91.
37. Funk S, Miller MM, Mishell Jr DR, Archer DF, Poindexter A, Schmidt J, et al. Safety and efficacy of Implanon, a single-rod implantable contraceptive containing etonogestrel. Contraception. 2005;71(5): 319–26.
38. Croxatto HB. Clinical profile of Implanon: a single-rod etonogestrel contraceptive implant. Eur J Contracept Reprod Health Care. 2000;5 Suppl 2:21–8.
39. Practice bulletin no. 114: management of endometriosis. Obstet Gynecol. 2010;116(1):223–36.
40. Lockhat FB, Emembolu JO, Konje JC. The efficacy, side-effects and continuation rates in women with symptomatic endometriosis undergoing treatment with an intra-uterine administered progestogen (levonorgestrel): a 3 year follow-up. Hum Reprod. 2005;20(3):789–93.
41. Petta CA, Ferriani RA, Abrao MS, Hassan D, Rosa ESJC, Podgaec S, et al. Randomized clinical trial of a levonorgestrel-releasing intrauterine system and a depot GnRH analogue for the treatment of chronic pelvic pain in women with endometriosis. Hum Reprod. 2005;20(7):1993–8.
42. Vercellini P, Frontino G, De Giorgi O, Pietropaolo G, Pasin R, Crosignani PG. Continuous use of an oral contraceptive for endometriosis-associated recurrent dysmenorrhea that does not respond to a cyclic pill regimen. Fertil Steril. 2003;80(3):560–3.
43. Vessey MP, Villard-Mackintosh L, Painter R. Epidemiology of endometriosis in women attending family planning clinics. BMJ. 1993;306(6871): 182–4.
44. Crosignani PG, Luciano A, Ray A, Bergqvist A. Subcutaneous depot medroxyprogesterone acetate versus leuprolide acetate in the treatment of endometriosis-associated pain. Hum Reprod. 2006;21(1):248–56.
45. Schlaff WD, Carson SA, Luciano A, Ross D, Bergqvist A. Subcutaneous injection of depot medroxyprogesterone acetate compared with leuprolide acetate in the treatment of endometriosis-associated pain. Fertil Steril. 2006;85(2):314–25.
46. Harada T, Momoeda M, Taketani Y, Hoshiai H, Terakawa N. Low-dose oral contraceptive pill for dysmenorrhea associated with endometriosis: a placebo-controlled, double-blind, randomized trial. Fertil Steril. 2008;90(5):1583–8.
47. Seracchioli R, Mabrouk M, Frasca C, Manuzzi L, Montanari G, Keramyda A, et al. Long-term cyclic and continuous oral contraceptive therapy and endometrioma recurrence: a randomized controlled trial. Fertil Steril. 2010;93(1):52–6.
48. Seracchioli R, Mabrouk M, Manuzzi L, Vicenzi C, Frasca C, Elmakky A, et al. Post-operative use of oral contraceptive pills for prevention of anatomical relapse or symptom-recurrence after conservative surgery for endometriosis. Hum Reprod. 2009; 24(11):2729–35.
49. Abou-Setta AM, Al-Inany HG, Farquhar CM. Levonorgestrel-releasing intrauterine device (LNG-IUD) for symptomatic endometriosis following surgery. Cochrane Database Syst Rev. 2006;4, CD005072.
50. Baird DD, Dunson DB, Hill MC, Cousins D, Schectman JM. High cumulative incidence of uterine leiomyoma in black and white women: ultrasound evidence. Am J Obstet Gynecol. 2003;188(1):100–7.
51. Practice Bulletin ACOG. Alternatives to hysterectomy in the management of leiomyomas. Obstet Gynecol. 2008;112(2 Pt 1):387–400.
52. Ross RK, Pike MC, Vessey MP, Bull D, Yeates D, Casagrande JT. Risk factors for uterine fibroids: reduced risk associated with oral contraceptives. Br Med J (Clin Res Ed). 1986;293(6543):359–62.
53. Marshall LM, Spiegelman D, Goldman MB, Manson JE, Colditz GA, Barbieri RL, et al. A prospective study of reproductive factors and oral contraceptive use in relation to the risk of uterine leiomyomata. Fertil Steril. 1998;70(3):432–9.
54. Wise LA, Palmer JR, Harlow BL, Spiegelman D, Stewart EA, Adams-Campbell LL, et al. Reproductive factors, hormonal contraception, and risk of uterine leiomyomata in African-American women: a prospective study. Am J Epidemiol. 2004;159(2):113–23.
55. Magalhaes J, Aldrighi JM, de Lima GR. Uterine volume and menstrual patterns in users of the levonorgestrel-releasing intrauterine system with idiopathic menorrhagia or menorrhagia due to leiomyomas. Contraception. 2007;75(3):193–8.
56. Kozak LJ, Owings MF, Hall MJ. National Hospital Discharge Survey: 2002 annual summary with detailed diagnosis and procedure data. Vital Health Stat. 2005;13(158):1–199.
57. Vessey M, Metcalfe A, Wells C, McPherson K, Westhoff C, Yeates D. Ovarian neoplasms, functional ovarian cysts, and oral contraceptives. Br Med J (Clin Res Ed). 1987;294(6586):1518–20.
58. Ory H. Boston Collaborative Drug Surveillance Program. Functional ovarian cysts and oral contraceptives. Negative association confirmed surgically. A cooperative study. JAMA. 1974;228:68–79.
59. Lanes SF, Birmann B, Walker AM, Singer S. Oral contraceptive type and functional ovarian cysts. Am J Obstet Gynecol. 1992;166(3):956–61.
60. Holt VL, Daling JR, McKnight B, Moore D, Stergachis A, Weiss NS. Functional ovarian cysts in relation to the use of monophasic and triphasic oral contraceptives. Obstet Gynecol. 1992;79(4):529–33.
61. Grimes DA, Godwin AJ, Rubin A, Smith JA, Lacarra M. Ovulation and follicular development associated with three low-dose oral contraceptives: a randomized controlled trial. Obstet Gynecol. 1994;83(1):29–34.

62. Christensen JT, Boldsen JL, Westergaard JG. Functional ovarian cysts in premenopausal and gynecologically healthy women. Contraception. 2002;66(3):153–7.
63. Grimes DA, Jones LB, Lopez LM, Schulz KF. Oral contraceptives for functional ovarian cysts. Cochrane Database Syst Rev. 2006;9, CD006134.
64. Tayob Y, Adams J, Jacobs HS, Guillebaud J. Ultrasound demonstration of increased frequency of functional ovarian cysts in women using progestogen-only oral contraception. Br J Obstet Gynaecol. 1985;92(10):1003–9.
65. Hidalgo MM, Lisondo C, Juliato CT, Espejo-Arce X, Monteiro I, Bahamondes L. Ovarian cysts in users of Implanon and Jadelle subdermal contraceptive implants. Contraception. 2006;73(5):532–6.
66. Turan C, Zorlu CG, Ugur M, Ozcan T, Kaleli B, Gokmen O. Expectant management of functional ovarian cysts: an alternative to hormonal therapy. Int J Gynaecol Obstet. 1994;47(3):257–60.
67. Johnson SR. Premenstrual syndrome, premenstrual dysphoric disorder, and beyond: a clinical primer for practitioners. Obstet Gynecol. 2004;104(4):845–59.
68. Sternfeld B, Swindle R, Chawla A, Long S, Kennedy S. Severity of premenstrual symptoms in a health maintenance organization population. Obstet Gynecol. 2002;99(6):1014–24.
69. Graham CA, Sherwin BB. The relationship between mood and sexuality in women using an oral contraceptive as a treatment for premenstrual symptoms. Psychoneuroendocrinology. 1993;18(4):273–81.
70. Yonkers KA, Brown C, Pearlstein TB, Foegh M, Sampson-Landers C, Rapkin A. Efficacy of a new low-dose oral contraceptive with drospirenone in premenstrual dysphoric disorder. Obstet Gynecol. 2005;106(3):492–501.
71. Freeman EW, Rickels K, Sondheimer SJ, Polansky M. Concurrent use of oral contraceptives with antidepressants for premenstrual syndromes. J Clin Psychopharmacol. 2001;21(5):540–2.
72. Foidart JM, Wuttke W, Bouw GM, Gerlinger C, Heithecker R. A comparative investigation of contraceptive reliability, cycle control and tolerance of two monophasic oral contraceptives containing either drospirenone or desogestrel. Eur J Contracept Reprod Health Care. 2000;5(2):124–34.
73. Edelman AB, Gallo MF, Jensen JT, Nichols MD, Schulz KF, Grimes DA. Continuous or extended cycle vs cyclic use of combined oral contraceptives for contraception. Cochrane Database Syst Rev. 2005;3, CD004695.
74. Lopez LM, Kaptein AA, Helmerhorst FM. Oral contraceptives containing drospirenone for premenstrual syndrome. Cochrane Database Syst Rev. 2012;2, CD006586.
75. Centers for Disease Control [Internet]. Atlanta: Centers for Disease Control: 2012 [cited 2013 Feb 11]. Available at www.cdc.gov/std/chlamydia.htm. 2012.
76. Centers for Disease Control [Internet]. Atlanta: Centers for Disease Control; 2014 [cited 2014 Jan 8]. Available at http://www.cdc/std/stats12/Surv2012.pdf. 2014.
77. Centers for Disease Control [Internet]. Atlanta: Centers for Disease Control: 2012 [cited 2013 May 22] Available at http://www.cdc.gov/nchhsstp/newsroom/docs/2012/HIV-Infections-2007-2010.pdf. 2012.
78. Cates Jr W. Review of non-hormonal contraception (condoms, intrauterine devices, nonoxynol-9 and combos) on HIV acquisition. J Acquir Immune Defic Syndr. 2005;38 Suppl 1:S8–10.
79. Farr G, Gabelnick H, Sturgen K, Dorflinger L. Contraceptive efficacy and acceptability of the female condom. Am J Public Health. 1994;84(12):1960–4.
80. Trussel J. Contraceptive Efficacy. In: Hatcher RA, editor. Contraceptive technology. 20th ed. New York: Ardent Media; 2011.
81. Henry-Suchet J. Hormonal contraception and pelvic inflammatory disease. Eur J Contracept Reprod Health Care. 1997;2(4):263–7.
82. Baeten JM, Nyange PM, Richardson BA, Lavreys L, Chohan B, Martin Jr HL, et al. Hormonal contraception and risk of sexually transmitted disease acquisition: results from a prospective study. Am J Obstet Gynecol. 2001;185(2):380–5.
83. Washington AE, Gove S, Schachter J, Sweet RL. Oral contraceptives, Chlamydia trachomatis infection, and pelvic inflammatory disease. A word of caution about protection. JAMA. 1985;253(15):2246–50.
84. Burkman RT. Oral contraceptives: current status. Clin Obstet Gynecol. 2001;44(1):62–72.
85. Morrison CS, Skoler-Karpoff S, Kwok C, Chen PL, van de Wijgert J, Gehret-Plagianos M, et al. Hormonal contraception and the risk of HIV acquisition among women in South Africa. AIDS. 2012;26(4):497–504.
86. Torok MR, Miller WC, Hobbs MM, Macdonald PD, Leone PA, Schwebke JR, et al. The association between oral contraceptives, depot-medroxyprogesterone acetate, and trichomoniasis. Sex Transm Dis. 2009;36(6):336–40.
87. Moreno V, Bosch FX, Munoz N, Meijer CJ, Shah KV, Walboomers JM, et al. Effect of oral contraceptives on risk of cervical cancer in women with human papillomavirus infection: the IARC multicentric case-control study. Lancet. 2002;359(9312):1085–92.
88. Marks M, Gravitt PE, Gupta SB, Liaw KL, Tadesse A, Kim E, et al. Combined oral contraceptive use increases HPV persistence but not new HPV detection in a cohort of women from Thailand. J Infect Dis. 2011;204(10):1505–13.
89. Nielsen A, Kjaer SK, Munk C, Osler M, Iftner T. Persistence of high-risk human papillomavirus infection in a population-based cohort of Danish women. J Med Virol. 2010;82(4):616–23.
90. Harris TG, Miller L, Kulasingam SL, Feng Q, Kiviat NB, Schwartz SM, et al. Depot-medroxyprogesterone acetate and combined oral contraceptive use and

cervical neoplasia among women with oncogenic human papillomavirus infection. Am J Obstet Gynecol. 2009;200(5):489.e1–8.
91. Syrjanen K, Shabalova I, Petrovichev N, Kozachenko V, Zakharova T, Pajanidi J, et al. Oral contraceptives are not an independent risk factor for cervical intraepithelial neoplasia or high-risk human papillomavirus infections. Anticancer Res. 2006;26(6C): 4729–40.
92. Longatto-Filho A, Hammes LS, Sarian LO, Roteli-Martins C, Derchain SF, Erzen M, et al. Hormonal contraceptives and the length of their use are not independent risk factors for high-risk HPV infections or high-grade CIN. Gynecol Obstet Invest. 2011;71(2):93–103.
93. International Collaboration of Epidemiological Studies of Cervical Cancer, Appleby P, Beral V, Berrington de Gonzalez A, Colin D, Franceschi S, et al. Cervical cancer and hormonal contraceptives: collaborative reanalysis of individual data for 16,573 women with cervical cancer and 35,509 women without cervical cancer from 24 epidemiological studies. Lancet. 2007;370(9599):1609–21.
94. Romer A, Shew ML, Ofner S, Gilliam ML, Martins SL, Fortenberry JD. Depot medroxyprogesterone acetate use is not associated with risk of incident sexually transmitted infections among adolescent women. J Adolesc Health. 2013;52(1):83–8.
95. Heffron R, Donnell D, Rees H, Celum C, Mugo N, Were E, et al. Use of hormonal contraceptives and risk of HIV-1 transmission: a prospective cohort study. Lancet Infect Dis. 2012;12(1):19–26.
96. Morrison CS, Chen PL, Kwok C, Richardson BA, Chipato T, Mugerwa R, et al. Hormonal contraception and HIV acquisition: reanalysis using marginal structural modeling. Aids. 2010;24(11): 1778–81.
97. Kleinschmidt I, Rees H, Delany S, Smith D, Dinat N, Nkala B, et al. Injectable progestin contraceptive use and risk of HIV infection in a South African family planning cohort. Contraception. 2007;75(6):461–7.
98. Myer L, Denny L, Wright TC, Kuhn L. Prospective study of hormonal contraception and women's risk of HIV infection in South Africa. Int J Epidemiol. 2007;36(1):166–74.
99. Jain AK. Hormonal contraception and HIV acquisition risk: implications for individual users and public policies. Contraception. 2012;86(6):645–52.
100. Rodriguez MI, Reeves MF, Caughey AB. Evaluating the competing risks of HIV acquisition and maternal mortality in Africa: a decision analysis. BJOG. 2012;119(9):1067–73.
101. Centers for Disease Control and Prevention. Update to CDC's U.S. Medical Eligibility Criteria for Contraceptive Use, 2010: revised recommendations for the use of hormonal contraception among women at high risk for HIV infection or infected with HIV. MMWR. 2012;61(24):449–52.
102. Farley TM, Rosenberg MJ, Rowe PJ, Chen JH, Meirik O. Intrauterine devices and pelvic inflammatory disease: an international perspective. Lancet. 1992;339(8796):785–8.
103. Grimes DA. Intrauterine device and upper-genital-tract infection. Lancet. 2000;356(9234):1013–9.
104. Stanback J, Shelton JD. Pelvic inflammatory disease attributable to the IUD: modeling risk in West Africa. Contraception. 2008;77(4):227–9.
105. Sufrin CB, Postlethwaite D, Armstrong MA, Merchant M, Wendt JM, Steinauer JE. Neisseria gonorrhea and Chlamydia trachomatis screening at intrauterine device insertion and pelvic inflammatory disease. Obstet Gynecol. 2012;120(6):1314–21.
106. Division of Reproductive Health NCfCDP, Health Promotion CfDC, Prevention. U.S. Selected Practice Recommendations for Contraceptive Use, 2013: adapted from the World Health Organization selected practice recommendations for contraceptive use, 2nd edition. MMWR Recomm Rep. 2013;62(RR-05):1–60.

Oncocontraception

14

Ashlesha Patel, Alicia Roston, Kelly Stempinski, Lindsay Zimmerman, Erica O'Neill, and Ashok R. Patel

Introduction

In 2009, approximately 719,000 women in the United States were newly diagnosed with various types of cancer [1]. With the recent advancements in cancer detection and treatment, survival rates are increasing for cancer patients. Over the past 30 years, the number of cancer survivors in the United States has increased to almost 14 million [1]. Today, approximately 4 in 100 women are cancer survivors [1].

Nearly 17 % of new cancer cases in women are diagnosed in the reproductive age [1]. The most common cancers diagnosed in women of childbearing age are breast, thyroid, melanoma, colorectal, and cervical [2]. Of these, breast is the most common malignancy site for women and is the second leading cause of cancer-related deaths in women [3]. Almost 90 % of women under 50 diagnosed with cancer are expected to survive beyond 5 years [4]. As more cancer patients survive due to the various advancements in screening and treatment modalities, quality of life issues, including reproductive health, increase in importance.

Research has indicated that fertility after treatment remains a major concern for many female cancer survivors [5]. Primary site and location of disease may impact reproductive potential directly or indirectly. Iatrogenic endocrine disruption and gonadal damage impact reproductive capacity. Furthermore, assessments of fertility and pregnancy risk are challenging. While fertility preservation for young cancer survivors has obtained research and public interest, reproductive health for women with cancer extends beyond fertility preservation. Sexuality and family planning ranging from contraception, preconception counseling, and optimization of present or future pregnancy comprise comprehensive reproductive health [6]. The full scope of reproductive health is often omitted from the discussion of cancer treatment planning at times to the detriment to the cancer survivor [7, 8].

Prioritization of pregnancy prevention often falls secondary to the primary focus of cancer survivorship [9]. Pregnancy prevention is a key component of reproductive health care which is suboptimally addressed for the vast majority of cancer survivors [10]. An unintended pregnancy has profound impact for the cancer survivor [1]. Issues of ambivalence regarding the pregnancy

A. Patel, M.D., M.P.H. (✉) • A. Roston, M.P.H.
K. Stempinski, M.P.H. • L. Zimmerman, M.P.H.
E. O'Neill, M.D., M.P.H.
Division of Family Planning Services, Department of Obstetrics and Gynecology, John H. Stroger, Jr. Hospital of Cook County, Chicago, IL, USA
e-mail: apatel2@cookcountyhhs.org; alicia.roston@gmail.com; kstempinski@cookcountyhhs.org; lpzimmerman@gmail.com; eoneill2@cookcountyhhs.org

A.R. Patel, M.D.
Rush Medical College, Chicago, IL, USA
e-mail: apatelfiji@sbcglobal.net

R.H. Allen and C.A. Cwiak (eds.), *Contraception for the Medically Challenging Patient*,
DOI 10.1007/978-1-4939-1233-9_14, © Springer Science+Business Media New York 2014

are not uncommon [11, 12]. A poorly timed pregnancy may be complicated by suboptimal maternal health, teratogenic exposures, deferment of cancer treatment, untoward fetal outcomes, or termination of pregnancy [13, 14]. While all women need access to contraception, the consequences of unintended pregnancy may be more severe in women with cancer [14]. When an unintended pregnancy results, priorities pertaining to cancer care may shift.

The provision of contraception for women diagnosed with cancer is challenging. In one study, 50 % of female cancer survivors indicated that their contraceptive management did not match future childbearing interest [14]. Medical risks associated with certain cancers may limit contraceptive options. Furthermore, comprehensive knowledge of contraceptive methods may be limited among oncologists, leaving many women at risk for unintended pregnancy [8, 15]. We have coined the term *oncocontraception* for the application of contraception within the context of cancer care. In this chapter, we will explore the facets of contraceptive care for the cancer survivor.

Oncocontraceptive Need

While there may be misconceptions regarding sexuality and reproductive interests, women with cancer often have the same reproductive interests as women without cancer [8, 13]. Focus on reproductive health needs, by providers and patients, is often overshadowed by the primary focus of cancer care. Women with cancer may falsely be perceived as asexual [13]; therefore, conversations surrounding childbearing interests do not occur. Furthermore, reproductive interests are not stagnant and may change as a woman transitions from cancer diagnosis and immediate therapies to long-term survival [13, 16].

Recommendations state that young women should be counseled about the long-term effects of cancer therapies, especially impaired fertility with cancer treatment [17]. However, studies suggest that only about half of those diagnosed with cancer during reproductive ages (age 15–44 years) receive such information from their providers [17]. Risks of infertility are recognized, and several guidelines have been developed to address the devastating outcome of undesired loss of fertility due to cancer treatment [18, 19].

With the common bias that cancer survivors are less sexually active and are at decreased perceived or actual fecundity, risk of undesired pregnancy has not yet been addressed with the same fervor as infertility [13]. Additionally, Partridge and colleagues found that women may tend to overestimate their risk of loss of fertility [5]. Unintended pregnancy rates in the United States are as high as 50 % of all pregnancies [20]. This rate is higher among women with chronic disease [21, 22]. Unintended pregnancy in the cancer survivor may be due to a number of factors. Factors may include patient ambivalence, lack of counseling regarding pregnancy risk, and lack of knowledge regarding appropriate methods of contraception [10–12].

Evidence indicates women with chronic disease may be less likely to receive counseling on contraception methods [23, 24]. A European study demonstrated that no adolescent cancer clinics had a policy regarding contraceptive management for adolescent patients [16]. In another study, two-thirds of women surveyed did not recall a discussion with providers regarding pregnancy as a health risk [17]. One study demonstrated that only 15 % of breast cancer patients received materials and 21 % contraceptive counseling prior to initiation of therapy [7]. Lack of knowledge and adherence to guidelines by health care providers often limits recommended contraceptive methods to barrier and fertility awareness methods (typical use failure rates of 15–85 %), leaving the patient at risk of unintended pregnancy [25, 26].

Regardless of childbearing interests, pregnancy within 1 year of cancer therapy completion would be considered suboptimal if surgical and medical treatments harmful to a pregnancy are utilized [27]. Although pregnancy may not worsen cancer outcomes, pregnancy may conflict with primary plan for cancer treatment [28, 29]. Additionally, deferment of pregnancy for hormonally mediated cancers is recommended for 2–5 years after diagnosis due to higher rates of recurrence [28]. Given these recommendations, the provision of long-term reversible contraception would be optimal. This, however, is rarely the case. Oncologists are ill equipped to offer long-term reversible methods. Additionally, ambivalence of the patient plays a factor [11]. Fear of loss of fertility may influence women to suboptimally contracept [5, 16].

Fertility Disruption for Women with Cancer

Further convoluting the contraceptive conversation is the uncertainty surrounding fecundity during and post-cancer treatment. Alteration of menstrual and ovulatory cycles is a common side effect of chemotherapy, localized radiation, and adjuvant therapy. Literature suggests that fertility rates may decrease between 10 and 50 % post-chemotherapy [27, 29, 30]. Factors that most influence ovarian function are type of chemotherapy and age of patient at the time of diagnosis. Some cancer therapy modalities induce amenorrhea. The absence of menstruation, however, does not necessarily indicate lack of ovarian function and fertility. Additionally, the possibility of spontaneous recovery of ovarian function has been observed following treatment [31]. After a short period of chemotherapy-induced amenorrhea, 50 % of women younger than 35 years resume menstruation. In older women, the risk of permanent amenorrhea is increased due to reduced ovarian reserve [32].

Endocrine Assessment

For patients who undergo chemotherapy, ovarian function should be reassessed periodically. This reassessment may serve dual purposes, guiding those who wish to maintain fertility as well as those who wish to prevent pregnancy. As menstrual activity is not a reliable index to assess ovarian function, various tests including follicle-stimulating hormone (FSH) level, inhibin A or B levels, or anti-Mullerian hormone (AMH) and vaginal ultrasonography assessment for number of antral follicles can be used [33, 34]. However, recent literature indicates the best biochemical indicators of ovarian reserve may be serum FSH and AMH levels [35, 36]. The knowledge of functional ovarian reserve may benefit patients prior to making important decisions regarding treatment, fertility preservation, and contraception [37]. Nevertheless, there remains confusion due to lack of consistent visible findings of ovulation/fertility (i.e., menstruation) or laboratory findings. Patients and providers make incorrect assumptions about fertility status and contraceptive need [36]. Given that there is no reliable marker of fertility, erring on the side of contraception, when pregnancy is undesired, is paramount.

Chemotherapy and Adjuvant Therapy

Gonadal damage due to chemotherapy is progressive, irreversible, and is directly influenced by the patients' age, type of the drug, as well as its cumulative dose [38]. When treated with chemotherapeutic agents, older women are more prone to develop permanent infertility due to already reduced ovarian reserve compared to younger women [39]. Cell cycle specific chemotherapeutic drugs have milder gonadotoxic effects whereas alkylating agents are associated with a high risk of infertility [18, 37, 39, 40] Category D chemotherapy drugs, such as busulfan, melphalan, cyclophosphamide, cisplatin, chlorambucil, mustine, carmustine, lomustine, vinblastine, cytarabine, and procarbazine, have been shown to affect fertility [41–46].

Many cancer therapies are Category D or X, which have demonstrated risk of fetal complications including birth defects. Category D drugs have demonstrated risk to the fetus, but potential benefits of these drugs outweigh the risks of fetal complications. However, Category X drugs are contraindicated in women diagnosed with cancer who are pregnant or will potentially be pregnant [47]. One study estimated that 6 % of pregnancies occur in women on a medication with a teratogenic risk (Category D) or teratogenic medication (Category X) [47, 48].

Tamoxifen, a selective estrogen receptor modulator and Category D drug, has several reproductive health implications [49]. In estrogen receptor positive breast cancer, tamoxifen reduces the recurrence of breast cancer and prolongs survival in women [50, 51]. Tamoxifen may stimulate the ovaries, induce ovulation, and increase the risk of pregnancy [52]. It additionally can induce fetal anomalies, and therefore is not recommended for women at risk for pregnancy [52–54]. Adjuvant therapies, such as tamoxifen, have recommended duration of use from 4.5 to 10 years, during which time pregnancy should be avoided [49].

It is important that women taking Category X medications are offered the most effective contraceptive methods. In a large, population based study, 11 % of the Category X drugs taken by women were antineoplastic. Of these women, 18 % were taking oral contraceptive pills (OCs). Women on Category X medications were no more adherent to oral contraceptive pills (OCs) than women not on Category X medications [55]. Possible hypotheses are lack of effectiveness of counseling or warning labels against pregnancy [55, 56]. Contraceptives requiring daily, weekly, or monthly adherence, with failure rates of 9–24 %, are not optimal in women taking Category X drugs [57].

Gonadotropin releasing hormone (GnRH) agonists (Category D/Category X) are used in conjunction with chemotherapy to prevent oocyte depletion [58]. Although GnRH agonists downregulate ovulatory function, once GnRH treatment is stopped they can upregulate the system, increasing the risk of unintended pregnancy [19, 59, 60]. Contraception should be implemented with GnRH agonist administration so that there is effective coverage at initiation and cessation of the GnRH agonist.

While teratogenic risk may be understood by clinicians and basic guidelines recommending contraception exist, mandated implementation of contraception is only required with the extremely teratogenic chemotherapeutic drug thalidomide (Category X) [61]. The Risk Evaluation and Mitigation Strategy (REMS) developed for thalidomide requires the provider to receive mandatory training on contraception and evidence of the patient using two contraceptive methods (one highly effective method and one back up coitally dependent method in case of primary method failure) [61].

Radiotherapy

The radiation dose used in cancer treatment ranges from 3,000 to7,000 centigray (cGy) [62]. These doses may destroy most human oocytes or a developing pregnancy. Radiation required to destroy half of human oocytes is estimated to be less than 200 cGy [63]. Gonadal damage due to this treatment may be temporary or permanent. It can occur either by direct exposure, as in pelvic or low abdominal irradiation, or by scattered radiation [64]. In young women with cancer desiring future childbearing, it is important to use gonadal protective precautions, such as shielding of the gonads or restricting the radiation field, to avoid direct ovarian irradiation [64].

In pregnancy, the accepted cumulative dose of radiation is 5 cGy. In the peri-implantation and organogenesis periods, radiation has an all or none effect, either destroying the developing fetus completely or having no effect. Radiation during pregnancy can cause embryonic death and congenital malformations, or there can be normal fetal development [65]. During the later fetal stages, a high dose of radiation exposure is known to affect brain development and cause mental retardation, growth impairment, and other abnormalities [62, 65].

Oncocontraception Conceptual Framework

Oncocontraception when offered to the cancer survivor must take a variety of factors into account. We describe three models of selecting appropriate contraceptive methods for the cancer survivor. Contraception may be categorized in the following ways to match the appropriate contraceptive to a given patient: (1) hormonal content, (2) medical eligibility-risk/benefit, and (3) efficacy and duration of method. An integration of these components is key to contraceptive optimization.

Decisions regarding contraceptive choice are generally based on patient preference and medical eligibility. Hormonal composition, duration of use, and efficacy additionally influence contraceptive selection. Based on principles of medical eligibility, compliance, and high effectiveness, both long-acting reversible contraceptives (LARC) and sterilization are important and underutilized methods in cancer patients. Short-term contraceptive methods, which include combined (estrogen and progestin) methods with various delivery systems, barrier, and behavioral methods, may be suboptimal for cancer patients due to decreased efficacy and compliance or hormones which may be relatively or absolutely contraindicated in cancer patients. Additionally, while some women will choose not to be sexually active, periodic abstinence requires contraceptive counseling as well. Table 14.1 highlights the contraceptive methods and associated failure rates as well as risks/benefits and method type.

Model 1: Hormonal Content

Considering contraception based on hormonal content is the most traditional framework. In this model, hormonal-based contraception is contraindicated for hormonally mediated cancers. Hormonal methods of contraception should be prescribed on an individual basis depending upon the type of cancer and medical history. These methods may be divided into combined methods (containing estrogen and progestin) and progestin-only methods.

Combined Hormonal Contraception

Combined hormonal contraception (CHC) includes the pill, transdermal patch, and vaginal ring, which are the most commonly used methods in the United States [66]. Having cancer is not a contraindication for CHC, except for malignancies where estrogen-based contraceptives are clearly contraindicated [25]. Estrogen and progesterone receptor positive cancers such as breast, endometrial, and other estrogen or progestin dependent tumors are absolute contraindications to use. In women with current or at increased risk for recurrent venous thromboembolism (VTE), CHC is absolutely contraindicated [67].

Progestin-Only Methods

Progestin-only methods may be delivered by daily pills, injections of depot medroxyprogesterone acetate (DMPA) every 3 months, the 3- and 5-year levonorgestrel intrauterine devices (LNG IUDs), and a 3-year etonogestrel implantable rod. The primary contraindication for these methods is estrogen or progesterone receptor-mediated breast cancer or other hormonally mediated cancers. For patients without hormonally mediated cancers, progestin-only hormonal contraceptives are still important options [68]. Safety-related issues are examined in Model 2.

Nonhormonal Methods

Cancer survivors are often left to use nonhormonal methods due to concerns of hormones and possible implications for cancer survivors. The copper intrauterine device (IUD) is a nonhormonal, reversible, and effective choice (0.8 % failure rate in the first year of use) [26], particularly for women with medical conditions who cannot take estrogen or progestin. There are minimal patient compliance issues with long-acting reversible contraception and the copper IUD can be used for up to 10 years. Natural methods such as withdrawal/periodic abstinence have little medical risk yet have high failure rates (22–24 %), particularly if the patient has irregular menstrual cycles with chemotherapy [26]. Barrier methods such as condoms, diaphragms, sponge, foams, and spermicides can be effective temporary contraceptive methods for highly motivated individuals [25]. Still, these are not the most effective contraceptive methods available with typical use failure rates of 12–28 %.

Sterilization is a common form of birth control in the United States [66]. Minilaparotomy, laparoscopic, or transcervical methods of tubal ligation or occlusion are available [69]. While various surgical approaches exist, they are generally safe and highly effective. For patients that are certain they have completed childbearing, tubal sterilization

Table 14.1 Contraceptive methods and relevance to the cancer patient

Contraceptive method	Long term	Failure rate with typical use	Failure rate with perfect use	Hormonal	Benefits	Risks/concerns	Application	Provision
Tier 1								
Male sterilization: vasectomy	Y	0.15 %	0.10 %	None	Permanent	Permanent, offers no protection against STIs and AIDS	Permanent	Provider Procedure
Female sterilization: tubal ligation (TL)	Y	0.50 %	0.50 %	None	Permanent	Permanent, offers no protection against STIs and AIDS	Permanent	Provider Procedure
Implant	Y	0.05 %	0.05 %	Progestin (etonogestrel)		Irregular bleeding, offers no protection against STIs and AIDS	Up to 3 years	Provider placed
Levonorgestrel IUDs	Y	0.20 %	0.20 %	Levonorgestrel (20 μg LNG/day; decreases progressively to 10 μg/day after 5 years	Decreased bleeding	Irregular or no bleeding, offers no protection against STIs and AIDS, rate of PID from IUD insertion 0–2 % in women without STIs and between 2 and 10 % in women with STIs[a]	Up to 3–7 years	Provider placed
Copper IUD	Y	0.80 %	0.60 %	None		Possible increased bleeding, offers no protection against STIs and AIDS, rate of PID from IUD insertion 0–2 % in women without STIs and between 2 and 10 % in women with STIs[a]	Up to 10–12 years	Provider placed
Tier 2								
DMPA	N	6 %	0.20 %	Medroxyprogesterone acetate	Amenorrhea	Decrease in bone mineral density, irregular bleeding initially, longer return to fertility, offers no protection against STIs and AIDS	Every 3 months	Provider provides
Ring	N	9 %	0.30 %	Ethinyl estradiol/ progestin(etonogestrel)	Cycle control	Increased risk of VTE, offers no protection against STIs and AIDS	Every 3–4 weeks	Prescription
Patch	N	9 %	0.30 %	Ethinyl estradiol/progestin (norelgestromin)	Cycle control	Increased risk of VTE, offers no protection against STIs and AIDS	Every week	Prescription
Combination pills	N	9 %	0.30 %	Ethinyl estradiol/progestin	Cycle control	Increased risk of VTE, offers no protection against STIs and AIDS	Daily	Prescription
Progestin-only pills	N	9 %	0.30 %	Progestin (norethindrone or norgestrel)	Cycle control	Offers no protection against STIs and AIDS	Daily	Prescription

Tier 3								
Diaphragms	N	12 %	6 %	None		Offers no protection against STIs and AIDS	Coitally dependent	Prescription
Cervical cap: nulliparous women	N	20 %	9 %	None		Offers no protection against STIs and AIDS	Coitally dependent	
Cervical cap: parous women	N	40 %	26 %	None		Offers no protection against STIs and AIDS	Coitally dependent	
Condom: male	N	18 %	2 %	None	If used properly, will reduce the risk of STIs, including AIDS		Coitally dependent	Over the counter
Condom: female	N	21 %	5 %	None	If used properly, will reduce the risk of STIs, including AIDS		Coitally dependent	Over the counter
Sponge: nulliparous women	N	12 %	9 %	None		Offers no protection against STIs and AIDS	Coitally dependent	Over the counter
Sponge: parous women	N	24 %	20 %	None		Offers no protection against STIs and AIDS	Coitally dependent	Over the counter
Fertility awareness-based methods	N	24 %	0.4–5 %	None		Offers no protection against STIs and AIDS	Coitally dependent	None
Tier 4								
Spermicides	N	28 %	18 %	None		Offers no protection against STIs and AIDS	Coitally dependent	None
Withdrawal	N	22 %	4 %	None		Offers no protection against STIs and AIDS	Coitally dependent	None

[a]Mohllajee AP, Curtis KM, Peterson HB. Does insertion and use of an intrauterine device increase the risk of pelvic inflammatory disease among women with sexually transmitted infection? A systematic review. Contraception. 2006;73:145–53

may be an appropriate method, specifically at the time of surgery for cancer treatment. Vasectomy is an important form of sterilization for patients with a stable male partner. This procedure carries lower risk of complications than female sterilization and should be discussed with women as an option for their partners [70].

Model 2: Medical Eligibility-Risk/Benefit

A second model of selection is based on medical eligibility and risk assessment. The Centers for Disease Control and Prevention (CDC) offers a resource to assist providers in assessing appropriateness of contraceptive methods for patients with medical conditions based on a risk-benefit analysis. In this set of guidelines, contraceptives are rated category 1 through 4:

1. No restriction
2. Advantages generally outweigh theoretical or proven risks
3. Theoretical or proven risks usually outweigh the advantages
4. Unacceptable health risk (method not to be used)

Cancer-related issues addressed by the CDC's US Medical Eligibility Criteria for Contraceptive Use (USMEC) are breast cancer, gestational trophoblastic disease, cervical cancer, endometrial cancer, ovarian cancer, hepatic cancer, VTE, and iron deficiency anemia [25].

Type of Cancer

Breast cancer is a category 4 contraindication for hormonal contraceptive methods, regardless of estrogen and progesterone receptor status. In women with no evidence of disease for 5 years, hormonal contraceptives become a category 3, a condition for which the theoretical or proven risks usually outweigh the advantages of using the method [67]. Insufficient evidence exists to determine if hormonal contraception is safe in women with estrogen and progesterone receptor negative breast cancer. It may be prudent to avoid hormonal contraception in breast cancer patients with nonhormonally mediated cancers since other options are available [71].

Cancer-Related Issues

Contraceptive choice may be influenced by existing medical issues related to cancer and treatment. Side effects of the contraception may alleviate or exacerbate underlying medical issues. Potential benefits for cancer patients with thrombocytopenia include reduction in uterine bleeding and cycle dependent symptoms. Side effects of contraceptives that impact cancer patients include thrombosis, insertion-related risk of infection, drug interactions, or malabsorption due to gastrointestinal-related issues. Each of these issues may be transient or chronic in nature and should be taken into account in regard to contraceptive selection.

Thrombocytopenia

Chemotherapy-induced thrombocytopenia may incite or exacerbate normal uterine bleeding. If the platelet nadir occurs at the time of scheduled menstrual bleeding, the amount and duration may be altered resulting in hemorrhage. Patients with transient thrombocytopenia may do well taking cyclic combined oral contraceptives if scheduled bleeding is not concurrent with platelet nadir [71]. If, however, the thrombocytopenia is prolonged or unpredictable, a course of continuous monophasic combined oral contraception may be of benefit [71]. Whether using cyclic or extended use combined oral contraceptives, patch, ring, implant, or the LNG IUD, women may experience less menstrual blood loss; however, extended use of these methods may increase irregular spotting or bleeding initially [26].

Long-term DMPA use may induce amenorrhea; however, initial use may cause irregular and excessive bleeding. In one study of thrombocytopenic cancer patients, DMPA induced amenorrhea in a significant proportion of participants (45 %); however, DMPA did not reduce the proportion of women reporting moderate to severe menstrual bleeding (20 %) [72]. There are concerns for hematoma formation with intramuscular injection during thrombocytopenic episodes; however, anecdotal evidence has not indicated this to be an issue [68]. The copper IUD can increase both duration and amount of bleeding, resulting in approximately 50 % more blood loss and, although hemoglobin levels do not change in healthy women, it should be used with caution in patients with thrombocytopenia [26].

Thrombosis

Cancer increases the risk of VTE by directly affecting thrombin production or indirectly activating the coagulation system [73]. A 4.1-fold increase in VTE risk has been reported in patients with cancer compared to the general population. This risk increases to 6.5-fold in individuals undergoing chemotherapy [74]. This risk is additionally increased by factors often associated with cancer, including advancement of disease, surgery, and age [75]. Estrogen-based contraceptives may further increase the risk of VTE due to changes in coagulation cascade (factor VII and factor X) and the fibrinolytic system [68]. Given the confluence of factors causing a hypercoagulable state, caution should navigate providers away from methods containing estrogen and towards other methods that might be equally effective with decreased risk. For women with current VTE or a history of VTE with active cancer, use of estrogen-containing oral contraceptives, ring, or patch is contraindicated [25].

Evidence suggests that progestin does not affect the coagulation cascade as estrogen does [25]. Labeling for norethindrone progestin-only oral contraceptives and the LNG IUD no longer include VTE as a contraindication. VTE remains listed as a contraindication on the label for norgestrel progestin-only pills and DMPA. However, the American College of Obstetricians and Gynecologists (ACOG) and the USMEC indicate that progestin-only methods may be appropriate for women with history of or at increased risk for VTE [25, 28].

Infection Risk

There is a theoretical concern of increased risk of infection with IUD use in women who may experience neutropenia during chemotherapy. A review of the literature does not demonstrate any evidence of an increased risk of IUD-induced reproductive tract infection in this population. Literature reviews of IUD utilization in women with ovarian cancer did not provide evidence that substantiated a risk of IUD-associated infection [76]. Similarly, women with HIV and women who have undergone organ transplant, both cohorts of immune-compromised individuals, have not been shown to have an increased risk of intrauterine infections associated with IUD use [25]. Overall, the net benefit of unintended pregnancy reduction likely outweighs this theoretical concern of IUD-associated infection with chemotherapy-induced neutropenia (see Chap. 9 for more information) [25].

Osteoporosis

The risk for osteoporosis is potentially increased in women treated with chemotherapy [77, 78]. Due to the potential of decreased bone mineral density with prolonged use, DMPA should be used cautiously in these women [25]. However, if it is the only method acceptable to the woman, then DMPA is not absolutely contraindicated as its effects are reversed after discontinuation [79]. Clinical judgment and patient counseling are essential. The implant has been known to alter radial and ulnar bone mineral density, but risk of fracture is unknown [80–82]. Surveillance and treatment for osteoporosis would be important for such patients [68]. Alternatively, use of estrogen-containing contraceptives may decrease or have no effect on the risk of osteoporosis [83, 84]. Nonhormonal methods will not affect the risk of osteoporosis (see Chap. 16 for more information).

Gastrointestinal Side Effects

Common side effects of certain cancers and chemotherapy are vomiting and mucositis. These side effects may reduce the absorption of oral contraceptives, which work through first-pass metabolism [16]. Recurrent infections and antibiotic use might alter hepatogastric circulation and impede absorption [71]. To avoid decreased efficacy with malabsorption, non-oral methods would be preferred.

Drug Interactions

Women with cancer often require many types of medication for primary or secondary treatment of cancer. Drug interactions are common and may reduce the efficacy of several contraceptive methods. Classes of contraception that require hepatic enzymatic pathways are often affected and conversely these contraceptives may impact other drug metabolism. While many anecdotal reports of oral contraceptive failure with antibiotic use exist, restrictions only exist for rifampin and rifabutin [68, 71]. Other categories of drugs that may interact with hormonal contraceptive methods are antacids (magnesium and aluminum types), analgesics, antifungals, anticonvulsants, antibiotics, and antiretrovirals as well as the herbal remedy St. John's wort [16, 68, 71]. Thus, contraceptive use should be closely monitored in the context of these medications (see Chap. 20).

Model 3: Duration and Efficacy

Duration of the Method

Contraceptive methods may be categorized in terms of short-acting and long-acting methods. Long-acting methods are characteristically defined by reduced dosing, increased compliance, and the highest available effectiveness. Long-term methods may be further delineated by reversible and nonreversible methods. Surgical irreversible methods of contraception, such as tubal sterilization, or partner vasectomy, should be considered for patients who have completed childbearing and are interested in a permanent method.

Contraceptive Effectiveness

Effectiveness is currently conceptualized in the WHO four tiered system (see Table 14.1). Tier 1 methods have the highest effectiveness and Tier 4 the lowest [57]. The key element of the tier differentiation is the difference between perfect use and typical use. While there may be women who use lower tier methods consistently, achieving near perfect use, most will fall into typical use patterns. Perfect use is most often achieved in the long-acting methods where compliance-related issues are minimized. Long-acting methods including sterilization, implants, and IUDs are the most effective methods of contraception with perfect use failure rates comparable to typical use failure rates ranging from 0.05 to 0.8 % (Tier 1) [57].

Tier 2 methods of contraception are the most commonly used in the United States and include progestin-only oral contraceptives, DMPA, and the combined hormonal oral contraceptives, patch and ring [85]. These methods offer 9 % typical use failure rates per 100 women-years [57]. While this tier offers a variety of delivery systems that may be appealing to women, the failure rate is still high for women with cancer who may need the most effective methods of contraception.

The lower tier methods include behavioral and barrier methods with typical use failure rates ranging between 12 and 28 % [57]. As these methods of contraception do not contain hormones, they are often incorrectly considered first line for the cancer patient despite effectiveness shortcomings. While many women utilized first and second tier contraceptive methods at the time of cancer diagnosis, once the diagnosis is made, they are often inappropriately relegated to Tier 3 and 4 contraceptive methods or permanent sterilization [27].

Emergency Contraception

Emergency contraception is an important backup method in case of contraceptive failure or non-use. Currently three methods of emergency contraception are available in the United States, levonorgestrel, ulipristal acetate, and the copper IUD. Emergency contraception use does not appear to be associated with VTE [68]. The levonorgestrel method is available in the United States without prescription for women. Recent data, however, suggest a decreased efficacy in women with increased weight [86]. Ulipristal acetate is also available and has demonstrated better efficacy than levonorgestrel and is effective up to 7 days after unprotected intercourse [87]. The ideal method in the appropriate patient is the copper IUD with the highest emergency contraceptive efficacy (99 %) also offering highly effective long-term contraceptive benefits [88].

Induced Abortion

Evidence suggests that female cancer survivors may be more likely to terminate an unintended pregnancy than matched control subjects [89, 90]. Preexisting or newly diagnosed malignancy was one of the leading causes of termination performed for maternal medical indication in one Australian study. The majority of malignancies were diagnosed during pregnancy; however, nearly one-third of these pregnancies occurred after cancer diagnosis. The study further demonstrated that the provision of contraception after termination was suboptimal, placing vulnerable women at risk for further unintended pregnancy [91]. Access to safe termination services is an essential component of reproductive health cancer care [12]. Pregnant women with cancer may have a great deal of ambivalence even with a desired pregnancy [11, 27]. Certainly in the case of an unintended pregnancy, women should be offered all options without judgment.

Special Issues

Tamoxifen Use and LNG IUD

While tamoxifen has protective effects on the breast, reducing the recurrence of breast cancer, it has negative effects of the endometrium, increasing risk of hyperplasia and endometrial cancer [49, 52, 53, 92]. The LNG IUD has a marked antiproliferative effect on the endometrium. Breast cancer patients on long-term tamoxifen may benefit from the LNG IUD because of its endometrial protection and contraceptive effect [93]. It is also associated with progressive reduction of menstrual duration and menstrual blood loss. LNG IUD can be considered in premenopausal women with breast cancer to prevent tamoxifen-induced endometrial changes; however, large prospective randomized trials are needed to confirm its benefit [94, 95]. One retrospective controlled cohort analysis of 79 premenopausal breast cancer patients demonstrated that women who were diagnosed with LNG IUD in place and maintained the method had an increased risk of breast cancer recurrence; therefore, further study is needed [96].

Sterilization Regret

As described earlier, women with cancer may be steered towards sterilization as a highly effective, nonhormonal, contraceptive solution for cancer survivors [27]. However, this method is considered permanent and prevents future childbearing. Depending on the study, approximately 0.9–26 % of women later regret their decision for tubal sterilization. The US Collaborative Review of Sterilization found the probability of sterilization regret to be 12.7 % with younger women (age less than 30 years) being at higher risk [97]. A decision for tubal sterilization made at the time of cancer diagnosis may be based on concerns about prognosis. Nevertheless, women who attain longevity of life may regain interest in childbearing. In some cases, tubal reversal surgery or in vitro fertilization may available; however, this is a costly process, not covered by insurance, with no guarantee of success [98]. Given the uncertainly of the future in newly diagnosed women, reversible contraceptives may be a better option. For women who are indeed certain of completion of childbearing, sterilization, particularly determined prior to cancer diagnosis, may be the correct choice.

Radiologic Testing

IUDs are safe with ultrasound and computed tomography (CT) scan. Most typical magnetic resonance imaging (MRIs) are safe for utilization for women who may require radiologic tests for cancer evaluation. The LNG IUD has Food and Drug Administration (FDA) labeling for use in up to 3 T MRIs and copper IUD has labeling for up to 1.5 T [99, 100]. Research in ex vivo and in vivo has been performed with the copper IUD demonstrating safety in MRI units using 3 T [100, 101]. As newer MRIs are developed, research will be necessary to prove safety of IUDs.

Solutions

Role of Oncologists in Providing Contraception or Referrals for Contraception

The majority of cancer survivors report never having been asked about contraception by their oncologist or health care provider [9]. Furthermore, physician recommendation has been demonstrated to be the best predictor of contraceptive compliance [102]. While reproductive health may be a challenging discussion, it is extremely important

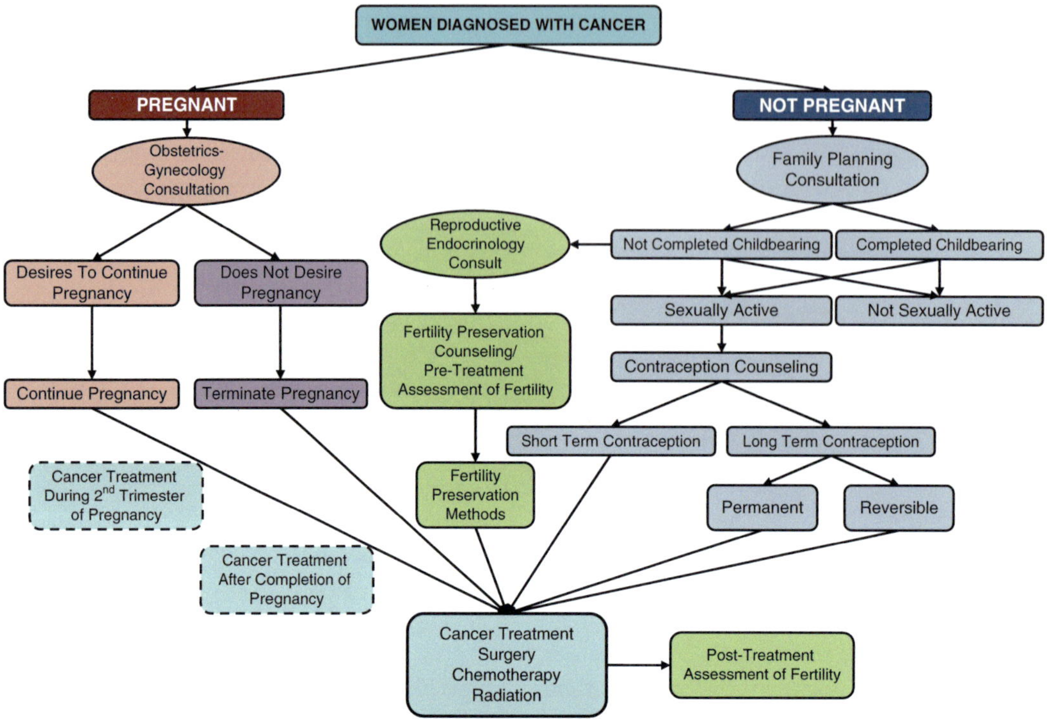

Fig. 14.1 Engendering reproductive health in oncologic survivorship algorithm

to cancer survivors, who do not often share sexual health concerns with their oncology team [8]. Leading organizations have guidelines to assist the oncology team navigating reproductive health issues. Many gynecologic and family planning providers and organizations can offer assistance and guidance. While the expectations of an oncology team may not be to provide contraceptive management, offering the appropriate referrals for reproductive health issues would be a feasible option.

Engendering Reproductive Health in Oncologic Survivorship (EROS) Algorithm

A simple tool, the EROS Algorithm (Fig. 14.1), can aid providers caring for cancer survivors to expediently optimize available and appropriate reproductive health care. The Cook County Health and Hospitals System Minority-Based Community Clinical Oncology Program (MBCCOP) in conjunction with the Division of Family Planning developed the algorithm to aid in the navigation of reproductive health management in newly diagnosed breast cancer survivors. In a pilot of this model, 100 % of women received reproductive health management consistent with the reproductive health interests of the women studied [103].

In this algorithm, cancer patients are initially thought of in terms of current pregnancy status. Currently pregnant patients are referred to an obstetrician for options counseling to discuss delaying treatment or termination. Women who are not pregnant (or after delivery/abortion) are further stratified by future childbearing interests. If women desire future pregnancy or are unsure of future childbearing interests, referral to fertility preservation specialists is advised. For all non-pregnant women, including those desiring future pregnancy and those who have completed childbearing, referral to a family planning specialist for oncocontraception counseling should be offered.

Conclusions from this pilot study demonstrated the success of the reproductive health algorithm in assisting providers in navigating patients towards appropriate oncocontraception, oncofertility, and onco-obstetrics. Further investigation to assess the utility of the reproductive health assessment and algorithm is underway.

General Principles to Adopt

- Perform periodic reproductive health assessments
- Utilization of the Engendering Reproductive Health in Oncologic Survivorship Algorithm
- Assume women at diagnosis of cancer may be interested in future childbearing, unless explicitly stated they have completed childbearing
- Assume fertility capability and contracept, rather than assume infertility and risk unintended pregnancy
- Tier 1 contraception methods should be offered as first-line contraception
- The copper IUD is an optimal method with high efficacy, reversibility, and no hormonal content
- Progestin-only methods are preferred over combination methods
- Implementation of Risk Evaluation and Mitigation Strategies for all Category D and X drugs

Resources

Organizations, such as the Centers for Disease Control and Prevention (CDC), American Cancer Society (ACS), National Comprehensive Cancer Network (NCCN), American Society of Clinical Oncologists (ASCO), Society for Family Planning (SFP), and American Society for Reproductive Medicine (ASRM), have recommendations regarding reproductive health in cancer. There is a paucity of literature in the area of reproductive health and the application of these guidelines in clinical practice.

Conclusion

Survivors of cancer desire to achieve many of the same reproductive life goals as women without cancer. Oncocontraception is a cornerstone of reproductive health along with oncofertility and sexuality. A multidisciplinary approach is necessary for optimal family planning. This chapter provides information, tools, and guidance to provide optimal choices to women to prevent pregnancy at the appropriate time. Along with other quality of life indicators, effective family planning will aid reproductive aged women in achieving survivorship goals.

References

1. De Moor JS, Mariotto AB, Parry C, Alfano CM, Padgett L, Kent EE, et al. Cancer survivors in the United States: prevalence across the survivorship trajectory and implications for care. Cancer Epidemiol Biomarkers Prev. 2013;22:561–70.
2. U.S. Cancer Statistics Working Group. United States cancer statistics: 1999–2010 incidence and mortality web-based report. Atlanta, GA: US Department of Health and Human Services, Centers for Disease Control and Prevention and National Cancer Institute; 2013.
3. American Cancer Society. Breast cancer facts & figures 2013–2014. Atlanta, GA: American Cancer Society Inc.; 2013.
4. Howlader NNA, Krapcho M, Garshell J, Neyman N, Altekruse SF, Kosary CL, et al., editors. SEER cancer statistics review. Bethesda, MD: National Cancer Institute; 1975–2013.
5. Partridge AH, Gelber S, Peppercorn J, Sampson E, Knudsen K, Laufer M, et al. Web-based survey of fertility issues in young women with breast cancer. J Clin Oncol. 2004;22:4174–83.
6. Schover LR. Sexuality and fertility after cancer. Hematol Am Soc Hematol Educ Progr. 2005;2005: 523–7.
7. Valle J, Clemons M, Hayes S, Fallowfield L, Howell A. Contraceptive use by women receiving chemotherapy for breast cancer. Breast. 1998;7:143–9.
8. Knapp CA, Quinn GP, Rapalo D, Woodworth L. Patient provider communication and reproductive health. Adv Exp Med Biol. 2012;732:175–85.
9. Quinn GP, Vadaparampil ST. Fertility preservation and adolescent/young adult cancer patients: physician communication challenges. J Adolesc Health. 2009;44:394–400.

10. Mitwally MF. Management of reproductive needs in cancer patients: clinical perspectives. Expert Rev Anticancer Ther. 2008;8:1589–95.
11. Schwarz EB, Lohr PA, Gold MA, Gerbert B. Prevalence and correlates of ambivalence towards pregnancy among nonpregnant women. Contraception. 2007;75:305–10.
12. Patel AA, Mini S, Sutaria RP, Schoenhage MB, Patel AR, Radeke EK, et al. Reproductive health issues in women with cancer. J Oncol Pract. 2008;4:101–5.
13. Murphy D, Klosky JL, Termuhlen A, Sawczyn KK, Quinn GP. The need for reproductive and sexual health discussions with adolescent and young adult cancer patients. Contraception. 2013;88:215–20.
14. Patel A, Sreedevi M, Malapati R, Sutaria R, Schoenhage MB, Patel AR, et al. Reproductive health assessment for women with cancer: a pilot study. Am J Obstet Gynecol. 2009;201:191e1-4.
15. Patel A, Schwarz EB. Cancer and contraception: release date May 2012 SFP guideline #20121. Contraception. 2012;86:191–8.
16. Laurence V, Rousset-Jablonski C. Contraception and cancer treatment in young persons. Adv Exp Med Biol. 2012;732:41–60.
17. Canada AL, Schover LR. Research promoting better patient education on reproductive health after cancer. J Natl Cancer Inst Monogr. 2005;2005:98–100.
18. Lee SJ, Schover LR, Partridge AH, Patrizio P, Wallace WH, Hagerty K, et al. American Society of Clinical Oncology recommendations on fertility preservation in cancer patients. J Clin Oncol. 2006; 24:2917–31.
19. Ethics Committee of the American Society for Reproductive Medicine. Fertility preservation and reproduction in cancer patients. Fertil Steril. 2005; 83:1622–8.
20. Guttmacher Institute. Contraceptive needs and services: national and state data, 2008 update. New York: Guttmacher Institute; 2010.
21. St James PJ, Younger MD, Hamilton BD, Waisbren SE. Unplanned pregnancies in young women with diabetes. An analysis of psychosocial factors. Diabetes Care. 1993;16:1572–8.
22. Holing EV, Beyer CS, Brown ZA, Connell FA. Why don't women with diabetes plan their pregnancies? Diabetes Care. 1998;21:889–95.
23. Schwarz EB, Maselli J, Gonzales R. Contraceptive counseling of diabetic women of reproductive age. Obstet Gynecol. 2006;107:1070–4.
24. Chuang CH, Chase GA, Bensyl DM, Weisman CS. Contraceptive use by diabetic and obese women. Womens Health Issues. 2005;15:167–73.
25. Centers for Disease Control and Prevention. U.S. medical eligibility criteria for contraceptive use, 2010. MMW Rep 2010;59.
26. Association of Reproductive Health Professionals (ARHP). Choosing a birth control method, 2011. Washington, DC: Association of Reproductive Health Professionals; 2011. p. 2011.
27. Schwarz EB, Hess R, Trussell J. Contraception for cancer survivors. J Gen Intern Med. 2009;24 Suppl 2:S401–6.
28. Helewa M, Levesque P, Provencher D, Lea RH, Rosolowich V, Shapiro HM. Breast cancer, pregnancy, and breastfeeding. J Obstet Gynaecol Can. 2002;24:164–80. quiz 81-4.
29. Cvancarova M, Samuelsen SO, Magelssen H, Fossa SD. Reproduction rates after cancer treatment: experience from the Norwegian radium hospital. J Clin Oncol. 2009;27:334–43.
30. Byrne J, Mulvihill JJ, Myers MH, Connelly RR, Naughton MD, Krauss MR, et al. Effects of treatment on fertility in long-term survivors of childhood or adolescent cancer. N Engl J Med. 1987;317: 1315–21.
31. Del Mastro L, Catzeddu T, Venturini M. Infertility and pregnancy after breast cancer: current knowledge and future perspectives. Cancer Treat Rev. 2006;32:417–22.
32. Chasle S, How CC. The effect of cytotoxic chemotherapy on female fertility. Eur J Oncol Nurs. 2003; 7:91–8.
33. Lie Fong S, Laven JS, Hakvoort-Cammel FG, Schipper I, Visser JA, Themmen AP, et al. Assessment of ovarian reserve in adult childhood cancer survivors using anti-Mullerian hormone. Hum Reprod. 2009;24:982–90.
34. Lutchman Singh K, Davies M, Chatterjee R. Fertility in female cancer survivors: pathophysiology, preservation and the role of ovarian reserve testing. Hum Reprod Update. 2005;11:69–89.
35. Gleicher N, Weghofer A, Barad DH. Anti-Mullerian hormone (AMH) defines, independent of age, low versus good live-birth chances in women with severely diminished ovarian reserve. Fertil Steril. 2010;94:2824–7.
36. Su HI, Sammel MD, Green J, Velders L, Stankiewicz C, Matro J, et al. Antimullerian hormone and inhibin B are hormone measures of ovarian function in late reproductive-aged breast cancer survivors. Cancer. 2010;116:592–9.
37. Rosendahl M, Andersen CY, La Cour Freiesleben N, Juul A, Lossl K, Andersen AN. Dynamics and mechanisms of chemotherapy-induced ovarian follicular depletion in women of fertile age. Fertil Steril. 2010;94:156–66.
38. Blumenfeld Z, Avivi I, Ritter M, Rowe JM. Preservation of fertility and ovarian function and minimizing chemotherapy-induced gonadotoxicity in young women. J Soc Gynecol Investig. 1999;6:229–39.
39. Abdallah RT, Muasher SJ. Surviving cancer, saving fertility-the promise of cryopreservation. Sexuality, reproduction and menopause. Sex Reprod Menopause. 2006;4:7–12.
40. Sönmezer M, Aytaç R, Demirel LC, Kurtay G. Mesenteric vein thrombosis in a pregnant patient heterozygous for the factor V (1691 G –>A) Leiden

mutation. Eur J Obstet Gynecol Reprod Biol. 2004; 114:234–5.

41. Howell S, Shalet S. Gonadal damage from chemotherapy and radiotherapy. Endocrinol Metab Clin North Am. 1998;27:927–43.
42. Fisher B, Dignam J, Mamounas EP, Costantino JP, Wickerham DL, Redmond C, et al. Sequential methotrexate and fluorouracil for the treatment of node-negative breast cancer patients with estrogen receptor-negative tumors: eight-year results from National Surgical Adjuvant Breast and Bowel Project (NSABP) B-13 and first report of findings from NSABP B-19 comparing methotrexate and fluorouracil with conventional cyclophosphamide, methotrexate, and fluorouracil. J Clin Oncol. 1996; 14:1982–92.
43. Goodwin PJ, Ennis M, Pritchard KI, Trudeau M, Hood N. Risk of menopause during the first year after breast cancer diagnosis. J Clin Oncol. 1999; 17:2365–70.
44. Lamb MA. Effects of chemotherapy on fertility in long-term survivors. Dimens Oncol Nurs. 1991; 5:13–6.
45. Longhi A, Macchiagodena M, Vitali G, Bacci G. Fertility in male patients treated with neoadjuvant chemotherapy for osteosarcoma. J Pediatr Hematol Oncol. 2003;25:292–6.
46. Simon B, Lee SJ, Partridge AH, Runowicz CD. Preserving fertility after cancer. CA Cancer J Clin. 2005;55:211–28. quiz 63-4.
47. Administration FD, editor. Content and format of labeling for human prescription drug and biological products; requirements for pregnancy and lactation labeling. Federal Register 2008;23. http://federalregister.gov/r/0910-AF11.
48. Andrade SE, Raebel MA, Morse AN, Davis RL, Chan KA, Finkelstein JA, et al. Use of prescription medications with a potential for fetal harm among pregnant women. Pharmacoepidemiol Drug Saf. 2006;15:546–54.
49. Delaware AstraZeneca Pharmaceuticals. NOLVADEX (Tamoxifen Citrate) [package insert]. Wilmington, DE: Delaware AstraZeneca Pharmaceuticals LP; 2004.
50. Early Breast Cancer Trialists' Collaborative Group. Tamoxifen for early breast cancer: an overview of the randomised trials. Lancet. 1998;351:1451–67.
51. Davies C, Pan H, Godwin J, Gray R, Arriagada R, Raina V, et al. Long-term effects of continuing adjuvant tamoxifen to 10 years versus stopping at 5 years after diagnosis of oestrogen receptor-positive breast cancer: ATLAS, a randomised trial. Lancet. 2013; 381:805–16.
52. Polin SA, Ascher SM. The effect of tamoxifen on the genital tract. Cancer Imaging. 2008;8:135–45.
53. Kedar RP, Bourne TH, Powles TJ, Collins WP, Ashley SE, Cosgrove DO, et al. Effects of tamoxifen on uterus and ovaries of postmenopausal women in a randomised breast cancer prevention trial. Lancet. 1994;343:1318–21.
54. Halakivi-Clarke L, Cho E, Onojafe I, Liao DJ, Clarke R. Maternal exposure to tamoxifen during pregnancy increases carcinogen-induced mammary tumorigenesis among female rat offspring. Clin Cancer Res. 2000;6:305–8.
55. Steinkellner A, Chen W, Denison SE. Adherence to oral contraception in women on category X medications. Am J Med. 2010;123:929–34e1.
56. Schwarz EB, Postlethwaite DA, Hung YY, Armstrong MA. Documentation of contraception and pregnancy when prescribing potentially teratogenic medications for reproductive-age women. Ann Intern Med. 2007;147:370–6.
57. Trussell J. Contraceptive failure in the United States. Contraception. 2011;83:397–404.
58. Takeda Pharmaceutical Company Limited. LUPRON DEPOT® (leuprolide acetate for depot suspension) [package insert]. Osaka: Takeda Pharmaceutical Company Limited; 2012.
59. Fossa SD, Dahl AA. Fertility and sexuality in young cancer survivors who have adult-onset malignancies. Hematol Oncol Clin North Am. 2008;22:291–303, vii.
60. Clowse ME, Behera MA, Anders CK, Copland S, Coffman CJ, Leppert PC, et al. Ovarian preservation by GnRH agonists during chemotherapy: a meta-analysis. J Womens Health (Larchmt). 2009;18: 311–9.
61. Celgene Corporation. Celgene risk evaluation and mitigation strategy. Berkeley Heights, NJ: Celgene Corporation; 2013.
62. Arnon J, Meirow D, Lewis-Roness H, Ornoy A. Genetic and teratogenic effects of cancer treatments on gametes and embryos. Hum Reprod Update. 2001;7:394–403.
63. Wallace WH, Thomson AB, Kelsey TW. The radiosensitivity of the human oocyte. Hum Reprod. 2003;18:117–21.
64. Meirow D, Nugent D. The effects of radiotherapy and chemotherapy on female reproduction. Hum Reprod Update. 2001;7:535–43.
65. Lishner M. Cancer in pregnancy. Ann Oncol. 2003;14 Suppl 3:31–6.
66. Daniels K, Mosher WD, Jones J. Contraceptive methods women have ever used: United States, 1982–2010. National health statistics reports, no 62. Hyattsville, MD: National Center for Health Statistics; 1982–2010. p. 2013.
67. American College of Obstetricians, Gynecologists Committee on Gynecologic Practice, Long-Acting Reversible Contraception Working Group. ACOG Committee opinion no. 450: increasing use of contraceptive implants and intrauterine devices to reduce unintended pregnancy. Obstet Gynecol. 2009; 114:1434–8.
68. ACOG. ACOG practice bulletin no. 73: use of hormonal contraception in women with coexisting medical conditions. Obstet Gynecol. 2006;107:1453–72.
69. Bartz D, Greenberg JA. Sterilization in the United States. Rev Obstet Gynecol. 2008;1:23–32.

70. Smith GL, Taylor GP, Smith KF. Comparative risks and costs of male and female sterilization. Am J Public Health. 1985;75:370–4.
71. Laurence V, Gbolade BA, Morgan SJ, Glaser A. Contraception for teenagers and young adults with cancer. Eur J Cancer. 2004;40:2705–16.
72. Meirow D, Rabinovici J, Katz D, Or R, Shufaro Y, Ben-Yehuda D. Prevention of severe menorrhagia in oncology patients with treatment-induced thrombocytopenia by luteinizing hormone-releasing hormone agonist and depo-medroxyprogesterone acetate. Cancer. 2006;107:1634–41.
73. Falanga A, Zacharski L. Deep vein thrombosis in cancer: the scale of the problem and approaches to management. Ann Oncol. 2005;16:696–701.
74. Heit JA, Silverstein MD, Mohr DN, Petterson TM, O'Fallon WM, Melton 3rd LJ. Risk factors for deep vein thrombosis and pulmonary embolism: a population-based case-control study. Arch Intern Med. 2000;160:809–15.
75. Lee AY, Levine MN. Venous thromboembolism and cancer: risks and outcomes. Circulation. 2003;107: I17–21.
76. Zapata LB, Whiteman MK, Marchbanks PA, Curtis KM. Intrauterine device use among women with ovarian cancer: a systematic review. Contraception. 2010;82:38–40.
77. Reid DM, Doughty J, Eastell R, Heys SD, Howell A, McCloskey EV, et al. Guidance for the management of breast cancer treatment-induced bone loss: a consensus position statement from a UK Expert Group. Cancer Treat Rev. 2008;34 Suppl 1:S3–18.
78. Ramaswamy B, Shapiro CL. Osteopenia and osteoporosis in women with breast cancer. Semin Oncol. 2003;30:763–75.
79. Gai L, Zhang J, Zhang H, Gai P, Zhou L, Liu Y. The effect of depot medroxyprogesterone acetate (DMPA) on bone mineral density (BMD) and evaluating changes in BMD after discontinuation of DMPA in Chinese women of reproductive age. Contraception. 2011;83:218–22.
80. Pongsatha S, Ekmahachai M, Suntornlimsiri N, Morakote N, Chaovisitsaree S. Bone mineral density in women using the subdermal contraceptive implant Implanon for at least 2 years. Int J Gynaecol Obstet. 2010;109:223–5.
81. Monteiro-Dantas C, Espejo-Arce X, Lui-Filho JF, Fernandes AM, Monteiro I, Bahamondes L. A three-year longitudinal evaluation of the forearm bone density of users of etonogestrel- and levonorgestrel-releasing contraceptive implants. Reprod Health. 2007;4:11.
82. Bahamondes L, Monteiro-Dantas C, Espejo-Arce X, Dos Santos Fernandes AM, Lui-Filho JF, Perrotti M, et al. A prospective study of the forearm bone density of users of etonorgestrel- and levonorgestrel-releasing contraceptive implants. Hum Reprod. 2006;21:466–70.
83. Bhalla AK. Management of osteoporosis in a premenopausal woman. Best Pract Res Clin Rheumatol. 2010;24:313–27.
84. Sim LA, McGovern L, Elamin MB, Swiglo BA, Erwin PJ, Montori VM. Effect on bone health of estrogen preparations in premenopausal women with anorexia nervosa: a systematic review and meta-analyses. Int J Eat Disord. 2010;43:218–25.
85. Martinez G, Daniels K, Chandra A. Fertility of men and women aged 15–44 years in the United States: National Survey of Family Growth. Natl Health Stat Report. 2006–2010;2012:1–28.
86. Glasier A, Cameron ST, Blithe D, Scherrer B, Mathe H, Levy D, et al. Can we identify women at risk of pregnancy despite using emergency contraception? Data from randomized trials of ulipristal acetate and levonorgestrel. Contraception. 2011;84:363–7.
87. Jadav SP, Parmar DM. Ulipristal acetate, a progesterone receptor modulator for emergency contraception. J Pharmacol Pharmacother. 2012;3:109–11.
88. Cheng L, Gulmezoglu AM, Oel CJ, Piaggio G, Ezcurra E, Look PF. Interventions for emergency contraception. Cochrane Database Syst Rev. 2004; 2004:Cd001324.
89. Green DM, Whitton JA, Stovall M, Mertens AC, Donaldson SS, Ruymann FB, et al. Pregnancy outcome of female survivors of childhood cancer: a report from the Childhood Cancer Survivor Study. Am J Obstet Gynecol. 2002;187:1070–80.
90. Winther JF, Boice Jr JD, Svendsen AL, Frederiksen K, Olsen JH. Induced abortions in Danish cancer survivors: a population-based cohort study. J Natl Cancer Inst. 2009;101:687–9.
91. Barrett HL, Lust K, Callaway LK, Fagermo N, Portmann C. Termination of pregnancy for maternal medical indications: failings in delivery of contraceptive advice? Aust N Z J Obstet Gynaecol. 2011; 51:532–5.
92. Wong AW, Chan SS, Yeo W, Yu MY, Tam WH. Prophylactic use of levonorgestrel-releasing intrauterine system in women with breast cancer treated with tamoxifen: a randomized controlled trial. Obstet Gynecol. 2013;121:943–50.
93. Gardner FJ, Konje JC, Abrams KR, Brown LJ, Khanna S, Al-Azzawi F, et al. Endometrial protection from tamoxifen-stimulated changes by a levonorgestrel-releasing intrauterine system: a randomised controlled trial. Lancet. 2000;356:1711–7.
94. FFPRHC. FFPRHC guidance (April 2004). The levonorgestrel-releasing intrauterine system (LNG-IUS) in contraception and reproductive health. J Fam Plann Reprod Health Care. 2004; 30:99–108. quiz 09.
95. ACOG. Practice ACoOaGCoG ACOG committee opinion. No 337: noncontraceptive uses of the levonorgestrel intrauterine system. Obstet Gynecol. 2006;107:1479–82.
96. Trinh XB, Tjalma WA, Makar AP, Buytaert G, Weyler J, van Dam PA. Use of the levonorgestrel-releasing intrauterine system in breast cancer patients. Fertil Steril. 2008;90:17–22.
97. Hillis SD, Marchbanks PA, Tylor LR, Peterson HB. Poststerilization regret: findings from the

United States collaborative review of sterilization. Obstet Gynecol. 1999;93:889–95.
98. Hirshfeld-Cytron J, Winter J. Laparoscopic tubal reanastomosis versus in vitro fertilization: cost-based decision analysis. Am J Obstet Gynecol. 2013;209:56.e1–6.
99. Teva Women's Health, Inc. ParaGard® T 380A intrauterine copper contraceptive [package insert]. Sellersville, PA: Teva Women's Health, Inc; 2013.
100. Correia L, Ramos AB, Machado AI, Rosa D, Marques C. Magnetic resonance imaging and gynecological devices. Contraception. 2012;85: 538–43.
101. Zieman M, Kanal E. Copper T380A IUD and magnetic resonance imaging. Contraception. 2007; 75:93–5.
102. Emans SJ, Grace E, Woods ER, Smith DE, Klein K, Merola J. Adolescents' compliance with the use of oral contraceptives. JAMA. 1987;257:3377–81.
103. Patel A, Radeke EK, Uy A, Zaren HA. Reproductive health algorithm. J Clin Oncol. 2011;29(Suppl 27; Abstr 263).

15 Contraception for Women with Endocrine Abnormalities

Carrie A. Cwiak and Allison Lange

Introduction

Endocrine abnormalities are linked with the reproductive system and the interplay between endogenous and exogenous hormones must be considered prior to contraceptive initiation. The most common endocrine abnormalities in reproductive-aged women are discussed in this chapter, including hyperthyroidism, hypothyroidism, and polycystic ovary syndrome (PCOS). Diabetes is becoming more prominent among women with PCOS and is addressed in a separate chapter (see Chap. 4). The complex hormonal mechanisms behind these conditions are addressed below, as well as any effects of contraception on specific disease characteristics.

Hyperthyroidism

Graves disease is the most common autoimmune disorder of the thyroid gland and the most common cause of hyperthyroidism. There is large variability in published epidemiologic reports as to the prevalence of hyperthyroidism. This is due to variable screening methods, nutritional iodine availability, and ethnic or geographical differences [1, 2]. Including all causes of hyperthyroidism, the 1977 Whickham survey from the UK demonstrated a prevalence of 1.1–1.6 % [2, 3], and it was assumed that the majority of these cases were Graves disease. Similarly, a 1997 meta-analysis estimated the overall prevalence of Graves disease in the USA to be 1 % [3].

Hormonal Alterations

Thyroid hormone disturbances are directly linked to changes in reproductive hormones. Sex hormone-binding globulin (SHBG), which transports steroid hormones throughout the body, increases in response to hyperthyroidism. Estrogen levels can also be 2–3 times higher in women with hyperthyroidism throughout their menstrual cycle. It is uncertain if this is due only to the increased SHBG or if there is actually an increase in free estrogen levels [4].

There are also changes in androgen levels in women with hyperthyroidism. Testosterone and androstenedione levels are increased due to higher production rates. Several studies have found that mean and maximum luteinizing hormone (LH) levels are also significantly increased throughout the menstrual cycle in these women. While these absolute levels increase, the pulsatile nature of their release is unchanged. With several weeks of treatment for hyperthyroidism, serum LH levels return to normal [5]. Studies have yet to elucidate the changes to follicle-stimulating hormone (FSH) seen in hyperthyroid women; they

C.A. Cwiak, M.D., M.P.H. (✉) • A. Lange, M.D.
Department of Gynecology and Obstetrics, Emory University School of Medicine, Atlanta, GA, USA
e-mail: ccwiak@emory.edu; Allison.lange@emory.edu

R.H. Allen and C.A. Cwiak (eds.), *Contraception for the Medically Challenging Patient*, DOI 10.1007/978-1-4939-1233-9_15, © Springer Science+Business Media New York 2014

may be elevated or remain normal. Nevertheless, most women with Graves disease are ovulatory.

Effects on Fertility

The onset of hyperthyroidism prior to puberty has been linked to delayed sexual maturation and menarche. However, some studies show only a nonsignificant trend toward an older mean age of menarche for hyperthyroid girls compared to healthy girls [6].

Amenorrhea has long been associated with hyperthyroidism. However, women may be more likely to experience irregular or heavy menstrual bleeding. This results from a variety of factors including the biochemical or the hormonal abnormalities, nutritional deficiencies, or mood imbalances that can accompany hyperthyroidism [7]. A 1993 case–control study by Joshi et al. compared 178 adolescents and adults with thyroid disease (hyperthyroidism, hypothyroidism, or goiter) to 49 healthy female controls and found that 65 % of women with hyperthyroidism had abnormal menstrual cycles compared to 12 % of healthy controls (p value <0.001) [8]. Abnormal bleeding patterns were most commonly lighter or less frequent menses, followed by heavier or more frequent menstrual bleeding. These menstrual disturbances were the first indication of thyroid abnormalities for 45 % of all cases identified, sometimes preceding diagnosis by several years. Of note, mean age of menarche was the same for cases and controls [8]. A 1994 case–control study of 214 Greek women aged 21–43 years found only a 21 % prevalence of menstrual disturbances in untreated hyperthyroid women compared with 8.4 % of age- and weight-matched controls. Again, abnormal bleeding patterns included lighter or less frequent menses, as well as heavier or more frequent menses; no women reported amenorrhea. Women with abnormal menstrual cycles had higher total T4 levels than those with normal cycles (268 nmol/L vs. 241 nmol/L, $p<0.05$), and all menstrual abnormalities resolved within 3 months of treatment. In contrast, total triiodothyronine (T3) levels have not shown correlation with menstrual irregularities. The authors suspected that better medical care and awareness of thyroid diagnoses allowed for earlier detection and less severe disease, leading to the lower prevalence of significant abnormalities compared to studies in the past [9].

However, amenorrhea or oligomenorrhea does not preclude fertility and need for contraception in hyperthyroid women wishing to avoid pregnancy. Few studies have specifically investigated hyperthyroid-related infertility. Most hyperthyroid women remain ovulatory. The study by Joshi et al. discovered that 5.8 % of hyperthyroid women had primary or secondary infertility compared to 2.4 % of controls ($p<0.05$) [8]. In a study by Poppe et al. of 438 women undergoing infertility treatment and 100 age-matched healthy controls, the risk of female-cause infertility in women with subclinical and overt hyperthyroidism was higher than that of fertile controls only for women who were positive for thyroid peroxidase antibodies (7 % vs. 1 %, $p=0.02$) [10].

Implications of Pregnancy

A commonly used treatment for hyperthyroidism is radioactive iodide. In those women treated with 10 mCi of R-I^{131}, the common dosing for hyperthyroidism, reproductive capacity is not affected and future children do not appear to be affected [11]. Women may still conceive after treatment, but it is typical to advise against pregnancy for at least 6 months after R-I^{131}. Therefore, use of an effective method of contraception until then should be strongly encouraged.

Maternal and neonatal outcomes of pregnancy in the setting of uncontrolled hyperthyroidism are directly related to the duration of poor control and the severity of disease. Hyperthyroidism is associated with spontaneous abortion, congestive heart failure, thyrotoxic storm, preeclampsia, preterm delivery, low birth weight, and stillbirth [4].

Data on Contraceptive Use

Increased estrogen levels, whether endogenous as with pregnancy or exogenous as with contraceptive or hormone therapy, increase serum levels of thyroid-binding globulin (TBG). Estrogen's effect on TBG is dose dependent and a result of decreased degradation and clearance due to the glycosylation of TBG. Since most T3 and T4 circulate bound to thyroid-binding globulin (TBG), albumin, lipoproteins, and transthyretin, the increase in serum concentration of TBG increases its ability to bind T3 and T4. This initially results in a lower absolute value of free circulating T3 and T4, in response to which the pituitary will produce more thyroid-stimulating hormone (TSH). In euthyroid women within 6–12 weeks of increased estrogen exposure, free T4 levels normalize though total T4 will be elevated once equilibrium is achieved [12]. The T3 uptake test will be increased as a result of the initial changes in TBG as it is a measure of unoccupied T4-binding sites. However, since free T4 levels remain normal in euthyroid women regardless of the change in TBG, free T4 can be used for diagnosis of suspected thyroid disease in women using estrogen-containing medications [13].

In euthyroid women using combined hormonal contraception (CHC), the effect of the estrogen component, ethinyl estradiol (EE), is counteracted by the progestin component, more so with increasing androgenic activity of the progestin. A Finnish study that followed 20 women 20–35 years old who used a combined oral contraceptive (COC) (30 μg EE/75 mg desogestrel) for three cycles noted a 101 % increase in TBG and a 44 % increase in total T4. Overall, TSH levels and response to thyrotropin-releasing hormone (TRH) were unchanged, and free T4, though slightly decreased, remained within normal limits [14].

In order to compare various estrogen and progestin types, one German study randomized 100 women 18–35 years of age to use one of the four low-dose COC formulations: 30 μg EE/2 mg dienogest (DNG), 20 μg EE/2 mg DNG, 10 μg EE/2 mg estradiol valerate (EV)/2 mg DNG, or 20 μg EE/1 mg levonorgestrel (LNG). Women in all four groups experienced a significant rise in TBG as early as the first cycle of use, which persisted throughout all six cycles of the study. This rise was significantly more so with the less androgenic DNG-containing COCs than with the LNG-containing COCs (50–60 % vs. 30 %, $p<0.05$) [15]. In further analysis of the same study, a 20–40 % increase in total T4 and T3 levels was noted in all six cycles, which tended to be more so with DNG compared to LNG, though the difference between progestins was not statistically significant. A significant rise in free T4 was only noted with the 10 μg EE/2 mg EV/2 mg DNG formulation (to 1.96 vs. the upper normal value of 1.8), suggesting that T4 changes with EE-containing COCs are not clinically relevant, but that EE plus EV may have more of an effect [16]. Adolescents experience similar changes. These effects on thyroid function do not appear to vary throughout the cycle [17], or differ with either triphasic [18] or continuous [19] COC formulations.

Non-oral CHC formulations have a similar effect. In a European trial of 77 women randomized to use either the contraceptive vaginal ring (15 μg EE/120 μg etonogestrel [ENG] daily release) or a COC (30 μg EE/150 μg LNG), median TSH was noted to be significantly increased in both groups 128 % by the third cycle and 110 % by the sixth cycle, though the median free T4 did not change in either group, indicating a lack of clinical effect [20]. A randomized controlled trial (RCT) of 19 reproductive-aged women compared the transdermal contraceptive patch (20 μg EE/150 μg norgestimate daily release) to a COC (35 μg EE/250 μg norgestimate) and found that the mean increase in TBG was significantly higher with the patch than with the COC (66 % vs. 52 %, $p<0.05$). This is likely due to the increased EE exposure women experience with the transdermal patch compared to a COC [21].

In contrast, use of intrauterine and progestin-only contraception does not affect TBG. In some comparative studies, women using the copper intrauterine device (Cu-IUD) have comprised the control group since the Cu-IUD is non-hormonal and therefore has no effect on thyroid function. An observational study conducted in the Netherlands followed adult women who were using COCs, the LNG-IUD, or the Cu-IUD. Over the 3 months of the study, TBG, TSH, and free T4 did not change for Cu-IUD or LNG-IUD users, while TBG and TSH increased in COC

Table 15.1 USMEC recommendations for the use of contraception in women with thyroid disorders

Guidelines for thyroid disorders	CHC	DMPA	Implant	LNG-IUD, POP	Cu-IUD
Simple goiter	1	1	1	1	1
Hyperthyroidism	1	1	1	1	1
Hypothyroidism	1	1	1	1	1

CHC combined hormonal contraception, *DMPA* depot medroxyprogesterone acetate, *LNG-IUD* levonorgestrel intrauterine device, *POP* progestin-only pill, *Cu-IUD* copper intrauterine device, *1*, a condition for which there is no restriction for use

users [22]. Eighty reproductive-aged women were randomized to receive either the ENG implant (Implanon, Merck, Whitehouse Station, NJ, USA) or the LNG implant (Norplant, no longer available in the USA) and then were followed for 24 months. Despite mild or transient increases in TBG, and total T4 and T3, all values remained within normal limits and were similar in both groups [23]. A 6-month observational study of 50 women who used progestin-only pills (POPs) containing 50 μg of norgestrel found no significant differences in mean total T4, T3 uptake, or TBG-binding capacity [24]. And a double-blind RCT comparing 30 μg LNG POPs and 75 μg desogestrel (DSG) POPs found no significant changes in TSH or free T4 associated with the use of either pill [25].

The risk of thyroid cancer does not appear to be increased with past contraceptive use. A case–control study in US adult women who were diagnosed with papillary, follicular, or mixed-type thyroid cancer found no significant association overall with ever use of COCs (RR 1.6, 95 % CI 0.98–2.5), including with COC use of long duration. The only significant association was with ever COC use and the subgroup of women with follicular cancer (RR 3.6, 95 % CI 1.1–12.8), though it was based on only 11 cases [26]. A Chinese prospective cohort study followed peri- and postmenopausal women for 7 years and found no association between ever use of COCs, IUDs, or tubal sterilization and thyroid cancer (hazard ratio 0.63, 95 % CI 0.38–1.04). This cohort included women at higher risk of thyroid cancer, including those with goiter [27].

There are no studies of contraceptive use in women with hyperthyroidism or goiter. For patients with thyroid disease, menstrual disorders may be a key determinant to guide contraceptive decision making and initiation. The primary treatment to regulate the menstrual cycle should be correction of the underlying thyroid abnormality. If a concurrent contraceptive is also needed, then a progestin-containing method (whether progestin-only or combined) should be prescribed to women who are anovulatory or amenorrheic to protect the uterine lining against unopposed estrogen exposure and subsequent development of endometrial hyperplasia. And as stated previously, women with hyperthyroidism may have endogenous estrogen levels 2–3 times higher than controls, so even eumenorrheic women may benefit from the endometrial protection of progestin-containing contraception. The use of the Cu-IUD is also associated with a decreased risk of endometrial cancer, but whether this protective effect is also experienced by hyperthyroid women is unknown. There is no data specific to women with hyperthyroidism to indicate a superior method for menstrual regulation. Anovulatory and amenorrheic hyperthyroid women may prefer to return to a pattern of monthly menstrual cycles provided by cyclic use of CHC or the Cu-IUD, or they may wish to continue the menstrual pattern they were accustomed to in their disease state by using CHC continuously or a progestin-only method. A discussion with the patient to determine the contraceptive method best suited to her lifestyle, reproductive health needs, and other coexisting medical problems is appropriate.

The Centers for Disease Control and Prevention (CDC) developed the US Medical Eligibility Criteria for Contraceptive Use (USMEC). For hyperthyroidism or simple goiter, the USMEC assigns a category 1 to all contraceptive methods, indicating that there is no need to restrict their use [28] (Table 15.1).

Hypothyroidism

Hypothyroidism is more common in women than men (by a 10:1 ratio) and is most often attributed to Hashimoto's disease. Hashimoto's has an incidence rate of approximately 3.5 per 1,000 women per year. The next most common cause of hypothyroidism is as a result of destructive treatment for thyrotoxicosis with an incidence of 0.6 per 1,000 women per year. There is a known increasing incidence of all hypothyroidism with advancing age: the probability of developing hypothyroidism is ten times greater for someone aged 75–80 years than 20–25 years (14 vs. 1.4 per 1,000 women per year) [4].

Hormonal Alterations

Women with hypothyroidism demonstrate decreased metabolic clearance of both androstenedione and estrone. Additionally, they have increased peripheral aromatization of androgens to estrogen [29]. Binding activity of SHBG is decreased, which also leads to increased unbound fractions of estradiol and testosterone. When a euthyroid state is achieved, these hormone alterations return to normal [30].

A delayed LH response has been reported in some women with hypothyroidism. When this occurs, serum prolactin (PRL) concentrations are often elevated. This is likely due to the hypothalamic response to low serum levels of thyroid hormone. The hypothalamic release of TRH stimulates TSH release from the pituitary. The increased levels of TRH inhibit dopamine, which in turn increases prolactin and decreases gonadotropin-releasing hormone (GnRH). Galactorrhea and infertility may develop, but this should resolve after thyroid treatment [31].

In animal studies, thyroid hormone (TH) levels have been shown to have an impact on reproductive function. Hypothyroidism has been shown to result in irregular estrous cycles and ovarian atrophy in rats. Thyroid receptors are found in rat uterine tissue, and administration of TH to mice has been shown to induce thickening of the endometrial stripe [4]. There are no similar studies in women, though indirect evidence is supposed as TH treatment improves fertility and abnormal uterine bleeding in hypothyroid women.

Effects on Fertility

As with hyperthyroidism, women with hypothyroidism may experience changes in both cycle length and amount of bleeding. Anovulation may result in amenorrhea or irregular menstrual bleeding. Alternatively, heavy menstrual bleeding may develop as a result of decreased levels of clotting factors VII, VIII, IX, and XI that can occur with thyroid dysfunction [32]. In the case–control study by Joshi et al. previously mentioned, 68 % of women with hypothyroidism complained of abnormal menstrual cycles compared to 12 % of healthy controls (p value <0.001) [8]. As with hyperthyroidism, abnormal bleeding patterns associated with hypothyroidism were most commonly lighter or less frequent menses, followed by heavier or more frequent menstrual bleeding. Whether the dysfunction was hyper- or hypothyroidism or goiter, menstrual disturbances were the first indication of thyroid abnormalities for 45 % of all cases identified, and mean age of menarche was the same for cases and controls [8]. Another study similarly found that 56 % of hypothyroid women presented with menstrual irregularities. Although the most common abnormality was lighter or less frequent menses, heavier or more frequent menstrual bleeding as well as amenorrhea were also noted [33].

There are limited studies investigating the impact of hypothyroidism on fertility. Most are poorly designed without controls and do not answer the question of the incidence of infertility in hypothyroid women. In considering the cause of infertility in women with hypothyroidism, altered peripheral metabolism of androgens and estrogen, hyperprolactinemia, defects in hemostasis, and abnormal pulsatile LH are all possible contributors. Joshi et al. found that 6.2 % of hypothyroid women had primary or secondary infertility compared to 2.4 % of controls ($p<0.05$) [8]. The case–control study by Poppe et al. noted that median TSH levels were higher among women with female-cause infertility compared to age-matched controls (1.3 mIU/L vs. 1.1 mIU/L, $p=0.005$), though the number of cases of hypothyroidism was not increased [10]. In addition to ovulatory control, hypothyroidism may hinder fertilization. A study by Cramer et al. of 509 US infertile women undergoing in vitro fertilization demonstrated that elevated serum TSH levels (2.5 mIU/L vs. 2.0 mIU/L) were predictive of fertilization failure (i.e., fertilization of less than 50 % of oocytes) ($p=0.05$) [34]. Nevertheless, the incidence of infertility in women with hypothyroidism is not universal, and so a discussion of contraceptive use with hypothyroid women wishing to avoid pregnancy is warranted. And as hormone levels normalize with treatment, spontaneous fertility increases toward baseline and menstrual cycles normalize.

Implications of Pregnancy

For those women with hypothyroidism who do conceive, proper control of thyroid levels is imperative for a good pregnancy outcome. The fetus is exposed to the same free T4 concentrations as the mother. Therefore, a decrease in maternal free T4 can have detrimental effects for fetal neurodevelopment in the first trimester, the sequelae of which would be impaired mental and motor function in childhood.

Spontaneous abortion and early fetal loss is known to be associated with hypothyroidism as well. This loss rate decreases once women are treated with thyroid hormone. Additionally, although studies are mixed, some have found higher rates of stillbirth, postpartum hemorrhages, preeclampsia, and cesarean sections in women with hypothyroidism [4]. A retrospective study of 114 women 16–39 years old found an early pregnancy loss rate of 31 % in women with uncontrolled hypothyroidism at the time of conception compared to 4 % in women who had achieved a euthyroid state with treatment prior to conception ($p<0.0001$) [35]. A prospective cohort of over 2,400 Dutch women found a small but significantly increased risk of all pregnancy loss in women with any doubling of TSH levels (OR 1.6, 95 % CI 1.04–2.47) [36]. Due to these potential complications, it is advised that women use effective contraception until their hypothyroidism is under control (i.e., TSH < 2.5 mIU/L). Even those women with aberrant menstrual cycles have the possibility of conceiving and would be at risk for unintended pregnancy and early pregnancy complications if not hormonally optimized.

Data on Contraceptive Use

Similar to hyperthyroidism, there are no studies of contraceptive use in women with hypothyroidism and conclusions can only be drawn from studies of euthyroid women. As previously noted, free T4 can be used for diagnosis of suspected thyroid disease in women using estrogen-containing medications [13], but to what extent the effect of CHC on TBG further alters free T4 or T3 is unknown. One study of 36 postmenopausal women using hormonal therapy (conjugated equine estrogens) compared euthyroid women to hypothyroid women taking thyroxine and found that in the hypothyroid women, FT4 levels did not completely normalize despite increases in thyrotropin-releasing hormone (TRH), necessitating increases in their thyroxine doses [37]. Due to the potential effect on TH requirements, follow-up of free T4 levels is recommended in hypothyroid women after the initiation of CHC. Since the use of intrauterine and progestin-only contraception does not affect TBG, thyroxine requirements and surveillance would not be expected to change during concomitant use.

For hypothyroid women with abnormal uterine bleeding, correction of the underlying TH abnormalities should be the primary concern in order to normalize hormonal alterations throughout the body. Treatment of anovulatory bleeding and amenorrhea is a particular concern in women with hypothyroidism since, as with other instances of hormonal imbalance, endometrial hyperplasia can develop due to prolonged estrogen exposure. This can be resolved with both TH treatment and administration of progestin-containing (either progestin-only or combined) contraceptive agents. And since women with hypothyroidism may have increased endogenous estrogen from peripheral aromatization, eumenorrheic women may also benefit from the endometrial protection of progestin-containing contraception. Whether the use of the Cu-IUD is as protective against the risk of endometrial cancer in hypothyroid women as it is in euthyroid women is unknown. There is no data specific to women with hypothyroidism to indicate a superior method for menstrual regulation. As with hyperthyroidism, a discussion with the patient to determine the contraceptive method best suited to her preferred bleeding pattern, lifestyle, reproductive health needs, and other coexisting medical problems is appropriate.

For hypothyroidism, the USMEC assigns a category 1 to all contraceptive methods, indicating that there is no need for restriction in their use [28] (see Table 15.1).

Polycystic Ovary Syndrome

Polycystic ovary syndrome (PCOS) is the most common endocrine disorder in women. The clinical characteristics of PCOS include oligo-ovulation or anovulation, hyperandrogenism, and the presence of polycystic ovaries. It has a prevalence of 6–10 % in the USA (as per National Institutes of Health (NIH) criteria) and can be as high as 15 % with wider diagnostic (i.e., Rotterdam) criteria [38]. The Rotterdam criteria were established as diagnostic measures in 2003 due to the variability of phenotypic presentation of the syndrome. These revised diagnostic criteria require the presence of two of the three key characteristics: oligo- or anovulation, clinical or biochemical signs of hyperandrogenism, and polycystic ovaries on ultrasound with exclusion of other etiologies [39].

Due to the erratic hormonal changes of adolescence, all three elements of the Rotterdam criteria should be documented in order to diagnose PCOS in teenagers. Oligomenorrhea or amenorrhea should be present for a minimum of 2 years after menarche, polycystic ovaries should be seen on ultrasound with increased ovarian size >10 cm^3, and laboratory hyperandrogenemia should be present, most commonly noted by an elevated serum testosterone level [40].

Hormonal Alterations

LH levels are increased in women with PCOS due to increased amplitude and frequency of LH pulses [41]. LH levels above the 95th percentile are seen in roughly 60 % of women with PCOS. When women who have recently ovulated are excluded from analysis, 95 % of women with PCOS demonstrate an elevated LH/FSH ratio. However, LH levels may be transiently normalized following ovulation. Levels are also lower in lean PCOS women [42]. Current research on the role of LH levels in PCOS and fertility is indeterminate and further work needs to be done before LH can be relied upon for diagnosis, treatment, or prognosis. Accordingly, neither the NIH nor the Rotterdam criteria include LH levels or LH/FSH ratio.

Hyperandrogenism is a key diagnostic factor in PCOS. While most patients demonstrate clinical signs of this aberration, primarily hirsutism or acne, some may only have serum evidence of hyperandrogenemia, while others have no overt abnormality. Hirsutism is found in roughly 70 % of women with PCOS and is a good clinical marker for hyperandrogenism regardless of ethnicity or body mass index. Androgens induce the transformation of thin vellus hair into course pigmented terminal hair. In women, elevated concentrations of androgens are needed to cause this change in typically masculine areas such as the face and chest. This process occurs in a gradual fashion and cannot be reversed once it occurs [38]. Measurement of free testosterone (*T*) or the free androgen index (the ratio of total *T* concentration to SHBG concentration) is the most sensitive serum method of assessing for hyperandrogenemia. There may be utility in obtaining a dehydroepiandrosterone sulfate (DHEA-S) level if there is a concern for an adrenal source of hyperandrogenism. However, free T levels are frequently inconsistent and therefore unreliable for diagnosis and surveillance of PCOS.

Effects on Fertility

As many as 95 % of adult women with PCOS have oligo- or amenorrhea. Amenorrheic women are more likely to have higher serum androgen levels and antral follicle counts compared to oligo- or eumenorrheic women. Although women with PCOS may have irregular or no menstrual cycles, they may ovulate spontaneously in up to 32 % of cycles and so are still at risk for unintended pregnancy if fertility is not desired or expected [38].

PCOS is a known risk factor for infertility. Women may be subfertile due to altered ovulatory function, oocyte quality, or endometrial receptivity. As in other phenotypic presentations of PCOS, this is variable and many women with PCOS can have ovulatory cycles as well as normal rates of implantation and fertilization. Irregular menstrual bleeding, amenorrhea, and obesity are more often associated with decreased fertility [43]. No matter their presentation, clinicians need to address the contraceptive needs of their patients with PCOS who wish to delay or prevent pregnancy. Once women become pregnant, it is believed that their risk of spontaneous abortion is similar to that of normal women. However, they have an increased incidence of gestational diabetes, hypertensive disorders, and small-for-gestational age babies. The health of these women should be optimized before any pregnancy is attempted [38].

Data on Contraceptive Use

There are no contraceptive methods that are contraindicated due to PCOS itself, and the USMEC does not address PCOS specifically. However, considerations that should be involved in contraceptive method selection depend on the features of the syndrome exhibited, including abnormal menstrual cycles, the effect of unopposed estrogen on the endometrium, androgenic symptoms, or obesity and insulin resistance. Symptoms of PCOS, including acne, hirsutism, irregular menses, amenorrhea, obesity, and subfertility, are major contributors to psychological morbidity or poor quality of life in these patients. Alleviating these factors should be considered when choosing a contraception method.

Combined oral contraceptives (COCs) are effective for menstrual cycle control in women with PCOS and are most often used for long-term contraception in these women. A 2007 review by Costello et al. included four RCTs in which women with PCOS were randomized to treatment with a COC vs. metformin, and two RCTs with a COC vs. COC/metformin combined therapy. Overall, metformin was significantly inferior to COCs in improving abnormal uterine bleeding (OR 0.08, 95 % CI 0.01–0.45). No data were available about the effect of either therapy on the long-term risk of endometrial cancer as none of the trials followed women for longer than 12 months [43].

Non-oral CHC, the transdermal patch and the vaginal ring, improve menstrual regularity as well. In addition, for a woman with PCOS who experiences abnormal uterine bleeding but minimal androgenic symptoms, any progestin-containing method (progestin-only or combined) can be used to protect the uterine lining against unopposed estrogen and the risk of endometrial hyperplasia. In this case, the highly effective long-term methods, such as the progestin implant or IUD, may be ideal options. The only studies of the LNG-IUD in women with PCOS include two case reports in which the LNG-IUD was effectively used as fertility-sparing treatment for complex endometrial hyperplasia with atypia [44] and well-differentiated early-stage endometrial cancer [45].

The use of CHC suppresses LH secretion which decreases ovarian androgen production. The estrogen component also increases serum levels of SHBG, which then decreases circulating free T levels. In addition, the progestin component competes for the androgen receptor and decreases adrenal androgen production. In addition, 5-alpha reductase activity in hair follicles and skin is decreased, the enzyme which converts testosterone to dihydrotestosterone. Therefore, for women with PCOS who have hyperandrogenism, CHC provides relief of androgenic symptoms. Most CHC methods marketed in the USA contain the same synthetic estrogen, EE. The progestin component varies and each class (i.e., generation) of progestins has its own androgenic potential. First- and second-generation progestins (norethindrone, norgestrel, and LNG) are more androgenic than third generation (DSG, norgestimate, DNG, and gestodene). However, when combined with EE, the overall effects of all CHCs are antiandrogenic. For example, the three COCs with Food and Drug Administration (FDA) approval for the treatment of acne all contain different progestins with different androgenic potential: norgestimate, norethindrone, and drospirenone.

Nevertheless, another alternative is to use a COC whose progestin has antiandrogenic activity, including cyproterone acetate, chlormadinone acetate (CMA), or drospirenone (DRSP). Small studies have shown improved androgen control compared to the other progestin components and so these medications might be better options for women with PCOS in whom androgenic symptoms are a primary concern. De Leo et al. randomized 40 women 18–36 years of age with PCOS to use 1 of 4 COC formulations: 30 µg EE/3 mg DRSP, 30 µg EE/2 mg CMA, 30 µg EE/75 µg gestodene, or 30 µg EE/150 µg DNG. All four groups experienced a drop in androgen levels, but the women taking COCs containing DRSP and CMA were associated with a significantly greater reduction in androgens and increase in SHBG ($p<0.05$) [46]. To investigate clinically relevant differences, Kriplani et al. randomized 60 women 16–40 years of age to either a COC containing 30 µg EE/3 mg DRSP or a COC containing 30 µg EE/150 µg DSG and measured acne and hirsutism scores both during 6 months of treatment and for 6 months after treatment. Use of both COCs resulted in a 33 % decrease in acne scores and this effect persisted 6 months posttreatment with the DRSP-containing COC. Only the DRSP-containing COC was associated with a significant decrease in hirsutism scores (36 %, $p=0.04$) that also persisted 6 months posttreatment [47].

The Costello review found COCs to be as effective as metformin in significantly alleviating clinical hirsutism and acne scores in women with PCOS, although only COCs were associated with a significant decrease in serum androgen levels [43]. A European trial by Battaglia et al. randomized 40 adult women with PCOS to use either a COC (30 µg EE/3 mg DRSP) or the contraceptive vaginal ring for 6 months. Both groups experienced a 300–400 % increase in SHBG. Accordingly, LH/FSH ratio, T level, free androgen index, and Ferriman-Gallwey score (a measure of hirsutism) were significantly decreased in both groups. The DRSP-containing COC was significantly more effective only in its effect on T level (1.1 nmol/L vs. 1.6 nmol/L, $p=0.029$) [48]. Ozdemir et al. randomized 79 adult women with PCOS to cyclic therapy either with a COC (30 µg EE/3 mg DRSP in a 21/7 pattern with 7 days of placebo) or oral provera (10 mg medroxyprogesterone acetate 10 days per month) for 6 months. Both therapies resulted in a significant decrease in LH, T, and free androgen index, but only the COC users experienced a significant increase in SHBG from baseline (49 µmol/L vs. 117 µmol/L). Accordingly, only COC users had a significant decrease in Ferriman-Gallwey score (10.4 vs. 7.5, $p=0.001$). Whether these changes are seen with contraceptive doses of progestins is unknown [49].

At least 6 months of hormonal treatment is needed to see a response in hirsutism [38], and continued treatment is needed to prevent recurrence. Although there is a limited effect of CHC on established hirsutism, these methods have shown benefit by decreasing progression and future hair growth as well as helping prevent pregnancy in those taking a combination of medications [50]. The combination of COCs and an antiandrogen to act at the hair follicle has also been used in an attempt to decrease hirsutism. Unfortunately, antiandrogens such as spironolactone, flutamide, and finasteride have not demonstrated an additional benefit over COCs alone [51]. There have not been long-term large clinical trials investigating the use of antiandrogens alone [50]. If they are used, these antiandrogens should not be given without adequate contraception due to the risk of teratogenicity.

There are theoretical concerns regarding the effects of hormonal contraception on the metabolic syndrome associated with PCOS. Forty percent of the US women with PCOS and hyperandrogenism have metabolic syndrome, defined as having at least three of the five cardiovascular and metabolic risk factors: elevated waist circumference, fasting plasma glucose, triglycerides, blood pressure, and reduced high-density lipoprotein [41]. Overall, the use of CHC does not appear to adversely affect these parameters. The Costello review reported that fasting levels of glucose and insulin did not change with COC treatment in the three RCTs that assessed that outcome. Risk of diabetes mellitus and cardiovascular disease could not be assessed as no studies followed women for longer than 12 months of use [43]. Similarly, the Ozdemir et al. trial noted that 6 months of a DRSP-containing COC had no significant adverse effect on fasting glucose or insulin, body mass index (BMI), waist-to-hip ratio (WHR), total cholesterol, triglycerides, or low-density lipoprotein [49]. And though the Battaglia trial found that total cholesterol and triglycerides increased with both the DRSP-containing COC and the contraceptive vaginal ring, levels remained within normal limits [48]. In contrast, a randomized trial of 55 adult women with PCOS compared the metabolic effects of a COC (20 μg EE/100 μg LNG) to the contraceptive vaginal ring (15 μg EE/ENG) and found that COC users had significantly increased insulin resistance ($p<0.04$) and decreased insulin sensitivity ($p<0.001$) after 5 months of use compared to baseline. Two of the women in the COC group developed impaired glucose tolerance. None of the ring users had changes in these parameters. Consistent with the other trials, there were no significant adverse changes noted in either group in BMI, WHR, total cholesterol, triglycerides, or low-density lipoprotein [52]. There are no studies of the transdermal patch in women with PCOS. Given these findings, the 2012 joint PCOS consensus committee of the European Society of Human Reproduction and Embryology (ESHRE) and the American Society for Reproductive Medicine (ASRM) concluded that the benefits of COC use outweigh the risks in most patients, but that women with PCOS may be more likely to have contraindications to their use that should be considered prior to initiation [38]. In addition, increased surveillance of glucose and lipid levels may be warranted after initiation of CHC.

Since women with PCOS and metabolic syndrome have multiple cardiovascular risk factors, progestin-only and intrauterine contraceptive methods can offer safer alternatives. There is less data on the use of these methods in women with PCOS. A study of the ENG implant in 13 nondiabetic women with PCOS showed increased insulin resistance though not impaired glucose tolerance after 6 months of use. BMI was also not affected [53]. The low progestin doses in the LNG-IUD and POPs would likely have no significant metabolic or blood pressure effects in these women [41]. And since it is nonhormonal, use of the Cu-IUD would not have any adverse effects on metabolic parameters. The Ozdemir trial in which women with PCOS were randomized to cyclic oral provera for menstrual regulation noted that oral provera does not appear to affect BMI, WHR, fasting glucose or insulin, or lipid levels [49]. However, the contraceptive progestin-only injection (150 mg depo-provera (DMPA)) delivered as an intramuscular injection every 3 months may lead to clinically significant changes in glucose tolerance and lipid levels in women with PCOS, especially with metabolic syndrome. The association of increased weight gain with DMPA for some women is also well known and may lead to a more adverse metabolic state. Therefore, DMPA should not be considered a first-line choice due to the potential deleterious effects on weight gain, fat distribution, and glucose tolerance, though its use is not contraindicated [41]. As with CHC, the patient's overall health, and in particular independent cardiovascular risk factors, should be considered prior to initiation. And increased surveillance of weight and glucose and lipid levels is recommended after initiation of DMPA.

Conclusion

Endocrine abnormalities are intimately connected to the reproductive system. Hypothyroidism and hyperthyroidism result in hormonal alterations that can lead to menstrual irregularities. This is often the first sign of the disorder in reproductive-aged women. There are no contraindications to any of the available contraceptive methods for either condition. Any hormonal method, due to the progestin component, would be beneficial for uterine protection in women with anovulatory bleeding or amenorrhea. Treating their thyroid abnormality is first line for improving menstrual irregularities, but any progestin-only or combination method would further improve bleeding patterns and counteract excess estrogen in the uterus.

Polycystic ovary syndrome is very common and seen in roughly 10 % of women. Special considerations in helping women with PCOS select appropriate contraceptive methods include the interplay of syndrome components. These women often demonstrate menstrual cycle abnormalities and may prefer the contraceptive benefit of cycle regulation. As in thyroid abnormalities, unopposed estrogen requires a progestin-containing method to prevent endometrial cancer. The typical method of contraception recommended for women with PCOS is CHC (COC, patch, or ring), which provides regulation of the menstrual cycle and decreased androgens. However, the highly effective, long-term progestin-only IUD or implant remains the first-line option for women who do not have significant androgenic symptoms. Finally, the possibility of coexisting metabolic syndrome should also be considered prior to prescribing contraception. In which case, the benefits of CHC still outweigh the risks in most patients, and intrauterine and most progestin-only are safe options. However, DMPA may not be appropriate for these women given its effects on weight gain, fat distribution, and glucose tolerance.

References

1. Furszyfer J, Kurland LT, McConahey WM, Woolner LB, Elveback LR. Epidemiologic aspects of Hashimoto's thyroiditis and Graves' disease in Rochester, Minnesota (1935–1967), with special reference to temporal trends. Metabolism. 1972;21(3):197–204. PubMed PMID: 5066850.
2. Tunbridge WM, Evered DC, Hall R, Appleton D, Brewis M, Clark F, et al. The spectrum of thyroid disease in a community: the Whickham survey. Clin Endocrinol. 1977;7(6):481–93. PubMed PMID: 598014.
3. Jacobson DL, Gange SJ, Rose NR, Graham NM. Epidemiology and estimated population burden of selected autoimmune diseases in the United States. Clin Immunol Immunopathol. 1997;84(3):223–43. PubMed PMID: 9281381.
4. Krassas GE, Poppe K, Glinoer D. Thyroid function and human reproductive health. Endocr Rev. 2010;31(5):702–55. PubMed PMID: 20573783.
5. Akande EO. The effect of oestrogen on plasma levels of luteinizing hormone in euthyroid and thyrotoxic postmenopausal women. J Obstet Gynaecol Br Commonw. 1974;81(10):795–803. PubMed PMID: 4419555.
6. Saxena KM, Crawford JD, Talbot NB. Childhood thyrotoxicosis: a long-term perspective. Br Med J. 1964;2(5418):1153–8. PubMed PMID: 14190483. Pubmed Central PMCID: 1816770.
7. Krassas G. The male and female reproductive system in thyrotoxicosis. In: Braverman Le UR, editor. Werner and Ingbar's the thyroid – a fundamental and clinical text. 9th ed. Philadelphia: Lippincott Williams & Wilkins; 2005. p. 621–8.
8. Joshi JV, Bhandarkar SD, Chadha M, Balaiah D, Shah R. Menstrual irregularities and lactation failure may precede thyroid dysfunction or goitre. J Postgrad Med. 1993;39(3):137–41. PubMed PMID: 8051643.
9. Krassas GE, Pontikides N, Kaltsas T, Papadopoulou P, Batrinos M. Menstrual disturbances in thyrotoxicosis. Clin Endocrinol. 1994;40(5):641–4. PubMed PMID: 8013145.
10. Poppe K, Glinoer D, Van Steirteghem A, Tournaye H, Devroey P, Schiettecatte J, et al. Thyroid dysfunction and autoimmunity in infertile women. Thyroid. 2002;12(11):997–1001. PubMed PMID: 12490077.
11. International Commission on Radiological Protection, Committee I. The evaluation of risks from radiation. Health Phys. 1966;12(2):239–302. PubMed PMID: 5331054.
12. Utiger RD. Estrogen, thyroxine binding in serum, and thyroxine therapy. N Engl J Med. 2001;344(23):1784–5. PubMed PMID: 11396448.
13. Sorger D, Schenk S, Schneider G. [Effects of various contraceptives on laboratory parameters in diagnosis of thyroid gland function with special reference to the free hormones FT4 and FT3]. Zeitschrift fur die gesamte innere Medizin und ihre Grenzgebiete. 1992;47(2):58–64. PubMed PMID: 1585690. Einflusse verschiedener Kontrazeptiva auf die Laborparameter der Schilddrusenfunktionsdiagnostik unter besonderer Berucksichtigung der freien Hormone FT4 und FT3.
14. Penttila IM, Makkonen M, Castren O. Thyroid function during treatment with a new oral contraceptive combination containing desogestrel. Eur J Obstet Gynecol Reprod Biol. 1983;16(4):269–74. PubMed PMID: 6232160.
15. Wiegratz I, Kutschera E, Lee JH, Moore C, Mellinger U, Winkler UH, et al. Effect of four different oral contraceptives on various sex hormones and serum-binding globulins. Contraception. 2003;67(1):25–32. PubMed PMID: 12521654.
16. Wiegratz I, Kutschera E, Lee JH, Moore C, Mellinger U, Winkler UH, et al. Effect of four oral contraceptives

on thyroid hormones, adrenal and blood pressure parameters. Contraception. 2003;67(5):361–6. PubMed PMID: 12742558.
17. Tuttlebee JW, Marsden JT. Thyroid function in oral contraception: is there cyclic variation? Ir Med J. 1983;76(2):80–1. PubMed PMID: 6841023.
18. Kuhl H, Gahn G, Romberg G, Althoff PH, Taubert HD. A randomized cross-over comparison of two low-dose oral contraceptives upon hormonal and metabolic serum parameters: II. Effects upon thyroid function, gastrin, STH, and glucose tolerance. Contraception. 1985;32(1):97–107.
19. Sanger N, Stahlberg S, Manthey T, Mittmann K, Mellinger U, Lange E, et al. Effects of an oral contraceptive containing 30 mcg ethinyl estradiol and 2 mg dienogest on thyroid hormones and androgen parameters: conventional vs. extended-cycle use. Contraception. 2008;77(6):420–5.
20. Duijkers I, Killick S, Bigrigg A, Dieben TO. A comparative study on the effects of a contraceptive vaginal ring NuvaRing and an oral contraceptive on carbohydrate metabolism and adrenal and thyroid function. Eur J Contracept Reprod Health Care. 2004;9(3):131–40. PubMed PMID: 15697102.
21. White T, Ozel B, Jain JK, Stanczyk FZ. Effects of transdermal and oral contraceptives on estrogen-sensitive hepatic proteins. Contraception. 2006;74(4):293–6. PubMed PMID: 16982228.
22. Raps M, Curvers J, Helmerhorst FM, Ballieux BE, Rosing J, Thomassen S, et al. Thyroid function, activated protein C resistance and the risk of venous thrombosis in users of hormonal contraceptives. Thromb Res. 2014;133(4):640–4. PubMed PMID: 24438944.
23. Biswas A, Viegas OA, Bennink HJ, Korver T, Ratnam SS. Effect of Implanon use on selected parameters of thyroid and adrenal function. Contraception. 2000;62(5):247–51. PubMed PMID: 11172795.
24. Goolden AW, Bateman DM, Pleehachinda R, Sanderson C. Thyroid-function tests in women taking norgestrel. Lancet. 1970;1(7647):624. PubMed PMID: 4190584.
25. Kivela A, Ruuskanen M, Agren U, Dieben T. The effects of two progestogen-only pills containing either desogestrel (75 microgram/day) or levonorgestrel (30 microgram/day) on carbohydrate metabolism and adrenal and thyroid function. Eur J Contracept Reprod Health Care. 2001;6(2):71–7.
26. McTiernan AM, Weiss NS, Daling JR. Incidence of thyroid cancer in women in relation to reproductive and hormonal factors. Am J Epidemiol. 1984;120(3):423–35. PubMed PMID: 6475918.
27. Dorjgochoo T, Shu XO, Li HL, Qian HZ, Yang G, Cai H, et al. Use of oral contraceptives, intrauterine devices and tubal sterilization and cancer risk in a large prospective study, from 1996 to 2006. Int J Cancer. 2009;124(10):2442–9. PubMed PMID: 19170208. Pubmed Central PMCID: 2666967.
28. Centers for Disease Control and Prevention. U.S. medical eligibility criteria for contraceptive use. MMWR. 2010;59(RR-4):1.
29. Longcope C, Abend S, Braverman LE, Emerson CH. Androstenedione and estrone dynamics in hypothyroid women. J Clin Endocrinol Metab. 1990;70(4):903–7. PubMed PMID: 2318947.
30. Gordon GG, Southren AL. Thyroid-hormone effects on steroid-hormone metabolism. Bull N Y Acad Med. 1977;53(3):241–59. PubMed PMID: 266410. Pubmed Central PMCID: 1807335.
31. Honbo KS, van Herle AJ, Kellett KA. Serum prolactin levels in untreated primary hypothyroidism. Am J Med. 1978;64(5):782–7. PubMed PMID: 645742.
32. Ansell JE. The blood in the hypothyroidism. In: Braverman LE, editor. Werner and Ingbar's the thyroid – a fundamental and clinical text. 7th ed. Philadelphia, PA: Lippincott-Raven; 1996. p. 821–5.
33. Scott Jr JC, Mussey E. Menstrual patterns in myxedema. Am J Obstet Gynecol. 1964;90:161–5. PubMed PMID: 14215872.
34. Cramer DW, Sluss PM, Powers RD, McShane P, Ginsburgs ES, Hornstein MD, et al. Serum prolactin and TSH in an in vitro fertilization population: is there a link between fertilization and thyroid function? J Assist Reprod Genet. 2003;20(6):210–5. PubMed PMID: 12877251. Pubmed Central PMCID: 3455321.
35. Abalovich M, Gutierrez S, Alcaraz G, Maccallini G, Garcia A, Levalle O. Overt and subclinical hypothyroidism complicating pregnancy. Thyroid. 2002;12(1):63–8. PubMed PMID: 11838732.
36. Benhadi N, Wiersinga WM, Reitsma JB, Vrijkotte TG, Bonsel GJ. Higher maternal TSH levels in pregnancy are associated with increased risk for miscarriage, fetal or neonatal death. Eur J Endocrinol. 2009;160(6):985–91. PubMed PMID: 19273570.
37. Arafah BM. Increased need for thyroxine in women with hypothyroidism during estrogen therapy. N Engl J Med. 2001;344(23):1743–9. PubMed PMID: 11396440.
38. Fauser BC, Tarlatzis BC, Rebar RW, Legro RS, Balen AH, Lobo R, et al. Consensus on women's health aspects of polycystic ovary syndrome (PCOS): the Amsterdam ESHRE/ASRM-sponsored 3rd PCOS consensus workshop group. Fertil Steril. 2012;97(1):28–38e25. PubMed PMID: 22153789.
39. Rotterdam EA-SPcwg. Revised 2003 consensus on diagnostic criteria and long-term health risks related to polycystic ovary syndrome (PCOS). Hum Reprod. 2004;19(1):41–7. PubMed PMID: 14688154.
40. Carmina E, Oberfield SE, Lobo RA. The diagnosis of polycystic ovary syndrome in adolescents. Am J Obstet Gynecol. 2010;203(3):201e1–5. PubMed PMID: 20435290.
41. Verhaeghe J. Hormonal contraception in women with the metabolic syndrome: a narrative review. Eur J Contracept Reprod Health Care. 2010;15(5):305–13. PubMed PMID: 20695771.
42. Taylor AE, McCourt B, Martin KA, Anderson EJ, Adams JM, Schoenfeld D, et al. Determinants of abnormal gonadotropin secretion in clinically defined women with polycystic ovary syndrome. J Clin Endocrinol Metab. 1997;82(7):2248–56. PubMed PMID: 9215302.

43. Costello MF, Shrestha B, Eden J, Johnson NP, Sjoblom P. Metformin versus oral contraceptive pill in polycystic ovary syndrome: a Cochrane review. Hum Reprod. 2007;22(5):1200–9. PubMed PMID: 17261574.
44. Ercan CM, Duru NK, Sakinci M, Alanbay I, Karasahin KE, Baser I. Successful twin pregnancy achieved by assisted reproductive technology in a patient with polycystic ovary syndrome with complex atypical endometrial hyperplasia treated with levonorgestrel-releasing intrauterine system. Gynecol Endocrinol. 2010;26(2):125–8. PubMed PMID: 20074021.
45. Fambrini M, Bargelli G, Peruzzi E, Buccoliero AM, Pieralli A, Andersson KL, et al. Levonorgestrel-releasing intrauterine system alone as primary treatment in young women with early endometrial cancer: case report. J Minim Invasive Gynecol. 2009;16(5):630–3. PubMed PMID: 19835809.
46. De Leo V, Di Sabatino A, Musacchio MC, Morgante G, Scolaro V, Cianci A, et al. Effect of oral contraceptives on markers of hyperandrogenism and SHBG in women with polycystic ovary syndrome. Contraception. 2010;82(3):276–80. PubMed PMID: 20705157.
47. Kriplani A, Periyasamy AJ, Agarwal N, Kulshrestha V, Kumar A, Ammini AC. Effect of oral contraceptive containing ethinyl estradiol combined with drospirenone vs. desogestrel on clinical and biochemical parameters in patients with polycystic ovary syndrome. Contraception. 2010;82(2):139–46. PubMed PMID: 20654754.
48. Battaglia C, Mancini F, Fabbri R, Persico N, Busacchi P, Facchinetti F, et al. Polycystic ovary syndrome and cardiovascular risk in young patients treated with drospirenone-ethinylestradiol or contraceptive vaginal ring. A prospective, randomized, pilot study. Fertil Steril. 2010;94(4):1417–25. PubMed PMID: 19591981.
49. Ozdemir S, Gorkemli H, Gezginc K, Ozdemir M, Kiyici A. Clinical and metabolic effects of medroxyprogesterone acetate and ethinyl estradiol plus drospirenone in women with polycystic ovary syndrome. Int J Gynaecol Obstet. 2008;103(1):44–9. PubMed PMID: 18635183.
50. Moghetti P, Toscano V. Treatment of hirsutism and acne in hyperandrogenism. Best Pract Res Clin Endocrinol Metab. 2006;20(2):221–34. PubMed PMID: 16772153.
51. Moghetti P, Tosi F, Tosti A, Negri C, Misciali C, Perrone F, et al. Comparison of spironolactone, flutamide, and finasteride efficacy in the treatment of hirsutism: a randomized, double blind, placebo-controlled trial. J Clin Endocrinol Metab. 2000;85(1): 89–94. PubMed PMID: 10634370.
52. Elkind-Hirsch KE, Darensbourg C, Ogden B, Ogden LF, Hindelang P. Contraceptive vaginal ring use for women has less adverse metabolic effects than an oral contraceptive. Contraception. 2007;76(5):348–56. PubMed PMID: 17963858.
53. Meyer C, Talbot M, Teede H. Effect of Implanon on insulin resistance in women with polycystic ovary syndrome. Austr N Z J Obstet Gynaecol. 2005;45(2): 155–8. PubMed PMID: 15760320.

16 Bone Health and Hormonal Contraception

Monica Dragoman, Andrew M. Kaunitz, and Michael R. McClung

Introduction

Hormonal contraceptives confer significant benefits to users. Not only do they offer effective and reversible protection against pregnancy, but women also derive a number of additional noncontraceptive health benefits from their use [1]. Hormonal contraception imparts some risks to users as well. Reports of reduced bone mineral density (BMD) with hormonal contraceptives have raised concerns about the risk for bone fracture both during use and following discontinuation. It is critical that health professionals understand the implications of BMD measures and fracture risk assessments in young women who receive hormonal contraception to insure that any screening and treatment decisions are grounded in evidence and reflect sound clinical judgment [2]. It is also important to balance the real risk for unintended pregnancy that accompanies use of less effective methods of contraception with the known and theoretical risk of fractures attributed to hormonal contraception use.

Nonhormonal contraceptive methods including permanent male and female sterilization, the copper intrauterine device (Cu-IUD), and barrier methods will not be addressed in this chapter, as there is no biologically plausible reason that they should impact bone health.

M. Dragoman, M.D., M.P.H. (✉)
Department of Obstetrics and Gynecology, Albert Einstein College of Medicine and Montefiore Medical Center, Bronx, NY, USA
e-mail: mdragoma@montefiore.org

A.M. Kaunitz, M.D., F.A.C.O.G.
Department of Obstetrics and Gynecology, University of Florida College of Medicine-Jacksonville, Jacksonville, FL, USA
e-mail: andrew.kaunitz@jax.ufl.edu

M.R. McClung, M.D.
Oregon Osteoporosis Center, Portland, OR, USA
e-mail: mmcclung@orost.com

Understanding Skeletal Growth and Development Across the Life Cycle

Bone is a dynamic tissue, continuously changing throughout life. These changes are key for skeletal growth and development and for regulating the body's mineral (e.g., calcium and phosphorus) stores. At any moment, the amount of bone tissue present represents the balance between the amount of bone formed during years of growth and the amount lost since that time. Sex steroids are among the most important of the many factors that contribute to both bone growth and bone loss in women [3]. Generally, bone's strength and density increase early in life until reaching a plateau, or peak bone mass; once peak bone mass is attained, the relationship between bone formation and resorption favors resorption, resulting in loss of bone mass over time.

R.H. Allen and C.A. Cwiak (eds.), *Contraception for the Medically Challenging Patient*,
DOI 10.1007/978-1-4939-1233-9_16, © Springer Science+Business Media New York 2014

Childhood is characterized by progressive accumulation of bone mass, generally in proportion to overall growth. Girls achieve about 80 % of their adult height and 40 % of their projected peak bone mass by age 7 [4]. Coincident with puberty, maximal rate of growth or peak height velocity occurs usually between the ages of 10 and 12. Over the next few years, approximately 50 % of a woman's peak bone mass is accrued, and peak bone mass is attained by the end of adolescence [5–11].

In healthy premenopausal women, BMD is stable or decreases very slowly (0.5 % per year in the proximal femur) [12–14]. Menopause is associated with a significant increase in the bone remodeling rate [15, 16]. This increase in bone remodeling persists for several years and is responsible for an interval of rapid bone loss. Beginning the year prior to final menses and continuing for about 5 years, the annual rate of bone loss is 1–2 %; most women lose between 10 and 20 % of bone mass across the menopausal transition [12–14, 17]. This period of rapid bone loss is accompanied by measurable deterioration in bone microarchitecture and a decline in bone strength [18, 19]. These changes contribute to fracture risk in early menopause and in later life.

Sex steroid production, linked to the female reproductive cycle, plays a profound role in regulating skeletal growth, development, and maintenance [3]. While the longitudinal and radial bone growth that occurs prior to menarche is reliant on the influence of growth hormone, insulin-like growth factors, cytokines, and other factors, sex steroid secretion at the time of puberty prompts accelerations in bone mineral acquisition and further growth that continues for approximately the next 10 years. The precipitous decline in ovarian hormone secretion at menopause is responsible for the rapid loss of bone mass occurring at this time. Though the dramatic rate of decline in bone mass accompanying the first years of menopause subsides, sex steroid deficiency underpins ongoing age-related bone loss.

Estrogen restrains osteoclastic activity. The complex mechanisms by which estrogen deficiency influences bone loss are increasingly understood; ultimately, decreased estrogen levels upregulate recruitment, activation, and decreased cell death of osteoclasts, which leads to bone resorption that outpaces new bone formation by osteoblasts [20]. Little is known about the independent effects of progesterone on bone; though in vitro studies suggest that endogenous progesterone may influence osteoblastic differentiation and activity [21]. Estrogen is the dominant sex steroid driving changes in bone health among women. Many studies demonstrate that hypoestrogenism results in decreased bone mass; this deficiency can be mediated by pathologic (e.g., primary hypothalamic amenorrhea), induced (e.g. use of progestin-only injectable contraception), or physiologic (e.g., menopause) suppression of ovarian estradiol production. Within these contexts, estrogen supplementation, both alone or in combination with progestins, can prevent or reverse declines in BMD among women with estrogen deficiency due to menopause or other causes [22–24].

Osteoporosis, Low Bone Mass, and Measures of Bone Mineral Density (BMD)

Osteoporosis is a disorder characterized by decreased bone mass and deterioration in bone microarchitecture resulting in poor bone quality; this can lead to fragility fractures at a variety of skeletal sites, most commonly the hip, spine, and wrists. Such fractures contribute to significant morbidity and mortality as well as high economic costs to society. In the United States (US), an estimated two million osteoporosis-related fractures occurred in 2005, associated with costs of 17 billion US dollars (USD), both expected to increase 50 % by 2025 as the population of elderly adults increases [25]. Due to the skeletal effects of estrogen deficiency, postmenopausal women are disproportionately affected by this disease; the Centers for Disease Control and Prevention (CDC) reports that 10 %, or 4.5 million, women over age 50 carry a diagnosis of osteoporosis compared to only 2 % of men of the same age [26].

Table 16.1 Ten-year probability of major osteoporotic fracture in postmenopausal women estimated by FRAX® using US Caucasian database (http://nof.org/hcp/clinicians-guide, Accessed March 14, 2014)[a]

Age	45	55	65	75	85
T-Score −1.5	2.9 %	6.3 %	8.4 %	11 %	13 %
T-Score −2.5	4.3 %	9.0 %	13 %	16 %	18 %

[a]*Note*: US National Osteoporosis Guidelines suggest pharmacological treatment for postmenopausal women with *T*-score values between −1 and −2.5 if 10-year probability of major osteoporotic fracture is 20 % or greater

Diagnostic criteria for osteoporosis in postmenopausal women, based on BMD measurements of the spine and hip by dual energy x-ray absorptiometry (DXA), have been provided by the World Health Organization (WHO) [27]. In postmenopausal women, BMD values at least 2.5 standard deviations (SD) below the average young adult female value (i.e., *T*-score ≤ −2.5) are consistent with osteoporosis. *T*-Score values between −1 and −2.5 are defined as low bone mass or osteopenia, while values ≥ −1 are described as normal BMD. In postmenopausal women, BMD is an important risk factor for fragility fracture, but the relationship between BMD and fracture risk is significantly modified by other risk factors, most importantly age and a history of previous fracture. The FRAX® calculator is the most validated and often used fracture risk assessment tool, combining clinical risk factors and BMD to estimate fracture risk in postmenopausal women [28–30]. Using FRAX®, the 10-year risk of a major osteoporotic fracture (hip, wrist, shoulder, or clinical spine fracture) can be calculated in postmenopausal women of different ages whose *T*-score value is −1.0 to −2.5 without other risk factors. Fracture risk is low in young postmenopausal women, even when BMD is consistent with osteoporosis (Table 16.1).

The WHO diagnostic criteria for osteoporosis and osteopenia are based on BMD and fracture risk in postmenopausal women. Because of this, these diagnostic criteria are not meant to be used in premenopausal women in whom normal BMD values, expressed as *T*-scores, are −2 to +2 [2, 31, 32]. In children and adolescents, comparisons with average age-matched values (*Z*-scores), rather than *T*-scores, are used to describe BMD values. Normal *Z*-score values are between −2 and +2. BMD *T*-scores of less than −2 in a premenopausal woman and *Z*-scores of less than −2 in an adolescent are described as low bone density, but the terms "osteoporosis" and "osteopenia" do not apply to such patients. FRAX® estimates of fracture risk are also not valid in premenopausal women or adolescents. Because fracture risk is so low in healthy premenopausal women, the relationship between BMD and fracture risk is relatively weak, and differences in BMD are associated with very small differences in absolute fracture risk. It would be very difficult to demonstrate that the small changes in BMD associated with hormonal contraceptive therapy significantly affect fracture risk.

Hormonal Contraception and Bone

Given the well-established relationship between hormonal status and bone health, understanding the impact that progestin-only and combined hormonal (estrogen and progestin) contraceptive methods may have on skeletal health is important. Particular concerns focus on the effects of exposure among adolescents who have not yet achieved peak bone mass and perimenopausal users at risk of impaired BMD recovery prior to the period of rapid bone loss accompanying menopause. Though changes in BMD have been observed during hormonal contraceptive use, the clinical relevance of these changes and their impact on risk for subsequent bone fracture remain controversial.

Unintended pregnancy is an important public health issue; nearly half of all pregnancies in the United States each year, or 3.4 million, are unintended [33]. Hormonal contraceptive methods are among the most popular and effective reversible modern methods of contraception available, with typical use failure rates ranging from less than 1 to 8 % [34, 35]. Evidence-based contraceptive decision making is key to ensuring that women's contraceptive choices are not unnecessarily limited, increasing the likelihood of less effective or no contraceptive use and subsequent unintended pregnancy. Further, any theoretical risks for bone fracture associated with hormonal contraceptive use must be balanced against real risks of pregnancy.

Progestin-Only Contraception

Progestin-only methods include oral (minipills), injectable, implantable, and intrauterine contraception. Since systemic exposure to the progestin agents in pills, implants, and intrauterine devices is relatively low, and serum estrogen levels remain within normal range during use [36–38], one might predict little effect on bone status. However, the progestin-only injectable, depot medroxyprogesterone acetate (DMPA), exposes women to higher doses of progestin and reduces ovarian estradiol production, resulting in lower systemic estradiol levels compared to normally cycling women [39–41]. Given the relative hypoestrogenism associated with DMPA use, changes in BMD might be anticipated.

Injectable Contraception (DMPA): BMD Changes in Adolescents

Prospective, longitudinal studies demonstrate decreases in BMD among adolescent DMPA users over time [42–51]. In this age group, changes in BMD reflect differences between losses observed among DMPA users and gains in BMD among nonusers. A prospective cohort study of 12- to 18-year olds using DMPA, combined oral contraceptives (COCs), or no contraception, compared BMD measurements at baseline and every 6 months through 2 years of follow-up [51]. At 12 months, DMPA users were noted to have decreases in BMD (mean percent changes in BMD: spine, −1.4 %; hip, −2.2 %), while non-contraceptive users gained (spine, +3.8 %; hip, +2.3 %); differences in the mean percent change of BMD across groups remained significant at 24 months. The calculations reflected adjustment for age, race/ethnicity, baseline BMD measurements, age at menarche, parity, previous hormonal contraceptive use, and lifestyle variables including smoking.

Age appears to be an important factor influencing changes in BMD. In a prospective study designed to evaluate BMD in a cohort of 16- to 33-year olds using DMPA, COC or non-hormonal contraception, DMPA users, aged 16–24 years, experienced more bone loss at the spine and hip than their older counterparts (lumbar spine: −4.2 vs. −3.2 %, $p<0.01$; femoral neck: −6.0 vs. −4.2 %, $p<0.01$) during 3 years of follow-up [48]. Studies have also suggested that the rate of BMD decline decreases with greater duration of DMPA use [42, 47, 48]. Cromer et al. reported that the rate of change in BMD at the spine was −1.4 % after year 1 and −0.1 % during year 2 among adolescent DMPA users [42].

While decreases in BMD are observed among adolescent DMPA users, existing evidence suggests that these declines are fully or substantially reversible 1–2 years after stopping DMPA injections (Fig. 16.1) [47, 48, 52]. A prospective, multicenter cohort study of 12- to 18-year-old adolescent DMPA users ($n=89$) reported BMD changes during up to over 4 years of DMPA use and up to nearly 6 years after discontinuation [52]. This study found that mean lumbar spine BMD recovered to baseline by 60 weeks following the last DMPA injection. At 240 weeks, 84 % of participants were noted to have lumbar spine measures that exceeded their pretreatment status, a mean 4.7 % increase in BMD over baseline. Full recovery of mean BMD was slower at the hip (240 weeks) and femoral neck (180 weeks). Age at initiation and duration of DMPA use do not appear to impair BMD gains after discontinuation [48]; however, greater losses of BMD during DMPA use (5 % or greater) may be associated with slower recovery [52].

Injectable Contraception (DMPA): BMD Changes in Premenopausal Adult Women

A number of studies demonstrate that premenopausal adult women experience declines in BMD with DMPA use. A systematic review published in 2006 identified 15 cross-sectional studies and 7 longitudinal studies evaluating BMD changes primarily in adult women (18 years and older) using DMPA [53]. While there was great variation in the magnitude and significance of reported changes in BMD among DMPA users across

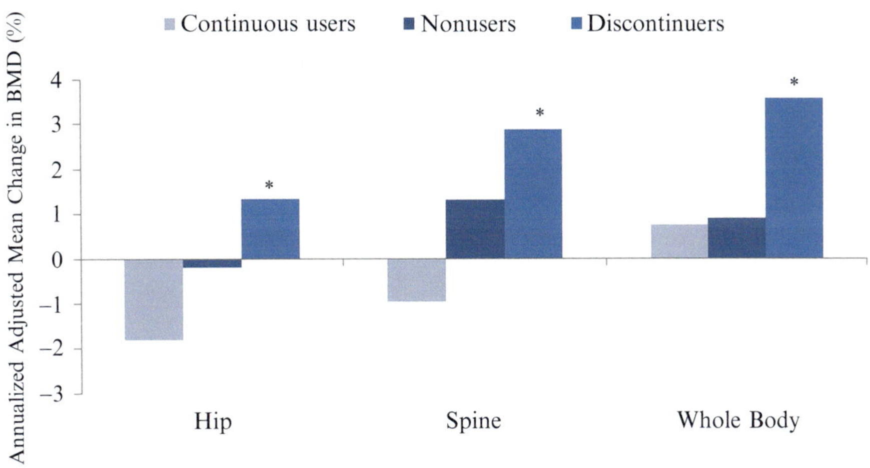

Fig. 16.1 Bone density changes in adolescent DMPA users (n=63), nonusers (n=84), and discontinuers (n=38) demonstrated that BMD among users was at least as high as nonusers at 12 months following DMPA discontinuation. *p<0.05 for discontinuers versus nonusers. Reprinted from Kaunitz AM. Update on hormonal contraception and bone density. Reviews in Endocrine and Metabolic Disorders 2011;12(2), with kind permission from Springer Science+Business Media

studies, any reported differences were almost uniformly attributed to decreases in BMD among DMPA users, while nonusers exhibited minimal changes from baseline BMD during surveillance [54–57]. Gai et al. reported similar findings in 2011. Eighty new DMPA initiators and 68 nonhormonal contraceptive users underwent scheduled assessments of BMD at the lumbar spine and femoral neck at baseline and every 12 months for 4 years. Declines in BMD were observed at the lumbar spine (mean percent change −5.52 %) and femoral neck (mean percent change −6.35 %) after 24 months of DMPA use, while nonusers exhibited no significant change from baseline [58]. Whether the rate of change in BMD varies by duration of use among adult women is unclear; some studies suggest that the degree of BMD loss decreases over time, while others report no difference [56, 57, 59].

A randomized, evaluator-blinded Phase 3 contraceptive trial investigated the percent change in BMD observed at the hip and lumbar spine among women between the ages of 18 and 35 years using different formulations of DMPA, 150 mg/1.0 mL intramuscularly (IM) (n=268) or 104 mg/0.65 mL subcutaneously (SC) (n=266) [41]. All women experienced some decrease in BMD during use of DMPA through up to 3 years of follow-up. In year 1, DMPA-SC users were noted to have less of a decrease in BMD compared to IM users for measures at the lumbar spine (−2.4 vs. −3.4 %, p=0.021), but statistically significant differences in declines in BMD between formulations were not noted at the hip. In years 2 and 3, the median percent changes in BMD among DMPA-SC and IM users were similar. The study suggests that the two formulations exert comparable effects on BMD over time.

BMD recovery is observed when adult premenopausal women stop using DMPA. A systematic review published in 2008 reported on results from one cross-sectional and four prospective cohort studies measuring changes in BMD upon DMPA discontinuation experienced by adult premenopausal women. Depending on measurement site and duration of follow-up, it concluded that any decreases in BMD are at least partially reversible with a return to levels at or near baseline [60]. A 7-year prospective age-matched cohort study recruited women between the ages of 25 and 35 who were new users of DMPA (n=248) or users of nonhormonal contraception (n=360) and measured BMD changes during up to 5 years of treatment and 2 years posttreatment [59]. During exposure to DMPA, declines in BMD at the hip (−5.16 %) and lumbar

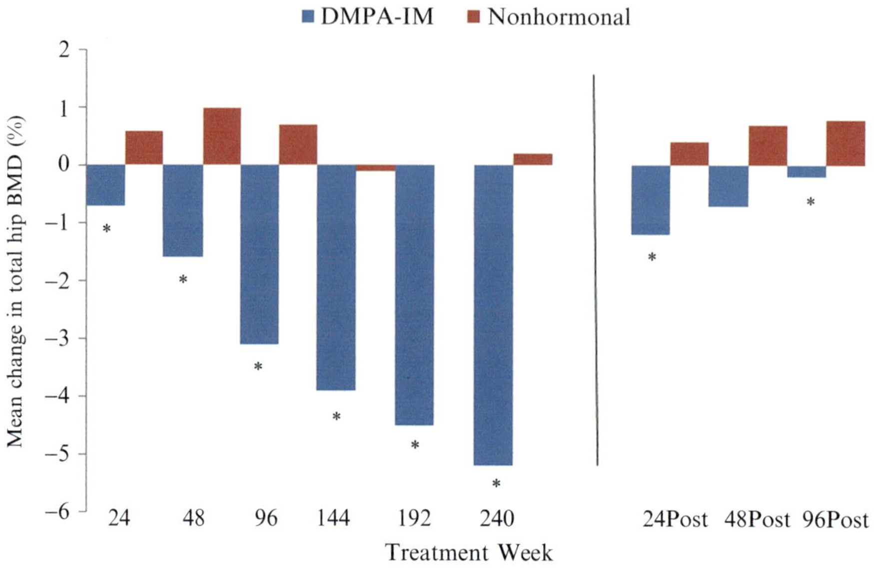

Fig. 16.2 Change in mean BMD at hip from baseline among DMPA and nonhormonal contraceptive users, ages 25–35 years, during treatment and after discontinuation. *$p<0.05$ between groups. Reprinted from Kaunitz AM, Miller PD, Rice VM, Ross D, McClung MR. Bone mineral density in women aged 25–35 years receiving depot medroxyprogesterone acetate: recovery following discontinuation. Contraception 2006;74(2):90–9, with permission from Elsevier

spine (−5.38 %) were consistent with other reports; at 96 weeks following DMPA discontinuation, the overall mean change in total hip BMD was noted to be −0.20 % ($n=25$) and −1.19 % ($n=41$) at the lumbar spine among past DMPA users compared to +0.84 % ($n=43$) and +0.47 % ($n=66$) among nonusers; these were statistically significant differences ($p<0.05$) (Fig. 16.2).

Injectable Contraception (DMPA): BMD Changes in Peri-/Postmenopausal Women

DMPA use during perimenopause, particularly up until the time of menopause, may theoretically increase risk of osteoporosis and fracture given the limited time for normalization of estradiol levels and BMD recovery upon discontinuation. A number of studies have reported on BMD measures among older women using DMPA. In a prospective cohort study of women ages 40–49 years, including 127 DMPA users (median duration of DMPA use 84 months) and 161 nonhormonal contraceptive users, no significant differences in BMD at the radius and ulna with and without adjustment for age were noted [61]. Similarly, a cross-sectional study evaluated BMD measures among 185 DMPA users in the United Kingdom. The authors noted that BMD among DMPA users aged 40–49 and 50–52 years in the study sample were similar to the population means for BMD among Caucasian women of the United Kingdom (UK), US, and Scandinavia [62]. A cross-sectional study of Chinese women (mean age 43 years) using DMPA for 5–15 years reported lower BMD among DMPA users compared to nonusers at the spine and hip [63]. A subgroup of 59 of these DMPA users was followed prospectively to determine changes in BMD during 3 years of observation. Although ongoing DMPA users did lose BMD over time, they actually lost less than what was projected for women not using hormonal contraception. Overall, no association between duration of DMPA use and changes in BMD were observed [64].

Sixteen women between the ages of 45 and 55 years, using DMPA for a minimum of 5 years and median duration of 12 years, discontinued at the time of menopause (5 with subsequent hormone therapy (HT) and 11 without). BMD changes in these long-term DMPA users were compared with changes in 15 never users (and no HT) who reached natural menopause during 3 years of follow-up [65]. Though BMD declined rapidly (6 % at hip and spine) in early menopause among never users, there was little change in BMD in DMPA users without HT. Former users of DMPA experienced increases in BMD at the spine and stable BMD at the hip on HT. It is possible that DMPA users avoid additional losses in BMD at menopause because their exposure preemptively induces a hypoestrogenic state with self-limited bone loss similar to the effects of natural menopause. Thus, DMPA users have already undergone bone loss due to hypoestrogenism, resulting in less bone loss during physiologic transition. Similar findings related to BMD changes in menopause among past perimenopausal users have been reported [66, 67].

Other Progestin-Only Contraception: BMD Changes

Though few studies have assessed BMD in women using progestin-only pills (POPs), implants, and IUDs, existing evidence suggests no differences among users compared to nonusers.

A prospective cohort study showed that breastfeeding women using POPs exhibited less BMD loss than breastfeeding women using barrier methods during the first 6 months postpartum. With weaning at 1 year, POP users gained 3 % BMD over baseline, while BMD in barrier method users was equivalent to baseline measurements. In comparison, women relying on formula feeding and barrier contraception had just over a 4 % increase in BMD from baseline [68].

One comparative study evaluated changes in BMD among women using either the etonogestrel implant or the Cu-IUD [69]. During 2 years of follow-up, there were no differences in BMD measures at the lumbar spine, femur, or distal radius. An uncontrolled study of levonorgestrel (LNG) and etonogestrel (ENG)—containing implant users in Brazil—demonstrated lower BMD at the midshaft of the ulna (LNG: −3.36 %, $p<0.01$; ENG: −3.75 %, $p<0.01$) but no difference at the distal radius after 18 months of implant use [70]. A cross-sectional study compared BMD in 50 Thai women using the implant for a minimum of 2 years (mean duration of use: 32.84±6.31 months) and 50 women not using hormonal contraception, with similar age, parity, and BMI at baseline [71]. Investigators observed no differences at the spine or femur, but reported BMD at the distal radius was lower in implant users (mean $BMD_{implant}$: 0.56±0.04 SD; mean $BMD_{control}$: 0.57±0.04 SD, $p=0.02$). Though this finding was statistically significant, this minimal difference may not be clinically meaningful.

Although prior reports assessing BMD in levonorgestrel intrauterine device (LNG IUD) users found no impact on BMD, a recent study found that use of the LNG IUD was associated with higher BMD [72–74]. Following conservative surgical treatment for endometriosis, women were randomized to DMPA or LNG IUD use with BMD measurements annually for 3 years. Compared with baseline levels, BMD increased at the hip (+2.56 %) and spine (+7.02 %) in the LNG IUD group [74].

Fracture Risk Associated with Progestin-Only Contraception

Most studies evaluating fractures among women exposed to progestin-only contraception report on risks among current and past users of DMPA. These reports have observed that DMPA use is associated with either no difference or a slightly increased risk for fracture [59, 75–78]. LNG IUD use may exert a protective effect, though small in magnitude [78].

Three recent studies relied on large national datasets to examine the association between fracture and DMPA or LNG IUD use [76–78]. Two of these were based on the same large UK database [76, 77]. The first of these, using case–control methodology, observed a higher risk of fracture associated with ever use of DMPA compared with never use (adjusted OR 1.44, 95 % CI 1.01–2.06) [76]. Using the same database, a second report employed a retrospective cohort analysis, and also observed that DMPA users had an increased risk for fracture (OR 1.41, 95 % CI 1.35–1.47) [77]. However, the investigators in this latter report noted that the elevated risk was present at baseline, *prior* to DMPA use, and therefore could not have been caused by DMPA [77]. A case–control analysis from Denmark also found that ever use of DMPA was associated with increased risk for fracture (adjusted OR 1.44, 95 % CI 1.01–2.06), but suggested that the subgroup of women choosing DMPA, 0.1 % of the study sample, were not representative of the larger Danish population, limiting interpretation of results [78]. Both the UK and the Danish studies raise the issue that women who choose DMPA are behaviorally different from women who choose other methods of contraception and hypothesize that fracture risk associated with DMPA exposure may in fact be due to unmeasured confounders in this group. For example, in the Danish study, the prevalence of alcoholism (a condition associated with fractures from motor vehicle and other accidents) in women using DMPA was 14 %, sevenfold higher than in women not using DMPA, and cases with fractures were some threefold more likely to be classified as alcoholics as control women [78].

The Danish study investigated risk for fracture among women of any age and included postmenopausal women, an age group at greatest risk for fracture, as well [78]. Of the three groups analyzed (under 25 years, 25–50 years, and over 50 years), only women aged over 50 years had an increased risk (OR 2.25, 95 % CI 1.14–4.42). However, data on contraceptive use was restricted to within 5 years prior to any event and no information on type of fracture was provided [78]. When other studies restricted analysis to axial and osteoporotic fractures, there was no association between fracture and DMPA among premenopausal users [76, 77]. The Danish study also reported a reduced risk for fracture among ever users of the LNG IUD (OR 0.75, 95 % CI 0.64–0.87) [78].

Progestin-Only Contraception: Recommendations

The CDC U.S. Medical Eligibility Criteria for Contraceptive Use (USMEC) [79] gives POPs and implants a Category 1 rating for women of all ages. DMPA has a Category 1 rating for women between the ages of 18 and 45, and a Category 2 rating for adolescents (menarche up to age 18) and perimenopausal women (over 45 years). The LNG IUD has a Category 2 rating for younger women (menarche up to 20 years) and a Category 1 rating for women 20 years and older; safety concerns are unrelated to issues of bone health (Table 16.2).

Combined Hormonal Contraception (CHC)

Combined hormonal methods include the combined oral contraceptive (COC), the transdermal patch, and vaginal ring. While formulations, regimens, and delivery systems for CHC continue to evolve, most currently available methods contain between 20 and 35 μg of ethinyl estradiol (EE), a potent synthetic estrogen, plus one of various progestin agents. Correct, consistent use of CHC results in effective inhibition of ovulation [80–82].

Table 16.2 Recommendations for the use of contraception by age [79]

Guidelines for age	LNG-IUD	Implants	DMPA	POP	CHC
(a) Menarche to <20 years	2				
(b) ≥20 years	1				
(a) Menarche to <18 years		1	2	1	
(b) 18–45 years		1	1	1	
(c) >45 years		1	2	1	
(a) Menarche to <40 years					1
(b) ≥40 years					2

1 A condition for which there is no restriction for use. *2* A condition for which the advantages of using a method generally outweigh the theoretical or proven risks. *3* A condition for which the theoretical or proven risks usually outweigh the advantages of using a method. *4* A condition that represents an unacceptable health risk if the contraceptive method is used

With ovarian suppression, endogenous production of estradiol decreases. However, systemic exposure to exogenous estrogens in CHC may counter endogenous estrogen deficiencies impacting bone health; a number of studies have demonstrated that women with hypoestrogenic conditions treated with CHC demonstrate increases in BMD [22, 83, 84].

Combined Oral Contraception: BMD Changes in Adolescents

Adolescents and young adults using COCs experience gains in BMD. While some studies document no differences, most report that these gains are typically less than those observed in nonusers, resulting in lower BMD in users [42, 48, 85–89]. It is possible that low-dose and very low-dose COC formulations are inadequate to support optimal bone acquisition during adolescence; however, the clinical implications of these observations are uncertain [85].

A large cohort study by Scholes et al. of adolescents between the ages of 14 and 18 analyzed changes in BMD during 24–36 months among users of COCs containing 30–35 μg EE or less than 30 μg EE and compared them to nonusers [87]. All groups gained BMD during follow-up, but adolescents using COC formulations with 30–35 μg EE were noted to have smaller mean percentage BMD gains than nonusers at the spine and whole body (+1.32 vs. +2.26 % and +1.45 vs. +2.03 %, respectively) that were statistically significant. Among new COC initiators, users of both COC formulations gained less BMD than nonusers at 30 months. Polatti et al. reported no changes in BMD among 19- to 22-year olds initiating COCs containing 20 μg EE, but nonusers experienced a 7.8 % increase in BMD in comparison during 5 years of surveillance [90]. Another cohort study evaluated BMD changes among postmenarchal adolescents between the ages 12 and 18 using either a COC with 20 μg EE or no method of contraception. While both groups gained BMD during 24 months of use, COC users experienced lower mean percent gains at the spine and femoral neck (+4.2 vs. +6.3 % and +3.0 vs. +3.8 %). The study was limited by high rates of attrition that varied across groups [42].

Twelve months after stopping use, past COC users gained less BMD than nonusers in the cohort study published by Scholes et al. [87]. A statistically significant difference in BMD gain 12 months after use was only observed at the spine when comparing nonusers and users of COC with 30–35 μg EE (1.72 vs. 0.51 %). In contrast with DMPA use, adolescents using COC do gain rather than lose BMD during use. More studies are needed to understand the effects of COC on BMD changes following discontinuation. Currently, it is unclear if failure to reach peak bone mass as a consequence of COC use during adolescence translates to an increased risk for fracture later in life [85, 91].

Combined Oral Contraception: BMD Changes in Premenopausal Adult Women

A systematic review and meta-analysis published in 2006 reported no differences in BMD among adult premenopausal COC users and nonusers [85]. Among the 11 studies included in the review, the authors identified two "good quality" studies supporting this conclusion. In one study, women underwent BMD assessments during COC or nonhormonal contraceptive use; 80 % of COC formulations contained 30–35 μg EE. No differences were noted in spine, femur, or whole body BMD at 36 months across groups. The investigators also examined whether COC use of varying duration (less than 2 years, 2–4 years, or greater than 4 years) impacted BMD and found no difference [92]. In the other study, women randomized to start COCs with either 20 or 15 μg EE had lumbar spine BMD similar to healthy controls at baseline and at 12 months; in addition, no group experienced a significant change in BMD over baseline during the study period [93]. Reports of more recent investigations record similar results [94, 95].

Combined Oral Contraception: BMD Changes in Peri-/Postmenopausal Women

Most comparative studies of COC use among perimenopausal and postmenopausal women demonstrate protective effects on bone; older reproductive age (greater than or equal to 40 years) women using COCs tend to gain or preserve BMD while nonusers experience typical age-related bone losses [96–104].

A series of prospective cohort studies evaluated BMD changes at various skeletal sites, including the spine, hip, heel, and radius, among oligomenorrheic perimenopausal women randomized to COC (20–30 μg EE) and calcium, or calcium supplementation alone for up to 2 years [97, 98, 100, 101]. Two of these studies also included nonrandomized normally menstruating women of the same age for comparison [97, 101]. Across studies, significant increases in BMD were noted in the oligomenorrheic COC users, while decreases were observed in the oligomenorrheic calcium users; BMD was stable in normally menstruating women using neither calcium nor COC.

Another study of similar design included oligomenorrheic perimenopausal women between the ages of 40 and 49 years who were randomized to receive 1 of 3 COC formulations containing 20 μg of EE and either levonorgestrel (LNG), desogestrel (DSG), or gestodene (GTD) [104]. Again, investigators included normally menstruating women of similar age as a nonrandomized comparison group. Twenty women in each of the five groups underwent BMD assessments at the lumbar spine at baseline and at 2 years. Oligomenorrheic women using any of the COC formulations were noted to have significantly increased BMD (COC_{DSG}: +2.3 %, COC_{LNG}: +1.6 %, COC_{GTD}: +1.0 %). BMD declined in oligomenorrheic women taking calcium alone (−2.3 %); eumenorrheic women maintained their BMD during surveillance.

Several studies have evaluated the influence of past use of COC on BMD changes among postmenopausal women. A cohort of Danish women recruited within 6 months to 3 years of menopause underwent baseline determination of bone mineral content (BMC) in the forearm followed by quarterly assessments over 2 years and a final measurement 12 years later; results were compared across women reporting ever use of COC (minimum 3 months) and never users [105]. At the completion of the study, the reported mean age of participants was 63 years. While ever users had higher BMC at baseline, no differences were noted after 12 years; previous lactation and parity did not affect results. The investigators also noted that past COC use tended to be associated with greater BMC loss compared with nonusers, but this difference was not statistically significant. A number of cross-sectional studies evaluating the effects of past COC use with exposures of varying duration found either increases or no difference in BMD compared to nonusers in women during and after menopause [106–110].

Other Combined Hormonal Contraception: BMD Changes

Very few studies have evaluated BMD changes associated with non-oral CHC, but existing evidence suggests that effects are similar to COC [111–113]. A pilot study was designed to compare differences in BMD among five adolescent transdermal patch initiators, age- and ethnicity-matched to adolescents not using hormonal contraception. Gains in BMD were greater among nonusers at 6 and 12 months with significant differences at the spine at 6 months and hip at 12 months after adjustment for multiple comparisons. Interpretation is limited by the small sample size [111].

BMD does not vary much during use of the transdermal patch and contraceptive vaginal ring by adult premenopausal women. Forty women between the ages of 23 and 34 years were randomized to start use of either the ring or patch and followed forward for 1 year; 20 healthy nonusers were also recruited as controls in this partially randomized controlled trial. No differences in BMD were noted from baseline or across groups [112]. Also, no differences in BMD measurements from baseline through 2 years of follow-up were observed in new contraceptive vaginal ring users participating in a prospective cohort study performed in Chile and the Netherlands [113]. Nonusers in the cohort had gains in BMD, but differences between groups were within 1 SD.

Fracture Risk Associated with Combined Hormonal Contraception

Studies of fracture risk associated with COC use have yielded inconsistent results. Most studies report no differences in risk among past COC users compared to never users, but some studies suggest mild protective or detrimental effects. No studies examine non-oral CHC and fracture incidence.

One of the best-designed studies tackling this issue to date reports no association between past COC use and risk for lifetime incident fractures [114]. The investigators performed a nested case–control study focused on Scottish participants in the Royal College of General Practitioners Oral Contraception Study. Over 600 cases with incident fractures reported between the ages of 20 and 87 years were each age-matched to two controls without fracture or history of fracture. The investigators excluded potential cases with skull or rib fractures and women with multiple fractures because of their possible association with trauma; they also excluded women with cancer or previous fracture. Ever users of COC did not have an increased risk for fracture compared to nonusers (adjusted OR: 1.05, 95 % CI, 0.86–1.29) in multivariable analyses adjusting for smoking, social class, parity, and use of HT. Likewise, duration of COC use did not influence fracture risk (adjusted OR: 1.23, 95 % CI, 0.22–7.02), and women in the sample reported using COC for a maximum of up to approximately 15 years. Fracture risk increased slightly as time since last COC use increased (less than 5 years: OR 1.06, 95 % CI 0.65–1.72; 5–9 years: OR 1.01, 95 % CI 0.62–1.65; 10 or more years: OR 1.55, 95 % CI 1.03–2.33), suggesting a proximal protective effect. There were no significant differences in fracture risk among ever and never users across age or fracture sites. Other large, population-based studies have similarly found no overall association between COC use and any fracture as well as with duration of COC exposure and fracture risk [76, 115–117]. When considering the association specifically between hip fractures and past COC use, studies report either no difference or decreased risks [118–120]. A case–control study from Sweden noted that postmenopausal hip fracture risk decreased as age at first COC use increased in comparison to never users (age over 39 years at first use: OR 0.69, 95 % CI 0.51–0.94) [118]. This finding correlates well with observed protective gains in BMD among perimenopausal COC users [96–104].

In contrast, several other cohort studies have reported slightly increased risks for fractures among ever versus never users of any COC [121–123]. When adjusted for age, social class, parity, and smoking status, ever users in a UK study had a greater likelihood of any fracture compared to nonusers (adjusted RR 1.3, 95 % CI 1.08–1.34). In this same study, women 50 years and older who used COC after age 35 had fracture rates similar to those of the same age who were never users [121]. Another study noted an increased relative risk for fracture with increasing duration of use (up to 97 months) when controlling for age (adjusted RR 1.2, 95 % CI 1.1–1.4) [122]. A large US cohort study noted no difference in fracture risk among ever versus never users of COC; further, women who used COCs for 5 years or less demonstrated slightly greater risk for fracture compared to women who used COCs for a longer duration and never users [123]. The analysis relied on self-report to ascertain COC use and fracture; there was potential for recall bias. More than half of reported spine fractures were poorly correlated with documentation in medical records. Moreover, fracture risk was not analyzed by age during COC use.

Combined Hormonal Contraception: Recommendations

The USMEC (79) gives COCs, patch, and ring a Category 1 rating for most reproductive age women (menarche up to 40 years), and a Category 2 rating for perimenopausal women (40 years and older) (see Table 16.2). Safety concerns among older adult women primarily reflect increasing risk for cardiovascular disease with increasing age rather than issues of bone health.

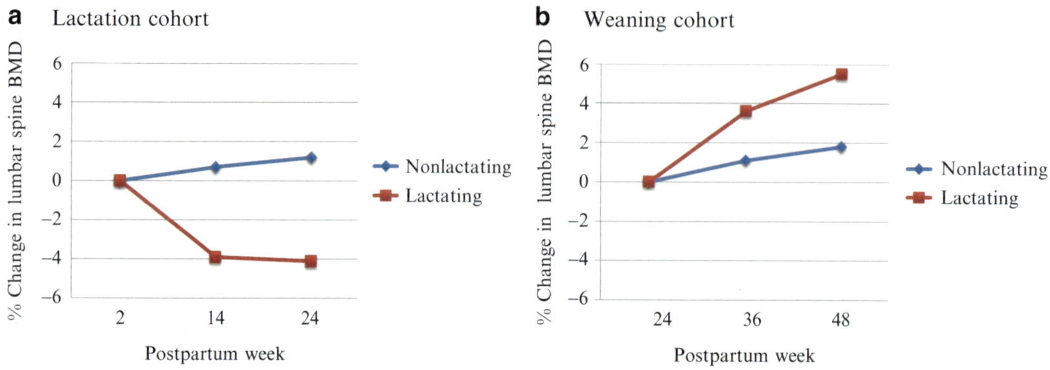

Fig. 16.3 (**a**) Mean percent change in BMD at lumbar spine among lactating women compared to nonlactating women through 24 weeks postpartum. (**b**) BMD recovery with weaning at 24 weeks postpartum among lactating women compared to BMD of nonlactating women through 48 weeks postpartum. Reprinted with permission from Kalkwarf HJ, Specker BL. Bone mineral loss during lactation and recovery after weaning. Obstet Gynecol 1995;86(1):26–32

Lactation and BMD

Postpartum breastfeeding offers a number of well-documented neonatal and maternal benefits in addition to providing a source of primary nutrition; a few examples include enhanced bonding, reductions in infant gastrointestinal and respiratory disorders, and reductions in maternal lifetime risk for breast and ovarian cancers [124]. Acknowledging the public health advantages related to lactation, a number of strategies to support a woman's choice to initiate and continue exclusive breastfeeding for optimal durations (a minimum of 6 months) have been endorsed [125–127].

Elevated circulating levels of prolactin necessary for lactation suppress ovulation by inhibiting pulsatile secretion of GnRH from the hypothalamus, resulting in reduced endogenous estradiol production [128, 129]. After weaning, serum prolactin levels decline and estradiol increases, followed by return of normal ovarian activity and first ovulation within 2 weeks to 1 month [130]. To safely and effectively rely on lactational amenorrhea for contraception, the following criteria must be met: (1) amenorrhea; (2) fully or nearly fully breastfeeding; (3) less than 6 months postpartum [131].

The transient hypoestrogenic state associated with lactation is associated with declines in BMD of 4–6 % after 6 months compared with nonlactating postpartum women, a change similar to what is observed among DMPA users [132, 133] (Fig. 16.3a, b). BMD recovers at least partially or completely with return of normal ovarian function [134–137]. Past breastfeeding is typically not associated with risk for osteoporosis later in life, and may in fact be associated with protection [138–140]. In a cross-sectional study evaluating BMD in a convenience sample of postmenopausal women 49 years and older presenting for DXA, women with a history of breastfeeding had higher BMD and lower prevalence of osteoporosis than women who had never breastfed [139].

Other Medical Conditions That May Affect Bone Health

Secondary osteoporosis describes a condition where a drug, underlying disease, or deficiency causes significant impairment to bone health [141]. In particular, chronic glucocorticoid therapy and conditions associated with prolonged immobilization and wheelchair confinement have been linked to increased risks of osteoporosis and fragility fracture [142, 143].

Bone health is among the safety considerations to be discussed as part of the contraceptive decision-making process for women with coexistent medical conditions that impair bone growth and development. An example of a patient in which contraceptive decision making is complicated is the woman with disabilities (e.g., spinal cord injury or cerebral palsy) associated with prolonged immobilization. Such women are at elevated risk for VTE as well as osteoporosis. For women with these disabilities, pregnancy and childbirth also pose extra risks. In addition, menstrual hygiene represents an important concern. Women should be offered the full range of medically appropriate effective contraceptive options to support their fertility desires, and the risks and benefits of each method should be weighed against the maternal and fetal risks associated with unintended pregnancy.

Long-term use of systemic glucocorticoid therapy represents a common and potent risk factor for fractures, with a 30–50 % chance of fragility fracture during long-term systemic use [144]. Increased fracture risk has been associated with chronic use of prednisone doses as small as 2.5–3 mg/day; continuous treatment with 10 mg of prednisone daily for 90 days or longer has been associated with a sevenfold increased risk in hip fractures compared with unexposed individuals [145]. Among various indications, these medications are mainstays in treatment for persistent asthma and allergy symptoms, other autoimmune disease, and organ transplantation [142]. Glucocorticoid exposure is also associated with risk of insulin resistance and diabetes as well as an increased risk for VTE [146, 147]. While bone health represents an important consideration for reproductive age women on chronic corticosteroids, the underlying condition necessitating glucocorticoid treatment along with other medication side effects should also be considered as part of the contraceptive decision-making process. Use of corticosteroids does not in itself contraindicate the use of any hormonal contraceptive method. Given that unintended pregnancy may exacerbate any or all of these concerns as well as their risks to fetal growth and development, women should be offered the most effective form of contraception available after careful consideration of the relative risks and benefits of each method.

Interventions to Promote Bone Health Among Hormonal Contraceptive Users

All reproductive age women, including those using hormonal contraception, should be advised on measures to support bone health. Ensuring adequate nutrition, sufficient calcium and vitamin D intake, and regular weight-bearing exercise is important for adolescents and women of all ages to reduce lifetime risk for osteoporosis [148, 149]. The recommended daily requirements for calcium and vitamin D vary by age and are informed by metabolic needs associated with normal bone growth and development across the life cycle [150]. Avoidance of smoking and excessive alcohol use also promotes bone health. Of note, regular long-term coffee exposure does not appear to increase risk for fracture later in life [151, 152]. Women with various medical conditions at risk for impaired skeletal health may require additional calcium and vitamin D supplementation, surveillance, and lifestyle modifications to prevent osteoporosis and fractures [153].

While healthy lifestyle choices may not necessarily curtail observed changes in BMD described among DMPA and other hormonal contraceptive users, there is value in promoting them as part of general health maintenance. Most American adults report inadequate calcium and vitamin D intake, with female adolescents reporting the lowest levels of all [154]. Less than half of adults and one-third of adolescents in the United States meet minimum criteria for adequate physical activity [155, 156].

Limited evidence demonstrates that low-dose estrogen or calcium supplementation provided to adolescent and adult DMPA users may limit bone loss during use [23, 46, 157]. The skeletal health impact of long-term estrogen supplementation in DMPA users has not been evaluated. The Society for Adolescent Medicine (SAM) recommends 1,300 mg calcium, 400 IU vitamin D supplementation, and exercise daily to all adolescents receiving DMPA [158]. The American Congress of Obstetricians and Gynecologists (ACOG) states that DMPA can be provided to women without requiring additional interventions, aside from routine preventive care [159].

A warning from the U.S. Food and Drug Administration (FDA) added to DMPA's labeling in 2004 suggests that BMD assessment may be appropriate for women considering long-term use of injectable contraception (see DMPA package label). In contrast with this guidance, data demonstrate that adolescent and adult DMPA users do not benefit from BMD assessments, with DXA or any other modality, before, during, or after use, regardless of duration [160]. No existing recommendations specify requirements for routine BMD screening of adolescent or premenopausal adult women based on DMPA exposure alone [32, 161–163]; furthermore, ACOG, the World Health Organization (WHO), and the Society of Obstetrics and Gynecology of Canada (SOGC) explicitly do not support routine BMD testing in DMPA users [159, 164].

Conclusion

Of all hormonal contraceptive methods, DMPA exerts the most pronounced effects on BMD, historically prompting the FDA to issue a black box warning in 2004 cautioning providers about long-term use of the method (more than 2 years) and recommending BMD evaluation with long-term use. In contrast to the alarm generated by the FDA warning, current evidence suggests that any observed decreases in BMD among DMPA users are typically within 1 SD of nonusers, transient, partially, or completely reversible, and associated with no elevation in subsequent risk of fracture. Various international and national professional organizations engaged in norm setting for reproductive health have questioned the FDA position and issued statements endorsing DMPA as an important contraceptive option for adolescents and women. Universally, these organizations (WHO, CDC, ACOG, SAM, SOGC) recognize that the benefits of DMPA use generally outweigh the mostly theoretical concerns about skeletal health, and that DMPA initiation and continuation should not be restricted [79, 158, 159, 164–166].

Other progestin-only and combined hormonal contraception appear to exert minimal impacts on skeletal health. Declines in BMD with lactation partially or completely recover after weaning, and lactation may be protective against future osteoporosis and fracture. Women with medical conditions or taking medications that alter bone health merit an individualized approach to contraceptive decision making in which benefits and risks of different methods are thoughtfully weighed. Regardless of contraceptive use, all women benefit from good nutrition, sufficient calcium and vitamin D intake, and regular physical exercise to insure healthy bones during their lifetime.

References

1. ACOG. ACOG practice bulletin no. 110: noncontraceptive uses of hormonal contraceptives. Obstet Gynecol. 2010;115(1):206–18.
2. Silverman SL, Calderon AD. The utility and limitations of FRAX: a US perspective. Curr Osteoporos Rep. 2010;8(4):192–7.
3. Clarke BL, Khosla S. Female reproductive system and bone. Arch Biochem Biophys. 2010;503(1):118–28.
4. Bass S, Delmas PD, Pearce G, Hendrich E, Tabensky A, Seeman E. The differing tempo of growth in bone size, mass, and density in girls is region-specific. J Clin Invest. 1999;104(6):795–804.
5. Baxter-Jones AD, Faulkner RA, Forwood MR, Mirwald RL, Bailey DA. Bone mineral accrual from 8 to 30 years of age: an estimation of peak bone mass. J Bone Miner Res. 2011;26(8):1729–39.
6. Recker RR, Davies KM, Hinders SM, Heaney RP, Stegman MR, Kimmel DB. Bone gain in young adult women. JAMA. 1992;268(17):2403–8.
7. Boot AM, de Ridder MA, van der Sluis IM, van Slobbe I, Krenning EP, Keizer-Schrama SM. Peak bone mineral density, lean body mass and fractures. Bone. 2010;46(2):336–41.
8. Cvijetic S, Colic Baric I, Keser I, Cecic I, Satalic Z, Blanusa M. Peak bone density in Croatian women: variations at different skeletal sites. J Clin Densitom. 2008;11(2):260–5.
9. Lorentzon M, Mellstrom D, Ohlsson C. Age of attainment of peak bone mass is site specific in Swedish men – the GOOD study. J Bone Miner Res. 2005;20(7):1223–7.
10. Matkovic V, Jelic T, Wardlaw GM, Ilich JZ, Goel PK, Wright JK, et al. Timing of peak bone mass in Caucasian females and its implication for the prevention of osteoporosis. Inference from a cross-sectional model. J Clin Invest. 1994;93(2):799–808.

11. Looker AC, Bolud LG, Hughes JP, Fan B, Shepherd JA, Sherman M. Total body bone area, bone mineral content and bone mineral density for individuals aged 8 and over: United States 1999–2006. Hyattsville, MD: National Center for Health Statistics; 2013.
12. Bainbridge KE, Sowers MF, Crutchfield M, Lin X, Jannausch M, Harlow SD. Natural history of bone loss over 6 years among premenopausal and early postmenopausal women. Am J Epidemiol. 2002; 156(5):410–7.
13. Recker R, Lappe J, Davies K, Heaney R. Characterization of perimenopausal bone loss: a prospective study. J Bone Miner Res. 2000;15(10): 1965–73.
14. Finkelstein JS, Brockwell SE, Mehta V, Greendale GA, Sowers MR, Ettinger B, et al. Bone mineral density changes during the menopause transition in a multiethnic cohort of women. J Clin Endocrinol Metab. 2008;93(3):861–8.
15. Recker R, Lappe J, Davies KM, Heaney R. Bone remodeling increases substantially in the years after menopause and remains increased in older osteoporosis patients. J Bone Miner Res. 2004;19(10): 1628–33.
16. Cauley JA, Danielson ME, Greendale GA, Finkelstein JS, Chang Y-F, Lo JC, et al. Bone resorption and fracture across the menopausal transition: the Study of Women's Health Across the Nation. Menopause (NY). 2012;19(11):1200–7.
17. Sirola J, Kroger H, Honkanen R, Jurvelin JS, Sandini L, Tuppurainen MT, et al. Factors affecting bone loss around menopause in women without HRT: a prospective study. Maturitas. 2003;45(3):159–67.
18. Akhter M, Lappe J, Davies K, Recker R. Transmenopausal changes in the trabecular bone structure. Bone. 2007;41(1):111–6.
19. Dufresne T, Chmielewski P, Manhart M, Johnson T, Borah B. Risedronate preserves bone architecture in early postmenopausal women in 1 year as measured by three-dimensional microcomputed tomography. Calcified Tissue Int. 2003;73(5):423–32.
20. Manolagas SC. Birth and death of bone cells: basic regulatory mechanisms and implications for the pathogenesis and treatment of osteoporosis. Endocr Rev. 2000;21(2):115–37.
21. Seifert-Klauss V, Prior JC. Progesterone and bone: actions promoting bone health in women. J Osteoporosis. 2010;2010:845180.
22. Castelo-Branco C, Vicente JJ, Pons F, Martinez de Osaba MJ, Casals E, Vanrell JA. Bone mineral density in young, hypothalamic oligoamenorrheic women treated with oral contraceptives. J Reprod Med. 2001;46(10):875–9.
23. Cundy T, Ames R, Horne A, Clearwater J, Roberts H, Gamble G, et al. A randomized controlled trial of estrogen replacement therapy in long-term users of depot medroxyprogesterone acetate. J Clin Endocrinol Metab. 2003;88(1):78–81.
24. Doren M, Nilsson JA, Johnell O. Effects of specific post-menopausal hormone therapies on bone mineral density in post-menopausal women: a meta-analysis. Hum Reprod. 2003;18(8):1737–46.
25. Burge R, Dawson-Hughes B, Solomon DH, Wong JB, King A, Tosteson A. Incidence and economic burden of osteoporosis-related fractures in the United States, 2005–2025. J Bone Miner Res. 2007; 22(3):465–75.
26. Looker AC, Statistics NCFH. Osteoporosis or low bone mass at the femur neck or lumbar spine in older adults, United States, 2005–2008. Hyattsville, MD: US Department of Health and Human Services, Centers for Disease Control and Prevention, National Center for Health Statistics; 2012.
27. Kanis J, McCloskey E, Johansson H. A reference standard for the definition of osteoporosis. Bone. 2008;42:467–75.
28. Kanis JA, Johnell O, Oden A, Dawson A, De Laet C, Jonsson B. Ten year probabilities of osteoporotic fractures according to BMD and diagnostic thresholds. Osteoporos Int. 2001;12(12):989–95.
29. McClung MR. The relationship between bone mineral density and fracture risk. Curr Osteoporos Rep. 2005;3(2):57–63.
30. Kanis JA, Oden A, Johansson H, Borgström F, Ström O, McCloskey E. FRAX® and its applications to clinical practice. Bone. 2009;44(5):734–43.
31. Watts NB, Ettinger B, LeBoff MS. FRAX facts. J Bone Miner Res. 2009;24(6):975–9.
32. Schousboe JT, Shepherd JA, Bilezikian JP, Baim S. Executive summary of the 2013 International Society for Clinical Densitometry Position Development Conference on bone densitometry. J Clin Densitom. 2013;16(4):455–66.
33. Finer LB, Zolna MR. Unintended pregnancy in the United States: incidence and disparities, 2006. Contraception. 2011;84(5):478–85.
34. Kost K, Singh S, Vaughan B, Trussell J, Bankole A. Estimates of contraceptive failure from the 2002 National Survey of Family Growth. Contraception. 2008;77(1):10–21.
35. Jones J, Mosher W, Daniels K. Current contraceptive use in the United States, 2006–2010, and changes in patterns of use since 1995. Natl Health Stat Rep. 2012;60:1–25.
36. Moghissi KS, Marks C. Effects of microdose norgestrel on endogenous gonadotropic and steroid hormones, cervical mucus properties, vaginal cytology, and endometrium. Fertil Steril. 1971; 22(7):424–34.
37. Xiao B, Zeng T, Wu S, Sun H, Xiao N. Effect of levonorgestrel-releasing intrauterine device on hormonal profile and menstrual pattern after long-term use. Contraception. 1995;51(6):359–65.
38. Bennink HJ. The pharmacokinetics and pharmacodynamics of Implanon, a single-rod etonogestrel contraceptive implant. Eur J Contracept Reprod Health Care. 2000;5 Suppl 2:12–20.
39. Mishell Jr DR. Pharmacokinetics of depot medroxyprogesterone acetate contraception. J Reprod Med. 1996;41(5 Suppl):381–90.

40. Jain J, Dutton C, Nicosia A, Wajszczuk C, Bode FR, Mishell Jr DR. Pharmacokinetics, ovulation suppression and return to ovulation following a lower dose subcutaneous formulation of Depo-Provera. Contraception. 2004;70(1):11–8.
41. Kaunitz AM, Darney PD, Ross D, Wolter KD, Speroff L. Subcutaneous DMPA vs. intramuscular DMPA: a 2-year randomized study of contraceptive efficacy and bone mineral density. Contraception. 2009;80(1):7–17.
42. Cromer BA, Bonny AE, Stager M, Lazebnik R, Rome E, Ziegler J, et al. Bone mineral density in adolescent females using injectable or oral contraceptives: a 24-month prospective study. Fertil Steril. 2008;90(6):2060–7.
43. Lara-Torre E, Edwards CP, Perlman S, Hertweck SP. Bone mineral density in adolescent females using depot medroxyprogesterone acetate. J Pediatr Adolesc Gynecol. 2004;17(1):17–21.
44. Cromer BA, Blair JM, Mahan JD, Zibners L, Naumovski Z. A prospective comparison of bone density in adolescent girls receiving depot medroxyprogesterone acetate (Depo-Provera), levonorgestrel (Norplant), or oral contraceptives. J Pediatr. 1996;129(5):671–6.
45. Busen NH, Britt RB, Rianon N. Bone mineral density in a cohort of adolescent women using depot medroxyprogesterone acetate for one to two years. J Adolesc Health. 2003;32(4):257–9.
46. Cromer BA, Lazebnik R, Rome E, Stager M, Bonny A, Ziegler J, et al. Double-blinded randomized controlled trial of estrogen supplementation in adolescent girls who receive depot medroxyprogesterone acetate for contraception. Am J Obstet Gynecol. 2005;192(1):42–7.
47. Scholes D, LaCroix AZ, Ichikawa LE, Barlow WE, Ott SM. Change in bone mineral density among adolescent women using and discontinuing depot medroxyprogesterone acetate contraception. Arch Pediatr Adolesc Med. 2005;159(2):139–44.
48. Berenson AB, Rahman M, Breitkopf CR, Bi LX. Effects of depot medroxyprogesterone acetate and 20-microgram oral contraceptives on bone mineral density. Obstet Gynecol. 2008;112(4):788–99.
49. Beksinska ME, Kleinschmidt I, Smit JA, Farley TM. Bone mineral density in a cohort of adolescents during use of norethisterone enanthate, depot-medroxyprogesterone acetate or combined oral contraceptives and after discontinuation of norethisterone enanthate. Contraception. 2009;79(5):345–9.
50. Zhang MH, Zhang W, Zhang AD, Yang Y, Gai L. Effect of depot medroxyprogesterone acetate on bone mineral density in adolescent women. Chin Med J (Engl). 2013;126(21):4043–7.
51. Cromer BA, Stager M, Bonny A, Lazebnik R, Rome E, Ziegler J, et al. Depot medroxyprogesterone acetate, oral contraceptives and bone mineral density in a cohort of adolescent girls. J Adolesc Health. 2004;35(6):434–41.
52. Harel Z, Johnson CC, Gold MA, Cromer B, Peterson E, Burkman R, et al. Recovery of bone mineral density in adolescents following the use of depot medroxyprogesterone acetate contraceptive injections. Contraception. 2010;81(4):281–91.
53. Curtis KM, Martins SL. Progestogen-only contraception and bone mineral density: a systematic review. Contraception. 2006;73(5):470–87.
54. Cundy T, Cornish J, Evans MC, Roberts H, Reid IR. Recovery of bone density in women who stop using medroxyprogesterone acetate. BMJ. 1994;308(6923):247–8.
55. Scholes D, LaCroix AZ, Ichikawa LE, Barlow WE, Ott SM. Injectable hormone contraception and bone density: results from a prospective study. Epidemiology. 2002;13(5):581–7.
56. Berenson AB, Breitkopf CR, Grady JJ, Rickert VI, Thomas A. Effects of hormonal contraception on bone mineral density after 24 months of use. Obstet Gynecol. 2004;103(5 Pt 1):899–906.
57. Clark MK, Sowers MR, Nichols S, Levy B. Bone mineral density changes over two years in first-time users of depot medroxyprogesterone acetate. Fertil Steril. 2004;82(6):1580–6.
58. Gai L, Zhang J, Zhang H, Gai P, Zhou L, Liu Y. The effect of depot medroxyprogesterone acetate (DMPA) on bone mineral density (BMD) and evaluating changes in BMD after discontinuation of DMPA in Chinese women of reproductive age. Contraception. 2011;83(3):218–22.
59. Kaunitz AM, Miller PD, Rice VM, Ross D, McClung MR. Bone mineral density in women aged 25–35 years receiving depot medroxyprogesterone acetate: recovery following discontinuation. Contraception. 2006;74(2):90–9.
60. Kaunitz AM, Arias R, McClung M. Bone density recovery after depot medroxyprogesterone acetate injectable contraception use. Contraception. 2008;77(2):67–76.
61. Beksinska ME, Smit JA, Kleinschmidt I, Farley TM, Mbatha F. Bone mineral density in women aged 40–49 years using depot-medroxyprogesterone acetate, norethisterone enanthate or combined oral contraceptives for contraception. Contraception. 2005;71(3):170–5.
62. Gbolade B, Ellis S, Murby B, Randall S, Kirkman R. Bone density in long term users of depot medroxyprogesterone acetate. Br J Obstet Gynaecol. 1998;105(7):790–4.
63. Tang OS, Tang G, Yip P, Li B, Fan S. Long-term depot-medroxyprogesterone acetate and bone mineral density. Contraception. 1999;59(1):25–9.
64. Tang OS, Tang G, Yip PS, Li B. Further evaluation on long-term depot-medroxyprogesterone acetate use and bone mineral density: a longitudinal cohort study. Contraception. 2000;62(4):161–4.
65. Cundy T, Cornish J, Roberts H, Reid IR. Menopausal bone loss in long-term users of depot medroxyprogesterone acetate contraception. Am J Obstet Gynecol. 2002;186(5):978–83.

66. Sanches L, Marchi NM, Castro S, Juliato CT, Villarroel M, Bahamondes L. Forearm bone mineral density in postmenopausal former users of depot medroxyprogesterone acetate. Contraception. 2008; 78(5):365–9.
67. Viola AS, Castro S, Marchi NM, Bahamondes MV, Viola CF, Bahamondes L. Long-term assessment of forearm bone mineral density in postmenopausal former users of depot medroxyprogesterone acetate. Contraception. 2011;84(2):122–7.
68. Caird LE, Reid-Thomas V, Hannan WJ, Gow S, Glasier AF. Oral progestogen-only contraception may protect against loss of bone mass in breast-feeding women. Clin Endocrinol (Oxf). 1994;41(6): 739–45.
69. Beerthuizen R, van Beek A, Massai R, Makarainen L, Hout J, Bennink HC. Bone mineral density during long-term use of the progestagen contraceptive implant Implanon compared to a non-hormonal method of contraception. Hum Reprod. 2000;15(1): 118–22.
70. Bahamondes L, Monteiro-Dantas C, Espejo-Arce X, dos Santos Fernandes AM, Lui-Filho JF, Perrotti M, et al. A prospective study of the forearm bone density of users of etonorgestrel-and levonorgestrel-releasing contraceptive implants. Hum Reprod. 2006;21(2):466–70.
71. Pongsatha S, Ekmahachai M, Suntornlimsiri N, Morakote N, Chaovisitsaree S. Bone mineral density in women using the subdermal contraceptive implant Implanon for at least 2 years. Int J Gynaecol Obstet. 2010;109(3):223–5.
72. Bahamondes L, Espejo-Arce X, Hidalgo MM, Hidalgo-Regina C, Teatin-Juliato C, Petta CA. A cross-sectional study of the forearm bone density of long-term users of levonorgestrel-releasing intrauterine system. Hum Reprod. 2006;21(5):1316–9.
73. Yang KY, Kim YS, Ji YI, Jung MH. Changes in bone mineral density of users of the levonorgestrel-releasing intrauterine system. J Nippon Med Sch. 2012;79(3):190–4.
74. Wong AYK, Tang LCH, Chin RKH. Levonorgestrel-releasing intrauterine system (Mirena®) and Depot medroxyprogesterone acetate (Depoprovera) as long-term maintenance therapy for patients with moderate and severe endometriosis: a randomised controlled trial. Aust N Z J Obstet Gynaecol. 2010;50(3):273–9.
75. Lappe JM, Stegman MR, Recker RR. The impact of lifestyle factors on stress fractures in female Army recruits. Osteoporos Int. 2001;12(1):35–42.
76. Meier C, Brauchli YB, Jick SS, Kraenzlin ME, Meier CR. Use of depot medroxyprogesterone acetate and fracture risk. J Clin Endocrinol Metab. 2010;95(11):4909–16.
77. Lanza LL, McQuay LJ, Rothman KJ, Bone HG, Kaunitz AM, Harel Z, et al. Use of depot medroxyprogesterone acetate contraception and incidence of bone fracture. Obstet Gynecol. 2013;121(3):593–600.
78. Vestergaard P, Rejnmark L, Mosekilde L. The effects of depot medroxyprogesterone acetate and intrauterine device use on fracture risk in Danish women. Contraception. 2008;78(6):459–64.
79. Centers for Disease Control and Prevention. U.S. medical eligibility criteria for contraceptive use, 2010. Recommendations and reports: morbidity and mortality weekly report. Recommendations and reports/Centers for Disease Control. MMWR. 2010; 59(4):1.
80. Westhoff CL, Torgal AH, Mayeda ER, Stanczyk FZ, Lerner JP, Benn EK, et al. Ovarian suppression in normal-weight and obese women during oral contraceptive use: a randomized controlled trial. Obstet Gynecol. 2010;116(2 Pt 1):275–83.
81. Sicat BL. Ortho Evra, a new contraceptive patch. Pharmacotherapy. 2003;23(4):472–80.
82. Westhoff CL, Torgal AH, Mayeda ER, Petrie K, Thomas T, Dragoman M, et al. Pharmacokinetics and ovarian suppression during use of a contraceptive vaginal ring in normal-weight and obese women. Am J Obstet Gynecol. 2012;207(1):39e1–6.
83. Seeman E, Szmukler GI, Formica C, Tsalamandris C, Mestrovic R. Osteoporosis in anorexia nervosa: the influence of peak bone density, bone loss, oral contraceptive use, and exercise. J Bone Miner Res. 1992;7(12):1467–74.
84. Hergenroeder AC, Smith EO, Shypailo R, Jones LA, Klish WJ, Ellis K. Bone mineral changes in young women with hypothalamic amenorrhea treated with oral contraceptives, medroxyprogesterone, or placebo over 12 months. Am J Obstet Gynecol. 1997;176(5):1017–25.
85. Martins SL, Curtis KM, Glasier AF. Combined hormonal contraception and bone health: a systematic review. Contraception. 2006;73(5):445–69.
86. Cibula D, Skrenkova J, Hill M, Stepan JJ. Low-dose estrogen combined oral contraceptives may negatively influence physiological bone mineral density acquisition during adolescence. Eur J Endocrinol. 2012;166(6):1003–11.
87. Scholes D, Hubbard RA, Ichikawa LE, LaCroix AZ, Spangler L, Beasley JM, et al. Oral contraceptive use and bone density change in adolescent and young adult women: a prospective study of age, hormone dose, and discontinuation. J Clin Endocrinol Metab. 2011;96(9):E1380–7.
88. Beksinska ME, Kleinschmidt I, Smit JA, Farley TM, Rees HV. Bone mineral density in young women aged 19–24 after 4–5 years of exclusive and mixed use of hormonal contraception. Contraception. 2009;80(2):128–32.
89. Pikkarainen E, Lehtonen-Veromaa M, Mottonen T, Kautiainen H, Viikari J. Estrogen-progestin contraceptive use during adolescence prevents bone mass acquisition: a 4-year follow-up study. Contraception. 2008;78(3):226–31.
90. Polatti F, Perotti F, Filippa N, Gallina D, Nappi RE. Bone mass and long-term monophasic oral con-

traceptive treatment in young women. Contraception. 1995;51(4):221–4.
91. Isley MM, Kaunitz AM. Update on hormonal contraception and bone density. Rev Endocr Metab Disord. 2011;12(2):93–106.
92. Reed SD, Scholes D, LaCroix AZ, Ichikawa LE, Barlow WE, Ott SM. Longitudinal changes in bone density in relation to oral contraceptive use. Contraception. 2003;68(3):177–82.
93. Nappi C, Di Spiezio Sardo A, Acunzo G, Bifulco G, Tommaselli GA, Guida M, et al. Effects of a low-dose and ultra-low-dose combined oral contraceptive use on bone turnover and bone mineral density in young fertile women: a prospective controlled randomized study. Contraception. 2003;67(5):355–9.
94. Sordal T, Grob P, Verhoeven C. Effects on bone mineral density of a monophasic combined oral contraceptive containing nomegestrol acetate/17beta-estradiol in comparison to levonorgestrel/ethinylestradiol. Acta Obstet Gynecol Scand. 2012;91(11):1279–85.
95. Gargano V, Massaro M, Morra I, Formisano C, Di Carlo C, Nappi C. Effects of two low-dose combined oral contraceptives containing drospirenone on bone turnover and bone mineral density in young fertile women: a prospective controlled randomized study. Contraception. 2008;78(1):10–5.
96. Shargil AA. Hormone replacement therapy in perimenopausal women with a triphasic contraceptive compound: a three-year prospective study. Int J Fertil. 1985;30(1):15, 18–28.
97. Gambacciani M, Spinetti A, Taponeco F, Cappagli B, Piaggesi L, Fioretti P. Longitudinal evaluation of perimenopausal vertebral bone loss: effects of a low-dose oral contraceptive preparation on bone mineral density and metabolism. Obstet Gynecol. 1994;83(3):392–6.
98. Gambacciani M, Spinetti A, Cappagli B, Taponeco F, Maffei S, Piaggesi L, et al. Hormone replacement therapy in perimenopausal women with a low dose oral contraceptive preparation: effects on bone mineral density and metabolism. Maturitas. 1994;19(2):125–31.
99. Volpe A, Amram A, Cagnacci A, Battaglia C. Biochemical aspects of hormonal contraception: effects on bone metabolism. Eur J Contracept Reprod Health Care. 1997;2(2):123–6.
100. Gambacciani M, Cappagli B, Ciaponi M, Benussi C, Genazzani AR. Hormone replacement therapy in perimenopause: effect of a low dose oral contraceptive preparation on bone quantitative ultrasound characteristics. Menopause. 1999;6(1):43–8.
101. Gambacciani M, Ciaponi M, Cappagli B, Benussi C, Genazzani AR. Longitudinal evaluation of perimenopausal femoral bone loss: effects of a low-dose oral contraceptive preparation on bone mineral density and metabolism. Osteoporos Int. 2000;11(6):544–8.
102. Taechakraichana N, Jaisamrarn U, Panyakhamlerd K, Chaikittisilpa S, Limpaphayom K. Difference in bone acquisition among hormonally treated postmenopausal women with normal and low bone mass. J Med Assoc Thai. 2001;84 Suppl 2:S586–92.
103. Taechakraichana N, Limpaphayom K, Ninlagarn T, Panyakhamlerd K, Chaikittisilpa S, Dusitsin N. A randomized trial of oral contraceptive and hormone replacement therapy on bone mineral density and coronary heart disease risk factors in postmenopausal women. Obstet Gynecol. 2000;95(1):87–94.
104. Gambacciani M, Cappagli B, Lazzarini V, Ciaponi M, Fruzzetti F, Genazzani AR. Longitudinal evaluation of perimenopausal bone loss: effects of different low dose oral contraceptive preparations on bone mineral density. Maturitas. 2006;54(2):176–80.
105. Hansen MA, Overgaard K, Riis BJ, Christiansen C. Potential risk factors for development of postmenopausal osteoporosis-examined over a 12-year period. Osteoporos Int. 1991;1(2):95–102.
106. Enzelsberger H, Metka M, Heytmanek G, Schurz B, Kurz C, Kusztrich M. Influence of oral contraceptive use on bone density in climacteric women. Maturitas. 1988;9(4):375–8.
107. Fortney JA, Feldblum PJ, Talmage RV, Zhang J, Godwin SE. Bone mineral density and history of oral contraceptive use. J Reprod Med. 1994;39(2):105–9.
108. Masaryk P, Lunt M, Benevolenskaya L, Cannata J, Dequeker J, Dohenhof C, et al. Effects of menstrual history and use of medications on bone mineral density: the EVOS study. Calcif Tissue Int. 1998;63(4):271–6.
109. Tuppurainen M, Kroger H, Saarikoski S, Honkanen R, Alhava E. The effect of previous oral contraceptive use on bone mineral density in perimenopausal women. Osteoporos Int. 1994;4(2):93–8.
110. Volpe A, Silferi M, Genazzani AD, Genazzani AR. Contraception in older woman. Contraception. 1993;47(3):229–39.
111. Harel Z, Riggs S, Vaz R, Flanagan P, Harel D, Machan JT. Bone accretion in adolescents using the combined estrogen and progestin transdermal contraceptive method Ortho Evra: a pilot study. J Pediatr Adolesc Gynecol. 2010;23(1):23–31.
112. Massaro M, Di Carlo C, Gargano V, Formisano C, Bifulco G, Nappi C. Effects of the contraceptive patch and the vaginal ring on bone metabolism and bone mineral density: a prospective, controlled, randomized study. Contraception. 2010;81(3):209–14.
113. Massai R, Makarainen L, Kuukankorpi A, Klipping C, Duijkers I, Dieben T. The combined contraceptive vaginal ring and bone mineral density in healthy premenopausal women. Hum Reprod. 2005;20(10):2764–8.
114. Memon S, Iversen L, Hannaford PC. Is the oral contraceptive pill associated with fracture in later life? New evidence from the Royal College of General Practitioners Oral Contraception Study. Contraception. 2011;84(1):40–7.
115. Mallmin H, Ljunghall S, Persson I, Bergstrom R. Risk factors for fractures of the distal forearm: a population-based case–control study. Osteoporos Int. 1994;4(6):298–304.

116. Vestergaard P, Rejnmark L, Mosekilde L. Oral contraceptive use and risk of fractures. Contraception. 2006;73(6):571–6.
117. Vestergaard P, Rejnmark L, Mosekilde L. Fracture risk in very young women using combined oral contraceptives. Contraception. 2008;78(5):358–64.
118. Michaelsson K, Baron JA, Farahmand BY, Persson I, Ljunghall S. Oral-contraceptive use and risk of hip fracture: a case–control study. Lancet. 1999;353(9163):1481–4.
119. Michaelsson K, Baron JA, Farahmand BY, Ljunghall S. Influence of parity and lactation on hip fracture risk. Am J Epidemiol. 2001;153(12):1166–72.
120. La Vecchia C, Tavani A, Gallus S. Oral contraceptives and risk of hip fractures. Lancet. 1999;354(9175):335–6.
121. Cooper C, Hannaford P, Croft P, Kay CR. Oral contraceptive pill use and fractures in women: a prospective study. Bone. 1993;14(1):41–5.
122. Vessey M, Mant J, Painter R. Oral contraception and other factors in relation to hospital referral for fracture. Findings in a large cohort study. Contraception. 1998;57(4):231–5.
123. Barad D, Kooperberg C, Wactawski-Wende J, Liu J, Hendrix SL, Watts NB. Prior oral contraception and postmenopausal fracture: a Women's Health Initiative observational cohort study. Fertil Steril. 2005;84(2):374–83.
124. Ip S, Chung M, Raman G, Chew P, Magula N, DeVine D, et al. Breastfeeding and maternal and infant health outcomes in developed countries. Evid Rep Technol Assess. 2007;153:1–186.
125. American Congress of Obstetricians and Gynecologists. ACOG Committee opinion no 361: Breastfeeding: maternal and infant aspects. Obstet Gynecol. 2007;109(2 Pt 1):479.
126. United States Department of Health and Human Services. The surgeon general's call to action to support breastfeeding. 2011. http://www.surgeongeneral.gov/library/calls/breastfeeding/factsheet.html.
127. Schanler RJ, Dooley S, Gartner LM, Krebs NF, Mass SB. Breastfeeding handbook for physicians. Washington, DC: American College of Obstetricians and Gynecologists; 2006.
128. Sauder S, Frager M, Case G, Kelch R, Marshall J. Abnormal patterns of pulsatile luteinizing hormone secretion in women with hyperprolactinemia and amenorrhea: responses to bromocriptine*. J Clin Endocrinol Metab. 1984;59(5):941–8.
129. Battin DA, Marrs RP, Fleiss PM, Mishell DR. Effect of suckling on serum prolactin, luteinizing hormone, follicle-stimulating hormone, and estradiol during prolonged lactation. Obstet Gynecol. 1985;65(6):785–8.
130. Speroff L, Darney PD. A clinical guide for contraception. Philadelphia, PA: Lippincott Williams & Wilkins; 2010.
131. Kennedy KI, Rivera R, McNeilly AS. Consensus statement on the use of breastfeeding as a family planning method. Contraception. 1989;39(5):477–96.
132. Kalkwarf HJ, Specker BL. Bone mineral loss during lactation and recovery after weaning. Obstet Gynecol. 1995;86(1):26–32.
133. Polatti F, Capuzzo E, Viazzo F, Colleoni R, Klersy C. Bone mineral changes during and after lactation. Obstet Gynecol. 1999;94(1):52–6.
134. Karlsson C, Obrant KJ, Karlsson M. Pregnancy and lactation confer reversible bone loss in humans. Osteoporos Int. 2001;12(10):828–34.
135. Chantry CJ, Auinger P, Byrd RS. Lactation among adolescent mothers and subsequent bone mineral density. Arch Pediatr Adolesc Med. 2004;158(7):650–6.
136. Honda A, Kurabayashi T, Yahata T, Tomita M, Takakuwa K, Tanaka K. Lumbar bone mineral density changes during pregnancy and lactation. Int J Gynaecol Obstet. 1998;63(3):253–8.
137. Lopez J, González G, Reyes V, Campino C, Diaz S. Bone turnover and density in healthy women during breastfeeding and after weaning. Osteoporosis Int. 1996;6(2):153–9.
138. Kalkwarf HJ. Lactation and maternal bone health. Adv Exp Med Biol. 2004;554:101–14.
139. Schnatz PF, Barker KG, Marakovits KA, O'Sullivan DM. Effects of age at first pregnancy and breastfeeding on the development of postmenopausal osteoporosis. Menopause. 2010;17(6):1161–6.
140. Canal-Macias ML, Roncero-Martin R, Moran JM, Lavado-Garcia JM, Costa-Fernandez Mdel C, Pedrera-Zamorano JD. Increased bone mineral density is associated with breastfeeding history in premenopausal Spanish women. Arch Med Sci. 2013;9(4):703–8.
141. Walker-Bone K. Recognizing and treating secondary osteoporosis. Nat Rev Rheumatol. 2012;8(8):480–92.
142. Buehring B, Viswanathan R, Binkley N, Busse W. Glucocorticoid-induced osteoporosis: an update on effects and management. J Allergy Clin Immunol. 2013;132(5):1019–30.
143. Giangregorio L, McCartney N. Bone loss and muscle atrophy in spinal cord injury: epidemiology, fracture prediction, and rehabilitation strategies. J Spinal Cord Med. 2006;29(5):489.
144. Compston J. Management of glucocorticoid-induced osteoporosis. Nat Rev Rheumatol. 2010;6(2):82–8.
145. Weinstein RS. Clinical practice. Glucocorticoid-induced bone disease. N Engl J Med. 2011; 365(1):62–70.
146. Johannesdottir SA, Horvath-Puho E, Dekkers OM, Cannegieter SC, Jorgensen JO, Ehrenstein V, et al. Use of glucocorticoids and risk of venous thromboembolism: a nationwide population-based case–control study. JAMA Intern Med. 2013;173(9):743–52.
147. Angelopoulos TP, Tentolouris NK, Bertsias GK, Boumpas DT. Steroid-induced diabetes in rheumatologic patients. Clin Exp Rheumatol. 2014;32(1): 126–30.
148. Bonjour JP, Kraenzlin M, Levasseur R, Warren M, Whiting S. Dairy in adulthood: from foods to nutri-

ent interactions on bone and skeletal muscle health. J Am Coll Nutr. 2013;32(4):251–63.
149. Bonjour JP. Dietary protein: an essential nutrient for bone health. J Am Coll Nutr. 2005;24(6 Suppl): 526S–36.
150. Ross AC, Taylor CL, Yaktine AL, Del Valle HB. Dietary reference intakes for calcium and vitamin D. Washington, DC: National Academies Press; 2011.
151. Baron JA, Farahmand BY, Weiderpass E, Michaelsson K, Alberts A, Persson I, et al. Cigarette smoking, alcohol consumption, and risk of hip fracture in women. Arch Intern Med. 2001;161(7):983–8.
152. Hallstrom H, Byberg L, Glynn A, Lemming EW, Wolk A, Michaelsson K. Long-term coffee consumption in relation to fracture risk and bone mineral density in women. Am J Epidemiol. 2013; 178(6):898–909.
153. Hudec SM, Camacho PM. Secondary causes of osteoporosis. Endocr Pract. 2013;19(1):120–8.
154. Bailey RL, Dodd KW, Goldman JA, Gahche JJ, Dwyer JT, Moshfegh AJ, et al. Estimation of total usual calcium and vitamin D intakes in the United States. J Nutr. 2010;140(4):817–22.
155. United States Department of Health and Human Services. Physical activity guidelines for Americans. 2008. http://www.health.gov/paguidelines/guidelines/.
156. Carlson SA, Fulton JE, Schoenborn CA, Loustalot F. Trend and prevalence estimates based on the 2008 physical activity guidelines for Americans. Am J Prevent Med. 2010;39(4):305–13.
157. Merki-Feld GS, Neff M, Keller PJ. A 2-year prospective study on the effects of depot medroxyprogesterone acetate on bone mass-response to estrogen and calcium therapy in individual users. Contraception. 2003;67(2):79–86.
158. Cromer BA, Scholes D, Berenson A, Cundy T, Clark MK, Kaunitz AM. Depot medroxyprogesterone acetate and bone mineral density in adolescents–the Black Box Warning: a Position Paper of the Society for Adolescent Medicine. J Adolesc Health. 2006; 39(2):296–301.
159. ACOG. ACOG Committee opinion no 415: depot medroxyprogesterone acetate and bone effects. Obstet Gynecol. 2008;112(3):727–30.
160. ACOG. ACOG practice bulletin no 129. Osteoporosis. Obstet Gynecol. 2012;120(3):718.
161. North American Menopause Society. Management of osteoporosis in postmenopausal women: 2006 position statement of the North American Menopause Society. Menopause (NY). 2006;13(3):340.
162. United States Preventive Task Force. Screening for osteoporosis: US preventive services task force recommendation statement. Ann Intern Med. 2011; 154(5):356.
163. World Health Organization. Prevention and management of osteoporosis: report of a WHO scientific group. Geneva: World Health Organization; 2003.
164. Canadian Contraception Consensus. Update on depot medroxyprogesterone acetate (DMPA). J Obstet Gynaecol Can. 2006;28(4):305–8.
165. d'Arcangues C. WHO statement on hormonal contraception and bone health. Contraception. 2006; 73(5):443–4.
166. World Health Organization. Medical eligibility criteria for contraceptive use. Geneva: World Health Organization; 2010.

17 Contraception for Women with Rheumatologic Disease

Kelly R. Culwell and Geraldine M. Navarro

Systemic lupus erythematosus (SLE) and rheumatoid arthritis (RA) are two of the most common rheumatologic diseases diagnosed in women. Both SLE and RA are frequently diagnosed in women of reproductive age and have significant implications for pregnancy, particularly if pregnancy occurs during periods of disease activity, major organ involvement, or while on teratogenic treatments. With improved knowledge of the risks of pregnancy, improved therapeutic modalities, and careful multidisciplinary monitoring, women with rheumatologic conditions can now have successful pregnancies. However, timing of pregnancy is critical to ensure the best possible outcomes, making preconceptional counseling and appropriate contraceptive options essential. In addition, women with rheumatologic disease, just like all other women, should have the ability to decide when and if to have children based on their own personal considerations, including health concerns.

Use of contraceptive methods in these conditions, particularly for SLE, has been controversial in the past, due to concerns regarding potential worsening of disease activity, increased risk for cardiovascular complications, or infection with certain methods in the setting of immunosuppressive treatment. The World Health Organization (WHO) added SLE to the conditions included in the Medical Eligibility Criteria for Contraceptive Use (MEC) in the fourth edition, published in 2010 [1], and RA was added as a new condition specific to the United States (US) context in the Centers for Disease Control and Prevention' (CDC) US adaptation of the MEC (USMEC) later that year [2]. In this chapter, the evidence and theoretical considerations behind these new recommendations will be presented along with recommendations for future research where gaps in our knowledge still exist.

Background on SLE and RA

Systemic lupus erythematosus is a complex, autoimmune disease characterized by pathogenic autoantibody formation, immune complex deposition, and multiple organ system involvement resulting in protean clinical manifestations. The disease can range from mild forms, with only skin disease and joint involvement, to severe neurological, renal, hematologic, pulmonary, and cardiac manifestations which can be life-threatening and with a variable disease course. Sixty-five percent of patients with SLE have

K.R. Culwell, M.D., M.P.H. (✉)
Planned Parenthood of the Pacific Southwest, San Diego, CA, USA
e-mail: krculwell@gmail.com

G.M. Navarro, M.D.
Division of Rheumatology, Department of Medicine, Ronald Reagan Medical Center, UCLA David Geffen School of Medicine, Porter Ranch, CA, USA
e-mail: geraldinemnavarro@gmail.com

R.H. Allen and C.A. Cwiak (eds.), *Contraception for the Medically Challenging Patient*, DOI 10.1007/978-1-4939-1233-9_17, © Springer Science+Business Media New York 2014

disease onset between the ages of 16 and 55 [3]. Twenty percent present before age 16 [4], and 15 % after the age 55 [5]. The reported prevalence rates of SLE in the population generally range from 20 to 70 per 100,000 [6].

Like SLE, RA is a chronic systemic autoimmune disorder in which complex genetic factors and environmental stimuli lead to synovial inflammation, which results in joint damage, deformities, and ultimately disability, and may shorten life-span [7, 8]. Patients with RA can also suffer from significant organ involvement leading to anemia, fatigue, skin nodules, neuropathy, ocular disease, splenomegaly, vasculitis, and pleuropericarditis [9]. Rheumatoid arthritis affects approximately 0.5–1 % of the population [10]. An estimated 1.3 million adults in the US have RA, with an estimated prevalence in women 2–3 times higher than men [11].

Classification Criteria

Classification criteria have been established for both SLE and RA. In 2012, the Systemic Lupus International Collaborating Clinics (SLICC) group revised and validated the American College of Rheumatology (ACR) SLE classification criteria [12]. SLE is diagnosed if the patient satisfies four of the clinical and immunologic criteria used in the SLICC classification system, including at least one clinical and one immunologic criterion, or if he or she has biopsy-proven nephritis compatible with SLE in the presence of antinuclear antibodies (ANAs) or anti-double-stranded DNA (anti-dsDNA) antibodies (Table 17.1) [12]. Clinical criteria include oral ulcers, acute and chronic cutaneous lupus, nonscarring alopecia, synovitis, serositis, hemolytic anemia, leucopenia or lymphopenia, thrombocytopenia, renal and neurologic involvement [12]. Immunologic criteria include the presence of the following: ANA, anti-dsDNA antibodies, anti-Smith antibodies, antiphospholipid antibodies, positive Direct Coombs test, or low complement levels [12].

In 2010, the American College of Rheumatology (ACR) and the European League Against Rheumatism (EULAR) revised the classification criteria for RA emphasizing characteristics that emerge early in the disease course for the purpose of classifying newly presenting patients with RA [13]. In the absence of an alternative diagnosis that better explains the synovitis, classification as definitive RA is based on the confirmed presence of synovitis in at least one joint and achievement of a total score of 6 or

Table 17.1 Classification criteria for systemic lupus erythematosus[a]

Clinical criteria
Acute cutaneous lupus
Chronic cutaneous lupus
Oral ulcers (palate, buccal, or tongue) OR nasal ulcers
Nonscarring alopecia
Synovitis involving two or more joints
Serositis—pleural or pericardial
Renal—urine protein to creatinine ratio or 24 h urine protein representing 500 mg protein/24 h OR red blood cell casts
Neurologic—seizures, psychosis, mononeuritis multiplex, myelitis, peripheral or cranial neuropathy, acute confusional state
Hemolytic anemia
Leukopenia <4,000/mm^3 at least once OR lymphopenia <1,000/mm^3 at least once
Thrombocytopenia <100,000/mm^3 at least once
Immunologic criteria
ANA level above laboratory reference range
Anti-dsDNA antibody level above laboratory reference range (or twofold the reference range if tested by ELISA)
Anti-Sm: presence of antibody to Sm nuclear antigen
Antiphospholipid antibody positivity as determined by any of the following: • Positive test result for lupus anticoagulant • False-positive test result for rapid plasma regain • Medium- or high-titer anticardiolipin antibody level (IgA, IgG, or IgM) • Positive test result for anti-β2 glycoprotein I (IgA, IgG, or IgM)
Low complement: low C3, C4, or CH50
Direct Coombs' test in the absence of hemolytic anemia

ANA antinuclear antibody, *anti-dsDNA* anti-double-stranded DNA, *ELISA* enzyme-linked immunosorbent assay, *Ig* immunoglobulin

[a]Adapted from the Systemic Lupus International Collaborating Clinics (SLICC) classification system, 2012 [12]. SLE is diagnosed if the patient satisfies 4 of the clinical and immunologic criteria used in the SLICC classification system, including at least one clinical and one immunologic criterion, or if he or she has biopsy-proven nephritis compatible with SLE in the presence of ANAs or anti-dsDNA antibodies. Criteria are cumulative and need not be present concurrently

Table 17.2 Classification criteria for rheumatoid arthritis[a]

Classification criteria[b]	Score
A. Joint involvement	
1 large joint	0
2–10 large joints	1
1–3 small joints (with or without involvement of large joints)	2
4–10 small joints (with or without involvement of large joints)	3
>10 joints (at least one small joint)	5
B. Serology (at least one test result is needed for classification)	
Negative RF AND negative anti-CCP	0
Low-positive RF OR low-positive anti-CCP	2
High-positive RF OR high-positive anti-CCP	3
C. Acute-phase reactants (at least one test result is needed for classification)	
Normal CRP AND normal ESR	0
Abnormal CRP OR abnormal ESR	1
D. Duration of symptoms	
<6 weeks	0
≥6 weeks	1

RF rheumatoid factor, *CCP* cyclic citrullinated peptide, *CRP* c-reactive protein, *ESR* erythrocyte sedimentation rate

[a]Adapted from the 2010 American College of Rheumatology/European League Against Rheumatism classification criteria for rheumatoid arthritis [13]

[b]Add score of categories A–D; a score of ≥6/10 is needed for classification of a patient as having definite RA

greater out of a possible score of 10 from the individual scores in four domains: number and site of involved joints, serologic abnormality, elevated acute-phase response, and symptom duration (Table 17.2) [13].

Cardiovascular Complications

Women with SLE and RA are at increased risk of cardiovascular disease (CVD). Premature atherosclerosis is a major comorbid condition in patients with SLE. Although with improved treatment the overall mortality in SLE has decreased, CVD remains a leading cause of death [14]. Young women with SLE have an estimated 50-fold increased risk of myocardial infarction compared with age- and sex-matched controls [15]. While SLE patients are subject to the same traditional risk factors as the general population, these factors do not adequately account for the significantly increased level of cardiovascular disease seen in SLE patients [16]. SLE-specific risk factors such as current disease activity, dose of corticosteroid, renal activity, and presence of lupus anticoagulant or anti-double-stranded DNA have also been implicated in the development of CVD [17].

Over the last two decades there has also been increasing evidence regarding CVD in RA patients. The prevalence of CVD in patients with RA is as high as in patients with type 2 diabetes mellitus [18], and patients with RA have a 1.5- to 2.0-fold increase in the risk of developing heart failure compared with healthy controls [19]. In RA, the risk of experiencing a cardiovascular event such as myocardial infarction or stroke is 3–4 times greater in women of reproductive age with RA compared to those without [20]. Risk factors such as dyslipidemia, hypertension, smoking, and obesity have been found in patients with RA in a similar frequency as in the general population [20, 21]. Although these risk factors contribute to the development of atherosclerosis in RA, their presence alone does not fully explain the increased CVD risk in RA patients [22, 23]. Since atherosclerosis is an inflammatory disease, the increased inflammatory state of patients with RA has been implicated in the increased CVD risk [24]. Other factors that are specific to RA, such as rheumatoid factor (RF) and anti-cyclic citrullinated peptide CCP positivity, joint erosions, extra-articular RA, joint damage, and physical inactivity have also been linked to the development of premature atherosclerosis in this condition [23]. Women with RA who are anti-CCP positive have been shown to have substantial excess mortality among postmenopausal women that is not explained by measured risk factors such as age, RF and ANA positivity, or use of RA treatment [25]. Lastly, CVD is frequently undertreated in patients with chronic diseases such as RA, which may also play a role in the increased risk of CVD in RA patients [18]. Some of the reasons for under treatment of CVD risk factors in RA may include patients' resistance to additional treatments and limited time during clinic visits for patients with complicated medical histories.

There may also be the perception that patients with reduced life expectancy may not benefit enough from preventive therapy [26].

Thromboembolism

Patients with SLE have an increased risk of arterial and venous thrombosis compared with the general population, with thrombosis being a major cause of death among SLE patients [27]. This risk for thromboembolism is further increased by the presence of persistently positive antiphospholipid antibodies [28, 29]. The risk of venous thromboembolism also appears to be increased two- to threefold in patients with RA compared with the general population [30, 31].

Antiphospholipid Antibodies and the Antiphospholipid Syndrome in Patients with SLE

Antiphospholipid syndrome (APS) is a disorder characterized by vascular thrombosis or poor pregnancy outcomes in the presence of antiphospholipid antibodies (aPLs) (Table 17.3). Antiphospholipid antibodies can be detected in about 1–5 % of asymptomatic healthy patients [32]. In SLE patients, about 40 % will have aPLs, though less than 40 % of these will have a thrombotic event [33]. These antibodies can also be found in patients with other rheumatic diseases, infections, malignancies, and with use of certain medications.

The revised Sapporo classification is used for the diagnosis of APS [34]. The criteria for diagnosis of APS specify both clinical and laboratory abnormalities. Clinical criteria include vascular thrombosis in any soft tissue or organ, or complications of pregnancy. Laboratory abnormalities may include elevated anticardiolipin (aCL) or anti-β-2 glycoprotein-I (anti-β-2 GPI) antibody titers by immunoassay, or detection of lupus anticoagulant (LA) by coagulation assays. The presence of these aPLs can be transient and could lead to misclassification. Therefore, classification of APS requires the persistence (at least 12 weeks apart) of aPLs and the clinical event and positive laboratory test should not be longer than 5 years apart (see Chap. 12).

Table 17.3 Revised classification criteria for antiphospholipid syndrome[a]

Clinical criteria[b]
1. Vascular thrombosis One or more clinical episodes of arterial, venous, or small vessel thrombosis, in any tissue or organ. Thrombosis must be confirmed by objective validated criteria (i.e., unequivocal findings of appropriate imaging studies or histopathology). For histopathologic confirmation, thrombosis should be present without significant evidence of inflammation in the vessel wall
2. Pregnancy morbidity (a) One or more unexplained deaths of a morphologically normal fetus at or beyond the tenth week of gestation, with normal fetal morphology documented by ultrasound or by direct examination of the fetus, or (b) One or more premature births of a morphologically normal neonate before the 34th week of gestation because of: (1) eclampsia or severe preeclampsia defined according to standard definitions , or (2) recognized features of placental insufficiency, or (c) Three or more unexplained consecutive spontaneous abortions before the tenth week of gestation, with maternal anatomic or hormonal abnormalities and paternal and maternal chromosomal causes excluded
Laboratory criteria[b]
One of the following
1. *Lupus anticoagulant (LA)* present in plasma, on two or more occasions at least 12 weeks apart, detected according to the guidelines of the International Society on Thrombosis and Haemostasis (Scientific Subcommittee on LAs/phospholipid-dependent antibodies)
2. *Anticardiolipin (aCL)* antibody of IgG and/or IgM isotype in serum or plasma, present in medium or high titer (i.e., >40 GPL or MPL, or >the 99th percentile), on two or more occasions, at least 12 weeks apart, measured by a standardized ELISA
3. *Anti-β-2 glycoprotein-I antibody (anti-β-2-GPI)* of IgG and/or IgM isotype in serum or plasma (in titer> the 99th percentile), present on two or more occasions, at least 12 weeks apart, measured by a standardized ELISA, according to recommended procedures

MPL IgM phospholipid units, *GPL* IgG phospholipid units
[a]Adapted from International consensus statement on an update of the classification criteria for definite antiphospholipid syndrome (APS) [34]
[b]Antiphospholipid antibody syndrome (APS) is present if at least one of the clinical criteria and one of the laboratory criteria that follow are met

Several studies have documented the clinical differences between primary APS and APS in women with SLE. In a European multisite study cohort of 1,000 patients with APS, deep venous thrombosis (DVT) was the most common presenting event. Primary APS patients were similar to APS patients with SLE, except that patients with APS associated with SLE had more arthritis, livedo reticularis, thrombocytopenia, and leucopenia [35]. In a cross-sectional study of consecutive patients in the Hopkins Lupus Center, in a total of 122 patients (84 % female, 74 % Caucasian) the prevalence of arterial thrombosis, venous thrombosis, and fetal loss was higher in APS associated with SLE than in primary APS (28 vs. 11 %, 36 vs. 10 %, and 29 vs. 10 %, respectively) [36].

Pregnancy in SLE and RA

Pregnancy in patients with SLE may be associated with several complications including maternal, obstetrical, and fetal complications. These pregnancies have higher rates of preterm delivery and decreased rates of live births, with almost one quarter of pregnancies in SLE patients resulting in pregnancy loss, defined in most studies to include spontaneous abortion and stillbirth [37–40]. More severe clinical manifestations of SLE such as active lupus nephritis may result in even higher percentage of fetal loss: 52 % compared with 11 % fetal loss in women with inactive lupus nephritis [41]. Due to the unpredictable nature of the disease and the increased risk of the disease flaring up during pregnancy, women with SLE had previously been advised to avoid pregnancy.

Women with SLE may experience uncomplicated pregnancies, provided they are able to optimally time the pregnancy. Several studies have shown that planned pregnancies in SLE patients have significantly better outcomes than unplanned ones [37, 42–44]. The prognosis for both mother and child is better when SLE is in remission; therefore, patients considering having children should be in remission or in a state of low disease activity and on stable medication for at least 6 months before conception. Preconception management is crucial to help women achieve a period of disease remission before pregnancy as well as to allow adjustment of therapy as all non-glucocorticoid immunosuppressive medications used to treat SLE (including methotrexate, mycophenolate mofetil, azathioprine, cyclosporine, tacrolimus, leflunomide, and cyclophosphamide) are teratogenic. Therefore, contraception is crucial at certain stages of disease and during immunosuppressive therapy that confers a risk to the developing fetus during pregnancy.

Women with APS and APS associated with SLE are prone to arterial as well as venous thrombosis and pregnancy itself is a procoagulant state. In APS pregnancies, there is an increased incidence of early onset preeclampsia, uteroplacental insufficiency causing intrauterine growth restriction (IUGR), placental abruption, and premature delivery. Recurrent fetal loss is more common in women with APS than in other women, and 40–50 % of these losses occur in the second and third trimesters [45]. The overall rate of live births in women with APS treated with heparin and aspirin is estimated to be 70 % [46]. In one study, women with APS during pregnancy had more than three times as many perinatal deaths as women without APS (20 % with APS vs. 6 % without APS) despite treatment with heparin and aspirin in the majority of the APS patients [37].

Pregnancy generally diminishes or eliminates symptoms in most patients with RA, though symptoms recur in up to 90 % of women after delivery [47]. Certain treatments for RA, such as methotrexate, are teratogenic. Women are advised to discontinue methotrexate at least 3 months prior to trying to conceive. Other common medications taken by women with RA include tumor necrosis factor inhibitors. Two of these (infliximab and adalimumab) are known to cross the placenta, but the risk to the developing fetus has been shown to be decreased when discontinued by the end of the second trimester. If clinically indicated, certolizumab can be used throughout pregnancy due to its minimal placental transfer [48].

Contraception in Women with SLE and RA

Previously, women with SLE have been discouraged from using hormonal methods of contraception primarily due to the concerns regarding increased disease activity and thrombosis [49, 50]. In addition, as noted above, people with SLE are at increased risk for cardiovascular diseases, such as atherosclerosis and hypertension. The possible presence of these concomitant conditions, which can impact the safety of contraceptive methods, must also be taken into account when helping a woman with SLE choose an appropriate contraceptive method. However, there is growing evidence that carefully planning for pregnancy to occur during times of disease quiescence improves maternal and fetal health outcomes. This further highlights the importance of counseling patients with SLE about contraception.

There are also concerns regarding the use of contraception in patients with RA. One of the concerns is the theoretical risk of infection with the use of an intrauterine device (IUD) particularly if a woman is on immunosuppressive treatments [51–53]. Given that bone loss is a serious complication of RA, there is also a concern regarding the effect of certain hormonal contraceptives on bone. Lastly, methods of contraception requiring self-insertion, like the contraceptive vaginal ring, may pose a problem to women who have joint deformities.

In the literature, women with serious medical conditions have been shown to receive less contraceptive counseling than women without chronic diseases [54–56]. In addition, they may be counseled against use of contraception, particularly hormonal contraception, because of concerns about the safety of these methods without consideration of the alternative risks of pregnancy.

In 2007, a cross-sectional survey of women with SLE in a referral clinic in the US found 55 % of women at risk for unintended pregnancy (not pregnant or trying to become pregnant and not using female or male sterilization for contraception) reported at least one occasion of unprotected intercourse in the previous 3 months with 23 % overall reporting having unprotected sex "most of the time" [57]. The most commonly used forms of contraception in this population were barrier methods (condoms 46 %, diaphragm 1 %), with low use of IUDs (4 %). This degree of IUD use is only slightly greater than the proportion of women in the US overall using IUDs for contraception in 2007 (3.5 %) [58]. No women surveyed reported the use of contraceptive implants or emergency contraception, while 24 % reported use of combined hormonal contraception (CHC).

Evidence on Safety of Contraceptive Use by Women with SLE and RA

Disease Activity

One of the main concerns for women with SLE using hormonal contraceptives has been disease activity. The high female-to-male ratio of patients with SLE during childbearing years has implicated estrogen in the development, and perhaps worsening, of SLE. In 2005, two randomized controlled trials were published which evaluated whether use of combined oral contraceptives (COCs) was associated with worsening SLE disease [59]. A single-blind, non-placebo, randomized controlled trial (RCT) from Mexico, randomized 54 women with SLE to COCs (30 μg ethinyl estradiol and 150 μg levonorgestrel), 54 to progestin-only pills (POPs, 30 μg levonorgestrel), and 54 to the copper (CuT380A) IUD [59]. There was no difference in global disease activity measured by the Systemic Lupus Erythematosus Disease Activity Index (SLEDAI) at any of the follow-up points in any of the groups over 1 year, including a separate analysis of patients with active disease at baseline. The probability of any flare or severe flares was not different among the three groups.

The second RCT (SELENA trial) was a double-blind, randomized, placebo controlled trial in which 183 women with inactive (76 %) or stable active (24 %) SLE were randomly assigned to receive either COCs (triphasic ethinyl estradiol at a dose of 35 μg plus norethindrone at a dose of 0.5–1 mg for 12 cycles of 28 days each; 91 women) or placebo (92 women) [60]. Subjects were excluded if they had diastolic blood pressure of more than 95 mmHg or systolic blood pressure of more than 145 mmHg on three determinations; a history of spontaneous DVT, arterial thrombosis, or pulmonary embolus; the presence of immunoglobulin (Ig) G, IgM, or IgA anticardiolipin antibodies (more than 40 IgG phospholipid units, 40 IgM phospholipid units, or 50 IgA phospholipid units, respectively), a demonstration of lupus anticoagulant by the dilute Russell's viper-venom time test, or both; or any other contraindication to CHCs [60].

The occurrence of a severe flare was infrequent in both groups: 7 of 91 subjects in the COC group (7.7 %) and 7 of 92 subjects in the placebo group (7.6 %) [60]. The 12-month severe flare rate was not different between the two groups, nor were any other measures of disease severity. While neither of these trials included women with very severe disease, the results indicate that at least for women with inactive or stable active disease, use of hormonal contraceptives does not seem to worsen disease activity. In addition, women in these studies were not excluded if they had severe disease in the past, even with renal involvement, as long as they were stable or had inactive disease at the time of enrollment.

Given that RA symptoms improve or disappear during pregnancy in nearly all women with RA, various studies have investigated the use of various COCs on disease activity in women with RA. Limited data suggest that COCs do not worsen disease activity in RA and may reduce symptoms, such as number of swollen joints in some patients [61]. Only one study has specifically evaluated disease activity during use of progestin-only therapy in women with RA. This was a non-comparative study to evaluate the potential effect of oral progesterone, 200–500 mg daily, on disease activity. This dose was chosen to mimic progesterone levels during pregnancy during which time many women experience a reduction in RA symptoms. However, there was no statistically significant difference in objective measurement of disease activity with this treatment [62].

Thromboembolism

Very few studies have evaluated hormonal contraceptive use and risk of thromboembolism in women with rheumatologic diseases. A case–control study of 157 participants (including 131 women) with positive aPLs (79 % of whom also had SLE) found a trend toward increased risk of thrombosis, particularly arterial in those with reported use of oral contraceptives (not specified whether COC or POP) [63]. None of the values were statistically significant but the study was not powered to look at this exposure. In a prospective cohort study of 65 women with SLE and positive aPLs, all women with a "history" of oral contraceptive (OC) use ($n=3$, not specified whether COC or POP and not specified whether any were current users) developed a thrombotic event whereas only 23 of the 62 women without history of OC use developed a thrombotic event [64]. In the SELENA trial [60], subjects were excluded if they had a history of thrombosis or the presence of IgG, IgM, or IgA anticardiolipin antibodies (more than 40 IgG phospholipid units, 40 IgM phospholipid units, or 50 IgA phospholipid units), a demonstration of lupus anticoagulant by the dilute Russell's viper-venom time test, or both. In the group that was randomized to receive COCs, there was one DVT and one clotted graft; in the placebo group, there was one DVT, one ocular thrombosis, and one superficial thrombophlebitis.

While it is certain that progestin only methods don't carry the same risk of thromboembolism as do methods containing estrogen, whether there is no risk or simply a lower risk of thromboembolism with progestin-only methods is not as clear. A recent meta-analysis of eight observational trials found that evidence on risk of thromboembolism with use of progestin-only methods was limited [65]. There appeared to be no increased risk with POPs or the levonorgestrel IUD, but that there may be an increased risk with progestin-only injectables. In the randomized trial by Sanchez-Guerrero et al., there were four episodes of thromboembolism, two in the COC group and two in the POP group, with none in the group assigned to the copper IUD [56]. All four of these patients were reported to have positive aPLs.

The incidence of thromboembolism was therefore 4.75/100 women-years in the COC group and 5.44/100 women-years in the POP group. This study was not powered to detect a difference in the outcome of thromboembolism between the groups. An additional cohort study evaluated the use of two progestin-only compounds by women with SLE: chlormadinone acetate (CMA) and cyproterone acetate (CPA) [66]. These medications are not labeled for use as contraceptives but are available and used for this purpose in France. Four patients in the study developed a venous or arterial thromboembolism: one deep vein thrombosis, one myocardial infarction, one peripheral arterial thrombosis, and one patient developed skin necrosis due to microthrombosis in the legs. All four patients were in the group treated with CPA. The incidence of venous thromboembolism was 33.5/100 women-years and the incidence of arterial thromboembolism was 67.3/100 women-years in women treated with CPA. However, the women in this study were a high risk for thromboembolic events. Nearly 30 % of the patients in the study had detectable aPLs, including 15 women with a history of venous thrombosis. In addition, nine patients in the study had a history of arterial thrombosis or myocardial infarction. Three out of the four patients who developed venous or arterial thrombosis in this study had other significant risk factors including prior thrombosis, obesity, smoking, and elevated aPLs. No venous or arterial thrombosis occurred with CMA use. Though the overall incidence of vascular events in the group who received CPA was not more than expected for these high-risk women, the fact that no women in the CMA group developed vascular complications may be due to the fact that CMA was only given to women in the study if they had not had a disease flare within the last year or if they developed side effects such as break-through bleeding with CPA. Therefore, women who received CPA in this study had more active disease at baseline and thus may have been at increased risk for vascular complications. Per the authors, the decision to start therapy with CPA for patients with more active disease was based on the fact that CPA has stronger antigonadotropic activity than CMA and therefore may lead to a greater hypoestrogenic state that might be more beneficial in women with more severe disease.

Immunosuppression and IUDs

Many patients with RA and SLE take immunosuppressive drugs. Women and their providers may be concerned about the risk of infection with IUD insertion if immunosuppressant medications are prescribed. It is reassuring that studies in women with other types of immunocompromised states, such as HIV, have not shown an increased risk of pelvic infection with IUD use [51, 53]. There is minimal evidence on use of IUDs by women with rheumatologic disease. No pelvic infections were seen in the 54 women with SLE who were randomized to receive the copper IUD (Cu-IUD) in the Sanchez-Guerrero trial [59]. There was a nonsignificant trend toward infection in this group that was presented in the study manuscript but this included two episodes of meningitis, two episodes of leg cellulitis, and one episode of herpes zoster. None of these infections are likely to have been due to the insertion or use of the IUD. In a secondary analysis of a retrospective cohort study, there were no pelvic infections during the use of the IUD in 28 women who had either a copper or copper and silver containing IUD inserted after the diagnosis of SLE [67].

Hormonal Contraception and Bone Health

Women with SLE or RA are at increased risk for osteoporosis, fractures, or avascular necrosis of bone, either from the disease itself or from long-term use of corticosteroid medication [68–70]. Therefore, the impact of hormonal contraception, particularly depot medroxyprogesterone acetate (DMPA) injectable contraception, on bone is a concern with use of these methods.

A prospective cohort study evaluated musculoskeletal complications among 407 women with SLE [68]. OC (not specified whether COC or POP) use was associated with decreased risk (OR 0.48, 95 % CI 0.28–0.81) of musculoskeletal damage in this study (defined as muscular atrophy or weakness, deforming arthritis, osteoporosis with fracture or vertebral collapse, avascular necrosis, osteomyelitis, and/or ruptured tendon) though no information on duration or timing of OC use with respect to the diagnosis of SLE was reported. A retrospective cohort study of 702 women with SLE evaluated the association of ever use (past or current) of OCs (not specified whether COC or POP) with fracture risk [70]. The authors reported that women who had never used OCs had a greater likelihood of fracture than those with a history of OC use (64 % of women without OC use had fracture, 53 % of women with ever use of OC had fracture; $p=0.03$). The USMEC does not comment on whether DMPA should be used with more caution in women with SLE who have musculoskeletal risk factors.

There is no data on use of hormonal contraception by women with RA looking at the outcome of bone health, including osteoporosis or fracture. Given that RA itself can cause osteoporosis and non-traumatic fracture, in addition to the frequency of corticosteroid use in this condition, the USMEC recommendation for DMPA use in women with RA is that the risks may outweigh the benefits (category 3) among women on long-term corticosteroid therapy with a history of, or risk factors for, non-traumatic fractures. This differs from the overall recommendations regarding DMPA and risk of bone loss in women without risk factors for development of osteoporosis as the bone loss demonstrated to occur with DMPA in low-risk women appears to be entirely reversible and has not been shown to be associated with risk of non-traumatic axial fracture [71, 72]. Otherwise, DMPA use for women with rheumatoid arthritis is classified as category 2 (benefits outweigh the risks).

Severe Thrombocytopenia

Mild thrombocytopenia (platelet counts between 100,000 and 150,000 μL^{-1}) has been noted in 25–50 % of patients with SLE, while severe thrombocytopenia (generally considered less than 50,000 μL^{-1}) occurs in only 10 % [73, 74]. There are several potential causes of thrombocytopenia in patients with SLE. Immune-mediated platelet destruction is most often the cause of thrombocytopenia in patients with SLE, but impaired platelet production can also be caused by the use of cytotoxic or immunosuppressive drugs.

The USMEC gives a category 3 recommendation (risks generally outweigh benefits) for DMPA and Cu-IUD initiation in women with SLE and severe thrombocytopenia based on the concern that these methods can cause irregular and/or heavier menstrual bleeding in the early months of use, which could exacerbate heavy menstrual bleeding that women with severe thrombocytopenia might experience. Continuation of these methods in women with SLE and severe thrombocytopenia is given a category 2 recommendation (benefits generally outweigh risks) as the risk of heavy menstrual bleeding is less likely with continued use of these methods.

In contrast, women with SLE who may also be at increased risk for heavy menstrual bleeding or hemorrhagic ovarian cysts due to treatment with anticoagulants or subsequent development of thrombocytopenia may benefit from treatment with hormonal contraceptives, including the levonorgestrel-releasing IUD (LNG-IUD). These methods may provide protection from these side effects of treatment or other complications of the disease, due to the effects of suppression of ovulation and decreased menstrual bleeding [75, 76]. No differentiation in the recommendations is made between initiation and continuation for the LNG IUD given that insertion of the IUD, including placement of a tenaculum, is unlikely to be a problem in women with thrombocytopenia.

Recommendations

Table 17.4 presents the recommendations for contraceptive use for women with SLE and RA from the USMEC [1]. The recommendations assign four categories to each medical condition/method combination with category 1 indicating no restriction on use of the method, category 2 indicating benefits generally outweigh proven or theoretical risks, category 3 indicating proven or theoretical risks generally outweigh benefits, and category 4 being an unacceptable health risk for use of the method in women with this condition. The methods addressed in the USMEC are CHC

Table 17.4 Recommendations for use of contraceptives by women with SLE and RA

Condition	CHC	POP	DMPA I	DMPA C	Implant	Cu-IUD I	Cu-IUD C	LNG-IUD	
Systemic lupus erythematosus									
(a) Positive (or unknown) antiphospholipid antibodies	4	3	3	3	3	1	1	3	
(b) Severe thrombocytopenia	2	2	3	2	2	3	2	2	
(c) Immunosuppressive treatment	2	2	2	2	2	2	1	2	
(d) None of the above	2	2	2	2	2	1	1	2	
						I	C	I	C
Rheumatoid arthritis									
(a) On immunosuppressive therapy	2	1	2/3[a]		1	2	1	2	1
(b) Not on immunosuppressive therapy	2	1	2		1	1		1	

United States medical eligibility for contraceptive use, 2010

CHC combined hormonal contraception, *POP* progestin-only pills, *DMPA* depo-medroxyprogesterone acetate, *Cu-IUD* copper intrauterine device, *LNG-IUD* levonorgestrel releasing intrauterine device, *I* initiation, *C* continuation

[a]DMPA use among women on long-term corticosteroid therapy with a history of, or with risk factors for, nontraumatic fractures is classified as category 3. Otherwise, DMPA use for women with rheumatoid arthritis is classified as category 2

(including low dose <35 μg ethinyl estradiol COC, combined contraceptive patch, and combined contraceptive vaginal ring), POP, DMPA, Implant (only the etonogestrel implant is in use in the US), Cu-IUD, and LNG-IUD. Recommendations for some methods are separated into initiation (*I*) versus continuation (*C*) indicating different risk/benefit ratios for initiating a method in a woman with a certain condition versus continuing the method once a woman has been diagnosed with the condition. While the recommendations for SLE were not changed from the recommendations in the WHO MEC, RA was a new condition added for the US context in the USMEC. The adaptation of the MEC in the UK also contains the same recommendations for SLE but does not include recommendations for RA [77].

Initiation of Contraception in Women with SLE/RA

The CDC recently published follow-up guidance to the USMEC entitled the Selected Practice Recommendations for Contraceptive Use (SPR) [78]. This document is adapted from the WHO SPR and provides guidance on how to provide contraceptive methods to women, including evaluation needed prior to starting and recommended follow-up for each contraceptive method. These recommendations apply primarily to otherwise healthy women using contraceptive methods but should be followed as minimum requirements for all women initiating contraception. Some key recommended evaluations prior to initiating contraceptive methods for all women include:

- Blood pressure (BP) measurement prior to initiation of CHC
- Bimanual pelvic and cervical examination prior to insertion of IUD
- Sexually transmitted infection (STI) screening at the time of insertion of IUD if indicated by risk factors

In addition, as with all women, a thorough assessment of past and current medical history to identify common concomitant conditions such as hypertension, coronary artery disease, and prior thrombotic events is indicated for women with SLE. When a woman has multiple medical conditions, the condition leading to the most restrictive category recommendation for use of the method should be used to determine her eligibility for that method. All recommendations in the USMEC assume that no other risk factors or conditions are present. When determining appropriateness of a method the provider should recognize that risks may be increased in the presence of multiple medical conditions. In women with SLE, inquiring about current SLE disease manifestations including anemia, thrombocytopenia, renal involvement, and current level of disease activity (of SLE) is useful in assessing risk of flare or other complications from initiation of hormonal contraception. Other key components of history in order to establish eligibility for contraceptive methods include smoking, migraine (with or without aura), liver disease, history or current breast cancer, diabetes, stroke, known thrombogenic mutations, complicated cardiac valvular disease, solid organ transplant, and current medications.

Required physical examination prior to initiation of contraceptive methods specific to women with SLE or RA is minimal beyond that which is recommended for all women in the US SPR (BP check for CHC, pelvic exam for IUD). For women with RA, assessment of manual dexterity should be done, particularly if the patient would like to initiate a method that requires self-insertion such as a vaginal ring, diaphragm, or female condom.

Laboratory evaluation prior to initiation of contraceptive methods should include assessment of aPLs status (anti-cardiolipin, anti-β-2 glycoprotein I antibodies, and lupus anticoagulant). Even if these antibodies have been previously tested and were negative, since these antibodies can fluctuate, it would be prudent to check aPLs status prior to initiation of contraception and yearly thereafter to assess for continued eligibility, particularly for CHC.

No other laboratory assessment is necessary prior to initiation of contraception in women with SLE or RA with the exception of a platelet count in women with signs of severe thrombocytopenia prior to initiation of DMPA or Cu-IUD. Otherwise, it is not necessary to obtain platelet counts prior to IUD insertion. Other tests may be recommended for individual patients based on disease-specific concerns but these plans should be developed on an individual basis with the rheumatologist involved in the patient's care.

Follow-up after initiation of contraceptive methods for women with SLE and RA should follow the recommendations for healthy women outlined in the US SPR. In addition, more frequent monitoring of blood pressure (such as every 3 months for the first year) in women with SLE or RA initiating a CHC is likely warranted. Women should be encouraged to return at any time to discuss side effects or other problems and when it is time to remove, replace, or refill their contraceptive method. Ideally, contraceptive care should be coordinated with the patient's primary rheumatologic care to assess individual needs for more intensive follow-up or monitoring.

Conclusion/Research Gaps

The primary risks from use of hormonal contraceptives in women with SLE involve thrombogenic risks, particularly in those women with positive aPLs. The best available evidence does not indicate a risk of worsening disease activity in women with inactive or stable active SLE who use hormonal contraceptives. As outlined in the WHO MEC and adaptations for the US and UK, with the exception of women at increased risk for thrombosis due to the presence of aPLs, the benefits of contraception outweigh the risks for most women with SLE.

Women with SLE are at most risk for adverse pregnancy outcomes if they become pregnant during a time of severe disease activity. Because the existing studies looking at impact of hormonal contraception on disease activity included only women with mild-moderate disease, it is unclear what impact hormonal contraceptives have in women with severe disease, and who are in the most need of effective contraception. Additional research focusing on outcomes of women with severe SLE with use of contraceptive methods would be helpful to establish a safe alternative to pregnancy for women during times of high disease activity. In addition, further data to establish whether progestin-only methods increase the risk of thrombosis in women with SLE, particularly those with positive aPLs or APS, would be useful to reassure providers and patients.

Though SLE patients with isolated but persistently positive aPLs appear to be at further risk of thrombosis, future studies that delineate the level at which these aPLs confer a risk for thrombosis would be helpful. Recognizing that patients with

APS and patients with positive aPLs may have different thrombotic risk profiles may assist clinicians in monitoring patients and further assessing the risks of thrombosis and the risks and benefits of hormonal contraceptives.

Women with RA are at most risk for adverse pregnancy outcomes if they become pregnant while using teratogenic medications. Overall, all contraceptive methods appear safe for most women with RA, with the exception of DMPA use in women with the greatest risk of osteoporosis (USMEC category 3). However, there is minimal evidence on safety of methods other than COCs in women with RA. Further research looking at the use of the most effective contraceptive options, including the contraceptive implant and IUDs in women with SLE and RA, particularly those with more severe disease, would help to provide additional evidence on the safety of these methods.

References

1. World Health Organization. Medical eligibility for contraceptive use. 4th ed. Geneva: World Health Organization; 2010.
2. Centers for Disease Control. US medical eligibility criteria for contraceptive use, 2010. Adapted from the World Health Organization medical eligibility criteria for contraceptive use. MMWR Recomm Rep. 2010;59(4):1–86.
3. Rothfield N. Clinical features of systemic lupus erythematosus. In: Kelley WN, Harris ED, Ruddy S, Sledge CB, editors. Textbook of rheumatology. Philadelphia, PA: WB Saunders; 1981.
4. Schaller J. Lupus in childhood. Clin Rheum Dis. 1982;8(1):219–28.
5. Ballou SP, Khan MA, Kushner I. Clinical features of systemic lupus erythematosus: differences related to race and age of onset. Arthritis Rheum. 1982;25(1): 55–60.
6. Pons-Estel GJ, Alarcón GS, Scofield L, Reinlib L, Cooper GS. Understanding the epidemiology and progression of systemic lupus erythematosus. Semin Arthritis Rheum. 2010;39(4):257–68.
7. Salliot C, Dougados M, Gossec L. Risk of serious infections during rituximab, abatacept and anakinra treatments for rheumatoid arthritis: meta-analyses of randomised placebo-controlled trials. Ann Rheum Dis. 2009;68(1):25–32.
8. Higashida J, Wun T, Schmidt S, Naguwa SM, Tuscano JM. Safety and efficacy of rituximab in patients with rheumatoid arthritis refractory to disease modifying antirheumatic drugs and anti-tumor necrosis factor-alpha treatment. J Rheumatol. 2005;32(11):2109–15.
9. Young A, Koduri G. Extra-articular manifestations and complications of rheumatoid arthritis. Best Pract Res Clin Rheumatol. 2007;21(5):907–27.
10. American College of Rheumatology Subcommittee. Guidelines. American College of Rheumatology Subcommittee on rheumatoid arthritis guidelines. Guidelines for the management of rheumatoid arthritis: 2002 update. Arthritis Rheum. 2002;46(2):328–46.
11. Helmick CG, Felson DT, Lawrence RC, Gabriel S, Hirsch R, Kwoh CK, et al. Estimates of the prevalence of arthritis and other rheumatic conditions in the United States. Part I. Arthritis Rheum. 2008;58(1):15–25.
12. Petri M, Orbai AM, Alarcón GS, Gordon C, Merrill JT, Fortin PR, et al. Derivation and validation of the systemic lupus international collaborating clinics classification criteria for systemic lupus erythematosus. Arthritis Rheum. 2012;64(8):2677–86.
13. Aletaha D, Neogi T, Silman AJ, Funovits J, Felson DT, Bingham CO, et al. Rheumatoid arthritis classification criteria: an American College of Rheumatology/European League Against Rheumatism collaborative initiative. Arthritis Rheum. 2010;62(9):2569–81.
14. Nossent J, Cikes N, Kiss E, Marchesoni A, Nassonova V, Mosca M, et al. Current causes of death in systemic lupus erythematosus in Europe, 2000–2004: relation to disease activity and damage accrual. Lupus. 2007;16(5):309–17.
15. Manzi S, Meilahn EN, Rairie JE, Conte CG, Medsger TA, Jansen-McWilliams L, et al. Age-specific incidence rates of myocardial infarction and angina in women with systemic lupus erythematosus: comparison with the Framingham Study. Am J Epidemiol. 1997;145(5):408–15.
16. Petri M. Hopkins lupus cohort 1999 update. Rheum Dis Clin North Am. 2000;26(2):199–213, v.
17. Magder LS, Petri M. Incidence of and risk factors for adverse cardiovascular events among patients with systemic lupus erythematosus. Am J Epidemiol. 2012;176(8):708–19.
18. van Halm VP, Peters MJ, Voskuyl AE, Boers M, Lems WF, Visser M, et al. Rheumatoid arthritis versus diabetes as a risk factor for cardiovascular disease: a cross-sectional study, the CARRE Investigation. Ann Rheum Dis. 2009;68(9):1395–400.
19. Crowson CS, Liao KP, Davis JM, Solomon DH, Matteson EL, Knutson KL, et al. Rheumatoid arthritis and cardiovascular disease. Am Heart J. 2013;166(4): 622–8.e1.
20. Solomon DH, Goodson NJ, Katz JN, Weinblatt ME, Avorn J, Setoguchi S, et al. Patterns of cardiovascular risk in rheumatoid arthritis. Ann Rheum Dis. 2006;65(12):1608–12.
21. del Rincón ID, Williams K, Stern MP, Freeman GL, Escalante A. High incidence of cardiovascular events in a rheumatoid arthritis cohort not explained by traditional cardiac risk factors. Arthritis Rheum. 2001; 44(12):2737–45.
22. del Rincón I, Freeman GL, Haas RW, O'Leary DH, Escalante A. Relative contribution of cardiovascular risk factors and rheumatoid arthritis clinical manifestations to atherosclerosis. Arthritis Rheum. 2005;52(11):3413–23.

23. Naranjo A, Sokka T, Descalzo MA, Calvo-Alén J, Hørslev-Petersen K, Luukkainen RK, et al. Cardiovascular disease in patients with rheumatoid arthritis: results from the QUEST-RA study. Arthritis Res Ther. 2008;10(2):R30.
24. Maradit-Kremers H, Nicola PJ, Crowson CS, Ballman KV, Gabriel SE. Cardiovascular death in rheumatoid arthritis: a population-based study. Arthritis Rheum. 2005;52(3):722–32.
25. Kuller LH, Mackey RH, Walitt BT, Deane KD, Holers VM, Robinson WH et al. Determinants of mortality among postmenopausal women in the women's health initiative who report rheumatoid arthritis. Arthritis Rheum. 2014;66(3):497–507.
26. Boers M, Dijkmans B, Gabriel S, Maradit-Kremers H, O'Dell J, Pincus T. Making an impact on mortality in rheumatoid arthritis: targeting cardiovascular comorbidity. Arthritis Rheum. 2004;50(6):1734–9.
27. Cervera R, Khamashta MA, Font J, Sebastiani GD, Gil A, Lavilla P, et al. Morbidity and mortality in systemic lupus erythematosus during a 10-year period: a comparison of early and late manifestations in a cohort of 1,000 patients. Medicine (Baltimore). 2003; 82(5):299–308.
28. Martinez-Berriotxoa A, Ruiz-Irastorza G, Egurbide MV, Garmendia M, Gabriel Erdozain J, Villar I, et al. Transiently positive anticardiolipin antibodies and risk of thrombosis in patients with systemic lupus erythematosus. Lupus. 2007;16(10):810–6.
29. Tektonidou MG, Laskari K, Panagiotakos DB, Moutsopoulos HM. Risk factors for thrombosis and primary thrombosis prevention in patients with systemic lupus erythematosus with or without antiphospholipid antibodies. Arthritis Rheum. 2009;61(1): 29–36.
30. Holmqvist ME, Neovius M, Eriksson J, Mantel Ä, Wållberg-Jonsson S, Jacobsson LT, et al. Risk of venous thromboembolism in patients with rheumatoid arthritis and association with disease duration and hospitalization. JAMA. 2012,308(13):1350–6.
31. Bacani AK, Gabriel SE, Crowson CS, Heit JA, Matteson EL. Noncardiac vascular disease in rheumatoid arthritis: increase in venous thromboembolic events? Arthritis Rheum. 2012;64(1):53–61.
32. Biggioggero M, Meroni PL. The geoepidemiology of the antiphospholipid antibody syndrome. Autoimmun Rev. 2010;9(5):A299–304.
33. Ruiz-Irastorza G, Crowther M, Branch W, Khamashta MA. Antiphospholipid syndrome. Lancet. 2010; 376(9751):1498–509.
34. Miyakis S, Lockshin MD, Atsumi T, Branch DW, Brey RL, Cervera R, et al. International consensus statement on an update of the classification criteria for definite antiphospholipid syndrome (APS). J Thromb Haemost. 2006;4(2):295–306.
35. Cervera R, Piette JC, Font J, Khamashta MA, Shoenfeld Y, Camps MT, et al. Antiphospholipid syndrome: clinical and immunologic manifestations and patterns of disease expression in a cohort of 1,000 patients. Arthritis Rheum. 2002;46(4):1019–27.
36. Danowski A, de Azevedo MN, de Souza Papi JA, Petri M. Determinants of risk for venous and arterial thrombosis in primary antiphospholipid syndrome and in antiphospholipid syndrome with systemic lupus erythematosus. J Rheumatol. 2009;36(6):1195–9.
37. Clowse ME, Magder LS, Witter F, Petri M. The impact of increased lupus activity on obstetric outcomes. Arthritis Rheum. 2005;52(2):514–21.
38. Petri M, Allbritton J. Fetal outcome of lupus pregnancy: a retrospective case-control study of the Hopkins lupus cohort. J Rheumatol. 1993;20(4): 650–6.
39. Georgiou PE, Politi EN, Katsimbri P, Sakka V, Drosos AA. Outcome of lupus pregnancy: a controlled study. Rheumatology (Oxford). 2000;39(9):1014–9.
40. Yasmeen S, Wilkins EE, Field NT, Sheikh RA, Gilbert WM. Pregnancy outcomes in women with systemic lupus erythematosus. J Matern Fetal Med. 2001; 10(2):91–6.
41. Moroni G, Ponticelli C. The risk of pregnancy in patients with lupus nephritis. J Nephrol. 2003;16(2): 161–7.
42. Lê Huong D, Wechsler B, Vauthier-Brouzes D, Seebacher J, Lefèbvre G, Blétry O, et al. Outcome of planned pregnancies in systemic lupus erythematosus: a prospective study on 62 pregnancies. Br J Rheumatol. 1997;36(7):772–7.
43. Rahman FZ, Rahman J, Al-Suleiman SA, Rahman MS. Pregnancy outcome in lupus nephropathy. Arch Gynecol Obstet. 2005;271(3):222–6.
44. Wagner SJ, Craici I, Reed D, Norby S, Bailey K, Wiste HJ, et al. Maternal and foetal outcomes in pregnant patients with active lupus nephritis. Lupus. 2009;18(4):342–7.
45. Geis W, Branch DW. Obstetric implications of antiphospholipid antibodies: pregnancy loss and other complications. Clin Obstet Gynecol. 2001;44(1): 2–10.
46. Esplin MS. Management of antiphospholipid syndrome during pregnancy. Clin Obstet Gynecol. 2001;44(1):20–8.
47. Ostensen M, Villiger PM. The remission of rheumatoid arthritis during pregnancy. Semin Immunopathol. 2007;29(2):185–91.
48. Nielsen OH, Loftus EV, Jess T. Safety of TNF-α inhibitors during IBD pregnancy: a systematic review. BMC Med. 2013;11:174.
49. Jungers P, Dougados M, Pélissier C, Kuttenn F, Tron F, Lesavre P, et al. Influence of oral contraceptive therapy on the activity of systemic lupus erythematosus. Arthritis Rheum. 1982;25(6):618–23.
50. Buyon JP, Petri MA, Kim MY, Kalunian KC, Grossman J, Hahn BH, et al. The effect of combined estrogen and progesterone hormone replacement therapy on disease activity in systemic lupus erythematosus: a randomized trial. Ann Intern Med. 2005;142(12 Pt 1):953–62.
51. Browne H, Manipalviratn S, Armstrong A. Using an intrauterine device in immunocompromised women. Obstet Gynecol. 2008;112(3):667–9.

52. Morrison CS, Sekadde-Kigondu C, Sinei SK, Weiner DH, Kwok C, Kokonya D. Is the intrauterine device appropriate contraception for HIV-1-infected women? BJOG. 2001;108(8):784–90.
53. Stringer EM, Kaseba C, Levy J, Sinkala M, Goldenberg RL, Chi BH, et al. A randomized trial of the intrauterine contraceptive device vs hormonal contraception in women who are infected with the human immunodeficiency virus. Am J Obstet Gynecol. 2007;197(2):144.e1–8.
54. Schwarz EB, Maselli J, Gonzales R. Contraceptive counseling of diabetic women of reproductive age. Obstet Gynecol. 2006;107(5):1070–4.
55. Guazzelli CA, Torloni MR, Sanches TF, Barbieri M, Pestana JO. Contraceptive counseling and use among 197 female kidney transplant recipients. Transplantation. 2008;86(5):669–72.
56. Chuang CH, Chase GA, Bensyl DM, Weisman CS. Contraceptive use by diabetic and obese women. Womens Health Issues. 2005;15(4):167–73.
57. Schwarz EB, Manzi S. Risk of unintended pregnancy among women with systemic lupus erythematosus. Arthritis Rheum. 2008;59(6):863–6.
58. Finer LB, Jerman J, Kavanaugh ML. Changes in use of long-acting contraceptive methods in the United States, 2007–2009. Fertil Steril. 2012;98(4):893–7.
59. Sánchez-Guerrero J, Uribe AG, Jiménez-Santana L, Mestanza-Peralta M, Lara-Reyes P, Seuc AH, et al. A trial of contraceptive methods in women with systemic lupus erythematosus. N Engl J Med. 2005; 353(24):2539–49.
60. Petri M, Kim MY, Kalunian KC, Grossman J, Hahn BH, Sammaritano LR, et al. Combined oral contraceptives in women with systemic lupus erythematosus. N Engl J Med. 2005;353(24):2550–8.
61. Farr SL, Folger SG, Paulen ME, Curtis KM. Safety of contraceptive methods for women with rheumatoid arthritis: a systematic review. Contraception. 2010; 82(1):64–71.
62. VIGNOS PJ, DORFMAN RI. Effect of large doses of progesterone in rheumatoid arthritis. Am J Med Sci. 1951;222(1):29–34.
63. Chopra N, Koren S, Greer WL, Fortin PR, Rauch J, Fortin I, et al. Factor V Leiden, prothrombin gene mutation, and thrombosis risk in patients with antiphospholipid antibodies. J Rheumatol. 2002; 29(8):1683–8.
64. Choojitarom K, Verasertniyom O, Totemchokchyakarn K, Nantiruj K, Sumethkul V, Janwityanujit S. Lupus nephritis and Raynaud's phenomenon are significant risk factors for vascular thrombosis in SLE patients with positive antiphospholipid antibodies. Clin Rheumatol. 2008;27(3):345–51.
65. Mantha S, Karp R, Raghavan V, Terrin N, Bauer KA, Zwicker JI. Assessing the risk of venous thromboembolic events in women taking progestin-only contraception: a meta-analysis. BMJ. 2012;345:e4944.
66. Chabbert-Buffet N, Amoura Z, Scarabin PY, Frances C, Lévy DP, Galicier L, et al. Pregnane progestin contraception in systemic lupus erythematosus: a longitudinal study of 187 patients. Contraception. 2011;83(3): 229–37.
67. Julkunen HA, Kaaja R, Friman C. Contraceptive practice in women with systemic lupus erythematosus. Br J Rheumatol. 1993;32(3):227–30.
68. Petri M. Musculoskeletal complications of systemic lupus erythematosus in the Hopkins lupus cohort: an update. Arthritis Care Res. 1995;8(3):137–45.
69. Haugeberg G, Ørstavik RE, Kvien TK. Effects of rheumatoid arthritis on bone. Curr Opin Rheumatol. 2003;15(4):469–75.
70. Ramsey-Goldman R, Dunn JE, Huang CF, Dunlop D, Rairie JE, Fitzgerald S, et al. Frequency of fractures in women with systemic lupus erythematosus: comparison with United States population data. Arthritis Rheum. 1999;42(5):882–90.
71. Lopez LM, Chen M, Mullins S, Curtis KM, Helmerhorst FM. Steroidal contraceptives and bone fractures in women: evidence from observational studies. Cochrane Database Syst Rev. 2012;8, CD009849.
72. Lanza LL, McQuay LJ, Rothman KJ, Bone HG, Kaunitz AM, Harel Z, et al. Use of depot medroxyprogesterone acetate contraception and incidence of bone fracture. Obstet Gynecol. 2013;121(3):593–600.
73. Nossent JC, Swaak AJ. Prevalence and significance of haematological abnormalities in patients with systemic lupus erythematosus. Q J Med. 1991;80(291): 605–12.
74. Keeling DM, Isenberg DA. Haematological manifestations of systemic lupus erythematosus. Blood Rev. 1993;7(4):199–207.
75. Pisoni CN, Cuadrado MJ, Khamashta MA, Hunt BJ. Treatment of menorrhagia associated with oral anticoagulation: efficacy and safety of the levonorgestrel releasing intrauterine device (Mirena coil). Lupus. 2006;15(12):877–80.
76. Schaedel ZE, Dolan G, Powell MC. The use of the levonorgestrel-releasing intrauterine system in the management of menorrhagia in women with hemostatic disorders. Am J Obstet Gynecol. 2005;193(4): 1361–3.
77. Faculty of Sexual and Reproductive Healthcare. UK medical eligibility criteria for contraceptive use (UKMEC 2009). 2009. http://www.fsrh.org/pdfs/UKMEC2009.pdf.
78. Division of Reproductive Health, National Center for Chronic Disease Prevention and Health Promotion, Centers for Disease Control and Prevention (CDC). US selected practice recommendations for contraceptive use, 2013: adapted from the World Health Organization selected practice recommendations for contraceptive use, 2nd edn. MMWR Recomm Rep. 2013;62(RR-05):1–60.

Contraception for Women with Gastrointestinal Disorders

18

Aparna Sridhar, Wendy Ho, Tram T. Tran, Angela Chen, and Anish Vinit Patel

Introduction

The gastrointestinal (GI) system serves two of the main functions of the human body: assimilating nutrients and eliminating waste. The diseases of the GI system can result from abnormalities within or outside of the gut and range in severity from those that produce mild symptoms and no long-term morbidity to those with intractable symptoms or adverse outcomes. Diseases may be localized to one organ or exhibit diffuse involvement at many sites. The most common symptoms of GI diseases, such as abdominal pain, heartburn, nausea, vomiting, altered bowel habits, and bleeding, can cause significant distress in day-to-day life. Women of reproductive age can suffer from variety of diseases due to alterations of gastrointestinal system. In addition, pregnancy alters the anatomy and physiology of GI tract. Therapy for many GI diseases must be altered during pregnancy. Women are encouraged to optimize their GI conditions prior to conception for best perinatal outcome. Thus, planned pregnancy after health optimization and maintenance of appropriate therapies bodes best for both the mother and her intended family.

This chapter aims to describe the scope of GI diseases among women of reproductive age and the scientific evidence behind contraception usage among women with some common GI diseases. Among the common GI diseases in women, we have focused on those conditions that are mentioned in the United States Medical Eligibility Criteria for Contraceptive Use published by the Centers for Disease Control and Prevention (USMEC) [1]. This chapter will include a brief description of common GI diseases in women of reproductive age, risks of pregnancy-related complications with these diseases, use and safety of contraception usage for each GI condition, and useful patient assessment tools.

A. Sridhar, M.D., M.P.H., F.A.C.O.G. (✉)
Department of Obstetrics and Gynecology, University of California Los Angeles, Los Angeles, CA, USA
e-mail: asridhar@mednet.ucla.edu

W. Ho, M.D., M.P.H.
Division of Digestive Diseases, Department of Medicine, University of California Los Angeles, Los Angeles, CA, USA
e-mail: wwho@mednet.ucla.edu

T.T. Tran, M.D.
Department of Gastroenterology, Liver Transplant, Cedars Sinai Medical Center, Los Angeles, CA, USA
e-mail: tram.tran@cshs.org

A. Chen, M.D., M.P.H.
Department of Obstetrics and Gynecology, David Geffen School of Medicine at UCLA, UCLA Health System, Los Angeles, CA, USA
e-mail: angelachen@mednet.ucla.edu

A.V. Patel, M.D.
Department of Internal Medicine, Cedars Sinai Medical Center, Los Angeles, CA, USA
e-mail: anish.patel@cshs.org

R.H. Allen and C.A. Cwiak (eds.), *Contraception for the Medically Challenging Patient*, DOI 10.1007/978-1-4939-1233-9_18, © Springer Science+Business Media New York 2014

Scope of the Problem

An overview of most common GI diseases with incidence, prevalence, and diagnosis is provided in this section.

Inflammatory Bowel Disease

Inflammatory bowel disease (IBD) is a group of conditions characterized by chronic immune activation and inflammation in the gastrointestinal tract. Ulcerative colitis and Crohn's disease are the two major forms of IBD. Ulcerative colitis affects the colon in a continuous and CIRCUMFERENTIAL manner, starting at the rectum and extending proximally. There is often a sharp demarcation between the diseased and normal segments of colon. In addition, the inflammation in ulcerative colitis is limited to the mucosal layer of the colon. On the other hand, Crohn's disease can affect any portion of the luminal GI tract, from the mouth to the anal canal, but it most commonly affects the distal small intestine and proximal colon. Inflammation in Crohn's disease is often discontinuous (skip lesions) and the inflammation can affect all layers of the intestine, from the mucosa to the serosa. Given the transmural involvement, advanced Crohn's disease can be associated with sinuses, fistulas, strictures, and walled-off abscesses.

IBD is most often diagnosed in patients 20–30 years of age with a second peak in diagnosis from 60–70 years of age. The symptoms of IBD reflect the area of the GI tract that is involved and can include fever, abdominal pain, diarrhea, rectal bleeding, tenesmus, and urgency. Crohn's disease patients may also have obstructive symptoms. Patients may also have extraintestinal manifestations of IBD including ankylosing spondylitis, sacroiliitis, erythema nodosum, pyoderma gangrenosum, Sweet's syndrome, primary sclerosing cholangitis, uveitis, and episcleritis. The incidence and prevalence of IBD is increasing. In a recent study, the incidence of ulcerative colitis in North America was found to be 19.2 cases/100,000 person-years and the incidence of Crohn's disease was found to be approximately 20.2 cases/100,000 person-years. The prevalence of ulcerative colitis in North America was 249/100,000 and that of Crohn's disease was 319/100,000 [2]. The incidence and prevalence are greater in North America and Europe and have been found to be lower in Asia and the Middle East.

Gallbladder Disease

Gallstones are very common, and it is estimated that 12 % of the United States (US) population has gallstones. Most cases of gallstone disease are silent, but 1/3 will eventually cause symptoms and complications. Female sex [3], age 40 and above [4], pregnancy, multiparity [5], and obesity [6] are risk factors for gallstone formation. Cholestasis can be caused by sepsis, medications, and biliary obstruction. Primary biliary cirrhosis and primary sclerosing cholangitis are two diseases that also cause cholestasis. In addition, cholestasis with hepatitis is also seen and is associated with viral hepatitis and medications. Medications that can cause cholestasis include sex steroids, anabolic steroids, amoxicillin-clavulanic acid, sulfonamides, griseofulvin, ketoconazole, tamoxifen, warfarin, ibuprofen, cyclosporine, and tacrolimus, among others. Cholestasis is caused by diminished bile flow, which includes bile acids, bilirubin, cholesterol, and trace elements. Instead of these substances being excreted through bile into the gut lumen, there is biliary stasis in the liver, which can lead to progressive liver damage, including biliary cirrhosis, portal hypertension, and liver failure. Decreased bile flow into the proximal small intestine can also cause impaired digestion and absorption of long-chain triglycerides and fat-soluble vitamins.

Viral Hepatitis

Viral hepatitis remains a global health issue with an estimated 1.25 million people in the US, and 350 million people worldwide chronically infected with hepatitis B [7]. In the case of hepatitis C, the prevalence of chronic infection ranges from low (less than 2.5 %) in North America and Europe, to intermediate (2.5–10 %) in South America and the Middle East, to high (greater than 10 %) in Africa [8]. There are no significant differences in the frequency of hepatitis A, B, and C, herpes simplex (HSV), cytomegalovirus (CMV), and Epstein Barr virus (EBV) in pregnant and nonpregnant individuals; cumulatively 40 % of jaundice cases in the US are caused by these entities [9].

Cirrhosis and Chronic Liver Failure

Cirrhosis and chronic liver failure together make up the 12th most common cause of death in the US in 2002, accounting for 9.5 deaths per 100,000 individuals. In the US, there were 36,000 hospital discharges related to cirrhosis and liver failure in 2000, and there were 17,935 persons with cirrhosis in 2005 waiting for a liver transplant. Approximately 40 % of patients with cirrhosis are asymptomatic [10].

The most common etiologies that cause cirrhosis include alcohol, chronic viral hepatitis, and nonalcoholic fatty liver disease (NASH). Cirrhosis is defined as a "progressive, diffuse, fibrosing and nodular condition that disrupts the normal architecture of the liver." Usually, it is estimated that at least 80 % of the liver parenchyma must be destroyed before someone manifests with liver failure. Hence cirrhosis is often initially a "silent disease" with most individuals remaining asymptomatic until liver failure and decompensation occurs. Early and well-compensated cirrhosis may present with anorexia, weight loss, and fatigue. As the disease progresses, one can present with ascites, spontaneous bacterial peritonitis, hepatic encephalopathy, or variceal bleeding [10].

Liver Tumors

Liver tumors are common in women of reproductive age. Hemangiomas are one of the most common liver tumors. There are benign vascular tumors found in 0.4–7.3 % of cases in the general population [11]. Another type of common liver tumor is the hepatic adenoma, which is also a benign liver tumor that occurs in women especially during their reproductive years. Some studies show an estimated incidence of hepatic adenoma of 1–1.3 per one million in those who have never used oral contraceptives, and 30–40 per one million in long-term users of oral contraceptives. It is postulated that estrogen or other steroids contribute to development of these rare adenomas. There is an overall 4.2 % risk of malignant transformation of adenomas [12].

Baseline Risks of GI Diseases in Pregnancy

Inflammatory Bowel Disease

Women with IBD have a higher risk of pregnancy complications compared to the general population, including early pregnancy loss, preterm birth, and complications of labor and delivery [13]. It is recommended that IBD disease be well controlled and in remission when a woman is considering pregnancy. The risk of an IBD flare in a woman who conceives while her IBD is in remission is similar to that of the nonpregnant patient. However, if a woman conceives during an active IBD flare, she has more than 50 % risk of persistent/worsening disease activity during the course of pregnancy [14]. Active disease at the time of conception is associated with a higher rate of early pregnancy loss. In addition, disease activity during pregnancy is associated with low birth weight and premature birth [15]. Therefore, women should be in remission while attempting to conceive and many women will need to stay on IBD medications in order to maintain remission through conception and pregnancy. However, they often have concerns about the safety of IBD drugs during conception and pregnancy (see the further discussion that follows). The key concept in managing a woman of childbearing age with IBD is that active disease, not treatment, poses the greatest risk to the fetus. Therefore, it is of utmost importance to keep the IBD in remission, both preconception and during pregnancy. Often, that means that women will need to be on therapy.

Since planned conception during a period of IBD remission rather than active disease is recommended, contraception in the IBD patient is very important. IBD frequently affects women during their childbearing years, and women with IBD need effective contraception to prevent unplanned pregnancy.

Gallbladder Disease

Pregnant women with gallstones are usually asymptomatic. However, symptomatic gallbladder disease is the second most common nonobstetrical abdominal emergency (after acute appendicitis) in pregnant women. In pregnancy, there is decreased gallbladder motility (from progesterone) and supersaturation of cholesterol in bile (from estrogen), which increases the risk of gallstone formation. Of note, estrogen hormonal therapy [16] also increases the risk of gallstone formation and combined oral contraceptive (COC) [17, 18] use slightly increases the risk of gallstone formation.

The primary symptom of biliary colic is epigastric or right upper quadrant abdominal pain that occurs 1–3 h after meals (classically fatty meals). Acute cholecystitis manifests as right upper quadrant abdominal pain with Murphy's sign (when examiner palpates gallbladder fossa under liver edge and patient takes a deep breath, the patient experiences pain and catches his/her breath), fever, and sometimes nausea and vomiting. Labs can show mild elevations of transaminases, alkaline phosphatase, or direct bilirubin. Significant elevations of these labs can be seen in choledocholithiasis, which can also cause pancreatitis with elevations of amylase and lipase. In suspected cholecystitis, ultrasound is the imaging test of choice, as it can show gallstones, gallbladder wall thickening in cholecystitis, and a sonographic Murphy's sign (abdominal pain and catching of breath observed with palpation of the gallbladder with the ultrasound probe), which is more accurate than the clinical Murphy's sign, since it confirms that the symptoms are due to palpation of the gallbladder. Computed tomography (CT) scan can also be used, although some gallstones which are isodense with bile are not visualized by CT scan. Initial episodes of biliary colic should be treated with supportive care. However, if the episodes are recurrent or if they are complicated by acute cholecystitis, choledocholithiasis, cholangitis, or biliary pancreatitis, hospitalization and prompt treatment with surgery or ERCP is needed. Pregnant women with symptomatic gallbladder disease who are treated surgically with cholecystectomy have better outcomes than those who are treated conservatively. Therefore, surgical treatment, preferably by laparoscopy in the second or early third trimester, is preferred [19, 20].

Liver Disease

Hepatitis

In the pregnant population, acute hepatitis A occurs in 1 per 1,000, while acute hepatitis B occurs in 2 per 1,000. Hepatitis E (HEV) infection is extremely rare in the US. However, it is endemic to populations in Asia, Africa, and Central America [9], and remains the most common cause of acute viral hepatitis worldwide [21] as well as being the most common viral cause of acute liver failure in pregnancy [22]. HSV, CMV, and EBV hepatitis are rare, and occur predominantly in individuals who are immunocompromised. Initial suspicion for viral hepatitis should be considered when any individual is noted to have transaminitis on laboratory testing. Additionally, risk factors such as multiple sexual partners, intravenous drug use, and contact with known infected individuals should increase suspicion for viral hepatitis. Acute hepatitis, if symptomatic, usually presents with nonspecific constitutional symptoms such as nausea, malaise, loss of appetite, or abdominal pain that are hard to differentiate from pregnancy induced nausea and vomiting. Findings of jaundice and abnormal liver function tests should prompt medical assessment in pregnancy. Chronic hepatitis may be more likely to be asymptomatic unless there is more advanced disease. Evaluation of acute hepatitis must include serologies for hepatitis A, B, and C (anti-HAV IgM, HBs Ag, anti-HBc IgM, and anti-HCV).

Pregnant women with chronic hepatitis B (HBV) are at risk of transmitting the virus to the fetus (vertical transmission). This is most common mode of transmission of HBV in endemic areas. Transmission can occur via the placenta (prenatal), during breastfeeding (postnatal), or during delivery. The mode of delivery does not appear to affect transmission risk, with similar rates seen with vaginal delivery and cesarean section [22]. Perinatal transmission of hepatitis B is highest in those individuals with acute hepatitis. Transmission rates are 50–80 % in patients with hepatitis B surface antigen positivity as these individuals have the highest levels of viral replication, 25 % compared to only 5 % in inactive carriers [9]. Additionally, HBV viral load is another significant risk factor for transmission, with high viral loads associated with an 80–90 % risk versus 10–30 % in those with undetectable viral load without immunoprophylaxis of the newborn [22]. Recent data suggest that in women with hepatitis B infection and high viral levels with HBV greater then 10X 8 copies/ml, perinatal transmission of hepatitis B may still be approximately 8%, even with appropriate immunoprophylaxis. Antiviral therapy in the third trimester may reduce this risk of transmission. Treatment of the pregnant woman with chronic HCV infection has previously been contraindicated due to low perinatal transmission rates and toxicity of medications including interferon and ribavirin. Even with new oral antiviral therapies for HCV becoming readily available, it is unlikely that therapy would be of urgent need to treat during pregnancy.

Cirrhosis

Pregnancy in women with cirrhosis is rare, as chronic liver disease, through hypothalamic–pituitary axis dysfunction and disturbed estrogen metabolism, typically results in anovulation, amenorrhea, and infertility [9, 22]. Should pregnancy occur, there are increased rare cases of early pregnancy loss, growth restriction (5 %), prematurity (39 %), and perinatal death (6 %) [23]. Physiologic changes include worsening portal hypertension due to increased blood volume as well as external compression of the inferior vena cava by the uterus. Patients with varices have an estimated 25 % risk of a bleeding episode, with the risk greatest in the second trimester (when portal pressures peak) and during delivery (with repeated Valsalva maneuvers) [8]. In the case of variceal bleeding, there is an associated mortality of 18 and 11 % for the woman and the fetus, respectively. Other risks include thrombocytopenia, rupture of splenic aneurysms (2.6 %), and placental abruption (7 %) related to coagulopathy and gestational hypertension [9, 23]. Cirrhotic patients are likely to experience a significant liver-related complication during pregnancy, and it may be safest to advise these patients against pregnancy [24]. The optimal management of pregnancy in women with cirrhosis is undefined. These cases must be comanaged by a high-risk obstetrician and a hepatologist. Currently, the American Association for the Study of Liver Disease (AASLD) recommends that all pregnant individuals with cirrhosis undergo screening for varices with an upper endoscopy in the second trimester (as this represents the time period when portal pressures increase and peak) [24]. The stress of pregnancy increases the risk of liver decompensation (up to 24 %), with a maternal mortality rate as high as 13–22 %, and fetal mortality of 12 % [25].

Liver Tumors

Liver masses identified during pregnancy are more commonly benign than malignant. These include hemangiomas, adenomas, focal nodal hyperplasia, angiomyolipoma, and lymphangiomatosis [11]. Most patients with liver tumors are asymptomatic and the tumors are often identified as an incidental finding on ultrasonographic examinations. In the case of symptomatic patients, they can present with right upper quadrant pain (usually due to intra-tumor bleeding) and elevated liver enzymes. This presentation can be difficult to differentiate from other more common etiologies of abdominal pain in pregnancy—preeclampsia, HELLP (Hemolysis, Elevated Liver enzymes, and Low Platelets) syndrome, gallbladder disease, or biliary pancreatitis. This can result in a diagnostic delay; however, with advanced imaging modalities, the time to diagnosis has improved [12, 26]. During pregnancy, there is a concern for liver tumor growth, with subsequent rupture and progression to hemorrhage. Acute onset of nausea, vomiting, right upper quadrant, or epigastric pain in any pregnant individual may be indicative of tumor enlargement and possible hemorrhage.

Individuals with hemangiomas usually have an indolent course, and though there is a risk of rupture during pregnancy, this risk does not appear to be different between pregnant and non-pregnant women [11]. Hepatic adenomas are sensitive to hormones, and are at a risk of hormone induced growth and rupture. These risks are exacerbated during pregnancy due to increased levels of steroid hormones. Some initial studies by Cobey et al. reported a maternal and fetal mortality of 44 and 38 %, respectively, in the event of a ruptured adenoma during pregnancy. The risk of rupture is greatest during the third trimester of pregnancy, likely due to high levels of accumulating estrogens and increase in vascularity of the liver with resulting growth of the adenoma [12]. The risk of bleeding is also high in the postpartum period, when sudden withdrawal of estrogens after delivery may cause a sudden regression of the tumor, resulting in hemorrhage [26]. Surgical management is recommended for large symptomatic tumors in the nonpregnant state. Other treatments include radio frequency ablation and selective arterial embolization. In pregnant women, close monitoring of the adenoma with ultrasound or magnetic resonance imaging (MRI) is recommended for surveillance of the size.

From the preceding descriptions of each disease it is very clear that pregnancy can pose serious risks to the health of mother and women with GI diseases.

Use of Contraception in Women with GI Diseases

With advances in medical treatment, women with chronic GI illnesses may live longer with better quality of life. Contraception becomes an integral component of the balancing act between their personal, professional, and reproductive life goals. Literature is lacking on the nature and extent to which family planning issues are discussed with patients who have GI disease. Most of the data on contraception use and counseling offered for women with GI diseases are from inflammatory bowel disease-related studies. A recent study published by Gawron et al. conducted a random sample chart review of women with IBD and identified that only 19 out of 100 patients had documentation of reproductive counseling and only 1 of 100 patients had a specific reference to use contraception to avoid unintended pregnancy [27]. Available data on women with IBD suggests that women rely on their gastroenterologist for counseling on IBD-related reproductive health concerns [28].

This likely demonstrates a large unmet need for contraception in women with gastrointestinal diseases, which have the potential to cause adverse pregnancy outcomes.

Risks of Contraception

The World Health Organization (WHO) has developed recommendations for use of specific contraceptive methods by women with specific medical conditions, entitled the Medical Eligibility Criteria for Contraceptive Use. The Centers for Disease Control and Prevention (CDC) created the US Medical Eligibility Criteria for Contraceptive Use (USMEC) for contraceptive use by modifying the WHO recommendations specifically for use in the US [1]. In the following sections, we will discuss the recommendations from the USMEC for contraceptive use among women with GI diseases. We will also identify other evidence (if available) to support the use of specific contraceptive methods among these women (Table 18.1).

Combined Hormonal Contraception (CHC)

The USMEC groups low-dose combined oral contraceptives (COCs) containing less than or equal to 35 μg of ethinyl estradiol, the combined hormonal patch, and combined vaginal ring as combined hormonal contraceptives (CHCs). Based on the available evidence, hormonal formulations, pharmacokinetic profiles, and safety of these methods are comparable to each other [29, 30]. For women with inflammatory bowel disease with no other risk factors for venous thromboembolism (VTE), USMEC recommends

Table 18.1 Contraception for women with gastrointestinal diseases[a]

Gastrointestinal diseases	CHC	POP	DMPA	Implant	Lng-IUD	Cu-IUD	Barrier
Inflammatory bowel disease	2/3	2	2	1	1	1	1
Gallbladder disease							
Symptomatic	2/3	2	2	2	2	1	1
Asymptomatic	2	2	2	2	2	1	1
History of cholestasis							
Pregnancy related	2	1	1	1	1	1	1
COC related	3	2	2	2	2	1	1
Viral hepatitis							
Acute or flare hepatitis	3/4	1	1	1	1	1	1
Carrier	1	1	1	1	1	1	1
Chronic	1	1	1	1	1	1	1
Cirrhosis							
Mild cirrhosis	1	1	1	1	1	1	1
Severe cirrhosis	4	3	3	3	3	1	1
Liver tumors							
Focal nodular hyperplasia of liver	2	2	2	2	2	1	1
Hepatocellular adenoma	4	3	3	3	3	1	1
Malignant hepatoma	4	3	3	3	3	1	1

CHC combined hormonal contraception, *POP* progesterone-only pills, *DMPA* depot medroxyprogesterone, *Lng-IUD* levonorgestrel intrauterine device, *Cu-IUD* copper intrauterine device, *Barrier* condom, spermicide, diaphragm, or cap

Key: 1 = A condition for which there is no restriction for the use of the contraceptive method. 2 = A condition for which the advantages of using the method generally outweigh the theoretical or proven risks. 3 = A condition for which the theoretical or proven risks usually outweigh the advantages of using the method. 4 = A condition that represents an unacceptable health risk if the contraceptive method is used

[a]Information adapted from Curtis KM, Tepper NK, Marchbanks PA. U.S. medical eligibility criteria for contraceptive use, 2010. Journal of Women's Health (2002). 2011 Jun;20(6):825–8. PubMed PMID: 21671772. Epub 2011/06/16. eng

that the benefits of using CHCs generally out weigh the risks (category 2). However, caution should be exercised when prescribing CHCs for women with IBD who have additional risk factors for VTE as the risks of use usually outweigh the benefits (category 3) [1]. Factors increasing the risk of VTE include extensive active disease, surgery, immobilization, and corticosteroid use. Risk of VTE and thrombosis in general are thought to be higher among women with IBD due to multiple interactions between acquired and inherited factors [31]. Thus, it is difficult to tease out the risk of VTE for women with IBD that is attributable to using CHCs. These recommendations are supported by the systematic review by Zapata et al. [32]. The review also highlights the fact that absorption of ethinyl estradiol (EE) and progestin may be impaired in women with inflammation or ulceration of intestinal mucosa and past bowel surgery (as in the severe cases of Crohn's disease). Based on the available evidence, there seems to be no relationship between COC use after diagnosis of IBD and relapse of the disease [33–36].

For women with asymptomatic gallbladder disease and symptomatic disease treated with cholecystectomy the USMEC recommends that the benefits of using CHCs generally outweigh the risks (category 2). For those who have medically treated disease or currently active gallbladder disease, the risk of worsening of the disease needs to be carefully considered before prescribing CHCs (category 3). Most of the data suggesting association between gallbladder diseases and COCs were found in earlier studies in which higher-dose EE formulations (50 μg) were used. A transient effect of COC use on the rate of gallbladder disease with a dose–effect relationship with EE was noted [17]. Over the course of the next few years, the progestin component (especially drospirenone) was hypothetically associated with gallbladder disease, although with no good scientific evidence. However, recent studies have shown that neither drospirenone nor levonorgestrel-containing COCs have any effect on increased risk of gallbladder disease compared to non-COC users [18, 37]. Although the exact mechanism is unknown, estrogen and 17-alkylated steroids can possibly induce cholestasis by causing changes in the bile acid transport protein expression or localization [38]. Thus, prior history of COC-related cholestasis predicts higher risk with subsequent hormonal use (category 3). For women with history of pregnancy-induced cholestasis, benefits of using COCs usually outweigh the risks (category 2).

Based on a systematic review evaluating the effects of combined hormonal contraceptive use among women with viral hepatitis and cirrhosis of liver [39] the World Health Organization (WHO) made some recommendations that are adapted in the USMEC. For women who have chronic hepatitis or who are carriers of the disease, there is no restriction to CHC use (category 1). For women with acute hepatitis, the risks of initiating CHCs generally outweigh the benefits, especially for severe disease (category 3/4). However, if a woman is already on a CHC, benefits of continuing the method during an acute flare generally outweigh the risks (category 2). For women with mild compensated liver cirrhosis, there is no restriction to the use of CHCs (category 1). However, CHCs should be avoided (category 4) in women with severe decompensated cirrhosis.

Benign liver tumors have been associated with long-term COC use. A role of sex steroids has been suggested on the incidence of focal nodular hyperplasia, given the female predominance of the disease. Higher baseline incidence of focal nodular hyperplasia has been suggested among women on COC (relative risk of ever COC use was 1.96) [40]. However, no rapid change in the size of adenoma was noted with COC use. Thus, USMEC suggests that benefits of using CHCs among women with focal nodular hyperplasia may outweigh the risks associated with it (category 2). Use of CHCs in women with hepatocellular adenoma or carcinoma is contraindicated [41]. USMEC recommends against use of CHCs among women with hepatocellular adenoma or malignant hepatoma (category 4). These liver tumors have been reported to be larger and more prone to hemorrhage and rupture in users of earlier generation COCs. This was attributed to vascular changes, ranging from minute areas of hemorrhage to small and diffuse liver hemangiomas [42].

Short-Term Progestin-Only Methods

Progestin-only pills (POPs) containing norethindrone, and depot medroxyprogesterone acetate (DMPA) injection are included in this category. A very scant body of literature exists about the safety of such formulations in women with GI diseases.

Progestin-Only Pills (POPS)

Similar to COCs, POPs may have reduced efficacy due to theoretical concern of malabsorption in women with severe small intestinal disease or small bowel surgery. Only one study was noted to have included POPs, and no adverse effects were noted with their use in women with IBD. However only 14 of 134 women in this study were using POPs and they did not have any different flare up rates compared to nonusers [33]. USMEC recommends the usage of POPs among women with IBD as benefits outweigh risks (category 2). For women with gallbladder disease, USMEC categorizes use of POPs as category 2 as well. In the study mentioned previously for COCs, both levonorgestrel and drospirenone use were compared (in COC formulations) with non-oral contraceptive use and no increased risk of gallbladder disease was noted [37]. However, no direct evidence exists with norethindrone formulations. Theoretically, a history of COC-related cholestasis might predict subsequent cholestasis with POP use. However, this has not been documented [1]. Thus, USMEC suggests that women with pregnancy-related cholestasis can use progestin-only methods without any restrictions (category 1) and even in those with COC-induced cholestasis the benefits of use generally outweigh the risks (category 2). For women with liver diseases, most of the evidence for the use of POPs comes from COC literature. USMEC suggests unrestricted use of POPs among women with acute and chronic hepatitis as well as mild compensated cirrhosis (category 1). Health care providers must exercise caution when prescribing these pills to women with compensated severe cirrhosis, and benign and malignant liver tumors as the risks usually outweigh the benefits (category 3).

Depot Medroxyprogesterone Acetate (DMPA)

The USMEC categories for the DMPA use for women with GI diseases (IBD, gallbladder disease, and liver diseases) are exactly the same as for POP use. Studies involving DMPA use among women with GI diseases are needed to strengthen the body of evidence. Women with inflammatory bowel disease are at higher risk for osteopenia and osteoporosis [43]. The use of corticosteroids contributes to the decline in bone loss; however, osteoporosis may develop in patients with inflammatory bowel disease independent of corticosteroid use [44, 45]. Given that long-term use of DMPA has been associated with decreased bone mineral density, USMEC cautions providers when using DMPA for a extended period of time among women with inflammatory bowel disease, though its use is assigned category 2 [46, 47].

Long-Acting Reversible Contraception (LARC)

The USMEC recommends use of long-acting reversible contraception (LARC) including hormonal intrauterine devices, copper intrauterine devices, and contraceptive implants among patients with inflammatory bowel disease without restrictions (category 1). There are no good studies to strengthen the evidence for usage of LARC methods among women with IBD. However, the intrauterine devices (IUDs) primarily prevent pregnancy by a combination of the foreign body effect and the specific medication (copper or levonorgestrel) that is released [48]. And so, the mechanism of action is independent of GI absorption of sex steroids, making them suitable for women with IBD. Two case reports described exacerbation of IBD among three women using the levonorgestrel IUD that occurred 5–25 days after insertion of the device. One of these reports did not document outcomes after removal. The second case report described gradual improvement in flare symptoms 3 months after removal of the IUD [49, 50]. Future studies should address the gaps in knowledge related to the safety and effectiveness of long-acting contraceptives for women with IBD.

For women with gallbladder disease, USMEC recommends unrestricted use of copper intrauterine device (category 1). Based on the same evidence as that of oral contraceptive use, USMEC suggests that it may be beneficial to use the levonorgestrel IUD or the contraceptive implant in situations where pregnancy poses serious risks (category 2). There appears to be no data on the use of LARC methods related to the safety and effectiveness for women with liver disease or liver tumors. The WHO expert working group reviewed the evidence to evaluate the medical eligibility criteria for hormonal contraceptive method usage for women with hepatitis and cirrhosis and the following recommendations (adapted in USMEC) were made [41]. Based on these recommendations, USMEC recommends unrestricted use of intrauterine devices and contraceptive implant for women with viral hepatitis and mild compensated cirrhosis (category 1). Although no direct evidence is available, USMEC cautions use of levonorgestrel IUD and contraceptive implant for women with severe decompensated cirrhosis, hepatocellular adenoma, and malignant hepatoma (category 3), though the copper IUD may be used (category 1) [1].

Barrier Methods

The barrier methods include male latex condoms, polyurethane male condoms and female condoms, spermicides, and diaphragm with spermicide or cervical cap. Male condoms can prevent pregnancy and many sexually transmitted infections, including human immunodeficiency virus (HIV). The US Medical Eligibility Criteria recommends no restriction for the use of barrier methods in women with inflammatory bowel disease, gallbladder disease, viral hepatitis, cirrhosis, or liver tumors. Because these barrier methods are nonhormonal, they rarely cause medical problems among users. Barrier methods with latex (male and female latex condoms) are contraindicated in women with latex allergy. The effectiveness of these methods however depends heavily on the skill level and experience of the user.

Emergency Contraception

Two dedicated emergency contraceptive pills available in the US are levonorgestrel (Plan B, Next Choice) and ulipristal acetate (Ella). In addition, the copper intrauterine device is effective as an emergency contraceptive when used within 5 days of unprotected intercourse. The USMEC has recommendations only for the use of levonorgestrel and COC pills as emergency contraception pills (although the COCs are not commonly used as emergency contraception). Although the copper IUD as emergency contraceptive is discussed in the USMEC, the guidelines are not specific to women with GI diseases. They do not include ulipristal acetate in the last set of recommendations published in 2010. For women with ulcerative colitis and Crohn's disease the USMEC recommends no restriction for the use of the emergency contraception pills (category 1). The advantage of using a one-time progestin dose in emergency contraception is considered beneficial even in women with severe liver disease including jaundice (category 2) compared to the risk of an unintended pregnancy complicating the medical condition. In the US, the labeling for levonorgestrel and ulipristal includes only one contraindication: known or suspected pregnancy. This is based on the review by the Committee on Safety of Medicines in the United Kingdom of all the adverse events that occurred during the first 13 years of COC pills usage as emergency contraception. Among four million uses, the review found 61 pregnancies and no serious GI side effects reported [51]. Review of safety of COC use among women with GI issues has already been reviewed in this chapter. The duration of emergency contraception use is less than that of regular use of COCs or progestin-only pills. Thus, USMEC suggests its use among women with GI issues would have minimal anticipated impact.

Surgical Sterilization

This includes tubal sterilization for females and vasectomy for males. Both of these are safe, effective, and permanent methods of contraception. A couple should be counseled about the permanent methods of contraception as options if they are done with childbearing.

Female Sterilization

Two most common methods for female sterilization in the US are postpartum tubal sterilization using a mini-laparotomy incision and interval tubal sterilization using a laparoscopic approach under general anesthesia. The third and relatively newer method of transcervical method of sterilization system called Essure is gaining popularity as well. Failure rates of tubal sterilization in females are comparable to those of long-acting reversible contraception [48]. In 1996 the Centers for Disease Control and Prevention (CDC) conducted a large prospective multicenter observational study of over 10,000 women undergoing trans-abdominal sterilization who were followed for up to 14 years. The study suggested that postpartum sterilization had the lowest cumulative pregnancy rates at 5 and 10 years compared to laparoscopic sterilization [52]. The long-term efficacy of transcervical sterilization method still needs to be fully assessed. High effectiveness, high acceptability, safety, and lack of significant side effects are some of the advantages of female sterilization methods. If a woman still has doubts about the future childbearing, sterilization should not be offered as restoring fertility after sterilization can be very difficult. Even though the surgical procedure of female sterilization is simple, it carries some risks that are specific to the type of sterilization procedure and anesthetic used.

Male Sterilization

Vasectomy has been proven to be one of the highly effective and most reliable contraceptive methods with first-year failure rate of 0.15 % [48]. In women with medical conditions that may have contraindications for the usage of different contraceptive methods, vasectomy of their partners should be considered. Vasectomy is almost always performed under local anesthesia using a no-scalpel approach. This is a safe, reliable technique with minimal side effects. However, the couple should be counseled that vasectomy is not immediately effective and women must use an adjunct contraceptive method until all sperm in the reproductive tract are cleared.

Challenges for Surgical Sterilization in Women with GI Diseases

Surgical sterilization can last anywhere from 30 min to 1 h. Most surgical sterilizations via laparotomy or laparoscopy are performed under general anesthesia. Transcervical sterilizations can be performed in an office-based setting with preoperative administration of ketorolac for pain control. If a woman with a known GI disease has gastrointestinal symptoms such as nausea, vomiting, diarrhea, or alterations in the electrolyte levels, prompt evaluation with preoperative endoscopies or imaging studies of gastrointestinal tract should be conducted prior to elective surgery. Otherwise, there are no major contraindications for women to undergo elective surgery.

Use of Contraceptive Methods for Management of Gynecologic Conditions

Many women use contraceptive methods for their non-contraceptive benefits. Gynecologists treat a variety of benign gynecological conditions using hormonal contraceptives. Treatments for menstrual cycle irregularity, heavy menstrual bleeding, dysmenorrhea, premenstrual syndrome, acne, fibroids, and pelvic pain due to endometriosis are some of the potential non-contraceptive benefits of contraceptive methods. USMEC document clarifies that their recommendations refer to the safety of contraceptive methods being used for contraceptive purposes. The recommendations do not consider the use of contraceptive methods for treatment of medical conditions as the eligibility criteria may differ in such circumstances. The framework of USMEC is helpful to identify the contraceptive choices that are safe in certain conditions. However, even for women with GI diseases, category 2 and category 3 recommendations may vary based on the gynecological need of the patient (see Chap. 13).

Medication Interactions

Role of Gastrointestinal System in the Absorption of Sex Steroids

The gastrointestinal system plays a major role in the absorption of oral contraceptive sex steroids. These hormones are absorbed from the small intestine and they undergo first-pass metabolism through the liver. More than half of the absorbed ethinyl estradiol is conjugated to form glucuronides and sulfate conjugates. The conjugated estrogen is returned to the small intestine through the gallbladder, and the bacteria in the large intestine will then enzymatically unconjugate these compounds. These newly unconjugated estrogens are absorbed from large intestine, and delivered to the liver for absorption, re-conjugation, and excretion. Sex steroids entering the circulation bypassing the oral route (ring, patch, intrauterine device, and implants) are also ultimately conjugated hepatically and excreted in the urine. When the EE from CHCs is in contact with the liver, it induces activation of cytochrome P450 enzymes. Pharmacokinetic studies done with high-dose (50 μg) CHCs suggested that absorption of these steroids did not differ significantly among women with mild ulcerative colitis and those with ileostomy (versus healthy controls) [53, 54].

Drugs most commonly used to treat women with GI diseases and their potential interactions with hormones are described in Table 18.2.

Table 18.2 Drugs most commonly used to treat GI diseases

Name of the drug	Pregnancy FDA category[a]	Interactions with hormonal birth control methods (if any)[b]
Aminosalicylates (sulfasalazine, mesalamine, and balsalazide)	B[c]	No potential interactions are noted with these medications and contraceptive hormones
Antibiotics (amoxicillin and clavulanic acid) for infections	B/C	No interactions are noted with oral contraceptive use and concomitant steroid use
Immunomodulators		
Methotrexate	X	No interactions are noted with oral contraceptive use and concomitant steroid use
6 Mercaptopurine	D	
Cyclosporine	C	Estrogen derivatives may enhance the hepatotoxic effects of cyclosporines, and drospirenone-containing contraceptives may enhance the hyperkalemic effect of cyclosporines. Caution should be exercised when using these drugs concomitantly [55]
Tacrolimus	C	Similar to cyclosporine, tacrolimus should not be used with drospirenone due to the fear of hyperkalemia [56]
Ribavirin	X	No interactions are noted with oral contraceptive use and concomitant steroid use

[a]Adapted from FDA pregnancy categories: A, Controlled Human Studies show no risk; B, No evidence of risk in studies; C, Risk cannot be ruled out; D, Positive evidence of risk; X, Contraindicated in pregnancy
[b]Interactions checked through *Launch Lexi-Interact™ Drug Interactions Program* (see "References")
[c]Product specific: The Asacol and Asacol HD brand of mesalamine is C, due to inactive ingredient dibutyl phthalate (DBP) in the enteric coating. Adverse effects in male rats were noted at doses greater than the recommended human dose. In addition, olsalazine is class C. The rest of the aminosalicylates are class B

Patient Assessment

History

Evaluation of a patient with gastrointestinal disease begins with a careful personal and family history. It is very important to recognize the timing of the symptoms. Acute infections, inflammation, ischemia, or toxic exposure can cause symptoms of shorter duration versus long standing symptoms, which may point towards neoplastic or chronic inflammatory diseases. Ingestion and defecation patterns and associated history of pain is key to elicit in the history. Recent travel history is important and prompts a search for enteric infection. Providers should also elicit detailed history of gastrointestinal bleeding in order to understand the location of the lesion. Medication history is very useful as some of the common medications can cause pain, altered bowel habits, and bleeding. Also, certain GI diseases are predominant in certain ethnic groups (e.g., celiac disease in women of northern European descent).

Following this, a comprehensive obstetric and gynecological history should be elicited. Pertinent gynecological history begins with detailed menstrual history (including documentation of last and previous menstrual period) and obstetric history (including the details of prior pregnancies) followed by history of vaginal or pelvic infections. In addition, providers should always remember that all women in reproductive age are candidates for preconception care. A reproductive life plan should be established that blends well with optimizing the medical condition as well as balancing the reproductive needs of the woman.

Physical Examination

The information from the history needs to be complemented with a thorough physical examination. As with any other condition, acute vital signs usually hint the need for immediate intervention. Fever suggests inflammation. Tachycardia and hypotension are present in those with significant GI blood loss. Complete abdominal examination should then be performed to identify presence of masses, ascites, or peritoneal signs (involuntary guarding, rigidity, or rebound). In women who desire intrauterine devices, pelvic examination to assess the size and position of the uterus is important.

Laboratory Tests

Women with chronic gastric, small intestinal, or pancreatic disease may have vitamin B 12 deficiency. Chronic mucosal blood loss may result in iron deficiency anemia. It may be worthwhile to check the complete blood count and levels of the micronutrients in such women, though this is not necessary before initiation of contraception. Blood testing also monitors medication therapy in some diseases, as with thiopurine metabolite levels in inflammatory bowel disease. Other tests and body fluids are sampled under certain circumstances. In women requesting initiation of birth control methods, pregnancy must be ruled out by thorough history as well as urine pregnancy test when indicated. Chlamydial and gonorrheal testing should be offered to women at risk for STIs who are considering intrauterine devices.

Contraception Method Initiation and Follow-Up

General principles for contraception initiation and maintenance are discussed in this section. These recommendations are mainly based on the United States Selected Practice Recommendations for Contraception Use published in 2013 [57]. Safety of the contraceptive method, availability of contraception method, and a responsible provider to initiate the method are key elements for choosing a particular method of contraception. Risk of sexually transmitted infection, HIV in particular, should be discussed with the patient. Consistent use of male latex condoms reduces the risk of HIV infection and other STIs and so dual protection should be offered in patients at risk for acquiring such infections. The CDC Selected Practice Recommendations highlight the importance of accurate assessment of pregnancy risk in a woman who is about to start a new contraceptive method. A contraceptive method can be initiated anytime a health care provider can reasonably certain that a woman is not pregnant. This is explained as the same day start (quick start) for hormonal contraceptive initiation. Health care providers can also offer emergency contraceptive pills if recent unprotected intercourse has been documented in the past 120 h (see Chap. 1).

Research Gaps

There is clear paucity of data to assess the frequency and content of reproductive counseling and contraception documentation for women with gastrointestinal and hepatobiliary diseases. More studies are needed to clearly state the unmet need for contraception education for specialists and primary care physicians who take care of these patients. Safety of combined hormonal contraceptives such as the contraceptive vaginal ring and patch needs to be better delineated with high quality research studies. Data for usage of LARC methods is also very sparse. More studies with larger number of patients are needed to confirm the safety of LARC methods among women with GI disease and fill the research gaps.

Conclusion

As women spend the majority of their reproductive years avoiding pregnancy, contraception counseling is an important aspect of care of women in reproductive age especially for women with chronic GI diseases. Regardless of intended family size and age at time of visit, unintended pregnancy can occur at any point in a woman's reproductive life. This highlights the need for continued counseling by health care providers, especially specialists with whom these women seek regular care.

References

1. World Health Organization. Medical eligibility criteria for contraceptive use: a WHO family planning cornerstone. Geneva: World Health Organization; 2010.
2. Molodecky NA, Soon IS, Rabi DM, Ghali WA, Ferris M, Chernoff G, et al. Increasing incidence and prevalence of the inflammatory bowel diseases with time, based on systematic review. Gastroenterology. 2012; 142(1):46–54.
3. The Rome Group for Epidemiology and Prevention of Cholelithiasis (GREPO). The epidemiology of gallstone disease in Rome, Italy. Part 1. Prevalence data in men. Hepatology. 1988;8(4):904–6.
4. Barbara L, Sama C, Morselli-Labate AM, et al. A ten year incidence of gallstone disease. The Sirmione study. J Hepatol. 1993;18 Suppl 1:S43.
5. Valdivieso V, Covarrubias C, Siegel F, Cruz F. Pregnancy and cholelithiasis: pathogenesis and natural course of gallstones diagnosed in early puerperium. Hepatology. 1993;17(1):1–4.
6. Stampfer MJ, Maclure KM, Colditz GA, Manson JE, Willett WC. Risk of symptomatic gallstones in women with severe obesity. Am J Clin Nutr. 1992; 55(3):652–8.
7. Keefe EB, Dieterich DT, Han SH, Jacobson IM, Martin P, Schiff ER, et al. A treatment algorithm for the management of chronic hepatitis B virus infection in the United States: an update. Clin Gastroenterol Hepatol. 2006;4:936–62.
8. Zaltron S, Spinetti A, Biasi L, Baiguera C, Castelli F. Chronic HCV infection: epidemiological and clinical relevance. BMC Infect Dis. 2012;12 Suppl 2:S2.
9. Hay JE. Liver disease in pregnancy. Hepatology. 2008;47:1067–76.
10. Heidelbaugh JJ, Bruderly M. Cirrhosis and chronic liver failure: part I diagnosis and evaluation. Am Fam Phys. 2006;74:756–62, 81.
11. Cobey FC, Salem RR. A review of liver masses in pregnancy and a proposed algorithm for their diagnosis and management. Am J Surg. 2004;187:181–91.
12. Van Aalten SM, Bröker ME, Busschbach JJ, de Koning HJ, de Man RA, Steegers EA, et al. Pregnancy and liver adenoma management: PALM study. BMC Gastroenterol. 2012;12:82.
13. Mahadevan U, Sandborn WJ, Li DK, Hakimian S, Kane S, Corley DA. Pregnancy outcomes in women with inflammatory bowel disease: a large community based study from Northern California. Gastroenterology. 2007;133:1106–12.
14. Caprilli R, Gassull MA, Escher JC, Moser G, Munkholm P, Forbes A, et al. European evidence based consensus on the diagnosis and management of Crohn's disease: special situations. Gut. 2006;55 suppl 1:i36–58.
15. Moleski SM, Choudhary C. Special considerations for women with IBD. Gastroenterol Clin North Am. 2011;40:387–98.
16. Racine A, Bijon A, Fournier A, Mesrine S, Clavel-Chapelon F, Carbonnel F, et al. Menopausal hormone therapy and risk of cholecystectomy: a prospective study based on the French E3N cohort. Can Med Assoc J. 2013;185(7):555–61.
17. Thijs C, Knipschild P. Oral contraceptives and the risk of gallbladder disease: a meta-analysis. Am J Public Health. 1993;83(8):1113–20.
18. Etminan M, Delaney JA, Bressler B, Brophy JM. Oral contraceptives and the risk of gallbladder disease: a comparative safety study. Can Med Assoc J. 2011; 183(8):899–904.
19. Dixon NP, Faddis DM, Silberman H. Aggressive management of cholecystitis during pregnancy. Am J Surg. 1987;154(3):292.
20. Date RS, Kaushal M, Ramesh A. A review of the management of gallstone disease and its complications in pregnancy. Am J Surg. 2008;196:599–608.
21. Scobie L, Dalton HR. Hepatitis E: source and route of infection, clinical manifestations and new developments. J Viral Hepat. 2013;20:1–11.
22. Joshi D, James A, Quaglia A, Westbrook RH, Heneghan MA. Liver disease in pregnancy. Lancet. 2010;375:594–605.
23. Shaheen AA, Myers RP. The outcomes of pregnancy in patients with cirrhosis: a population based study. Liver Int. 2010;30(2):275–83.
24. Westbrook RH, Yeoman AD, O'Grady JG, Harrison PM, Devlin J, Heneghan MA. Model for end stage liver disease score predicts outcome in cirrhotic patient during pregnancy. Clin Gastroenterol Hepatol. 2011;9:694–9.
25. Sinha S, Kumar M. Pregnancy and chronic hepatitis B virus infection. Hepatol Res. 2010;40:31–48.
26. Noels JE, van Aalten SM, van der Windt DJ, Kok NF, de Man RA, Terkivatan T, et al. Management of hepatocellular adenoma during pregnancy. J Hepatol. 2011;54:553–8.
27. Gawron LM, Hammond C, Keefer L. Documentation of reproductive health counseling and contraception in women with inflammatory bowel diseases. Patient Educ Couns. 2014;94(1):134–7. doi:10.1016/j.pec.2013.09.013. Epub 2013 Sep 27.
28. Mountifield R, Bampton P, Prosser R, Muller K, Andrews JM. Fear and fertility in inflammatory bowel disease: a mismatch of perception and reality affects family planning decisions. Inflamm Bowel Dis. 2009;15(5):720–5. PubMed PMID: 19067431. Epub 2008/12/11. eng.
29. Veres S, Miller L, Burington B. A comparison between the vaginal ring and oral contraceptives. Obstet Gynecol. 2004;104(3):555–63. PubMed PMID: 15339769. Epub 2004/09/02. eng.
30. Devineni D, Skee D, Vaccaro N, Massarella J, Janssens L, LaGuardia KD, et al. Pharmacokinetics and pharmacodynamics of a transdermal contraceptive patch and an oral contraceptive. J Clin Pharmacol. 2007;47(4):497–509.
31. Koutroumpakis EI, Tsiolakidou G, Koutroubakis IE. Risk of venous thromboembolism in patients with inflammatory bowel disease. Semin Thromb Hemostas. 2013;39(5):461–8. PubMed PMID: 23629820. Epub 2013/05/01. eng.

32. Zapata LB, Paulen ME, Cansino C, Marchbanks PA, Curtis KM. Contraceptive use among women with inflammatory bowel disease: a systematic review. Contraception. 2010;82(1):72–85. PubMed PMID: 20682145.
33. Cosnes J, Carbonnel F, Carrat F, Beaugerie L, Gendre JP. Oral contraceptive use and the clinical course of Crohn's disease: a prospective cohort study. Gut. 1999;45(2):218–22. PubMed PMID: 10403733. Pubmed Central PMCID: PMC1727605. Epub 1999/07/14. eng.
34. Sutherland LR, Ramcharan S, Bryant H, Fick G. Effect of oral contraceptive use on reoperation following surgery for Crohn's disease. Digest Dis Sci. 1992;37(9):1377–82. PubMed PMID: 1505289. Epub 1992/09/01. eng.
35. Timmer A, Sutherland LR, Martin F. Oral contraceptive use and smoking are risk factors for relapse in Crohn's disease. The Canadian Mesalamine for Remission of Crohn's Disease Study Group. Gastroenterology. 1998;114(6):1143–50. PubMed PMID: 9618650. Epub 1998/06/10. eng.
36. Wright JP. Factors influencing first relapse in patients with Crohn's disease. J Clin Gastroenterol. 1992;15(1): 12–6. PubMed PMID: 1500656. Epub 1992/07/01. eng.
37. Jick S, Pennap D. Drospirenone- and levonorgestrel-containing oral contraceptives and the risk of gallbladder disease. Contraception. 2012;86(3):220–3.
38. Yang K, Kock K, Sedykh A, Tropsha A, Brouwer KL. An updated review on drug-induced cholestasis: mechanisms and investigation of physicochemical properties and pharmacokinetic parameters. J Pharm Sci. 2013;102(9):3037–57. PubMed PMID: 23653385.
39. Kapp N, Tilley IB, Curtis KM. The effects of hormonal contraceptive use among women with viral hepatitis or cirrhosis of the liver: a systematic review. Contraception. 2009;80(4):381–6. PubMed PMID: 19751861. Epub 2009/09/16. eng.
40. Heinemann LA, Weimann A, Gerken G, Thiel C, Schlaud M, DoMinh T. Modern oral contraceptive use and benign liver tumors: the German Benign liver tumor case–control study. Eur J Contracept Reprod Health Care. 1998;3(4):194–200. PubMed PMID: 10036602. Epub 1999/02/26. eng.
41. Kapp N, Curtis KM. Hormonal contraceptive use among women with liver tumors: a systematic review. Contraception. 2009;80(4):387–90. PubMed PMID: 19751862. Epub 2009/09/16 eng.
42. Conter RL, Longmire Jr WP. Recurrent hepatic hemangiomas. Possible association with estrogen therapy. Ann Surg. 1988;207(2):115–9. PubMed PMID: 2829759. Pubmed Central PMCID: PMC1493383. Epub 1988/02/01. eng.
43. Miznerova E, Hlavaty T, Koller T, Toth J, Holociova K, Huorka M, et al. The prevalence and risk factors for osteoporosis in patients with inflammatory bowel disease. Bratisl Lek Listy. 2013;114(8):439–45. PubMed PMID: 23944617. Epub 2013/08/16. eng.
44. Valentine JF, Sninsky CA. Prevention and treatment of osteoporosis in patients with inflammatory bowel disease. Am J Gastroenterol. 1999;94(4):878–83. PubMed PMID: 10201450. Epub 1999/04/14. eng.
45. Cravo M, Guerreiro CS, dos Santos PM, Brito M, Ferreira P, Fidalgo C, et al. Risk factors for metabolic bone disease in Crohn's disease patients. Inflamm Bowel Dis. 2010;16(12):2117–24. PubMed PMID: 20848459. Epub 2010/09/18. eng.
46. Berenson AB, Breitkopf CR, Grady JJ, Rickert VI, Thomas A. Effects of hormonal contraception on bone mineral density after 24 months of use. Obstet Gynecol. 2004;103:899–906.
47. Clark MK, Sowers MR, Nichols S, Levy B. Bone mineral density changes over two years in first-time users of depot medroxyprogesterone acetate. Fertil Steril. 2004;82:1580–6.
48. Hatcher R. Contraceptive technology. 20th ed. Bridging the Gap Communications: Atlanta, GA; 2011.
49. Wakeman J. Exacerbation of Crohn's disease after insertion of a levonorgestrel intrauterine system: a case report. J Fam Plann Reprod Health Care. 2003;29(3):154. Faculty of Family Planning & Reproductive Health Care, Royal College of Obstetricians & Gynaecologists. PubMed PMID: 12885311. Epub 2003/07/30. eng.
50. Cox M, Tripp J, Blacksell S. Clinical performance of the levonorgestrel intrauterine system in routine use by the UK family planning and reproductive health research network: 5-year report. J Fam Plann Reprod Health Care. 2002;28(2):73–7. Faculty of Family Planning & Reproductive Health Care, Royal College of Obstetricians & Gynaecologists. PubMed PMID: 12396776. Epub 2002/10/25. eng.
51. Glasier A. Emergency postcoital contraception. N Engl J Med. 1997;337(15):1058–64.
52. Peterson Hb, Xia Z, Hughes JM, Wilcox LS, Tylor LR, Trussell J. The risk of pregnancy after tubal sterilization: findings from the US collaborative review of sterilization. 19960617 DCOM-19960617(0002-9378 (Print)). eng.
53. Grimmer SF, Back DJ, Orme ML, Cowie A, Gilmore I, Tjia J. The bioavailability of ethinyloestradiol and levonorgestrel in patients with an ileostomy. Contraception. 1986;33(1):51–9. PubMed PMID: 3082591. Epub 1986/01/01. eng.
54. Nilsson LO, Victor A, Kral JG, Johansson ED, Kock NG. Absorption of an oral contraceptive gestagen in ulcerative colitis before and after proctocolectomy and construction of a continent ileostomy. Contraception. 1985;31(2):195–204. PubMed PMID: 3921310. Epub 1985/02/01. eng.
55. Deray G, le Hoang P, Cacoub P, Assogba U, Grippon P, Baumelou A. Oral contraceptive interaction with cyclosporin. Lancet. 1987;1(8525):158–9. PubMed PMID: 2879990. Epub 1987/01/17. eng.
56. Astellas Pharma US, Inc. Prescribing information Prograf (tacrolimus). Deerfield, IL: Astellas Pharma US Inc.; 2009.
57. Centers for Disease Control. U.S. selected practice recommendations for contraceptive use, 2013: adapted from the World Health Organization selected practice recommendations for contraceptive use, 2nd ed. MMWR Recomm Rep. 2013;62 (RR-05):1–60. PubMed PMID: 23784109. Epub 2013/06/21. eng.

Contraception in the Perimenopause

19

Julie M. Sroga and Michael A. Thomas

Introduction

Menopause occurs after 1 year of amenorrhea which typically happens in the late fourth and fifth decades of a woman's life, with the average age occurring at 51 years [1]. The years preceding menopause, known as perimenopause, encompass the change from regular ovulatory cycles to cessation of menses. During the perimenopause, changes in the menstrual cycle can occur. Menstrual cycle length increases approximately 2–8 years prior to menopause, with anovulation becoming increasingly common [2]. Although cycles can be irregular at this time and often are greater than 40 days, as many as 25 % can still be ovulatory despite these irregularities [3].

Perimenopausal signs and symptoms are associated with changes in hormonal levels that result from a declining follicular pool [4, 5]. Several longitudinal studies have reported changes in hormonal levels during the perimenopause including elevated follicular stimulating hormone levels (FSH) and decreased inhibin levels (inhibin-A and inhibin-B). A decrease in inhibin-B is often the first change noted during the menopausal transition resulting directly from the decreasing follicular pool since preantral follicles are the main source of inhibin-B. This decline in inhibin-B releases the negative feedback on FSH. Both normal and decreased corpus luteum production of progesterone have been reported during the menopausal transition. Estradiol levels have been shown to be normal or slightly increased [6–8] with androgen levels being normal or decreased independent of sex hormone binding globulin (SHBG) levels [9, 10]. High levels of estrogen are more commonly a feature of the early perimenopause with lower levels found just prior to menstrual cessation [6, 11]. Anti-Müllerian hormone levels also decrease during the transition from the reproductive years to menopause, becoming undetectable approximately 5 years prior to menopause [12].

Women progressing through the menopausal transition may complain of a variety of symptoms that are related to these hormonal changes. The symptoms most frequently seen include disturbances in menstrual pattern, vasomotor symptoms, and atrophic conditions [10]. Menstrual changes can include anovulation, reduced or increased menstrual flow, shorter or lengthened cycles, and finally amenorrhea. Vasomotor symptoms (VMS), including hot flashes, night sweats, and palpitations, may vary in intensity and frequency but can begin as mild and worsen as the woman completes the transition to menopause. Finally, vaginal atrophy can result in

J.M. Sroga, M.D. • M.A. Thomas, M.D. (✉)
Section of Reproductive Endocrinology and Infertility, Department of Obstetrics and Gynecology, University of Cincinnati College of Medicine, West Chester, OH, USA
e-mail: Julie.sroga@uc.edu; thomasma@ucmail.uc.edu

R.H. Allen and C.A. Cwiak (eds.), *Contraception for the Medically Challenging Patient*,
DOI 10.1007/978-1-4939-1233-9_19, © Springer Science+Business Media New York 2014

a degree of symptoms including dyspareunia, pruritus, and urinary complaints such as urgency and cystitis [10].

Rationale for Contraception in the Perimenopause

Fertility Control

Even though fertility declines with advancing maternal age, about one-quarter of menstrual cycles remain ovulatory, putting this population of women at risk for pregnancy. Women between ages 35 and 39 have a fertility rate of approximately 335 per 1,000 which decreases to 25 per 1,000 in women over 45, in comparison to 400 per 1,000 for women under 35 [13]. Women of advanced maternal age are also at increased risk of pregnancy related complications including spontaneous abortions, fetal malformations, aneuploidy, preeclampsia and other hypertensive disorders, gestational diabetes, preterm labor, and preterm birth [14]. In 2008, 12 % of all induced abortions occurred in women over 35 years of age. Approximately, 7.8 per 1,000 occurred in women 35–39 years and 2.7 per 1,000 occurred in women aged 40 and older [15]. Therefore, in this population, women who are currently sexually active or are considering being so require and should receive counseling regarding safe and effective methods of contraception.

Symptom Relief

Menstrual disturbances affect many women during this transition often involving unpredictable and heavy bleeding. Several decades ago these symptoms were frequently treated surgically with hysterectomy [16]. Hormonal contraceptives offer today's clinicians an alternative to surgical intervention. Combined hormonal contraceptives (CHCs) and progestin-only regimens (levonorgestrel IUD, etonogestrel implant, DMPA injectable, and progestin-only pills) are all options for perimenopausal women to control menstrual bleeding unless contraindications exist.

Approximately 80 % of women in perimenopause will suffer from VMS [16], and these symptoms may significantly affect the quality of life in these women. VMS begin in the perimenopause and persist for variable lengths of time but median durations of 4 and 10 years have been reported [17]. Estrogen-containing hormonal contraceptive regimens can offer effective and safe treatment of vasomotor symptoms if severe [18]. One study found that over a 3-year observational study, 90 % of women using COC had improvement of VMS compared to 40 % of non-users [19]. Another study compared two different COC regimens and documented a reduction in VMS from 88 % of women pre-treatment to 17–26 % of women 6 months post-therapy [20]. Other non-hormonal treatment options such as antidepressants or gabapentin may improve VMS in some women [21, 22]. The various herbal treatments or supplements have not proven consistently to be beneficial [23]. Therefore, if no contraindication to estrogen is present, then combined hormonal contraceptives would be of benefit in symptomatic perimenopausal patients who need contraception.

Noncontraceptive Benefits

Combined oral contraceptives (COC) have been shown to significantly reduce the risk of endometrial and ovarian cancer. Endometrial cancer risk, including all major histologic subtypes (adenocarcinoma, adenoacanthoma, and adenosquamous cancers), decreases by about 50 % after 12 months of COC use [24–28]. This protective effect is greatest after at least 3 years of use and can persist for more than 15–20 years after discontinuing the medication [24, 29]. All monophasic COC preparations at doses under 50 μg have demonstrated this uterine protective effect; however, limited data exists on multiphasic regimens [24, 26, 30]. In perimenopausal women, irregular and anovulatory bleeding combined with peripheral sources of estrogen (adipose tissue) place patients at risk of endometrial hyperplasia and cancer; therefore, COCs are a good option in this population for prevention.

The progestin component of COC blocks any estrogenic stimulation of the endometrial lining, thus preventing hyperplasia and conversion to endometrial cancer. Ovarian cancer risk reduction is one of the most important benefits of COC since this type of cancer is often diagnosed in late stages and so is frequently fatal. A 40 % reduction in developing epithelial (all histologic subtypes) ovarian cancer is seen in COC users over nonusers [26, 28, 31–37]. Risk reduction increases with duration of use and can persist for more than 20 years after discontinuation. Users with as little as 3–6 months of use have shown benefit, but COC use for greater than 3 years is needed for significant impact.

Women who have been diagnosed with certain gynecological conditions including endometriosis, adenomyosis, and uterine fibroids may have clinical symptoms such as pelvic pain and heavy uterine bleeding that persist until menopause is reached [38, 39]. Historically once childbearing was complete or perimenopause occurred, these conditions were treated surgically with hysterectomy with or without bilateral salpingoophorectomy. Hormonal contraceptives, including combined (estrogen–progestin) or progestin-only regimens can help reduce uterine blood flow until menopause is reached, avoiding surgery in these patients. In addition, ovarian suppression with these hormonal regimens can improve pain symptoms in women with endometriosis, again avoiding surgery and preserving the ovaries which can continue to provide hormone production (although reduced) after menopause (see Chap. 13).

Osteoporosis is a common bone disease in the elderly and is a major health concern. After the age of 35, women lose bone at a rate of 0.7 % per year, which then increases to 1–1.5 % per year after menopause [39, 40]. A decrease in estrogen production during perimenopause and menopause accounts for this accelerated loss. In a hypoestrogenic environment, osteoclastic activity predominates, resulting in increased bone resorption and less bone formation causing a lower bone mineral density (BMD) [10]. In perimenopausal women, particularly those over 40 years of age, estrogen-containing contraceptives can significantly increase BMD even at low doses [41, 42]. A review of 13 studies assessing the effect of low-dose COC (20 mcg ethinyl estradiol) use on BMD found that 9 of the 13 studies indicated an increase in BMD, 4 showed no difference, but no study found a decrease. Therefore, the authors conclude that there is fair (category B) evidence that COC use is favorable on BMD [41]. A randomized control trial by Gambacciani et al. comparing different COC found that BMD decreased in oligomenorrheic perimenopausal women during the observation period but that COC use demonstrated an increase in BMD in both normal cycling and perimenopausal women [42]. However, studies have failed to demonstrate a decreased fracture risk with COC in perimenopausal women [43, 44] (see Chap. 16).

Discontinuation of Contraception

Most women will be able to use contraception safely until they are assured of menopause. The decision of when to stop a contraception method must evaluate the benefits of the method, health risks resulting from its use as age increases, diminishing risk of pregnancy, and availability of alternative method (Table 19.1). Contraception may be discontinued by all women above the age of 55. The frequency of ovulation or chance of spontaneous pregnancy is essentially zero at this age [1]. There are no reliable tests to confirm the loss of fertility in women [45]. The use of FSH levels to define menopause is challenging in that fluctuations are common and become more variable as menstrual irregularity increases. A single serum FSH level may be elevated with an accompanying low estradiol in menopausal ranges, but another random sample may be in normal premenopausal ranges [46]. One study reported that a random serum FSH >25 IU/L is characteristic of the late menopausal transition [47], but measurements of serum FSH during the late menopausal transition are not routinely recommended because of their variability. Therefore, clinical signs and symptoms should be used to make the diagnosis of perimenopause and menopause.

Table 19.1 When women can stop using contraceptives

	Advice on stopping contraception	
Contraceptive Method	Age < 50 years	Age ≥ 50 years
Non-hormonal	May stop contraception after 2 years of amenorrhea	May stop contraception after 1 year of amenorrhea
Progestin-only methods: intrauterine device, implant, injection, pill	Can be continued up to age 55	Can be continued up to age 55 *OR* Switch to non-hormonal method and stop after 1 year of amenorrhea
Estrogen-containing methods: Ring, patch, pill	Can be continued up to age 50 or higher if no cardiovascular risk factors	Can be continued up to age 55 if no cardiovascular risk factors *OR* Switch to non-hormonal method and stop after 1 year of amenorrhea

FSH and estradiol hormone levels can be helpful as an adjunct in some situations (e.g., women without a uterus) but should not be relied upon alone for the diagnosis of menopause.

According to the United States Medical Eligibility Criteria for Contraceptive Use (USMEC), there are no contraceptive methods that are contraindicated based on age alone (Table 19.2) [48]. However, there are some medical conditions more common in older women that may make some contraceptive methods inappropriate and women should be assessed for these conditions before contraception is prescribed. In women older than 50 years using estrogen-containing contraceptives, contraception should be continued at least 1 year following the final menstrual period; if less than 50 years, continuation of contraception for 2 years after the final menstrual cycle is recommended [1]. Estrogen-containing contraceptives should be discontinued in women who develop cardiovascular risk factors and an alternative contraceptive should be selected if the patient is not menopausal. This includes patients with stroke, hypertension, diabetes, vascular disease, or ischemic heart disease.

Other forms of contraception including the progestin-only pill, etonogestrel contraceptive implant (Implanon/Nexplanon, Merck, Whitehouse Station, NJ, USA), depot medroxyprogesterone acetate (DMPA) (Depo-Provera, Pfizer Inc., New York, NY, USA), the copper T380A IUD (ParaGard, Teva, Israel), and the levonorgestrel intrauterine device (Mirena/Skyla, Bayer Healthcare Pharmaceuticals, Wayne, NJ, USA) can be used until menopause is diagnosed or age 55. Of note, any women with a hormone sensitive tumor would need to discontinue hormonal contraception at the time of diagnosis. This would include any hormonal contraceptives, including progestin-only, in women with estrogen or progesterone receptor positive cancers such as breast cancer [48].

Table 19.2 US medical eligibility criteria for contraceptive use categories based on age

Method	Age range (years)	USMEC
Combined hormonal contraception	≥40	Benefits outweigh risks
Progestin-only pill	≥40	No restriction
Progestin implant	≥40	No restriction
DMPA	≥40–45 >45	No restriction Benefits outweigh risks
Copper IUD	≥40	No restriction
LNG-IUD	≥40	No restriction

DMPA depot medroxyprogesterone acetate, *LNG-IUD* levonorgestrel intrauterine device

Not all women who discontinue hormonal contraceptives will need to be transitioned to hormone therapy (HT). HT is recommended for moderate to severe vasomotor symptoms where symptoms are impacting the woman's quality of life [10]. When discontinuing hormonal contraception, the patient and her health care provider should assess the need for HT, and if needed, a regimen containing estrogen and progestin (if she has an intact uterus) of the lowest hormonal dose and shortest duration should be selected [17].

Contraceptive Options in Perimenopausal Women

Older women still have a variety of contraceptive options available for use that are both safe and effective (Table 19.3). Contraception should be individualized to a patient's lifestyle and individual preferences, but should also be selected based on the patient's medical history, physical exam (i.e., blood pressure and BMI for CHC and pelvic exams for IUD), and prior contraceptive experience [45]. A patient should be counseled on all contraceptive options that are available to her as well as be counseled on risks and benefits of each method. Risks and contraindications to certain contraceptives may be different than in a younger woman. Health care providers should be aware of these differences to ensure appropriate contraceptive counseling.

Table 19.3 Contraceptive options and considerations in the older population

Method	Considerations in older women
Combined oral contraceptives, transdermal patch, and vaginal ring	Older women have higher risk of myocardial infarction, stroke, and venous thromboembolism and estrogen containing regimens may increase this risk
Depot medroxyprogesterone acetate	Suppresses bone turnover, often produces prolonged amenorrhea
Progestin-only pill	Produces unpredictable bleeding, requires daily time specific pill taking
Etonogestrel implant	Produces irregular bleeding and amenorrhea
Copper IUD	Can produce cause heavier menstrual flow and longer menstrual cycles. If inserted after age 40, can be left in place until menopause.
Levonorgestrel IUD	May improve heavy and painful menses but may rarely cause hormonal side effects including breast pain, acne, mood changes. If inserted after age 45, can be left in place until menopause.
Barrier methods	Use in new relationships despite age and other methods of contraception to protect against sexually transmitted infections

Intrauterine Devices

Both the levonorgestrel IUD (LNG-IUD) and copper IUD are highly effective (0.6 and 0.1 % failure rates, respectively) and safe to use in most perimenopausal women. Though the LNG-IUD is associated with a warning for a potential increase in breast cancer risk, a retrospective study demonstrated no increased risk with this device [49]. A 3-year smaller LNG-IUD is now available that has been studied and shown effective (failure rate of 0.9 %). The copper IUD has very few contraindications and is approved for 10 years of use. The LNG-IUD comes in two sizes and can be used up to 3 or 5 years depending on which device is inserted. Both LNG-IUDs have a number of noncontraceptive benefits that could be useful in the perimenopausal woman although there is no data evaluating the smaller LNG-IUD in this population. Women in the perimenopause are at higher risk of anovulatory bleeding episodes, and both versions of the LNG-IUD offer a beneficial suppressive effect on the endometrial lining, which is attributed to a progestin-induced decidualization of the endometrium [50]. Though spotting or light bleeding can occur after LNG-IUDs are initially inserted, these irregularities often dissipate after 3–6 months, resulting in amenorrhea in 20–50 % of users by the second year of use [51]. Noncontraceptive benefits include a decrease in menstrual blood loss, dysmenorrhea, and de novo endometrial polyp formation in breast cancer patients using tamoxifen [52].

Sterilization

As a couple ages, the use of either male or female sterilization as their primary form of contraception increases. In the USA, the use of vasectomy (16.8 %) and female sterilization (45.8 %) was highest in women between the ages of 40 and 44 years [53]. After age 30, the number of couples choosing sterilization increases as their planned family size becomes complete. Therefore, as her fertility declines, the risk of regret after sterilization is also reduced [54]. The investigators also noted that women under the age of 30 years had regret as high as 20.3 % within 14 years of their tubal ligation, whereas women from 31 to 44 years only expressed a rate of regret at 5.9 % [55].

Though various techniques of tubal sterilization are available, the majority of women in the perimenopausal age group undergo a laparoscopic tubal ligation which is performed with cautery of or applying a clip to the mid-portion of the Fallopian tubes. Tubal sterilization may also be performed at the time of the last pregnancy during cesarean delivery or immediately after vaginal delivery, but the perimenopausal women is usually well beyond her last pregnancy therefore an interval method is more commonly utilized. Importantly, failure rates 8–14 years after tubal ligation decreases as a woman ages [56]. This is most likely due to the rate of natural fertility decline as a woman gets older.

Hysteroscopic tubal occlusion with nickel–titanium coil microinserts (Essure, Bayer Healthcare Pharmaceuticals, Wayne, NJ, USA) can be performed as an office or hospital outpatient procedure. The placement of microinserts into the tubal ostia can be performed in most women regardless of medical condition or obesity. A hysteroscope is placed through the cervix and the inserts are easily guided into the ostia. However, the microinserts are not effective immediately. It takes up to 3 months to allow tissue growth around the inserts to permanently occlude the tubal ostia. A hysterosalpinogram should be performed after this 3-month time frame before this method can be relied on for contraception.

Combined Hormonal Contraceptives

Combination contraceptive agents contain both an estrogen (typically ethinyl estradiol) and a progestin component. These medications were first introduced in the USA in the early 1960s and originally contained much higher doses of both hormonal components compared to the pills that are currently approved. Combined contraceptives can be administered orally, transdermally, or vaginally. All of these medications can be safely utilized by perimenopausal women who are healthy and nonsmokers. Nevertheless, the risk of VTE increases with increasing age [57]. This also likely applies to the combined hormonal patch and vaginal ring (see Chap. 12). Since rates of both venous and arterial events with estrogen-containing methods are still lower than during pregnancy, these methods have no upper age limit for use [58]. However, the USMEC "top tier" methods (IUDs, implants, sterilization) are preferred for women of older reproductive age for their superior effectiveness and lack of association with cardiovascular events [59].

As discussed above, no matter the route of administration, combination contraceptives confer more than pregnancy prevention in this patient population. As women enter the perimenopause, they can develop cycle irregularities and anovulatory bleeding problems. The use of these combination agents act to decrease abnormal uterine bleeding (menorrhagia, metrorrhagia), which will also decrease anemia. Combined methods also offer a reduction in dysmenorrhea and pelvic pain, the formation of functional ovarian cysts, vasomotor symptoms (hot flashes, night sweats, vaginal dryness), and help to maintain bone density. The risks of cardiovascular disease, including hyperlipidemia and hypertension, increase as a woman ages. The estrogen component of combination contraceptives can worsen cardiovascular disease and hypertension. Therefore, perimenopausal women initiating or continuing combination contraceptives should have periodic screening of blood pressure, weight, and fasting lipid levels as part of their health care maintenance [10].

Progestin-Only Contraceptives

Progestin-only contraceptives contain no estrogen and can be administered orally, as a long-acting injection (DMPA), or an implantable rod (etonogestrel implant). As progestin-only contraceptive methods do not appear to increase the risk of venous thromboembolism (VTE), they represent safe options for women who are at higher risk for cardiovascular events, whether due to age, obesity, or medical comorbidities like diabetes mellitus and hypertension. Because of the lack of estrogen in these progestin-only agents, menstrual irregularities may occur. Any of these options may cause unpredictable spotting, light continuous bleeding, or amenorrhea. Patients should be counseled prior to use about the likely possibility of a change in their normal bleeding pattern.

Emergency Contraception

Options for emergency contraception (EC) for perimenopausal women are no different than in younger women and these include levonorgestrel (LNG)-only pill, ulipristal acetate (UPA), and the copper IUD [60–63]. LNG-only regimens include a dosing regimen of 0.75 mg given twice 12 h apart or 1.5 mg given once. These regimens are available without a prescription, have approximately 85 % reduction in risk for pregnancy, and are most effective if taken within 72 h of unprotected coitus. Efficacy and contraindications are similar in perimenopausal women and younger patients [63]. UPA is a second-generation selective progesterone receptor modulator (SPRM) that directly interferes with progesterone activity in target tissues [64, 65]. Currently, UPA is approved for EC in a single 30 mg dose up to 120 h following unprotected intercourse. It is more effective than levonorgestrel emergency contraception when used within 24 h or up to 5 days after unprotected sexual intercourse [66]. Unlike levonorgestrel, UPA prevents follicle rupture after the luteinizing-hormone surge [67]. One meta-analysis showed that ulipristal acetate almost halved the risk of pregnancy compared with LNG in women who received emergency contraception within 120 h after sexual intercourse (odds ratio [OR], 0.55; 95 % confidence interval [CI], 0.32–0.93) [66]. Women 36 and older were included in the trials of UPA with no plausible difference in efficacy in perimenopausal women.

The copper IUD is the most effective emergency contraceptive and is a good alternative for women who desire long-term contraception or women with a contraindication to hormonal regimens. Insertion of a copper IUD should be performed within 5 days after ovulation or during the preovulatory phase. Failure rates are approximately 0.1 % in women of all ages, and contraindications are also similar across all ages and include uterine anomalies and active cervicitis or pelvic infection [63].

Barrier Methods

Condoms (male or female) and diaphragms can be used in perimenopausal women without any concern for any preexisting medical problems. However, both of these devices have higher failure rates in typical users compared to hormonal methods or IUDs. Though diaphragms are used infrequently by women of all ages, the use of these barrier methods also demand timing with coitus and some degree of manual dexterity to insert the device into the vagina.

Conclusion

Perimenopausal women will experience hormonal changes during the transition from reproductive age to menopause, and during this time they may suffer from various symptoms resulting from these changes. Although the chance of becoming pregnant declines with increasing age, women are still at risk for pregnancy and pregnancy-related complications during perimenopause. Therefore, medical providers should discuss the various contraceptive options with their perimenopausal patients who are sexually active. The choice of contraceptive should be individualized to the patient's needs so that it may provide both contraceptive effectiveness and noncontraceptive benefit when needed.

References

1. Gebbie AE, Hardman SM. Contraception in the perimenopause—old and new. Menopause Int. 2010;16(1):33–7. PubMed PMID: 20424284.
2. Treloar AE, Boynton RE, Behn BG, Brown BW. Variation of the human menstrual cycle through reproductive life. Int J Fertil. 1967;12(1):77–126. PubMed PMID: 5419031.

3. O'Connor KA, Ferrell R, Brindle E, Trumble B, Shofer J, Holman DJ, et al. Progesterone and ovulation across stages of the transition to menopause. Menopause. 2009;16(6):1178–87. PubMed PMID: 19568209. Pubmed Central PMCID: 2783957.
4. Richardson SJ, Senikas V, Nelson JF. Follicular depletion during the menopausal transition: evidence for accelerated loss and ultimate exhaustion. J Clin Endocrinol Metab. 1987;65(6):1231–7. PubMed PMID: 3119654.
5. Gougeon A, Ecochard R, Thalabard JC. Age-related changes of the population of human ovarian follicles: increase in the disappearance rate of non-growing and early-growing follicles in aging women. Biol Reprod. 1994;50(3):653–63. PubMed PMID: 8167237.
6. Defey D, Storch E, Cardozo S, Diaz O, Fernandez G. The menopause: women's psychology and health care. Soc Sci Med. 1996;42(10):1447–56. PubMed PMID: 8735901.
7. Olshansky SJ, Carnes BA, Cassel CK. The aging of the human species. Sci Am. 1993;268(4):46–52. PubMed PMID: 8446881.
8. Fries JF, Crapo LM. Vitality and aging. San Francisco: Freeman; 1981.
9. Duke RC, Speidel JJ. The 1991 Albert Lasker Public Service Award. Women's reproductive health. A chronic crisis. JAMA. 1991;266(13):1846–7. PubMed PMID: 1890715.
10. Fritz MA, Speroff L. Clinical gynecologic endocrinology and infertility. 8th ed. Philadelphia, PA: Lippincott, Williams & Wilkins; 2011.
11. Dennerstein L, Smith AM, Morse C, Burger H, Green A, Hopper J, et al. Menopausal symptoms in Australian women. Med J Aust. 1993;159(4):232–6. PubMed PMID: 8412889.
12. Sowers MR, Eyvazzadeh AD, McConnell D, Yosef M, Jannausch ML, Zhang D, et al. Anti-Mullerian hormone and inhibin B in the definition of ovarian aging and the menopause transition. J Clin Endocrinol Metab. 2008;93(9):3478–83. PubMed PMID: 18593767. Pubmed Central PMCID: 2567855.
13. Heffner LJ. Advanced maternal age—how old is too old? N Engl J Med. 2004;351(19):1927–9. PubMed PMID: 15525717.
14. Bayrampour H, Heaman M, Duncan KA, Tough S. Advanced maternal age and risk perception: a qualitative study. BMC Pregnancy Childbirth. 2012;12:100. PubMed PMID: 22988825. Pubmed Central PMCID: 3490979.
15. Parker K. Abortion Survelliance—United States 2008 2011 [cited 2013 December 23]. http://www.cdc.gov/mmwr/preview/mmwrhtml/ss6015a1.htm?s_cid=ss6015a1_w.
16. Hardman SM, Gebbie AE. Hormonal contraceptive regimens in the perimenopause. Maturitas. 2009;63(3):204–12. PubMed PMID: 19524378.
17. ACOG Practice Bulletin No. 141: Management of menopausal symptoms. Obstet Gynecol. 2014;123(1):202–16. PubMed PMID: 24463691.
18. Kaunitz AM. Clinical practice. Hormonal contraception in women of older reproductive age. N Engl J Med. 2008;358(12):1262–70. PubMed PMID: 18354104.
19. Shargil AA. Hormone replacement therapy in perimenopausal women with a triphasic contraceptive compound: a three-year prospective study. Int J Fertil. 1985;30(1):15, 8–28. PubMed PMID: 2862116.
20. Saure A, Planellas J, Poulsen HK, Jaszczak P. A double-blind, randomized, comparative study evaluating clinical effects of two sequential estradiol-progestogen combinations containing either desogestrel or medroxyprogesterone acetate in climacteric women. Maturitas. 2000;34(2):133–42. PubMed PMID: 10714908.
21. Archer DF, Seidman L, Constantine GD, Pickar JH, Olivier S. A double-blind, randomly assigned, placebo-controlled study of desvenlafaxine efficacy and safety for the treatment of vasomotor symptoms associated with menopause. Am J Obstet Gynecol. 2009;200(2):172 e1–10. PubMed PMID: 19110224.
22. Brown JN, Wright BR. Use of gabapentin in patients experiencing hot flashes. Pharmacotherapy. 2009;29(1):74–81. PubMed PMID: 19113798.
23. Low Dog T. Menopause: a review of botanical dietary supplements. Am J Med. 2005;118(Suppl 12B):98–108. PubMed PMID: 16414334.
24. Combination oral contraceptive use and the risk of endometrial cancer. The Cancer and Steroid Hormone Study of the Centers for Disease Control and the National Institute of Child Health and Human Development. JAMA. 1987;257(6):796–800. PubMed PMID: 3027423.
25. Schlesselman JJ. Oral contraceptives and neoplasia of the uterine corpus. Contraception. 1991;43(6):557–79. PubMed PMID: 1868733.
26. Vessey MP, Painter R. Endometrial and ovarian cancer and oral contraceptives—findings in a large cohort study. Br J Cancer. 1995;71(6):1340–2. PubMed PMID: 7779735. Pubmed Central PMCID: 2033840.
27. Schlesselman JJ. Risk of endometrial cancer in relation to use of combined oral contraceptives. A practitioner's guide to meta-analysis. Hum Reprod. 1997;12(9):1851–63. PubMed PMID: 9363696.
28. Salazar-Martinez E, Lazcano-Ponce EC, Gonzalez Lira-Lira G, Escudero-De los Rios P, Salmeron-Castro J, Hernandez-Avila M. Reproductive factors of ovarian and endometrial cancer risk in a high fertility population in Mexico. Cancer Res. 1999;59(15):3658–62. PubMed PMID: 10446978.
29. Jick SS, Walker AM, Jick H. Oral contraceptives and endometrial cancer. Obstet Gynecol. 1993;82(6):931–5. PubMed PMID: 8233267.
30. Sherman ME, Sturgeon S, Brinton LA, Potischman N, Kurman RJ, Berman ML, et al. Risk factors and hormone levels in patients with serous and endometrioid uterine carcinomas. Mod Pathol. 1997;10(10):963–8. PubMed PMID: 9346174.
31. The reduction in risk of ovarian cancer associated with oral-contraceptive use. The Cancer and Steroid Hormone Study of the Centers for Disease Control

and the National Institute of Child Health and Human Development. N Engl J Med. 1987;316(11):650–5. PubMed PMID: 3821795.
32. Hankinson SE, Colditz GA, Hunter DJ, Spencer TL, Rosner B, Stampfer MJ. A quantitative assessment of oral contraceptive use and risk of ovarian cancer. Obstet Gynecol. 1992;80(4):708–14. PubMed PMID: 1407899.
33. Whittemore AS, Harris R, Itnyre J. Characteristics relating to ovarian cancer risk: collaborative analysis of 12 US case-control studies. II. Invasive epithelial ovarian cancers in white women Collaborative Ovarian Cancer Group. Am J Epidemiol. 1992; 136(10):1184–203. PubMed PMID: 1476141.
34. Wittenberg J, Cook LS, Rossing MA, Weiss NS. Reproductive risk factors for mucinous and non-mucinous epithelial ovarian cancer. Epidemiology. 1999;10(6):761–3. PubMed PMID: 10535792.
35. Ness RB, Grisso JA, Klapper J, Schlesselman JJ, Silberzweig S, Vergona R, et al. Risk of ovarian cancer in relation to estrogen and progestin dose and use characteristics of oral contraceptives. SHARE Study Group Steroid Hormones and Reproductions. Am J Epidemiol. 2000;152(3):233–41. PubMed PMID: 10933270.
36. Royar J, Becher H, Chang-Claude J. Low-dose oral contraceptives: protective effect on ovarian cancer risk. Int J Cancer. 2001;95(6):370–4. PubMed PMID: 11668519.
37. Collaborative Group on Epidemiological Studies of Ovarian C, Beral V, Doll R, Hermon C, Peto R, Reeves G. Ovarian cancer and oral contraceptives: collaborative reanalysis of data from 45 epidemiological studies including 23,257 women with ovarian cancer and 87,303 controls. Lancet. 2008;371(9609): 303–14. PubMed PMID: 18294997.
38. Schindler AE. Non-contraceptive benefits of oral hormonal contraceptives. Int J Endocrinol Metab. 2013;11(1):41–7. PubMed PMID: 23853619. Pubmed Central PMCID: 3693657.
39. Matkovic V, Jelic T, Wardlaw GM, Ilich JZ, Goel PK, Wright JK, et al. Timing of peak bone mass in Caucasian females and its implication for the prevention of osteoporosis. Inference from a cross-sectional model. J Clin Invest. 1994;93(2):799–808. PubMed PMID: 8113412. Pubmed Central PMCID: 293933.
40. Recker RR, Davies KM, Hinders SM, Heaney RP, Stegman MR, Kimmel DB. Bone gain in young adult women. JAMA. 1992;268(17):2403–8. PubMed PMID: 1404797.
41. Kuohung W, Borgatta L, Stubblefield P. Low-dose oral contraceptives and bone mineral density: an evidence-based analysis. Contraception. 2000;61(2): 77–82. PubMed PMID: 10802271.
42. Gambacciani M, Cappagli B, Lazzarini V, Ciaponi M, Fruzzetti F, Genazzani AR. Longitudinal evaluation of perimenopausal bone loss: effects of different low dose oral contraceptive preparations on bone mineral density. Maturitas. 2006;54(2):176–80. PubMed PMID: 16332417.
43. Cooper C, Hannaford P, Croft P, Kay CR. Oral contraceptive pill use and fractures in women: a prospective study. Bone. 1993;14(1):41–5. PubMed PMID: 8443001.
44. Vessey M, Mant J, Painter R. Oral contraception and other factors in relation to hospital referral for fracture. Findings in a large cohort study. Contraception. 1998;57(4):231–5. PubMed PMID: 9649913.
45. Division of Reproductive Health NCfCDP, Health Promotion CfDC, Prevention. U.S. Selected Practice Recommendations for Contraceptive Use, 2013: adapted from the World Health Organization selected practice recommendations for contraceptive use, 2nd ed. MMWR recommendations and reports : morbidity and mortality weekly report recommendations and reports/Centers for Disease Control. 2013;62(RR-05):1–60. PubMed PMID: 23784109.
46. Hee J, MacNaughton J, Bangah M, Burger HG. Perimenopausal patterns of gonadotrophins, immunoreactive inhibin, oestradiol and progesterone. Maturitas. 1993;18(1):9–20. PubMed PMID: 8107620.
47. Freeman EW, Sammel MD, Gracia CR, Kapoor S, Lin H, Liu L, et al. Follicular phase hormone levels and menstrual bleeding status in the approach to menopause. Fertil Steril. 2005;83(2):383–92. PubMed PMID: 15705379.
48. Centers for Disease C, Prevention. U S. Medical Eligibility Criteria for Contraceptive Use, 2010. MMWR Recommendations and reports : morbidity and mortality weekly report recommendations and reports/Centers for Disease Control. 2010;59(RR-4):1–86. PubMed PMID: 20559203.
49. Dinger J, Bardenheuer K, Minh TD. Levonorgestrel-releasing and copper intrauterine devices and the risk of breast cancer. Contraception. 2011;83(3):211–7. PubMed PMID: 21310281.
50. Nilsson CG. Comparative quantitation of menstrual blood loss with a d-norgestrel releasing IUD and a Nova-T-copper device. Contraception. 1977;15(4): 379–87. PubMed PMID: 880815.
51. Hidalgo M, Bahamondes L, Perrotti M, Diaz J, Dantas-Monteiro C, Petta C. Bleeding patterns and clinical performance of the levonorgestrel-releasing intrauterine system (Mirena) up to two years. Contraception. 2002;65(2):129–32. PubMed PMID: 11927115.
52. Wong AW, Chan SS, Yeo W, Yu MY, Tam WH. Prophylactic use of levonorgestrel-releasing intrauterine system in women with breast cancer treated with tamoxifen: a randomized controlled trial. Obstet Gynecol. 2013;121(5):943–50. PubMed PMID: 23635729.
53. Mosher WD, Martinez GM, Chandra A, Abma JC, Wilson SJ. Advance data from vital and health statistics, no 350. Hyattsville, MD: National Center for Health Statistics; 2004.
54. Wilcox LS, Chu SY, Eaker ED, Zeger SL, Peterson HB. Risk factors for regret after tubal sterilization: 5 years of follow-up in a prospective study. Fertil Steril. 1991;55(5):927–33. PubMed PMID: 2022271.

55. Hillis SD, Marchbanks PA, Tylor LR, Peterson HB. Poststerilization regret: findings from the United States Collaborative Review of Sterilization. Obstet Gynecol. 1999;93(6):889–95. PubMed PMID: 10362150.
56. Peterson HB, Xia Z, Hughes JM, Wilcox LS, Tylor LR, Trussell J. The risk of pregnancy after tubal sterilization: findings from the U.S. Collaborative Review of Sterilization. Am J Obstet Gynecol. 1996;174(4):1161–8.
57. Heinemann LA, Dinger JC. Range of published estimates of venous thromboembolism incidence in young women. Contraception. 2007;75(5):328–36. PubMed PMID: 17434013.
58. Centers for Disease Control and Prevention. U.S. Medical Eligibility Criteria for Contraceptive Use, 2010. MMWR. 2010;59(RR-4).
59. Johns Hopkins Bloomberg School of Public Health/Center for Communication Programs and World Health Organization. Family planning: a global handbook for providers. Geneva: World Health Organization; 2011.
60. Morris JM, Van Wagenen G. Post-coital oral contraception. Caribb Med J. 1966;28(1–4):22–5. PubMed PMID: 12255249.
61. Haspels AA. The "morning-after pill"—a preliminary report. IPPF Med Bull. 1969;3(3):6. PubMed PMID: 12275493.
62. Yuzpe AA, Thurlow HJ, Ramzy I, Leyshon JI. Post coital contraception—a pilot study. J Reprod Med. 1974;13(2):53–8. PubMed PMID: 4844513.
63. Cheng L, Gulmezoglu AM, Piaggio G, Ezcurra E, Van Look PF. Interventions for emergency contraception. Cochrane Database Syst Rev. 2008;2, CD001324. PubMed PMID: 18425871.
64. Richardson AR, Maltz FN. Ulipristal acetate: review of the efficacy and safety of a newly approved agent for emergency contraception. Clin Ther. 2012;34(1):24–36. PubMed PMID: 22154199.
65. Bouchard P, Chabbert-Buffet N, Fauser BC. Selective progesterone receptor modulators in reproductive medicine: pharmacology, clinical efficacy and safety. Fertil Steril. 2011;96(5):1175–89. PubMed PMID: 21944187.
66. Glasier AF, Cameron ST, Fine PM, Logan SJ, Casale W, Van Horn J, et al. Ulipristal acetate versus levonorgestrel for emergency contraception: a randomised non-inferiority trial and meta-analysis. Lancet. 2010;375(9714):555–62. PubMed PMID: 20116841. Epub 2010/02/02. eng.
67. Brache V, Cochon L, Jesam C, Maldonado R, Salvatierra AM, Levy DP, et al. Immediate preovulatory administration of 30 mg ulipristal acetate significantly delays follicular rupture. Hum Reprod. 2010;25(9):2256–63. PubMed PMID: 20634186. Epub 2010/07/17. eng.

20 Medication Interactions with Contraceptives

Rachel Perry, Rebecca H. Stone, and Sadia Haider

Background

Scope of the Problem

Women with chronic diseases frequently rely on medical therapies for short- or long-term management of disease or disease-related symptoms. In addition, the use of prescription medication is increasing among the general population, with 49 % using at least one prescription drug in the past month in the years 2007–2010 compared to 38 % in 1988–1994. Women aged 18–44 have had a similar increase in prescription drug use, from 41 to 48 % over the same time period. The use of multiple medications is also escalating among reproductive age women, with 12 % taking three or more prescription drugs in the past month [1]. Some women with chronic disease may be represented in this latter group.

Pregnancies occurring among women with chronic disease may have implications for disease progression or increased rate of pregnancy complications [2–5]. Medications for chronic disease may allow women to optimize their health prior to attempting conception, such as anti-glycemic agents to achieve glycemic control for women with diabetes. Drug interactions with contraception, therefore, are particularly salient for the woman with chronic disease, as any interactions may potentially impact the effectiveness of contraception (leading to unintended pregnancy, which may have different implications for women with chronic disease than otherwise healthy women) or, conversely, the effectiveness of the medication designed to control the disease state. Additionally, medical therapies may be known teratogens, and decreasing risk of unplanned conception is important. In addition, women with chronic disease may turn to natural, nonprescription products such as botanicals or dietary supplements. Approximately, 17 % of US adults had used a natural product (excluding vitamins/minerals) in the past year, according to the 2007 National Health Interview Survey [1]. Finally, although not a drug interaction per se, the provider should understand that increased pill burden may decrease adherence to medication regimens [6], which may have implications for contraceptive counseling.

R. Perry, M.D.
Department of Obstetrics and Gynecology, University of Illinois Hospital and Health Sciences System, Chicago, IL, USA
e-mail: rachelp@uic.edu

R.H. Stone, Pharm.D., B.C.P.S.
College of Pharmacy, University of Illinois Hospital and Health Sciences System, University of Illinois at Chicago, Chicago, IL, USA
e-mail: stonereb@uic.edu

S. Haider, M.D., M.P.H. (✉)
Department of Obstetrics and Gynecology, University of Illinois at Chicago, Chicago, IL, USA
e-mail: sadiah@uic.edu

R.H. Allen and C.A. Cwiak (eds.), *Contraception for the Medically Challenging Patient*, DOI 10.1007/978-1-4939-1233-9_20, © Springer Science+Business Media New York 2014

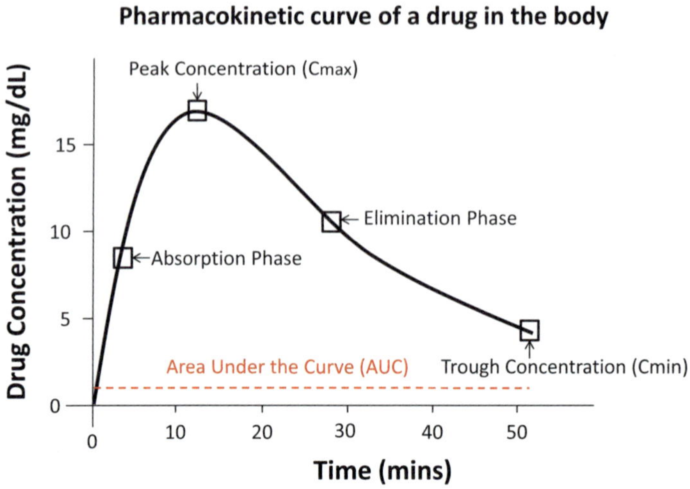

Fig. 20.1 Pharmacokinetic curve of a drug in the body demonstrating the area under the curve as a function of drug concentration (mg/dL) in the body over time (minutes)

Understanding Pharmacokinetics

Pharmacokinetics is the movement of drugs through the body. It includes the processes of absorption, distribution, metabolism, and excretion. Co-administered medications, among other factors, may affect the pharmacokinetics of a given drug. The amount of drug reaching the systemic circulation is referred to as its bioavailability. For example, the bioavailability for orally administered drugs is expressed as:

$$\text{Bioavailability} = \left(\text{AUC oral} / \text{AUC intravenous}\right) \times 100,$$

where AUC refers to "area under the curve," an estimate of total drug exposure over a given period of time (Fig. 20.1).

For orally administered combined oral contraceptives (COCs), the bioavailability is 40 % on average for the estrogen component [7–9], which consists of ethinyl estradiol (EE) for the majority of COCs marketed in the USA. Two additional estrogen formulations are available, but are less frequently prescribed. Mestranol, an alternative estrogen component that is metabolized to EE, is available in two 50 mcg COC formulations; however, this dose of EE is rarely used in clinical practice. Estradiol valerate is only available in Natazia, the first four-phase COC marketed in the USA. Currently, there is not a generic formulation available, and a 2011 Cochrane Review recommends monophasic products as first line since there is insufficient evidence to determine if quadriphasic and monophasic products differ in efficacy, bleeding pattern, and side effects [10]. Progestins, which are synthetic derivatives that mimic the action of endogenous progesterone, are the primary contraceptive components of COCs, and are used in progestin-only pills (POPs) and other progestin-only methods. The bioavailability of these synthetic agents depends on the class of progestin used, with a range of 65 % to greater than 90 % [11]. Approximately a dozen progestins have been used in COCs in the USA and are categorized into one of four "generations" [12]. The first generation was derived from testosterone (Estranes) and 17 hydroxyprogesterone (Pregnanes) in the 1960s and 1970s with a primary design target of antigonadotropic activity. The subsequent generations were developed in pursuit of an "ideal progestin" with more potent progestational and antiestrogenic actions on the endometrium in conjunction with less androgenic, estrogenic, or glucocorticoid effects such as acne, decreased high-density lipoprotein-C (HDL-C), bloating, and water retention. The second-generation progestins, norgestrel and levonorgestrel, are Gonanes derived from testosterone, while the third generation is composed of the gonane derivatives gestodene, norgestimate, desogestrel, and its active metabolite etonogestrel. Currently, fourth-generation progestins

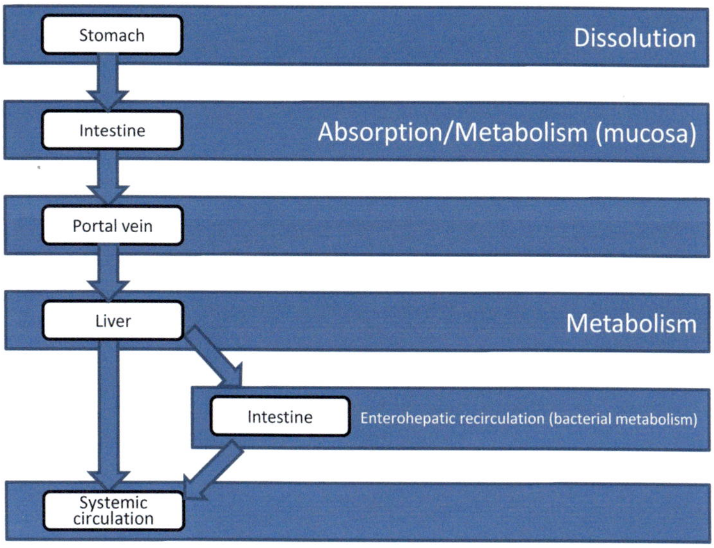

Fig. 20.2 Steps in the absorption and metabolism of ethinyl estradiol. Adapted from Contraception, 82/4, Edelman AB, Cherala G, Stanczyk FZ, Metabolism and pharmacokinetics of contraceptive steroids in obese women: a review, 314–323, Copyright 2010, with permission from Elsevier

available in the USA include drospirenone and dienogest. Drospirenone is derived from spironolactone, and exhibits antimineralocorticoid and antiandrogenic activity [13]. Dienogest, which is only available in Natazia, is structurally related to testosterone but also exhibits antiandrogenic and antiestrogenic properties [13]. Effectiveness does not vary by type of progestin, though side effects may differ [14].

Orally administered contraceptive steroids undergo hepatic first-pass metabolism. After the COC is ingested, it dissolves in the stomach and is absorbed across the wall of the small intestine. Some EE is conjugated to an inactive metabolite in the jejunal mucosa, which accounts for 65 % of its first-pass metabolism. Depending on the progestin, it may be conjugated to form an inactive metabolite by intestinal bacteria. The mixture of conjugated and unconjugated steroids is then transported to the liver through the portal vein, where both EE and progestins are metabolized by cytochrome P450 (CYP) enzymes and that fraction of both steroids that remains unmetabolized is transported into the systemic circulation as bioavailable drug.

Inactive conjugates of EE are then excreted in the bile, at which point some authors have suggested that the original EE compound may be liberated by gut bacteria and reabsorbed, thereby possibly increasing its bioavailability [15]. This concept is termed enterohepatic recirculation. However, the extent to which enterohepatic recirculation is clinically significant for EE metabolism in humans is disputed. In a small study of women status post-ileostomy (and thus elimination of bacteria implicated in metabolism), the bioavailability of EE was no different from controls [16]. Progestins do not have the capacity to undergo enterohepatic recirculation, and their specific pharmacokinetics depend on the type and chemical structure [11]. For COCs containing mestranol rather than EE, metabolism is essentially identical to EE, after a rapid demethylation [15]. While the average bioavailability of oral EE is 40 %, there is considerable individual variation, with a range of 20–65 % [15] (Fig. 20.2).

Nonoral routes of administration for combined contraceptive steroids include the vaginal (ring) and transdermal (patch). Nonoral routes of administration of progestin-only contraceptives include subcutaneous (implant), intramuscular or subcutaneous (depot medroxyprogesterone acetate—DMPA), and intrauterine (levonorgestrel intrauterine device—LNG-IUD). Though

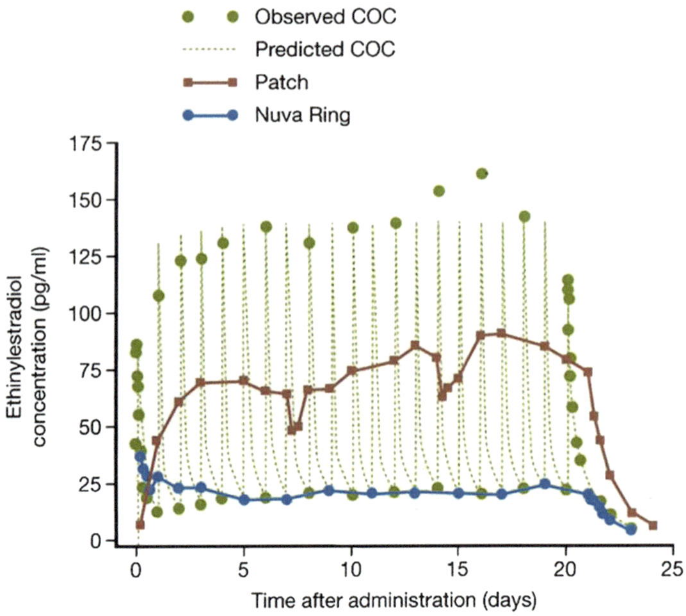

Fig. 20.3 Concentration-time curves for ethinyl estradiol for three routes of administration. Reprinted from Contraception, 72/3, van den Heuvel MW, van Bragt AJM, Alnabawy AKM, Kaptein MCJ, Comparison of ethinyl estradiol pharmacokinetics in three hormonal contraceptive formulations: the vaginal ring, the transdermal patch, and an oral contraceptive, 168–174, Copyright 2005, with permission from Elsevier

the pharmacokinetics of each of these methods vary by route, but all share the absence of first-pass metabolism. The levels of systemic progestin in the implant and DMPA are high enough to suppress ovulation [17–19], while the LNG-IUD works through local action and has the lowest systemic absorption of progestin compared to all routes [20–22].

Levels of EE also vary by route of administration, and the comparative levels of EE are shown in Fig. 20.3. Given the unique characteristics of each of the progestins, a similar comparison of progestin levels by route of administration is not available.

Mechanisms of Drug Interaction for Contraceptive Steroids

Drugs may interact in a synergistic or antagonistic fashion. The combination of synthetic estrogen and progestin is an example of a synergistic interaction; the ability of the combination of drugs to suppress gonadotropins together is greater than either drug alone [23]. Most drug interactions of clinical significance for contraceptive steroids, however, are antagonistic. Drug interactions between contraceptive steroids and noncontraceptive drugs may potentially affect levels of contraceptive drug or levels of noncontraceptive drug. This may lead to subtherapeutic or supratherapeutic levels of either drug and lead to lowered efficacy (for antagonistic interactions) or adverse drug effects (for synergistic interactions).

The first drug interaction with oral contraception was reported in 1971 when Reimers and Jezek reported increased intermenstrual bleeding among women taking COCs and rifampin for tuberculosis [24]. Further studies showed an increase in pregnancies among women taking rifampin compared to the accepted failure rate of COCs [7, 25–27]. Most drug interactions with contraceptive steroids involve drugs that induce or inhibit cytochrome P450 3A4 isoenzymes and affect the hepatic metabolism of estrogens and progestins. Drugs that induce CYP may increase the rate of hepatic degradation of contraceptive steroids, leading to a lower bioavailability and potential loss of contraceptive effect. In studies of drug interactions, a significant change in the AUC for Drug A when combined with Drug B compared to Drug A and placebo indicates that there is an interaction between Drug A and Drug B.

Though the effect on hepatic metabolism is the main mechanism by which contraceptive steroid drug interactions are mediated, several other mechanisms are possible, including (1) reduction in amount of steroid absorbed; (2) increased serum protein binding of steroid hormone; (3) decreasing gut bacteria such that enterohepatic recirculation is affected. However, data from available studies suggest that these mechanisms do not affect contraceptive steroid metabolism in a clinically relevant way.

Special Circumstances

With a growing obesity epidemic in the USA, there is an emergent need for research on the pharmacokinetics of contraceptive steroids as well as other drugs in the obese population. Limited research explores whether obesity affects the metabolism and bioavailability of contraceptive steroids, which may have implications for both contraceptive effectiveness and drug interactions. Most efficacy studies of steroidal contraceptives exclude women over 130 % of ideal body weight. One study of orally administered EE/LNG did include women with greater than 130 % ideal body weight, and the half-life, and subsequently the time to reach steady state, was double in obese versus non-obese women [28]. Another study found lower AUC and maximum plasma concentration for EE among obese women compared to non-obese women who were given EE/LNG COCs, although steady state was not reached in this study [29]. A study of subcutaneous DMPA (DMPA-SC) among normal weight, obese, and extremely obese women showed lower levels of MPA among the obese compared to the non-obese subjects, with the lowest levels in the extremely obese subjects [30]. The clinical significance of these differences in steroid pharmacokinetics for obese women is not yet understood, and further research is necessary.

Nonhormonal Contraception

Clinicians should consider the copper IUD as an effective alternative to hormonal methods of contraception. The copper IUD is a long-acting, highly effective method with high continuation rates that relies on local release of copper ions for its effect, and therefore does not interact with medications [31].

Medication Classes

Antibiotics/Antimycobacterials

Rifampin and rifabutin, two antimycobacterial drugs in the rifamycin class, affect the hormone levels of combined hormonal contraceptives, POPs, and etonogestrel implants through induction of the CYP 3A4 enzyme [32]. Rifampin and rifabutin (and combination drugs Rifamate and Rifater) are inducers of CYP 3A4 and increase degradation of EE and progestins, to the extent that unintended pregnancies may occur [24, 26, 32, 33]. Women should be encouraged to consider DMPA or an IUD if long-term use of these agents is required [32]. Pharmacokinetic studies of other broad-spectrum antibiotic classes (aminoglycosides, cephalosporins, macrolides, and penicillins) have not been proven in pharmacokinetic studies to interact with combined hormonal contraceptives or progestin-only methods [32] (Table 20.1).

Table 20.1 Studies showing no effect of broad-spectrum antibiotic use on pharmacokinetics of combined oral contraceptives, ring, or patch

Antibiotic	Year	Author
Ampicillin 500 mg BID	1980	Joshi et al.
Ampicillin 500 mg TID	1982	Back et al.
Ampicillin 250 mg QID	1980	Friedman et al.
Amoxicillin 875 mg BID[a]	2005	Dogterom et al.
Ciprofloxacin 500 mg BID	1998	Schloten et al.
Ciprofloxacin 500 mg BID	1991	Maggiolo et al.
Clarithromycin 250 mg BID	1991	Back et al.
Doxycycline 100 mg BID	1991	Neely et al.
Doxycycline 100 mg BID[a]	2005	Dogterom et al.
Metronidazole 400 mg TID	1980	Joshi et al.
Ofloxacin 200 mg BID	1996	Csemiczky et al.
Temafloxacin 600 mg BID	1991	Back et al.
Tetracycline 500 mg TID	1991	Murphy

[a]Patch and ring

However, some controversy over the possible interaction of broad-spectrum antibiotics with contraceptive steroids has historically involved the theory that if gut flora is depleted, EE conjugates do not undergo enterohepatic recirculation and the amount of bioavailable steroid is reduced. However, the data supporting this theory is based on retrospective case series and small observational series. A large case-crossover study of 1,330 patients with COC failure from a large national registry showed no relationship between antibiotic use and pregnancy. However, this study lacked power to detect pregnancy resulting from COC failure [27]. In a review of the evidence, Dickinson reported that given the relatively high rate of COC failure under typical use, it might be impossible to identify an increased risk even if one existed [34]. The US Medical Eligibility Criteria for Contraceptive Use (USMEC) ranks broad-spectrum antibiotic use as a category 1 condition for use of all combination hormonal methods (COC, patch, and ring), while rifampin and rifabutin are category 3 [32].

Antifungals

Medications in the antifungal class azoles have an inhibitory effect on CYP 3A4 and can increase the bioavailability of contraceptive steroids. While there should be no concern about decreased contraceptive efficacy, adverse events may theoretically occur. The most common antifungal in the azole group among reproductive-aged women is fluconazole, often given orally for vaginal yeast infection. Fluconazole is thought to be a weak inhibitor of CYP 3A4, and the increases in the EE component of COCs seen in studies are unlikely to be of clinical significance [35, 36]. Voriconazole, however, was found in one study to increase EE and norethindrone bioavailability to a greater degree, and co-administration may also increase levels of voriconazole. Therefore, patients using this medication with systemic contraceptive steroids should be monitored for adverse events related to both medications [37]. Antifungals are category 1 in the USMEC.

Antiretrovirals

Treatment options for patients with HIV have evolved dramatically since its emergence in the 1980s. Therapy is based on treatment with highly active antiretroviral therapy (HAART), and continues to evolve with development of new agents and formulations of these drugs. Antiretroviral (ARV) classes that are recommended for first-line treatment and most frequently utilized are the nucleoside reverse transcriptase inhibitors (NRTI), non-nucleoside reverse transcriptase inhibitors (NNRTI), protease inhibitors (PI), and integrase inhibitors (INSTI). Contraceptive steroids and many ARVs are metabolized by the CYP P450 system, predisposing these agents to drug interactions in a patient population with complex medication regimens [38]. Clinical trial information that is available regarding hormonal contraception and ARVs is based on limited pharmacokinetic studies with small sample sizes and short durations of exposure [38]. Additionally, the primary outcome for most of these studies is change in drug serum level; however contraceptive drug serum levels do not directly translate to clinical effects. For example, there is no literature correlating a specific decrease in drug serum level with a clinically significant contraceptive failure such as an unplanned pregnancy. One study did analyze serologic evaluation of ovulation [39]; however, the majority of studies did not evaluate measures such as serum hormone levels or pelvic ultrasounds to detect ovulation [38]. Of the ARV agents, CYP 450 interactions between PIs and COCs demonstrated the most significant effect on EE and progestin AUCs, followed by NNRTIs, as shown in Table 20.2 [38]. Efavirenz is the most commonly used NNRTI, and in addition to decreasing sex steroids in COCs, it has also significantly decreased progestin levels following administration of LNG emergency contraception. There are currently no data evaluating LNG emergency contraception with concurrent PI use. Additionally, there are no studies evaluating drug interactions between ulipristal acetate and ARVs; however, this agent is metabolized by CYP3A4 enzymes and may have altered serum concentrations when used with CYP3A4 inducers

Table 20.2 Interactions between hormonal contraception and antiretroviral therapy[a]

Drug class	Sex steroid area under the curve (AUC) percent change: EE	Progestin	DMPA	Etonogestrel implant	LNG-IUD	LNG emergency contraception
NRTI	No change	No change	0–↑1 %	No AUC data[b]	No change	No AUC data
NNRTI	↓22–↑22 %	↓5–↓64 %	0–↑1 %			↓48 %
PI	↓55–↑48 %	↓18–↑110 %	No change			No AUC data
INSTI	↓2 %	↑14 %	No change			No AUC data

EE ethinyl estradiol, *DMPA* depot medroxyprogesterone acetate, *LNG* levonorgestrel, *NRTI* nucleoside reverse transcriptase inhibitors, *NNRTI* non-nucleoside reverse transcriptase inhibitors, *PI* protease inhibitors, *INSTI* integrase inhibitors

[a]Adapted from [33]

[b]No AUC data for ENG implant. However, there have been six case reports of pregnancies with the NNRTI efavirenz and the ENG implant during the latter half of the 3-year post-insertion period

or inhibitors such as ARVs [40]. Interestingly, while there are also no AUC data evaluating etonogestrel arm implants and HAART therapy, there are six case reports of pregnancy in patients who had the etonogestrel implant and who were also taking triple ART therapy containing the NNRTI efavirenz. These women all had the implant inserted between 1.5 and 3 years prior, placing them in the latter half of the therapeutic window. It is not recommended to use NNRTIs or PIs in conjunction with combined hormonal contraception (CHC) or etonogestrel implants. Limited data suggest emergency contraception should be used with caution in the setting of NNRTIs or PIs while there are no studies evaluating ulipristal acetate in this setting; however, these methods may be utilized if other first-line methods are not accessible, preferably in conjunction with barrier methods. The LNG-IUD and DMPA demonstrated no change in hormone levels with these agents, and are acceptable for use with PIs and NNRTIs, as is the copper IUD. INSTIs and NRTIs do not appear to have a significant effect on sex steroid concentrations, and are safe to use with all contraceptive options. Of note, individuals infected with human immunodeficiency virus (HIV) are recommended to use condoms with every act of intercourse to prevent transmission and potential mutation of virus, regardless of other concurrent contraceptive agents (see Table 20.2).

Antimalarials

There are no suspected drug interactions or studies evaluating interactions with chloroquine, atovaquone-proguanil, or mefloquine and any of the contraceptives. One study demonstrated that there is no interaction between quinine and oral contraceptives [41].

Anticonvulsants

The anticonvulsants are commonly used for epilepsy as well as many other indications in current practice, including treatment for migraines, depression, neuropathic pain, and drug dependency. As a drug class it has been well documented that anticonvulsants can have significant interactions with contraceptive hormones, with the first report appearing in the literature in 1972 [42, 43]. Two types of clinically significant interactions may occur with concurrent contraceptive and anticonvulsant use: those that reduce the effectiveness of contraceptives, and those that influence the metabolism of anticonvulsants.

Contraceptive hormones are metabolized by CYP450 enzymes in the liver, and many anticonvulsants are strong inducers of CYP3A enzymes, which together may accelerate the hepatic metabolism of hormonal contraceptives regardless of the route of administration. This decreased duration and intensity of contraceptive action may lead to increased ovulation and pregnancy rates [43]. The magnitude of this effect varies with individual anticonvulsant agents, since some may be potent inducers of CYP 3A4 enzymes (notably carbamazepine, oxcarbazepine, phenobarbital, phenytoin, primidone), while others have moderate (topiramate), weak, or no effects (Table 20.3). There are many reports in the literature of

Table 20.3 Interactions between hormonal contraception and antiepileptic therapy[a]

Antiepileptic drug	Brand	Serum hormone levels		Antiepileptic levels
Potent CYP inducers		*Ethinyl estradiol*	*Progestin*	
Carbamazepine	Tegretol	↓ EE	↓LNG	No data
Oxcarbazepine	Trileptal	↓ EE	↓LNG	No data
Phenobarbital	Generic	↓ EE	↓LNG	No data
Phenytoin	Dilantin	↓ EE	↓LNG	No data
Primidone	Mysoline	No data	No data	No data
Moderate CYP inducers				
Topiramate	Topamax	↓ EE	No Δ NOR	No data
Weak CYP inducers				
Felbamate	Felbatol	↓ EE	↓GSD	No data
Gabapentin	Neurontin	No Data	No Data	No data
Levetiracetam	Keppra	No Δ EE	No Δ LNG	No data
Tiagabine	Gabitril	No Δ EE	No Δ LNG	No data
Vigabatrin	Sabril	No Δ EE	No Δ LNG	No data
Zonisamide	Zonegran	No Δ EE	No Δ NOR	No data
Lacosamide		No Δ EE	No Δ LNG	No data
Ethosuximide	Zarontin	No Δ COC	No data	No data
Pregabalin	Lyrica	No Δ COC	No data	No data
Undergo glucuronidation				
Lamotrigine	Lamictal	No Δ EE	↓LNG	↓ w/COCs No data w/patch No data w/ring
Valproic Acid	Depakote Depakene	No Δ EE	No Δ LNG	↓ w/COCs ↓ w/patch No data w/ring

EE ethinyl estradiol, *LNG* levonorgestrel, *GSD* gestodene, *NOR* norethisterone, *COCs* combined oral contraceptives
[a]Adapted from Contraception, 83/1, Gaffield ME, Culwell KR, Lee CR, The use of hormonal contraception among women taking anticonvulsant therapy, 16–29, Copyright 2011, with permission from Elsevier

unintended pregnancy with concurrent use of moderate or potent CYP3A inducers and estrogen-containing contraceptives, and three reports of pregnancy in the only trial evaluating POPs [43]. Therefore, women requiring these agents while using CHC or POPs should be switched to more effective methods or add a second method [32, 43]. There have been three reports of unintended pregnancy with progestin implants (two Norplant, one Implanon), and one report of pregnancy with a LNG-IUD [43, 44]. The USMEC recommends women who require a moderate or potent CYP3A4 inducing anticonvulsant consider switching to a more effective method than the etonogestrel implant or add a second method [32]. Since there is only a single report of pregnancy with the LNG-IUD, and no pregnancy reports or demonstrated pharmacokinetic interaction with DMPA or the copper IUD, these agents are recommended as first line by the USMEC [32].

The metabolism of anticonvulsants may be affected by another specific mechanism of drug clearance, glucuronidation. The estrogen component in contraceptives may induce glucuronidation, which can significantly decrease levels of anticonvulsants metabolized by this route such as lamotrigine and valproic acid [43]. While EE is an inducer of glucuronidation, a portion of EE metabolism is also completed via glucuronidation; however, this has not been evaluated in clinical trials and does not appear to affect contraceptive hormone levels [43]. When used with CHC, lamotrigine doses may need to be adjusted due to the significant decrease in antiepileptic drug levels (41–64 %) [12, 43]. While there are also decreases in lamotrigine levels with LNG use, they are less significant; therefore, dose adjustments are likely not needed when using POPs, DMPA, implants, or IUDs with this agent [43]. For clinical recommendations, see Chap. 8.

Triptans

Concurrent use of triptan agents with CHC has been shown to reduce the clearance of triptans, demonstrated by a reduced naratriptan clearance of 32 % when used with an oral contraceptive [45]; however, there are no documented cases of triptan toxicity in conjunction with hormonal contraceptives. Dosing changes are not recommended unless the patient experiences adverse effects related to increased triptan exposure. There are no restrictions on use of POPs, DMPA, implants, or IUDs with triptans.

Diabetes Agents

While EE and some progestins may affect plasma glucose and reduce insulin sensitivity, studies show that COCs, ring, implant, and DMPA in modern doses do not affect these parameters in any clinically meaningful way [46–48]; thus doses of diabetic medications do not need to be adjusted for a woman using hormonal contraceptives.

Certain thiazolidinediones may affect the metabolism of contraceptive steroids. Troglitazone (Rezulin), which was removed from the US market in 2001 due to cases of liver failure, is a CYP 3A4 inducer, which decreased the bioavailability of both EE and norethindrone by approximately 30 % [49]. However, the thiazolidinedione rosiglitazone (Avandia) is metabolized by another CYP enzyme, and it has been found that co-administration with EE and norethindrone did not affect the pharmacokinetics of either steroid hormone [50]. While no studies have been done on contraceptive hormones and the third member of this class, pioglitazone (Actos), it is metabolized by CYP 3A4 [51], so co-administration with contraceptive steroids could theoretically lead to decreased bioavailability of the steroid hormones.

Glucagon-like peptide receptor agonists slow gastric emptying, among other effects, which has implications for metabolism of orally administered drugs such as COCs or POPs. One study examined a COC containing EE and levonorgestrel administered 1 h before versus 30 min after exenatide (Byetta) injection and found a reduction in maximum concentration (Cmax) for the contraceptive steroids in the post-injection group but no difference in AUC [52]. Regardless, it is recommended that exenatide users who also use medications relying on threshold concentrations for efficacy (such as COCs) take these medications at least 1 h prior to exenatide injection [53]. The prescribing information for the other medication in this class, liraglutide (Victoza), states "caution should be used when oral medications are concomitantly administered" [54].

No studies have been completed to evaluate the interaction of contraceptive steroids with second-generation sulfonylureas (glipizide, glyburide, glimepiride), biguanides (metformin), alpha glucosidase inhibitors (acarbose, miglitol), DPP-4 inhibitors (saxagliptin, sitagliptin), meglitinides (nateglinide, mitiglinide), or amylin agonists (pramlintide).

Thyroid Agents

In women using contraceptive hormones that are systemically absorbed, the binding of T3 and T4 is increased due to the effect of hormones on hepatic globulin synthesis (increased thyroid binding globulin). Thus the total level of thyroid hormone is increased but not the free fraction [55, 56]. There are no reported interactions with T3 or T4 preparations (such as levothyroxine), thionamides, or iodinated agents with contraceptive hormones.

Autoimmune Agents

Immunosuppressants such as cyclosporine, sirolimus, and tacrolimus are metabolized by the CYP 3A4 system. Concurrent use with CHC may inhibit the metabolism of these agents and increase their concentrations, which may lead to adverse effects [57–59]. Since estrogens are metabolized by CYP 3A4, these immunosuppressants may also increase levels of EE with corresponding side effects [59]. Patients may be monitored for both immunosuppressant level changes and symptoms of estrogen excess if CHC is initiated. If CHC is discontinued, then close monitoring of the patients immunosuppressant level may be considered to evaluate the need for dose adjustment.

There is a theoretical concern that immunosuppressive agents may interfere with the inflammatory reaction produced by IUDs in the endometrium, but there are no studies evaluating this potential interaction [59]. It has been suggested that macrophages play a significant role in the local inflammatory reaction produced by IUDs, and immunosuppressants are believed to have minimal effect on macrophage activity. However, there is no interaction between these immunosuppressive agents and the LNG or copper ions in IUD systems [59]. There are no studies evaluating POPs, DMPA, or implants with these immunosuppressive agents.

Psychiatric Agents

The most commonly used agents for depression in the USA are selective serotonin reuptake inhibitors (SSRIs). At this time there are no studies evaluating drug interactions between these agents; however there are reports of a theoretical interaction regarding concurrent use of citalopram and estrogen. In vitro data indicate that EE is an inhibitor of CYP 2C19, and recommendations for citalopram indicate since it is a substrate for CYP 2C19, the maximum citalopram dose should be 20 mg/day in patients receiving CYP 2C19 inhibitors due to dose-dependent QT interval prolongation [60]. There are no documented cases of this interaction, and currently no empiric dose changes are recommended due to interactions between COC and SSRI use. There are no clinical trials evaluating serotonin-norepinephrine reuptake inhibitors (SNRIs) and contraceptives.

Combined hormonal contraception (CHC) may increase the effect of tricyclic antidepressants (TCAs) by inhibiting their hepatic metabolism, and the patient should be monitored for symptoms of TCA toxicity if CHC is initiated [58–61]. Additionally, the concentration of monoamine oxidase inhibitors (MAOIs) significantly increases with use of CHC due to inhibition of first-pass metabolism. In one small trial with eight subjects, selegeline levels increased by approximately 20 times normal serum levels with COC use [62]. There are no studies evaluating the use of MAOIs with the vaginal ring or patch. Use of MAOIs should be avoided or the dose decreased to avoid adverse effects, including hypertensive reactions, when CHC is initiated. There are no studies evaluating MAOIs with progestin-only products.

There is a theoretical interaction indicating CHC may decrease the blood serum concentration of some antipsychotics. Ethinyl estradiol is an inhibitor of CYP 1A2 enzymes, which metabolize chlorpromazine, clozapine, thioridazine, and olanzapine and may therefore increase the levels of these antipsychotics [63]. In a case report, one woman taking a COC and clozapine experienced elevated clozapine plasma levels and side effects, both of which resolved upon discontinuation of her COC [64]. However, a recent study evaluating olanzapine with CHC or progestin-only contraceptives found no clinically relevant changes in olanzapine serum concentrations. This study found decreased levels of olanzapine metabolites with CHC; however, this was not clinically significant [65]. There are no dose adjustments recommended for patients taking antipsychotics and CHC or POPs; however, it may be beneficial to monitor patients for adverse reactions related to increased antipsychotic concentrations with concurrent use of CHC.

Benzodiazepine clearance is inhibited by EE and may yield increased serum concentrations [66, 67]; however, one study demonstrated that a low-dose estrogen formulation COC did not significantly influence the clearance of alprazolam [68]. This interaction with hormonal contraceptives may not be limited to EE alone: another study evaluated triazolam with concurrent use of progesterone (Prometrium, 100 or 200 mg) and found the effects of triazolam were increased and extended [67]. Patients starting hormonal contraceptives should be monitored for increased effects of benzodiazepine use.

There are no perceived interactions or studies evaluating interactions between any of the psychiatric agents and DMPA, LNG implants, or IUDs.

Antihypertensives

Antihypertensives and EE do not demonstrate any clinically significant interaction with standard dosing. While some clinical trials have demonstrated decreased clearance of the beta blocker metoprolol [69, 70] and metabolites from the calcium channel blocker nifedipine [71], there was no clinically significant change in blood pressure due to this inhibition of CYP 3A4 activity. Other antihypertensives such as angiotensin-converting enzyme (ACE) inhibitors, angiotensin receptor blockers, diuretics, and nitrates are not documented to have any type of clinically significant interaction with EE.

While first-, second-, and third-generation progestins do not interact with any of the antihypertensive agents, the fourth-generation progestin drospirenone acts as an antimineralocorticoid and can interact with other potassium-sparing drugs. One study found very little effect in potassium levels in healthy women taking drospirenone in conjunction with spironolactone [72]. However, agents such as ACE inhibitors, angiotensin-II antagonists, potassium sparing diuretics, and aldosterone antagonists may cause hyperkalemia, which may be exacerbated when used with drospirenone, especially in the setting of renal impairment. Providers may consider checking serum potassium levels in these patients within the first month of therapy [73].

Anticoagulants

It is well established that estrogens increase the risk of thrombosis; therefore, contraceptives containing estrogens are typically avoided in patients who require anticoagulation. The limited data evaluating concurrent vitamin K antagonist and hormonal contraceptive use includes a case report series noting an increased anticoagulant effect with COCs [74], a single case report with varying international normalized ratio (INR) effects in response to combined followed by progestin-only contraceptives [75], and a case report with increased anticoagulant effect following use of a levonorgestrel emergency contraceptive [76]. If concurrent use of warfarin and hormonal contraception is required, it is recommended to monitor INR more closely while therapy is initiated. Antiplatelet agents may decrease EE concentrations but do not appear to alter progestin concentrations when taken with COCs. This was demonstrated by ticagrelor, an antiplatelet agent metabolized by CYP 3A4/5, which decreased ethinyl estradiol exposure by 20 % with a COC [77]. However, interaction with antiplatelet agents is not thought to be clinically significant because the effect on EE metabolism is relatively small and the primary contraceptive benefit is provided by the progestin component of COCs.

Heparins and low molecular weight heparins do not interact with oral contraceptives. It is unknown if newer anticoagulant classes such as the direct thrombin inhibitors (dabigatran, argatroban, etc.) and direct factor Xa inhibitors (rivaroxaban, apixaban) are affected by oral hormonal contraceptives.

Progestin-only methods such as DMPA, LNG implants, or IUDs are preferred in patients requiring anticoagulation. There are no known interaction between these agents and any of the anticoagulant classes.

Gastrointestinal Agents

There is no evidence for interaction between contraceptive steroids and antacids. In a study of 12 women co-administered antacid and COC there was no change in the total bioavailability of either steroid compared to baseline [78].

A randomized, placebo-controlled study showed that COC co-administered with lansoprazole did not affect the bioavailability of contraceptive steroids [79], suggesting that proton-pump inhibitors do not interact with contraceptive hormones. There are no studies that evaluate contraception interaction with the other commonly used drug class for gastrointestinal reflux disease, H2-receptor blockers.

For medications for the management of inflammatory bowel disease (IBD), see autoimmune agents.

There is no evidence of interactions between antidiarrheals and contraceptives.

Respiratory System Agents

There is no evidence suggesting interaction between commonly used medications for asthma, including bronchodilators, beta 2 adrenergic agonists, or inhaled corticosteroids and contraceptive steroids. Theophylline, a medication rarely used due to a narrow therapeutic window, has been shown to interact with COCs whereby clearance of theophylline is reduced, increasing the risk of theophylline toxicity [80]. If a patient is taking theophylline, consideration should be given to nonhormonal methods or the levonorgestrel IUD.

One medication for treatment of pulmonary arterial hypertension, bosentan, has shown to interact with COCs. Bosentan (Tracleer) decreased the AUC of norethindrone and EE in one study, which suggests that nonhormonal methods or LNG-IUD may be preferable to systemic steroids for patients taking bosentan [81].

Other commonly used respiratory agents such as antitussives, mucolytics, and decongestants do not interact with contraceptive steroids.

Lipid-Lowering Agents

The most common lipid-lowering agents utilized in practice today are statins. Due to the possible teratogenicity of these agents, they should only be taken by sexually active women of childbearing age if they are using contraception. Atorvastatin and rosuvastatin have been shown to increase the area AUC of EE 20–26 % and progesterone by 15–34 % [82]. It is likely that CYP 3A4 metabolism is involved in this interaction with most of the statins, but there are likely additional factors since rosuvastatin does not demonstrate CYP 3A4 induction but still caused an increase in EE AUC. However, this increase of EE and progestin with statins is not clinically significant, and no dose change is required unless the patient experiences side effects from excess EE or progestin. The package insert of bile acid sequestrants recommends that oral drugs that have not been studied with these agents, including oral contraceptives, be taken 1 h before or 4 h after to prevent absorption interference [83]. There are no suspected interactions or studies evaluating CHC or POPs with any other lipid-lowering agents, including fibrates, ezetimibe, nicotinic acid, or omega 3 fatty acids.

There are no known interactions between any of the lipid-lowering agents and DMPA, etonogestrel implants, or IUDs.

Analgesics

There is no evidence for interaction between most common analgesics, including acetaminophen (APAP), narcotics, muscle relaxants, or aspirin, with contraceptive steroids. The package insert of drospirenone-containing contraceptives states that concurrent use with NSAIDS may have additive effects on serum potassium, and may warrant potassium monitoring during the first month of concurrent therapy. However, the one clinical trial found no evidence of hyperkalemia with concurrent drospirenone and indomethacin use [72, 84].

Common Supplements

St. Johns wort is a known inducer CYP 3A4, 2E1, and 2C19, which predisposes it to interact with COCs. Studies have demonstrated increased intermenstrual bleeding with COCs that is indicative of reduced plasma concentrations of both EE and progestin [85–87], and there is one case report of unwanted pregnancy [88]. Due to less US Food and Drug Administration (FDA) oversight with dosing and availability of herbal supplements, in conjunction with these potential drug interactions, it is recommended to avoid St. Johns wort with both estrogen-containing and progestin-only contraceptives. There are no studies evaluating interactions with DMPA, etonogestrel implants, and IUDs.

Research Gaps and Clinical Implications

This chapter provides a comprehensive summary of possible drug interactions with hormonal contraception based on the existing evidence; however, further research is needed in areas where evidence is lacking. Specific areas of need for additional research include ARV therapy (particularly regimens that include efavirenz and implanon, as well as emergency contraception and PIs), use of contraception with benzodiazepines, and oral contraceptive use with all forms of newer anticoagulant therapy (i.e., thrombin inhibitors and direct factor Xa inhibitors). As described throughout the chapter, long-acting reversible methods of contraception (LARC), like the IUDs in the majority of clinical situations and the implant in most clinical situations, have limited drug interactions. The limited drug interactions coupled with the high efficacy of LARC methods make them an optimal choice for most women, especially those with chronic disease. Clinicians should emphasize the safety of LARC methods, their efficacy, and the lack of need for adding additional medications to existing daily medication regimens when counseling women with chronic diseases.

References

1. National Center for Health Statistics (2013) Health, United States, 2012: with special feature on Emergency Care, Hyattsville, MD.
2. Misra DP, Grason H, Weisman C. An intersection of women's and perinatal health: the role of chronic conditions. Wom Health Issues. 2000;10(5):256–67.
3. Khairy P, Ouyang DW, Fernandes SM, Lee-Parritz A, Economy KE, Landzberg MJ. Pregnancy outcomes in women with congenital heart disease. Circulation. 2006;113(4):517–24.
4. Vellanki K. Pregnancy in chronic kidney disease. Adv Chronic Kidney Dis. 2013;20(3):223–8.
5. American College of Obstetricians and Gynecologists. ACOG Practice Bulletin No. 125: chronic hypertension in pregnancy. Obstet Gynecol. 2002;119(1):396–407.
6. Ickovics JR, Meisler AW. Adherence in AIDS clinical trials: a framework for clinical research and clinical care. J Clin Epidemiol. 1997;50(4):385–91.
7. Back DJ, Breckenridge AM, Crawford FE, MacIver M, Orme ML, Rowe PH, et al. An investigation of the pharmacokinetics of ethynylestradiol in women using radio-immunoassay. Contraception. 1979;20(3):263–73.
8. Humpel M, Nieuweboer B, Wendt H, Speck U. Investigations of pharmacokinetics of ethinyloestradiol to specific consideration of a possible first-pass effect in women. Contraception. 1979;19(4):421–32.
9. Back DJ, Breckenridge AM, MacIver M, Orme M, Purba HS, Rowe PH, et al. The gut wall metabolism of ethinyloestradiol and its contribution to the pre-systemic metabolism of ethinyloestradiol in humans. Br J Clin Pharmacol. 1982;13(3):325–30.
10. Van Vliet HA, Raps M, Lopez LM, Helmerhorst FM. Quadriphasic versus monophasic oral contraceptives for contraception. Cochrane Database Syst Rev. 2011;(11):CD009038. doi(11):CD009038.
11. Stanczyk FZ. All progestins are not created equal. Steroids. 2003;68(10–13):879–90.
12. Hatcher RA, Trussel J, Nelson AL, editors. Contraceptive technology. 20th ed. New York, NY: Ardent Media; 2011.
13. Sitruk-Ware R. New progestagens for contraceptive use. Hum Reprod Update. 2006;12(2):169–78.
14. Lawrie TA, Helmerhorst FM, Maitra NK, Kulier R, Bloemenkamp K, Gulmezoglu AM. Types of progestogens in combined oral contraception: effectiveness and side-effects. Cochrane Database Syst Rev. 2011;(5):CD004861. doi(5):CD004861.
15. Hanker JP. Gastrointestinal disease and oral contraception. Am J Obstet Gynecol. 1990;163(6 Pt 2):2204–7.
16. Grimmer SF, Back DJ, Orme ML, Cowie A, Gilmore I, Tjia J. The bioavailability of ethinyloestradiol and levonorgestrel in patients with an ileostomy. Contraception. 1986;33(1):51–9.
17. Mäkäräinen L, van Beek A, Tuomivaara L, Asplund B, Coelingh BH. Ovarian function during the use of a single contraceptive implant: implanon compared with Norplant. Fertil Steril. 1998;69(4):714–21.
18. Mishell DRJ. Pharmacokinetics of depot medroxyprogesterone acetate contraception. J Reprod Med. 1996;41(5 Suppl):381–90.
19. Halpern V, Combes SL, Dorflinger LJ, Weiner DH, Archer DF. Pharmacokinetics of subcutaneous depot medroxyprogesterone acetate injected in the upper arm. Contraception. 2014;89(1):31–5.
20. Rivera R, Yacobson I, Grimes D. The mechanism of action of hormonal contraceptives and intrauterine contraceptive devices. Am J Obstet Gynecol. 1999; 181(5 Pt 1):1263–9.
21. Mechanism of action, safety and efficacy of intrauterine devices. Report of a WHO Scientific Group. World Health Organ Tech Rep Ser. 1987;753:1–91.
22. Nilsson CG, Lahteenmaki PL, Luukkainen T, Robertson DN. Sustained intrauterine release of levonorgestrel over five years. Fertil Steril. 1986;45(6):805–7.

23. Fraser IS, Jansen RP. Why do inadvertent pregnancies occur in oral contraceptive users? Effectiveness of oral contraceptive regimens and interfering factors. Contraception. 1983;27(6):531–51.
24. Reimers D, Jezek A. The simultaneous use of rifampicin and other antitubercular agents with oral contraceptives. Prax Pneumol. 1971;25:255–62.
25. Joshi JV, Joshi UM, Sankholi GM, Krishna U, Mandlekar A, Chowdhury V. A study of interaction of low-dose combination oral contraceptive with ampicillin and metronidazole. Contraception. 1980;22:643–52.
26. Bolt HM, Bolt M, Kappus H. Interaction of rifampicin treatment with pharmacokinetics and metabolism of ethinyloestradiol in man. Acta Endocrinol. 1977;85: 189–97.
27. Toh S, Mitchell AA, Anderka M, de Jong-van den Berg LT, Hernandez-Diaz S, National Birth Defects Prevention Study. Antibiotics and oral contraceptive failure—a case-crossover study. Contraception. 2011; 83(5):418–25.
28. Edelman AB, Carlson NE, Cherala G, Munar MY, Stouffer RL, Cameron JL, et al. Impact of obesity on oral contraceptive pharmacokinetics and hypothalamic-pituitary-ovarian activity. Contraception. 2009;80(2): 119–27.
29. Westhoff CL, Torgal AH, Mayeda ER, Pike MC, Stanczyk FZ. Pharmacokinetics of a combined oral contraceptive in obese and normal-weight women. Contraception. 2010;81(6):474–80.
30. Segall-Gutierrez P, Taylor D, Liu X, Stanzcyk F, Azen S, Mishell DRJ. Follicular development and ovulation in extremely obese women receiving depo-medroxyprogesterone acetate subcutaneously. Contraception. 2010;81(6):487–95.
31. Hubacher D, Reyes V, Lillo S, Pierre-Louis B, Zepeda A, Chen PL, et al. Preventing copper intrauterine device removals due to side effects among first-time users: randomized trial to study the effect of prophylactic ibuprofen. Hum Reprod. 2006;21(6):1467–72.
32. WHO. Medical eligibility criteria for contraceptive use. 4th ed. Geneva: WHO; 2009. http://www.who.int/reproductivehealth/publications/family_planning/9789241563888/en/index.html.
33. Back DJ, Breckenridge AM, Crawford FE, Hall JM, MacIver M, Orme ML, et al. The effect of rifampicin on the pharmacokinetics of ethynylestradiol in women. Contraception. 1980;21:135–43.
34. Dickinson BD, Altman RD, Nielsen NH, Sterling ML, Council on Scientific Affairs, American Medical Association. Drug interactions between oral contraceptives and antibiotics. Obstet Gynecol. 2001;98(5 Pt 1):853–60.
35. Sinofsky FE, Pasquale SA. The effect of fluconazole on circulating ethinyl estradiol levels in women taking oral contraceptives. Am J Obstet Gynecol. 1998; 178(2):300–4.
36. Hilbert J, Messig M, Kuye O, Friedman H. Evaluation of interaction between fluconazole and an oral contraceptive in healthy women. Obstet Gynecol. 2001;98(2): 218–23.
37. Andrews E, Damle BD, Fang A, Foster G, Crownover P, LaBadie R, et al. Pharmacokinetics and tolerability of voriconazole and a combination oral contraceptive co-administered in healthy female subjects. Br J Clin Pharmacol. 2008;65(4):531–9.
38. Robinson JA, Jamshidi R, Burke AE. Contraception for the HIV-positive woman: a review of interactions between hormonal contraception and antiretroviral therapy. Infect Dis Obstet Gynecol. 2012;2012:890160.
39. Scholler-Gyure M, Kakuda TN, Woodfall B, Aharchi F, Peeters M, Vandermeulen K, et al. Effect of steady-state etravirine on the pharmacokinetics and pharmacodynamics of ethinylestradiol and norethindrone. Contraception. 2009;80(1):44–52.
40. Ella Tablets (ulipristal acetate) [package insert]. Parsippany, NJ: Watson Pharma, Inc; 2012.
41. Wanwimolruk S, Kaewvichit S, Tanthayaphinant O, Suwannarach C, Oranratnachai A. Lack of effect of oral contraceptive use on the pharmacokinetics of quinine. Br J Clin Pharmacol. 1991;31(2):179–81.
42. Kenyon IE. Unplanned pregnancy in an epileptic. Br Med J. 1972;1(5801):686–7.
43. Gaffield ME, Culwell KR, Lee CR. The use of hormonal contraception among women taking anticonvulsant therapy. Contraception. 2011;83(1):16–29.
44. Haukkamaa M. Contraception by Norplant subdermal capsules is not reliable in epileptic patients on anticonvulsant treatment. Contraception. 1986;33(6):559–65.
45. Amerge Tablets (Naratriptan) [package insert]. Research Triangle Park, NC: GlaxoSmithKline; 2013.
46. Sitruk-Ware R, Nath A. Metabolic effects of contraceptive steroids. Rev Endocr Metab Disord. 2011; 12(2):63–75.
47. Grigoryan OR, Grodnitskaya EE, Andreeva EN, Chebotnikova TV, Melnichenko GA. Use of the NuvaRing hormone-releasing system in late reproductive-age women with type 1 diabetes mellitus. Gynecol Endocrinol. 2008;24(2):99–104.
48. Diab KM, Zaki MM. Contraception in diabetic women: comparative metabolic study of Norplant, depotmedroxyprogesterone acetate, low dose oral contraceptive pill and CuT380A. J Obstet Gynaecol Res. 2000;26(1):17–26.
49. Loi CM, Stern R, Koup JR, Vassos AB, Knowlton P, Sedman AJ. Effect of troglitazone on the pharmacokinetics of an oral contraceptive agent. J Clin Pharmacol. 1999;39(4):410–7.
50. Inglis AM, Miller AK, Culkin KT, Finnerty D, Patterson SD, Jorkasky DK, et al. Lack of effect of rosiglitazone on the pharmacokinetics of oral contraceptives in healthy female volunteers. J Clin Pharmacol. 2001;41(6):683–90.
51. Lebovitz HE. Differentiating members of the thiazolidinedione class: a focus on safety. Diabetes Metab Res Rev. 2002;18 Suppl 2:S23–9.
52. Kothare PA, Seger ME, Northrup J, Mace K, Mitchell MI, Linnebjerg H. Effect of exenatide on the pharmacokinetics of a combination oral contraceptive in healthy women: an open-label, randomised, crossover trial. BMC Clin Pharmacol. 2012;12:8. 6904-12-8.

53. Byetta [package insert]. Princeton, NJ: Bristol-Meyers Squibb Company; 2013. http://packageinserts.bms.com/pi/pi_byetta.pdf.
54. Victoza [package insert]. Plainsboro, NJ: Novo Nordisk Inc.; 2013. http://www.novo-pi.com/victoza.pdf.
55. Loriaux DL, Wild RA. Contraceptive choices for women with endocrine complications. Am J Obstet Gynecol. 1993;168(6 Pt 2):2021–6.
56. Wiegratz I, Kutschera E, Lee JH, Moore C, Mellinger U, Winkler UH, et al. Effect of four oral contraceptives on thyroid hormones, adrenal and blood pressure parameters. Contraception. 2003;67(5):361–6.
57. Deray G, le Hoang P, Cacoub P, Assogba U, Grippon P, Baumelou A. Oral contraceptive interaction with cyclosporin. Lancet. 1987;1(8525):158–9.
58. Hansten PD, Horn JR. Cytochrome P450 enzymes and drug interactions, table of cytochrome P450 substrates, inhibitors, inducers and P-glycoprotein, with footnotes. In: The top 100 drug interactions—a guide to patient management. 2008 edition. Freeland, WA: H&H Publications; 2008. p. 142–157.
59. Paulen ME, Folger SG, Curtis KM, Jamieson DJ. Contraceptive use among solid organ transplant patients; a systematic review. Contraception. 2010; 82(1):102–12.
60. Chang SY, Chen C, Yang Z, Rodrigues AD. Further assessment of 17alpha-ethinyl estradiol as an inhibitor of different human cytochrome P450 forms in vitro. Drug Metab Dispos. 2009;37(8):1667–75.
61. Somani SM, Khurana RC. Mechanism of estrogen-imipramine interaction. JAMA. 1973;223(5):560.
62. Laine K, Anttila M, Helminen A, Karnani H, Huupponen R. Dose linearity study of selegiline pharmacokinetics after oral administration: evidence for strong drug interaction with female sex steroids. Br J Clin Pharmacol. 1999;47(3):249–54.
63. Talib HJ, Alderman EM. Gynecologic and reproductive health concerns of adolescents using selected psychotropic medications. J Pediatr Adolesc Gynecol. 2013;26(1):7–15.
64. Gabbay V, O'Dowd MA, Mamamtavrishvili M, Asnis GM. Clozapine and oral contraceptives: a possible drug interaction. J Clin Psychopharmacol. 2002; 22(6):621–2.
65. Haslemo T, Refsum H, Molden E. The effect of ethinylestradiol-containing contraceptives on the serum concentration of olanzapine and *N*-desmethyl olanzapine. Br J Clin Pharmacol. 2011;71(4):611–5.
66. Stoehr GP, Kroboth PD, Juhl RP, Wender DB, Phillips JP, Smith RB. Effect of oral contraceptives on triazolam, temazepam, alprazolam, and lorazepam kinetics. Clin Pharmacol Ther. 1984;36(5):683–90.
67. Babalonis S, Lile JA, Martin CA, Kelly TH. Physiological doses of progesterone potentiate the effects of triazolam in healthy, premenopausal women. Psychopharmacology (Berl). 2011;215(3):429–39.
68. Scavone JM, Greenblatt DJ, Locniskar A, Shader RI. Alprazolam pharmacokinetics in women on low-dose oral contraceptives. J Clin Pharmacol. 1988; 28(5):454–7.
69. Kendall MJ, Jack DB, Quarterman CP, Smith SR, Zaman R. Beta-adrenoceptor blocker pharmacokinetics and the oral contraceptive pill. Br J Clin Pharmacol. 1984;17 Suppl 1:87S–9.
70. Kendall MJ, Quarterman CP, Jack DB, Beeley L. Metoprolol pharmacokinetics and the oral contraceptive pill. Br J Clin Pharmacol. 1982;14(1):120–2.
71. Balogh A, Gessinger S, Svarovsky U, Hippius M, Mellinger U, Klinger G, et al. Can oral contraceptive steroids influence the elimination of nifedipine and its primary pryidine metabolite in humans? Eur J Clin Pharmacol. 1998;54(9–10):729–34.
72. Bird ST, Pepe SR, Etminan M, Liu X, Brophy JM, Delaney JA. The association between drospirenone and hyperkalemia: a comparative-safety study. BMC Clin Pharmacol. 2011;11:23.
73. Yasmin [package insert]. Wayne, NJ: Bayer HealthCare Pharmaceuticals Inc.; 2012. http://www.accessdata.fda.gov/drugsatfda_docs/label/2012/021098s019lbl.pdf.
74. de Teresa E, Vera A, Ortigosa J, Pulpon LA, Arus AP, de Artaza M. Interaction between anticoagulants and contraceptives: an unsuspected finding. Br Med J. 1979;2(6200):1260–1.
75. Zingone MM, Guirguis AB, Airee A, Cobb D. Probable drug interaction between warfarin and hormonal contraceptives. Ann Pharmacother. 2009; 43(12):2096–102.
76. Ellison J, Thomson AJ, Greer IA, Walker ID. Drug points: apparent interaction between warfarin and levonorgestrel used for emergency contraception. BMJ. 2000;321(7273):1382.
77. Butler K, Teng R. Effect of ticagrelor on the pharmacokinetics of ethinyl oestradiol and levonorgestrel in healthy volunteers. Curr Med Res Opin. 2011;27(8): 1585–93.
78. Joshi JV, Sankolli GM, Shah RS, Joshi UM. Antacid does not reduce the bioavailability of oral contraceptive steroids in women. Int J Clin Pharmacol Ther Toxicol. 1986;24(4):192–5.
79. Fuchs W, Sennewald R, Klotz U. Lansoprazole does not affect the bioavailability of oral contraceptives. Br J Clin Pharmacol. 1994;38(4):376–80.
80. Roberts RK, Grice J, McGuffie C, Heilbronn L. Oral contraceptive steroids impair the elimination of theophylline. J Lab Clin Med. 1983;101(6):821–5.
81. van Giersbergen PL, Halabi A, Dingemanse J. Pharmacokinetic interaction between bosentan and the oral contraceptives norethisterone and ethinyl estradiol. Int J Clin Pharmacol Ther. 2006;44(3):113–8.
82. Simonson SG, Martin PD, Warwick MJ, Mitchell PD, Schneck DW. The effect of rosuvastatin on oestrogen & progestin pharmacokinetics in healthy women taking an oral contraceptive. Br J Clin Pharmacol. 2004;57(3):279–86.
83. Welchol tablets (colesevelam hydrochloride) [package insert]. Parsippany, NJ: Daiichi Sankyo, Inc.; 2013.
84. Schütt B, Kunz M, Blode H. Coadministration of estradiol/drospirenone and indomethacin does not cause hyperkalemia in healthy postmenopausal

women: a randomized open-label crossover study. J Clin Pharmacol. 2007;47(6):774–81.

85. Pfrunder A, Schiesser M, Gerber S, Haschke M, Bitzer J, Drewe J. Interaction of St John's wort with low-dose oral contraceptive therapy: a randomized controlled trial. Br J Clin Pharmacol. 2003;56(6): 683–90.
86. Murphy PA, Kern SE, Stanczyk FZ, Westhoff CL. Interaction of St. John's Wort with oral contraceptives: effects on the pharmacokinetics of norethindrone and ethinyl estradiol, ovarian activity and breakthrough bleeding. Contraception. 2005; 71(6):402–8.
87. Borrelli F, Izzo AA. Herb-drug interactions with St John's wort (Hypericum perforatum): an update on clinical observations. AAPS J. 2009;11(4):710–27.
88. Schwarz UI, Buschel B, Kirch W. Unwanted pregnancy on self-medication with St John's wort despite hormonal contraception. Br J Clin Pharmacol. 2003; 55(1):112–3.

Appendix: CDC Medical Eligibility Criteria for Contraceptive Use 2010: Summary Chart

Summary Chart of U.S. Medical Eligibility Criteria for Contraceptive Use

Key:	
1	No restriction (method can be used)
2	Advantages generally outweigh theoretical or proven risks
3	Theoretical or proven risks usually outweigh the advantages
4	Unacceptable health risk (method not to be used)

Updated June 2012. This summary sheet only contains a subset of the recommendations from the US MEC. For complete guidance, see: http://www.cdc.gov/reproductivehealth/unintendedpregnancy/USMEC.htm

Most contraceptive methods do not protect against sexually transmitted infections (STIs). Consistent and correct use of the male latex condom reduces the risk of STIs and HIV.

Condition	Sub-condition	Combined pill, patch, ring	Progestin-only pill	Injection	Implant	LNG–IUD	Copper -IUD
		I | C	I | C	I | C	I | C	I | C	I | C
Age		Menarche to <40=1 ≥40=2	Menarche to <18=1 18-45=1 >45=1	Menarche to <18=2 18-45=1 >45=2	Menarche to <18=1 18-45=1 >45=1	Menarche to <20=2 ≥20=1	Menarche to <20=2 ≥20=1
Anatomic abnormalities	a) Distorted uterine cavity					4	4
	b) Other abnormalities					2	2
Anemias	a) Thalassemia	1	1	1	1	1	2
	b) Sickle cell disease‡	2	1	1	1	1	2
	c) Iron-deficiency anemia	1	1	1	1	1	2
Benign ovarian tumors	(including cysts)	1	1	1	1	1	1
Breast disease	a) Undiagnosed mass	2*	2*	2*	2*	2	1
	b) Benign breast disease	1	1	1	1	1	1
	c) Family history of cancer	1	1	1	1	1	1
	d) Breast cancer‡						
	i) current	4	4	4	4	4	1
	ii) past and no evidence of current disease for 5 years	3	3	3	3	3	1
Breastfeeding (see also Postpartum)	a) < 1 month postpartum	3*	2*	2*	2*		
	b) 1 month or more postpartum	2*	1*	1*	1*		
Cervical cancer	Awaiting treatment	2	1	2	2	I: 4 | C: 2	I: 4 | C: 2
Cervical ectropion		1	1	1	1	1	1
Cervical intraepithelial neoplasia		2	1	2	2	2	1
Cirrhosis	a) Mild (compensated)	1	1	1	1	1	1
	b) Severe‡ (decompensated)	4	3	3	3	3	1
Deep venous thrombosis (DVT) /Pulmonary embolism (PE)	a) History of DVT/PE, not on anticoagulant therapy						
	i) higher risk for recurrent DVT/PE	4	2	2	2	2	1
	ii) lower risk for recurrent DVT/PE	3	2	2	2	2	1
	b) Acute DVT/PE	4	2	2	2	2	2
	c) DVT/PE and established on anticoagulant therapy for at least 3 months						
	i) higher risk for recurrent DVT/PE	4*	2	2	2	2	2
	ii) lower risk for recurrent DVT/PE	3*	2	2	2	2	2
	d) Family history (first-degree relatives)	2	1	1	1	1	1
	e) Major surgery						
	(i) with prolonged immobilization	4	2	2	2	2	1
	(ii) without prolonged immobilization	2	1	1	1	1	1
	f) Minor surgery without immobilization	1	1	1	1	1	1
Depressive disorders		1*	1*	1*	1*	1*	1*
Diabetes mellitus (DM)	a) History of gestational DM on	1	1	1	1	1	1
	b) Non-vascular disease						

(continued)

R.H. Allen and C.A. Cwiak (eds.), *Contraception for the Medically Challenging Patient*,
DOI 10.1007/978-1-4939-1233-9, © Springer Science+Business Media New York 2014

Condition	Sub-condition	Combined pill, patch, ring		Progestin-only pill		Injection		Implant		LNG-IUD		Copper-IUD	
		I	C	I	C	I	C	I	C	I	C	I	C
Diabetes mellitus (cont.)	(i) non-insulin dependent	2		2		2		2		2		1	
	(ii) insulin dependent‡	2		2		2		2		2		1	
	c) Nephropathy/ retinopathy/ neuropathy‡	3/4*		2		3		2		2		1	
	d) Other vascular disease or diabetes of >20 years' duration‡	3/4*		2		3		2		2		1	
Endometrial cancer‡		1		1		1		1		4	2	4	2
Endometrial hyperplasia		1		1		1		1		1		1	
Endometriosis		1		1		1		1		1		2	
Epilepsy	(see also Drug Interactions)	1*		1*		1*		1*		1		1	
Gallbladder disease	a) Symptomatic												
	(i) treated by cholecystectomy	2		2		2		2		2		1	
	(ii) medically treated	3		2		2		2		2		1	
	(iii) current	3		2		2		2		2		1	
	b) Asymptomatic	2		2		2		2		2		1	
Gestational trophoblastic	a) Decreasing or undetectable ß-hCG levels	1		1		1		1		3		3	
disease	b) Persistently elevated ß-hCG levels or malignant disease‡	1		1		1		1		4		4	
Headaches	a) Non-migrainous	1*	2*	1*	1*	1*	1*	1*	1*	1*	1*	1*	
	b) Migraine												
	i) without aura, age<35	2*	3*	1*	2*	2*	2*	2*	2*	2*	2*	1*	
	ii) without aura, age≥35	3*	4*	1*	2*	2*	2*	2*	2*	2*	2*	1*	
	iii) with aura, any age	4*	4*	2*	3*	2*	3*	2*	3*	2*	3*	1*	
History of bariatric surgery‡	a) Restrictive procedures	1		1		1		1		1		1	
	b) Malabsorptive procedures	COCs: 3 P/R: 1		3		1		1		1		1	
History of cholestasis	a) Pregnancy-related	2		1		1		1		1		1	
	b) Past COC-related	3		2		2		2		2		1	
History of high blood pressure during pregnancy		2		1		1		1		1		1	
History of pelvic surgery		1		1		1		1		1		1	
HIV	High risk	1		1		1*		1		2	2	2	2
	HIV infected (see also Drug Interactions)‡	1*		1*		1*		1*		2	2	2	2
	AIDS (see also Drug Interactions)‡	1*		1*		1*		1*		3	2*	3	2*
	Clinically well on therapy	**If on treatment, see Drug Interactions**								2	2	2	2
Hyperlipidemias		2/3*		2*		2*		2*		2*		1*	
Hypertension	a) Adequately controlled hypertension	3*		1*		2*		1*		1		1	
	b) Elevated blood pressure levels (properly taken measurements)												
	(i) systolic 140-159 or diastolic 90-99	3		1		2		1		1		1	
	(ii) systolic ≥160 or diastolic ≥100‡	4		2		3		2		2		1	
	c) Vascular disease	4		2		3		2		2		1	
Inflammatory bowel disease	(Ulcerative colitis, Crohn's disease)	2/3*		2		2		1		1		1	
Ischemic heart disease‡	Current and history of	4		2	3	3		2	3	2	3	1	
Liver tumors	a) Benign												
	i) Focal nodular hyperplasia	2		2		2		2		2		1	
	ii) Hepatocellular adenoma‡	4		3		3		3		3		1	
	b) Malignant‡	4		3		3		3		3		1	

(continued)

Condition	Sub-condition	Combined pill, patch, ring		Progestin-only pill		Injection		Implant		LNG–IUD		Copper-IUD	
		I	C	I	C	I	C	I	C	I	C	I	C
Malaria		1		1		1		1		1		1	
Multiple risk factors for arterial cardiovascular disease	(such as older age, smoking, diabetes and hypertension)	3/4*		2*		3*		2*		2		1	
Obesity	a) ≥30 kg/m^2 body mass index (BMI)	2		1		1		1		1		1	
	b) Menarche to <18 years and ≥ 30 kg/m^2 BMI	2		1		2		1		1		1	
Ovarian cancer‡		1		1		1		1		1		1	
Parity	a) Nulliparous	1		1		1		1		2		2	
	b) Parous	1		1		1		1		1		1	
Past ectopic pregnancy		1		2		1		1		1		1	
Pelvic inflammatory disease	a) Past, (assuming no current risk factors of STIs)												
	(i) with subsequent pregnancy	1		1		1		1		1	1	1	1
	(ii) without subsequent pregnancy	1		1		1		1		2	2	2	2
	b) Current	1		1		1		1		4	2*	4	2*
Peripartum cardiomyopathy‡	a) Normal or mildly impaired cardiac function												
	(i) < 6 months	4		1		1		1		2		2	
	(ii) ≥ 6 months	3		1		1		1		2		2	
	b) Moderately or severely impaired cardiac function	4		2		2		2		2		2	
Postabortion	a) First trimester	1*		1*		1*		1*		1*		1*	
	b) Second trimester	1*		1*		1*		1*		2		2	
	c) Immediately post -septic abortion	1*		1*		1*		1*		4		4	
Postpartum (see also Breastfeeding)	a) < 21 days	4		1		1		1					
	b) 21 days to 42 days												
	(i) with other risk factors for VTE	3*		1		1		1					
	(ii) without other risk factors for VTE	2		1		1		1					
	c) ≥ 42 days	1		1		1		1					
Postpartum (in breastfeeding or non-breastfeeding women, including post-cesarean section)	a) < 10 minutes after delivery of the placenta									2		1	
	b) 10 minutes after delivery of the placenta to < 4 weeks									2		2	
	c) ≥ 4 weeks									1		1	
	d) Puerperal sepsis									4		4	
Pregnancy		NA*		NA*		NA*		NA*		4*		4*	
Rheumatoid arthritis	a) On immuno suppressive therapy	2		1		2/3*		1		2	1	2	1
	b) Not on immunosuppressive therapy	2		1		2		1		1		1	
Schistosomiasis	a) Uncomplicated	1		1		1		1		1		1	
	b) Fibrosis of the liver ‡	1		1		1		1		1		1	
Severe dysmenorrhea		1		1		1		1		1		2	
Sexually transmitted infections (STIs)	a) Current purulent cervicitis or chlamydial infection or gonorrhea	1		1		1		1		4	2*	4	2*
	b) Other STIs (excluding HIV and hepatitis)	1		1		1		1		2	2	2	2
Sexually transmitted infections (cont.)	c) Vaginitis (including trichomonas vaginalis and bacterial vaginosis)	1		1		1		1		2	2	2	2
	d) Increased risk of STIs	1		1		1		1		2/3*	2	2/3*	2
Smoking	a) Age < 35	2		1		1		1		1		1	
	b) Age ≥ 35, < 15 cigarettes/day	3		1		1		1		1		1	
	c) Age ≥ 35, ≥15 cigarettes/day	4		1		1		1		1		1	

(continued)

Condition	Sub-condition	Combined pill, patch, ring I	Combined pill, patch, ring C	Progestin-only pill I	Progestin-only pill C	Injection I	Injection C	Implant I	Implant C	LNG-IUD I	LNG-IUD C	Copper-IUD I	Copper-IUD C
Solid organ transplantation‡	a) Complicated	4		2		2		2		3	2	3	2
	b) Uncomplicated	2*		2		2		2		2		2	
Stroke‡	History of cerebrovascular accident	4		2	3	3		2	3	2		1	
Superficial venous thrombosis	a) Varicose veins	1		1		1		1		1		1	
	b) Superficial thrombophlebitis	2		1		1		1		1		1	
Systemic lupus erythematosus‡	a) Positive (or unknown) antiphospholipid antibodies	4		3		3	3	3		3		1	1
	b) Severe thrombocytopenia	2		2		3	2	2		2*		3*	2*
	c) Immunosuppressive treatment	2		2		2	2	2		2		2	1
	d) None of the above	2		2		2	2	2		2		1	1
Thrombogenic mutations‡		4*		2*		2*		2*		2*		1*	
Thyroid disorders	Simple goiter/ hyperthyroid/hypothyroid	1		1		1		1		1		1	
Tuberculosis‡ (see also Drug Interactions)	a) Non-pelvic	1*		1*		1*		1*		1		1	
	b) Pelvic	1*		1*		1*		1*		4	3	4	3
Unexplained vaginal bleeding	(suspicious for serious condition) before evaluation	2*		2*		3*		3*		4*	2*	4*	2*
Uterine fibroids		1		1		1		1		2		2	
Valvular heart disease	a) Uncomplicated	2		1		1		1		1		1	
	b) Complicated‡	4		1		1		1		1		1	
Vaginal bleeding patterns	a) Irregular pattern without heavy bleeding	1		2		2		2		1	1	1	
	b) Heavy or prolonged bleeding	1*		2*		2*		2*		1*	2*	2*	
Viral hepatitis	a) Acute or flare	3/4*	2	1		1		1		1		1	
	b) Carrier/Chronic	1	1	1		1		1		1		1	
Drug Interactions													
Antiretroviral therapy	a) Nucleoside reverse transcriptase inhibitors	1*		1		1		1		2/3*	2*	2/3*	2*
	b) Non-nucleoside reverse transcriptase inhibitors	2*		2*		1		2*		2/3*	2*	2/3*	2*
	c) Ritonavir-boosted protease inhibitors	3*		3*		1		2*		2/3*	2*	2/3*	2*
Anticonvulsant therapy	a) Certain anticonvulsants (phenytoin, carbamazepine, barbiturates, primidone, topiramate, oxcarbazepine)	3*		3*		1		2*		1		1	
	b) Lamotrigine	3*		1		1		1		1		1	
Antimicrobial therapy	a) Broad spectrum antibiotics	1		1		1		1		1		1	
	b) Antifungals	1		1		1		1		1		1	
	c) Antiparasitics	1		1		1		1		1		1	
	d) Rifampicin or rifabutin therapy	3*		3*		1		2*		1		1	

I = initiation of contraceptive method; C = continuation of contraceptive method; NA = Not applicable

* Please see the complete guidance for a clarification to this classification:www.cdc.gov/reproductivehealth/unintendedpregnancy/USMEC.htm

‡ Condition that exposes a woman to increased risk as a result of unintended pregnancy.

Index

R.H. Allen and C.A. Cwiak (eds.), *Contraception for the Medically Challenging Patient*, DOI 10.1007/978-1-4939-1233-9, © Springer Science+Business Media New York 2014

Made in the USA
Monee, IL
12 September 2026

62976353R00238